Health the Basics

Fifth Edition

Rebecca J. Donatelle

Oregon State University

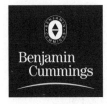

Benjamin Cummings

San Francisco Boston New York
Cape Town Hong Kong London Madrid Mexico City
Montreal Munich Paris Singapore Sydney Tokyo Toronto

Publisher: *Daryl Fox*
Sponsoring Editor: *Deirdre McGill*
Project Editor: *Susan Teahan*
Development Editor: *Alice E. Fugate*
Publishing Assistant: *Michelle Cadden*
Managing Editor, Production: *Wendy Earl*
Development Manager: *Claire Brassert*
Production Editor: *Sharon Montooth*
Cover and Text Design: *Kathleen Cunningham*
Art Coordinator: *Bradley Burch*
Photo Researcher: *Diane Austin*
Copy Editor: *Sally Peyrefitte*
Proofreader: *Martha Ghent*
Compositor: *GTS Graphics*
Manufacturing Buyer: *Stacey Weinberger*
Marketing Manager: *Sandra Lindelof*

Cover Art: *Copyright© Heidi Younger. All rights reserved.*

Library of Congress Cataloging-in-Publication Data
Donatelle, Rebecca J., 1950–
    Health: the basics / Rebecca J. Donatelle.—5th ed.
      p.   cm.
    Includes bibliographical references and index.
    ISBN 0-8053-5326-7
      1. Health.   I. Title.
    RA776.D663 2002
    613—dc21   2002025995

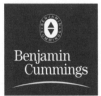

ISBN 0-8053-5326-7
2 3 4 5 6 7 8 9 10–BAM–06 05 04 03

www.aw.com/bc

PREFACE

As we enter the early years of a new millennium, health has become a hot topic. Whether trying to improve appearance, lose weight, exercise more, feel better, enhance interpersonal relationships, or avoid disease-causing pathogens that lurk in the environment, more and more people are tuned in to health issues and topics.

Not too long ago, disease and illness were seen as phenomena people had little power over. People who became sick from an infectious disease either weathered the illness and recovered or, in all too many cases, died. Few choices were available in foods, medicines, and services, and, consequently, health care decisions usually focused on cleanliness, avoiding known hazards, and staying away from others who were sick.

In sharp contrast, today's health-conscious individuals have choices surrounding health that their grandparents could not have imagined: pharmacies loaded with prescription and over-the counter drugs, health food stores with thousands of products that claim to promote wellness and prevent illness, Yellow Pages filled with doctors and alternative practitioners to choose from, grocery stores and fast-food restaurants packed with every imaginable food, and transportation moving people to and from the deepest recesses of the planet in a matter of hours. Books, television, computers, and other media-driven sources are constantly luring consumes into buying miracle products. Talk show hosts offer formulas for relationship success, sexual prowess, and a slew of other behaviors that promise happier and healthier living.

While being bombarded with marketing choices, individuals have to deal with the threat of both real and imagined adversaries. Violent acts are played out on the nightly news and in newspaper headlines. Divorce statistics seem to spell doom and gloom for the American family. Obesity, soaring drug use and abuse, epidemic depression and mental illness, increasing rates of infectious and noninfectious diseases, threats from emerging and resurging diseases, tales of environmental destruction, and a host of other bad news topics seem to permeate the culture.

Juxtaposed against the threats to health are advances in medical research, new opportunities for personal choice, increased attention to policies designed to preserve health and protect against harm, and improved strategies for promoting health and preventing premature disease and disability. Technologies continue to be developed, with concomitant improvements in diagnosis of disease and treatment occurring daily. At no time in history has it been more evident that by taking action, an individual can prevent illness and prolong a productive, fully functional life. Regardless of whether changes in public policy and community and corporate behavior are necessary to help improve health status, this much is true: The better individuals prepare themselves to make wise decisions, and the more community leaders and representatives of the health care system work together to help achieve and maintain excellent health status, the more likely that everyone's quality of life will improve.

Each new class of college students represents a more savvy group of health connoisseurs, complete with its own, unique perspectives on health. An astounding, often contradictory and confusing array of health information is available through the simple click of a mouse, the routine turn on of the television, or the casual perusal of a magazine. Because there is no one recipe for achieving health, it is important to consider the various opinions and options available to determine what information is the most scientifically defensible and which poses the least amount of risk to wellness.

After over 30 years of teaching public health students from a wide range of health and other disciplines and after working on several editions of this book, I continue to be excited about the tremendous opportunities that students today have to *make a difference* to their health, the health of their loved ones, and the health of others. Part of my goal in writing this book is to help students be better "change agents" as they view the health controversies of today and those that will shape their future—not just in the arena of personal health behaviors, but also in the larger realm of policy changes and community behaviors, which ultimately can assist the global population in living smarter, longer, and better. In short, this book is designed not just to teach health facts but to present health as a much broader concept, something that everyone desires and deserves. By understanding the factors that contribute to health risk, exploring concepts provided in this text, contemplating action plans that might serve to reduce risk, and utilizing the technological tools provided, students can take the first steps in accessing better health.

NEW TO THE FIFTH EDITION

As in the previous edition, I am committed to excellence in the fifth edition of *Health: The Basics*. The fifth edition represents one of the largest overall revisions undertaken to date, one which involved line-by-line updates reflecting cutting-edge research to describe the discoveries, controversies, issues, and realities of today's personal health marketplace. As is the tradition in *Health: The Basics,* new and uncharted territory in health is covered, with major enhancements in the following areas:

- **Expanded coverage in Chapter 2, "Psychosocial Health,"** of the mind–body connection and spirituality helps students understand how their state of mind can influence their personal health. The chapter includes an explanation of what spirituality means, how other cultures view and value the spiritual dimension of health, and the importance of spirituality to overall health and well-being.
- **New sections in Chapter 5, "Healthy Relationships and Sexuality,"** including "Communicating: A Key to Good

Relationships," "Communicating How You Feel," and "Improving Communication/Improving Relationships," provide students with valuable interpersonal skill strategies for improving communication with partners, family, friends, and colleagues.

- **Extended coverage of violence, terrorism, and bioterrorism in Chapter 4, "Violence and Abuse" and Chapter 14, "Infectious and Noninfectious Conditions"** will assist students in determining violence and disease risk levels as well as methods for risk reduction. New sections include "Terrorism: Increased Risk from Multiple Sources" and "Bioterrorism: The New Global Threat." In addition, new Health in a Diverse World boxes are included: "World Post Traumatic Stress: The Aftermath of Terror" and "Bioterrorism: A Pandora's Box?"

- **Significant expansion of coverage in Chapter 11, "Personal Fitness,"** offers students the latest information on flexibility, strength, and endurance exercises, including related health benefits and risks. The chapter includes several new sections: "Flexibility: Stretching and Well-Being," "Yoga, Tai Chi, and Pilates," "Improving Muscular Strength and Endurance," "Gender Differences in Weight Training," and "The Benefits of Strength Training."

- **Comprehensive coverage of cardiovascular disease** has been added, with an entire chapter (Chapter 12) dedicated to the topic. New sections include "Syndrome X," "Reducing Intake of Standard Fats," "Modifying Other Dietary Habits," "Gender Bias in CVD Research?" and "Cardiac Rehabilitation."

- **More in-depth coverage of cancer** has also been added, with a complete chapter (Chapter 13) on the disease that offers new sections: "Variations in Rates," "Smoking and Cancer Risk," "Obesity and Cancer Risk," "Cancer of the Pancreas," and "Talking with Your Doctor about Cancer."

- **A new chapter (Chapter 18), "Complementary and Alternative Medicine: New Choices and Responsibilities for Healthwise Consumers,"** offers ground-breaking information that reflects the National Institutes of Health for Complementary and Alternative Medicine major domains: alternative medical systems, mind–body interventions, biologically based therapies, manipulative and body-based interventions, and energy therapies. I am excited about the opportunity to provide a first chance for students to receive an unbiased, scientifically defensible, critical look at various CAM options. As some CAM techniques become more widely used and gain scientific validity, others will continue to be steeped in controversy, so it is crucial that students have a starting place for making informed decisions.

- **New feature series have been added: Women's Health/Men's Health** boxes, which explore unique gender-specific issues and concerns facing men and women; **Assess Yourself** boxes, which offer hands-on tools for examining personal behaviors that impact health; and **New Horizons in Health** boxes, which offer late-breaking health news and high-interest journal pieces.

Maintaining a Standard of Excellence

With every edition of *Health: The Basics,* the challenge has been to make the book better than before and to provide information and material that will surpass the competition at every level. The fact that there are many fine health texts on the market today makes the task even more difficult. As such, I have painstakingly considered our reviewer feedback, student comments, focus group discussions, and the broader health marketplace in designing a book that reflects the **3 Rs** for a successful book: *relevance*—reflects real-world issues and problems that students can identify with and have special meaning/importance to them; *reliability*—reflects cutting edge consensus research from several reliable and valid research studies; *readability*—captures the attention of today's techno-influenced students with nonjudgmental writing that engages them and inspires them to read on.

Of equal importance to the above are the pedagogical standards that have been built upon with each successive edition of *Health: The Basics:*

- Chapter 1, "Promoting Healthy Behavior Change," establishes a dual approach used throughout the text: the individual and social context of health and disease and the importance of health to society as a whole.

- To assist students in their efforts to achieve health, the book provides a foundation of information and thought-provoking questions to help students think about specific, negative health behaviors and what strategies might promote behavior change. Additionally, students are challenged to think how their actions may impact others now and in the future. The text guides students through their own health evolution. Rather than just advising students on how to behave in a particular manner, the text emphasizes behavior choice by presenting students with various health options.

- Pedagogical aids such as the What Do You Think? chapter opener scenarios and the Taking Charge chapter closing sections encourage students to apply information acquired from the chapter to their own lives.

- A broad approach to diversity, both within the United States and in the global community, is incorporated throughout the text, emphasizing the fact that health discussions can no longer be limited to populations that reside inside United States borders, but must encompass the potential impact of health policies and behaviors on other nations, cultures, ideologies, and perspectives.

- The roles of community, health policies, and health services in disease prevention and health promotion are integrated throughout the text. The public health approach is often ignored in health texts in favor of a pure individual focus. Optimum health changes will occur only in environments that are conducive to change, in which individuals are informed and can maximize resources to make long-term behavior changes. The underlying philosophy concerning the capacity for change is incorporated throughout the text and highlighted in the Checklist for Change section of each chapter.

- Within a strong pedagogical framework, the importance of building health behavior skills is emphasized and integrated consistently throughout the text. Readers will learn specific applications to their own lives in every chapter through the Assess Yourself, Reality Check, and Skills for Behavior Change boxes offered throughout the text.

SPECIAL FEATURES

Each chapter of *Health: The Basics* includes several of the following special features in various combinations. These features are designed to help students think about healthy behavior skills and how to apply concepts found in the boxes to their everyday lives.

- **Skills for Behavior Change** boxes focus on practical strategies that students can use to improve their personal health and reduce their risks from harmful health behaviors.
- **Assess Yourself** boxes are designed to provide quick, general indicators of personal health status in various areas, which students may consider when initiating behavior change.
- **Reality Check** boxes focus attention on potential risks and safety issues, often as they relate to college-aged students. Statistical information and trends help students recognize risks as they relate to particular behaviors and outcomes.
- **Health in a Diverse World** boxes are designed to increase awareness and appreciation for individual and cultural differences. They promote acceptance of diversity on college campuses and help students adjust to an increasingly diverse world. In particular, these boxes focus on health implications and issues for diverse populations.
- **Women's Health/Men's Health** boxes are designed to help students better understand some of the unique aspects of men's and women's health, as well as the challenges faced by each group as they attempt to achieve optimal health.
- **Consumer Health** boxes focus on health issues that relate to consumer skills by promoting a broad scope of awareness about the health market and hitting on particular consumer issues.
- **New Horizons in Health** boxes report on late-breaking health news and topics of recent concern. They show students that health is a dynamic and constantly changing field.

LEARNING AIDS

- Each chapter is introduced with **Chapter Objectives** to alert students to the key concepts to be covered in upcoming material.

- Designed to prompt discussions that are relevant to the chapter and that apply to students' experiences, **What Do You Think? scenarios** introduce each chapter.
- Groups of **What Do You Think? questions** that encourage students to think critically are highlighted and strategically placed throughout each chapter.
- To emphasize and support understanding of material, pertinent health terminology are boldfaced in the text and defined in the **running glossary** appearing at the bottom of text pages.
- Appearing at the end of each chapter **Accessing Your Health on the Internet** provides descriptions of relevant Internet websites, including organizations such as the World Health Organization (WHO), Centers for Disease Control and Prevention (CDC), WebMD, and the Mayo Clinic.
- At the end of each chapter, the **Taking Charge** section summarizes content while encouraging students to apply what they have learned at both the personal and community levels.

STUDENT SUPPLEMENTS

Available with *Health: The Basics,* fifth edition is a comprehensive set of ancillary materials designed to enhance learning:

- *Take Charge of Your Health! Self-Assessment Workbook with Review and Practice Tests.* Featuring chapter overviews, worksheets, review questions, and practice tests with answers, the workbook is to be used in conjunction with the text to enable students to acquire a broader understanding of health issues and obtain a clearer picture of their overall health.
- **Companion website for *Health: The Basics,* Fifth Edition** at http://www.aw.com/donatelle contains many excellent features for both instructors and students: "Accessing Your Health on the Internet" links, flashcards, practice quizzes, audio and video clips, self-assessment and critical thinking activities, and an instructor's section with PowerPoint® lecture presentation slides.
- **StudentBody 101** website, accredited by Health on the Net (HON), focuses on alcohol, drugs, stress, fitness, nutrition, tobacco, and sexuality and facilitates active learning by posting current journal articles, self-assessments, online discussions, and personalized behavior change tips.
- *Study Guide for StudentBody 101* provides several activities to ensure maximum use of the website StudentBody 101.
- *Behavior Change Log Book* is a tool that makes discovering unhealthy behaviors, tracking daily nutritional intake, and creating long-term personal nutrition and fitness programs easy, offering labs, worksheets, behavior contracts, assessments, and more.
- *Health on the Net 2002* offers the most valuable Internet writing resources and demonstrates how to perform

research online with course-specific URLs and writing guidelines for Modern Language Association (MLA) and American Psychological Association (APA) styles.

INSTRUCTOR SUPPLEMENTS

A full resource package accompanies *Health: The Basics* to assist the instructor with classroom preparation and presentation:

- **Instructor's Resource Manual with Media Guide** is an excellent teaching tool, providing classroom activities, chapter objectives, lecture outlines, and companion website resources to reinforce chapter concepts and develop effective student learning. To help integrate media, the manual also includes an interactive teaching companion.
- **Test Bank** (in both print and computer versions) offers comprehensive testing material with multiple choice, short-answer, true/false, matching, and essay questions for each chapter. The computer version, TestGen 4.0/QuizMaster 3.0, is presented on a dual platform CD-ROM for Macintosh and PC users.
- **PowerPoint® presentation slides** include all figures and tables from the book and lecture outlines that may be customized for lecture presentation.
- **Transparency acetates** contain all figures and tables from the text in full-color.
- **Instructor's Guide to StudentBody101** provides tips for using journal articles and online resources offered on StudentBody101.com in conducting discussion sessions, assigning writing activities, spurring debates, and encouraging self-assessment.

ACKNOWLEDGMENTS

After writing several editions of *Health: the Basics,* there is only one thing that I am certain of: It NEVER gets any easier. In fact, as the Internet expands our ability to seek out new information and explore different and unique aspects of the world of health, my job as an author becomes even more challenging. The complexities and considerations of publishing a book are too numerous to detail here; however, it boils down to having a solid group of professionals to work with. I have been very fortunate in having a wonderful and competent group of professionals to assist me in my writing journey at each step of the process. From the excellent initial efforts of Joe Header and Ted Boolean of Prentice Hall, to the continued professionalism of Allyn and Bacon editors Suzy Spivey and Joe Burns, to the recent acquisition by editorial staff at Benjamin Cummings, I have always worked with people who believed in the project and had a sincere interest in making *Health: The Basics* the BEST in a marketplace filled with good health texts. I am especially grateful to my new Sponsoring Editor, Deirdre McGill, who assembled a wonderful group of editorial staff to help make the transition to

Benjamin Cummings one of the best experiences that I have had to date in working with a publisher of college level texts. A special thank-you goes to my Project Editor, Susan Teahan, who helped guide the day to day revisions of this text and who was able to keep the project moving with a level of expertise, patience, and level-headedness that I have yet to experience in this market. My appreciation also goes to Publishing Assistant Michelle Cadden, for preparing the manuscript and overseeing the text supplements. I would like to acknowledge the wonderful editorial assistance provided by Alice E. Fugate, who did a remarkable job in a short time frame to develop a revised version of the book that surpasses all previous editions. In addition, I would like to thank my Production Editor, Sharon Montooth, for her invaluable assistance in final book development and refinement. Another dedicated group of professionals I would like to thank are the marketing and sales force, particularly Marketing Manager Sandra Lindelof, who spent countless hours making sure *Health: The Basics* got into instructors' hands. Although I have worked with many fine individuals in my years of writing, I believe that the Benjamin Cummings group is among the finest that I have worked with to date. I would like to thank each and every one of the Benjamin Cummings staff for making this text so successful.

In addition to the Benjamin Cummings staff, many colleagues, students, and staff members have provided invaluable feedback, ideas, reviews, assistance, and encouragement over the years, allowing me to meet the demands of rigorous publishing deadlines. Your input, suggestions and overall contributions have helped develop a text that meets the needs of today's students. I could not have written a book like *Health: The Basics* without each and every one of you. Thank you!

Contributions to the Fifth Edition

In particular, I'd like to thank Dr. Patricia Ketcham of Oregon State University for her work on the substance abuse and reproductive health chapters of this text. Pat's contribution to these chapters has been key to the ongoing success of *Health: The Basics* since the first edition in 1988. Her past work as Director of Health Promotion at the University of Iowa and her current instruction at Oregon State University have provided the text with a unique and important vision of student life and issues.

Reviewers for the Fifth Edition of *Health: The Basics*

The expertise of many professionals is necessary to create a finished work that represents the best available health information source for college level students. Clearly, *Health: The Basics* continues to be an evolving work in progress incorporating the help of many fine minds in ensuring a quality product. Each new edition builds on the combined expertise of many colleagues throughout the country who are dedicated to the education and positive behavioral change of students and the health of the population as a whole. My thanks go to the following reviewers who have helped us with this admirable tradition:

M. Betsy Bergen, Ph.D., Kansas State University; Ashok Malik, College of San Mateo; Mary Duquin, University of Pittsburgh; Bridget Driscoll, California State Fullerton; Terry Wessel, James Madison University; Barbara Day Lockhart, Brigham Young University; Dr. Jenny Yi, University of Houston; Rusty Wright, University of Arkansas at Little Rock; John Borogno, College of the Sequoias; David White, Eastern Carolina University; Jill Black, Ph.D., Cleveland State University; Michael Lee, Joliet Junior College; Gary L. Wilson, The Citadel Military College of South Carolina; Debra Tavasso, Eastern Carolina University; Dr. Roland Lamarine, Chico State University

Rebecca J. Donatelle
Health & Kinesiology
Benjamin Cummings
1301 Sansome Street
San Francisco, California 94111

Brief Contents

Contents

Chapter 6
Birth Control, Pregnancy, and Childbirth: Managing Your Fertility   128

Part III Avoiding or Overcoming Harmful Habits

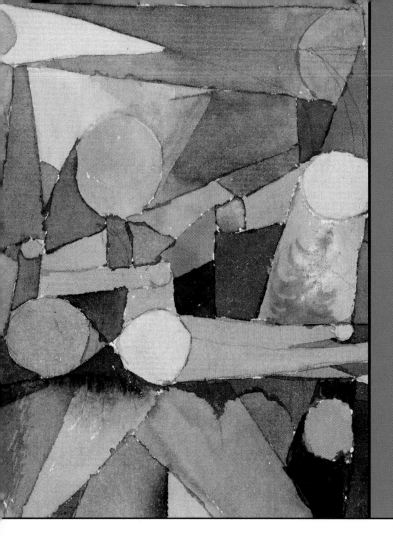

Promoting Healthy Behavior Change

objectives

* Discuss health in terms of historical perspectives and its multidimensional elements. Note the importance of a health-promoting lifestyle in preventing premature disease and disability.

* Discuss the health status of Americans, the factors that contribute to health, and the importance of *Healthy People 2000, Healthy People 2010,* and the Agency for Health Care, Research, and Quality (AHRQ) guidelines in establishing national goals for promoting health and preventing premature death and disability.

* Evaluate the role of gender in health status, health research, and health training.

* Provide a rationale for focusing on current risk behaviors as a means of influencing current and future health status.

* Examine how predisposing factors, beliefs, attitudes, and significant others affect a person's behavior changes.

* Assess behavior-change techniques, and learn how to apply them to personal situations.

* Apply decision-making techniques to behavior changes.

Concerned about your health? You are not alone. At no time in U.S. history have so many government agencies, educational systems, community groups, businesses, and health care organizations been so concerned about health or invested so many resources to influence daily health habits. On a daily basis, you are challenged to "Just do it," "Be all you can be," "Drink your milk," "Eat cruciferous vegetables," "Protect the environment," and exercise, exercise, exercise! Policy makers restrict smoking in public, require detailed labeling on foods, and legislate a host of other policies designed to protect health. Friends and family members comment on your weight. For some people, a need to be thought of as healthy or part of the "in crowd" prompts a seemingly endless stream of chatter about the latest workout, current percentage of body fat, or details about diet. All this leaves us wondering, Has our society gone too far in "hyping" health? How can the average person figure out which information is accurate and which is bogus?

Given the national preoccupation with health, it should be easy for people to get healthy, stay healthy, and live a long and productive life. However, many indicators provide evidence of our collective difficulties in achieving these goals. Consider these points:

- Several national studies indicate that U.S. citizens are becoming more obese and more unfit each year.[1]
- Sales of high-fat foods, red meats, butter, and other products, which had been on the decline, are seeing an unprecedented rise.[2]
- At popular restaurant chains, salad bars, low-fat grilled items, and portion control are becoming less popular as consumers opt for SUPER-sized burgers and MONSTER meals.

- Cigarette smoking among our nation's young has declined, but some groups of young people, particularly young women, continue to smoke at high rates.[3]
- Depression, other mental health problems,[4] some infectious diseases, and other preventable ailments are on the rise.

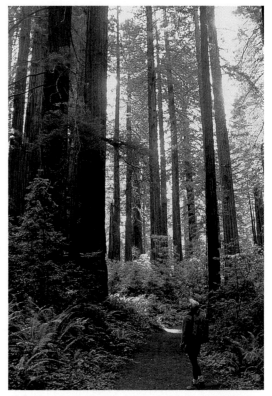

Today, health and wellness mean taking a positive, proactive attitude toward life and living it to its fullest.

- Diabetes rates among young adults are skyrocketing—up over 30 percent in the past decade.[5]
- Increasing numbers of Americans lack access to basic health care.[6]

Why is being healthy so challenging for so many of us? What can we do to overcome these challenges, make better decisions about our behaviors, and become wiser, more responsible health consumers? There are no easy answers, because health is influenced by myriad factors—some that we can control, some that we can't. But the good news is that many people have found the skills and motivation to look objectively at where they are, plan carefully, and make decisions that improve their life and health. Have you ever wondered how a friend managed to lose weight and start kayaking and running in triathlons, when you can't seem to lose an ounce and climbing a flight of stairs leaves you panting for breath? Or why another friend seems to thrive under pressure, while it makes you break down into a screaming fit or tears? Why do so many good intentions to become healthier remain only intentions, without progressing to action?

This book is not designed to provide a foolproof recipe for achieving health or answer all of your questions. It *is* designed to provide fundamental knowledge about many health topics, to help you utilize personal and community resources to create your own health profile, and to challenge you to think more carefully before making decisions that affect your health. This book also provides information about how policies, programs, the media, and socioeconomic status influence health, both directly and indirectly.

Health decisions should be based on the best available research and should be consistent with who you are, your values and beliefs, and who you want to become. Although health is not always totally within your control, some behavior choices that affect your health *are*. The choices you make can enhance your health today, as well as reduce future health risks. For those risk factors that are beyond your control, you must learn to react, adapt, respond appropriately, and use a reasoned, rather than purely emotional, rationale for your choices. By making informed, rational decisions, you can improve both the quality and the length of your own life and perhaps exert a positive influence on those around you.

Putting Health in Perspective

Although we use the term **health** almost unconsciously, few people understand what it really means. For some, *health* simply means the antithesis of sickness. To others, it means being in good physical shape and able to resist illness. Still others use terms such as **wellness** or *well-being* to include a wide array of factors that seem to lead to positive health status. Why all of these variations? In part, the differences are due to an increasingly enlightened way of viewing health that has taken shape over time. In addition, as our collective understanding of illness has improved, so has our ability to understand the many nuances of health. Our progress to

current understanding about health has evolved over centuries, and we have a long way to go in achieving a truly comprehensive view of this complex subject.

Health: Yesterday and Today

Prior to the 1800s, a person who wasn't sick was regarded as not only lucky, but also healthy. When deadly epidemics such as bubonic plague, pneumonic plague, influenza, tuberculosis, and cholera killed millions of people, survivors were believed to be of hearty, healthy stock, and they congratulated themselves on their good fortune. Poor health was often associated with poor hygiene and unsanitary conditions, and certain stigmas were attached to households that harbored any of these illnesses. Not until the late 1800s did researchers discover that victims of these epidemics were not simply unhealthy or dirty. Rather, they were victims of environmental factors (microorganisms found in contaminated water, air, and human waste) which made them sick and over which they often had little control. Public health officials moved swiftly to address these problems, and as a result, the term *health* became synonymous with *good hygiene*. Colleges offered courses in health and hygiene; these were the predecessors of the course you are taking today.

Investigation into the environment as the primary cause of disease continued into the 1900s as outbreaks of tuberculosis, pneumonia, and influenza surged in many regions of the world. People who made it through the first few years of life without succumbing to an infectious disease usually were able to survive to "old age." Keep in mind, however, that the average life expectancy in 1900 was only 47 years. Continued improvements in sanitation brought dramatic changes in life expectancy, and the development of vaccines and antibiotics added even more years to the average life.

By the 1940s, progressive thinkers in public health began to note that there was more to health than hygiene or disease. At an international conference in 1947 focusing on global health issues, the World Health Organization (WHO) took the landmark step of trying to clarify what *health* truly meant: "Health is the state of complete physical, mental, and social well-being, not just the absence of disease or infirmity."[7] For the first time, the concept of health came to mean more than not being ill.

Not until the 1960s, however, did scientists successfully argue that health included much more than physical, social, or mental elements of life. Other elements, such as environmental, spiritual, emotional, and intellectual aspects, helped define whether a person was truly capable of optimal

Health Dynamic, ever-changing process of achieving individual potential in the physical, social, emotional, mental, spiritual, and environmental dimensions.

Wellness The achievement of the highest level of health possible in each of several dimensions.

functioning. In addition, these new voices argued that it isn't just length of life or the number of disease-free years that matters, but rather achieving your potential for a happy, healthy, and productive life.

Today, because most childhood diseases are preventable or curable and because massive public health efforts are aimed at reducing the spread of infectious diseases, many people are living well into their 70s and 80s. According to **mortality** (death rate) statistics, people are now living longer than at any time in our history. **Morbidity** (illness) rates also indicate that people less frequently contract the common infectious diseases that devastated previous generations. However, longer life and less frequent disease are not proof that people are indeed *healthier*.

> ### What do you think?
> *René Dubos, the renowned bacteriologist who developed many key philosophies about health, is credited with saying, "Measure your Health by your sympathy with Morning and Spring."* ☀ *What do you think Dubos meant by this statement?* ☀ *Discuss how well your own health measures up when weighed against this criterion.*

The Evolution Toward Wellness

René Dubos, biologist and philosopher, aptly summarized the thinking of his contemporaries by defining *health* as "a quality of life, involving social, emotional, mental, spiritual, and biological fitness on the part of the individual, which results from adaptations to the environment."[8] The concept of adaptability, or the ability to successfully cope with life's ups and downs, became a key element of the overall health definition. Eventually the term *wellness* became popular and not only included the previously mentioned elements, but also implied that there were levels of health in each category. To achieve *high-level wellness,* a person moved progressively higher on a continuum of positive health indicators. Those who failed to achieve these levels might move to the illness side of the continuum. Today, *health* and *wellness* are often used interchangeably to mean the dynamic, ever-changing process of trying to achieve one's potential in each of several interrelated dimensions. These dimensions typically include those presented in Figure 1.1.

> **Mortality** Death rate.
>
> **Morbidity** Illness rate.
>
> **Activities of Daily Living (ADLs)** Performance of tasks of everyday living, such as bathing, and walking up the stairs.

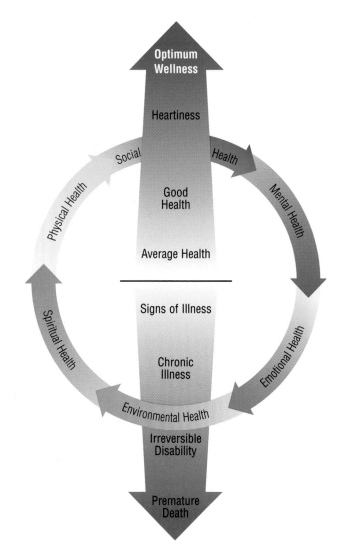

Figure 1.1
The Dimensions of the Health and Wellness Continuum

- *Physical health.* This dimension includes characteristics such as body size and shape, sensory acuity and responsiveness, susceptibility to disease and disorders, body functioning, physical fitness, and recuperative abilities. Newer definitions of physical health also include our ability to perform normal **activities of daily living (ADLs),** or those tasks that are necessary to normal existence in today's society. Being able to get out of bed in the morning, being able to bend over to tie your shoes, and other usual daily tasks are examples of ADLs.
- *Intellectual health.* This dimension refers to the ability to think clearly, to reason objectively, to analyze critically, and to use "brain power" effectively to meet life's challenges. It means learning from successes and mistakes and making sound, responsible decisions that take into consideration all aspects of a situation.
- *Social health.* This dimension refers to the ability to have satisfying interpersonal relationships: interactions with others, adaptation to various social situations, and daily behaviors.

- *Emotional health.* This dimension refers to the feeling component—to express emotions when it is appropriate, to control them when it is not, and to avoid expressing them in an inappropriate manner. Feelings of self-esteem, self-confidence, self-efficacy, trust, love, and many other emotional reactions and responses are all part of emotional health.
- *Environmental health.* This dimension refers to an appreciation of the external environment and the role individuals play in preserving, protecting, and improving environmental conditions.
- *Spiritual health.* This dimension may involve a belief in a supreme being or a specified way of living prescribed by a particular religion. Spiritual health also includes the feeling of unity with the environment—a feeling of oneness with others and with nature—and a guiding sense of meaning or value in life. It also may include the ability to understand and express one's purpose in life; to feel a part of a greater spectrum of existence; to experience love, joy, pain, sorrow, peace, contentment, and wonder over life's experiences; and to care about and respect all living things.

A well individual might display the following characteristics:

- A realistic sense of self, including personal capabilities and limitations
- An appreciation of all living things, no matter how ugly or beautiful, how unique or different, or how great or small
- A willingness to understand imperfection, to forgive others' mistakes, and to grow from personal mistakes or shortcomings
- The ability to laugh, to cry, and to genuinely "feel" emotions without getting lost in emotional upsets
- The ability to function at a reasonable level physiologically
- The ability to maintain and support healthy relationships with family, friends, intimate partners, and strangers
- An appreciation for one's role in preserving and protecting the environment
- A sense of satisfaction with life and an appreciation for the stages of the life experience
- A zest for living, coupled with a curiosity about what each new encounter and each new day will bring
- A respect for self, as well as a respect for others
- A realistic perspective about life's challenges and the skills to cope with life's stresses and challenges
- A balance in all things

Many people believe that wellness can best be achieved by adopting a *holistic* approach, which emphasizes the integration of and balance among mind, body, and spirit. Achieving wellness means attaining the optimum level of wellness for a given person's unique set of limitations and strengths. A physically disabled person may function at his or her optimum level of performance; enjoy satisfying interpersonal relationships; maintain emotional, spiritual, and intellectual health; and have a strong interest in environmental concerns. In contrast, those who spend hours lifting weights to perfect the size and shape of each muscle but pay little attention to nutrition may *look* healthy, but they may not maintain

a good balance in all areas of health. Although we often consider physical attractiveness and other external trappings in measuring the overall health of a person, appearance and physical performance are actually only two signs of wellness, indicating little about the other dimensions.

What do you think?

Based on the wellness dimensions discussed here, what are some of your strengths in each dimension? ✳ What are some of your deficiencies in each dimension? ✳ What one or two things can you do to enhance your strong areas? ✳ To improve on your weaknesses?

New Directions for Health

In 1990, in response to the many indications that Americans were not as healthy as they should be, the U.S. Surgeon General proposed a national plan for promoting health among individuals and groups. Known as *Healthy People 2000,* the plan outlined a series of long-term objectives. Many communities worked toward achieving these goals; nevertheless, by the new millennium as a nation we still had a long way to go.

Healthy People 2000 and *2010* and Other Initiatives

A new plan, *Healthy People 2010,* takes the initiative to the next level. *Healthy People 2010* is a nationwide program with two broad goals: (1) eliminate health disparities, and (2) increase the life span and quality of life. The plan includes 28 focus areas, each representing a public health priority such as nutrition, tobacco use, substance abuse, access to quality health services, and common health conditions, for example, heart disease and diabetes.

For each focus area, the plan presents specific objectives for the nation to achieve during the next decade. For instance, nutrition data show that only 42 percent of Americans aged 20 and older are at their healthy weight; the goal is to raise that number to 60 percent. In the focus area of physical activity and fitness, 40 percent of Americans aged 18 and older do not engage in any leisure-time physical activity. The objective is to reduce this number to 20 percent by 2010.[9]

In the public sector, the Agency for Health Care Research and Quality (AHRQ) offers additional direction for national health care efforts through its *AHRQ Guidelines,* a set of objectives for health care providers to meet in specific areas of practice. Other government agencies and research centers also address specific health concerns. An example is *Best Practices for Comprehensive Tobacco Control Programs,* a publication that recommends budgets and treatment guidelines to curb smoking.[10]

How Healthy Are You?

Rate your health status in each of the following dimensions by circling the number that best describes you.

	Very Unhealthy	Somewhat Unhealthy	Somewhat Healthy	Very Healthy
Physical Health	1	2	3	4
Social Health	1	2	3	4
Emotional Health	1	2	3	4
Environmental Health	1	2	3	4
Spiritual Health	1	2	3	4
Intellectual Health	1	2	3	4

How healthy do you think you are? Which area(s), if any, could you work on improving? Now indicate how often you think the following statements describe you.

PHYSICAL HEALTH

	Rarely, If Ever	Sometimes	Most of the Time	Always
1. I maintain a desirable weight.	1	2	3	4
2. I engage in vigorous exercises, such as brisk walking, jogging, swimming, or running, for at least 30 minutes per day, 3–4 times per week.	1	2	3	4
3. I do exercises designed to strengthen my muscles and joints.	1	2	3	4
4. I warm up and cool down by stretching before and after vigorous exercise.	1	2	3	4
5. I feel good about the condition of my body.	1	2	3	4
6. I get 7–8 hours of sleep each night.	1	2	3	4
7. My immune system is strong, and I am able to avoid most infectious diseases.	1	2	3	4
8. My body heals itself quickly when I get sick or injured.	1	2	3	4
9. I have lots of energy and can get through the day without being overly tired.	1	2	3	4
10. I listen to my body; when there is something wrong, I seek professional advice.	1	2	3	4

SOCIAL HEALTH

	Rarely, If Ever	Sometimes	Most of the Time	Always
1. When I meet people, I feel good about the impression I make on them.	1	2	3	4
2. I am open and honest, and I get along well with other people.	1	2	3	4
3. I participate in a wide variety of social activities and enjoy being with people who are different from me.	1	2	3	4
4. I try to be a "better person" and work on behaviors that have caused problems in my interactions with others.	1	2	3	4

How Healthy Are You?

	Rarely, If Ever	Sometimes	Most of the Time	Always
5. I get along well with the members of my family.	1	2	3	4
6. I am a good listener.	1	2	3	4
7. I am open and accessible to a loving and responsible relationship.	1	2	3	4
8. I have someone I can talk to about my private feelings.	1	2	3	4
9. I consider the feelings of others and do not act in hurtful or selfish ways.	1	2	3	4
10. I consider how what I say might be perceived by others before I speak.	1	2	3	4

EMOTIONAL HEALTH

	Rarely, If Ever	Sometimes	Most of the Time	Always
1. I find it easy to laugh about things that happen in my life.	1	2	3	4
2. I avoid using alcohol as a means of helping me forget my problems.	1	2	3	4
3. I can express my feelings without feeling silly.	1	2	3	4
4. When I am angry, I try to let others know in nonconfrontational and nonhurtful ways.	1	2	3	4
5. I am not a chronic worrier and do not tend to be suspicious of others.	1	2	3	4
6. I recognize when I am stressed and take steps to relax through exercise, quiet time, or other activities.	1	2	3	4
7. I feel good about myself and believe others like me for who I am.	1	2	3	4
8. When I am upset, I talk to others and actively try to work through my problems.	1	2	3	4
9. I am flexible and adapt or adjust to change in a positive way.	1	2	3	4
10. My friends regard me as a stable, emotionally well-adjusted person.	1	2	3	4

ENVIRONMENTAL HEALTH

	Rarely, If Ever	Sometimes	Most of the Time	Always
1. I am concerned about environmental pollution and actively try to preserve and protect natural resources.	1	2	3	4
2. I report people who intentionally hurt the environment.	1	2	3	4
3. I recycle my garbage.	1	2	3	4
4. I reuse plastic and paper bags and tin foil.	1	2	3	4
5. I vote for pro-environment candidates in elections.	1	2	3	4

Continued on page 8

How Healthy Are You?

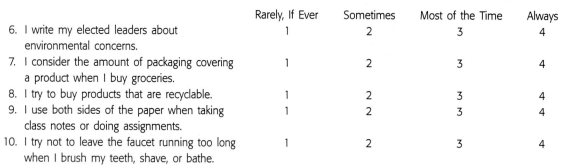

	Rarely, If Ever	Sometimes	Most of the Time	Always
6. I write my elected leaders about environmental concerns.	1	2	3	4
7. I consider the amount of packaging covering a product when I buy groceries.	1	2	3	4
8. I try to buy products that are recyclable.	1	2	3	4
9. I use both sides of the paper when taking class notes or doing assignments.	1	2	3	4
10. I try not to leave the faucet running too long when I brush my teeth, shave, or bathe.	1	2	3	4

SPIRITUAL HEALTH

	Rarely, If Ever	Sometimes	Most of the Time	Always
1. I believe life is a precious gift that should be nurtured.	1	2	3	4
2. I take time to enjoy nature and the beauty around me.	1	2	3	4
3. I take time alone to think about what's important in life—who I am, what I value, where I fit in, and where I'm going.	1	2	3	4
4. I have faith in a greater power, be it a God-like force, nature, or the connectedness of all living things.	1	2	3	4
5. I engage in acts of caring and good will without expecting something in return.	1	2	3	4
6. I feel sorrow for those who are suffering and try to help them through difficult times.	1	2	3	4
7. I feel confident that I have touched the lives of others in a positive way.	1	2	3	4
8. I work for peace in my interpersonal relationships, in my community, and in the world at large.	1	2	3	4
9. I am content with who I am.	1	2	3	4
10. I experience life to the fullest.	1	2	3	4

INTELLECTUAL HEALTH

	Rarely, If Ever	Sometimes	Most of the Time	Always
1. I think about consequences before I act.	1	2	3	4
2. I learn from my mistakes and try to act differently the next time.	1	2	3	4
3. I follow directions or recommended guidelines and act in ways likely to keep myself and others safe.	1	2	3	4
4. I consider the alternatives before making decisions.	1	2	3	4

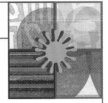

How Healthy Are You?

	Rarely, If Ever	Sometimes	Most of the Time	Always
	1	2	3	4
5. I am alert and ready to respond to life's challenges in ways that reflect thought and sound judgment.	1	2	3	4
6. I tend to let my emotions get the better of me and I act without thinking.	1	2	3	4
7. I actively learn all I can about products and services before making decisions.	1	2	3	4
8. I manage my time well rather than let time manage me.	1	2	3	4
9. My friends and family trust my judgment.	1	2	3	4
10. I think about my self-talk (the things I tell myself) and then examine the evidence to see if my perceptions and feelings are sound.	1	2	3	4

PERSONAL CHECKLIST

Now, total your scores in each of the health dimensions and compare it to the ideal score. Which areas do you need to work on? How does your score compare with how you rated yourself in the first part of the questionnaire?

	Ideal Score	Your Score
Physical Health	40	_____
Social Health	40	_____
Emotional Health	40	_____
Environmental Health	40	_____
Spiritual Health	40	_____
Intellectual Health	40	_____

WHAT YOUR SCORES MEAN

Scores of 35–40: Outstanding! Your answers show that you are aware of the importance of this area to your health. More important, you are putting your knowledge to work for you by practicing good health habits. As long as you continue to do so, this area should not pose a serious health risk. It's likely that you are setting an example for your family and friends to follow. Although you received a very high score on this part of the test, you may want to consider areas where your scores could be improved.

Scores of 30–35: Your health practices in this area are good, but there is room for improvement. Look again at the items you answered that scored 1 or 2 points. What changes could you make to improve your score? Even a small change in behavior can help you achieve better health.

Scores of 20–30: Your health risks are showing! Find information about the risks you are facing and why it is important to change these behaviors. Perhaps you need help in deciding how to make the changes you desire. Assistance is available in this book, from your professor, and from student health services at your school.

Scores below 20: You may be taking serious and unnecessary risks with your health. Perhaps you are not aware of the risks and what to do about them. In this book you will find the information you need to help you improve your scores and your health.

Source: Adapted from U.S. Health and Human Services, *Health Style: A Self-Test* (Washington, DC: Public Health Service, 1981).

Although *Healthy People 2000* was viewed as a landmark public health measure, many health authorities in the field criticized the document because they felt its goals were unreachable and because there was neither national financial support nor a clear plan for achieving the goals. Because less than 5 percent of our national budget is allocated for prevention and historically we have spent most of our health care dollars on treatment, achieving these goals may be difficult.

Health Promotion

The objectives from the *Healthy People* documents prompted action through social, environmental, policy-related, and community-based programming to promote health and prevent premature disability. In addition, a new emphasis on assisting individuals in their pursuit of specific behavior changes began to emerge. However, changing behavior without help is not easy. The term **health promotion** describes the educational, organizational, procedural, environmental, social, and financial supports that help individuals and groups reduce negative health behaviors and promote positive change.

Health promotion programs identify healthy people who are engaging in **risk behaviors,** or behaviors that increase susceptibility to negative health outcomes, and motivate them to change their actions. Effective stop-smoking programs, for instance, don't simply say, "Just do it." Instead, they provide information about risk behaviors and possible consequences to smokers and the victims of their sidestream smoke (educational support); they encourage smokers to participate in smoking cessation classes and employers to allow time off for worker attendance, or they set up buddy systems to help smokers (organizational support); they establish rules governing smokers' behaviors and supporting their decisions to change, such as banning smoking in the workplace and removing cigarettes from vending machines (environmental support); and they provide incentives to motivate people to participate (financial support).[11]

Health promotion programs also encourage those with sound health habits to maintain them. By attempting to modify behaviors, increase skills, change attitudes, increase

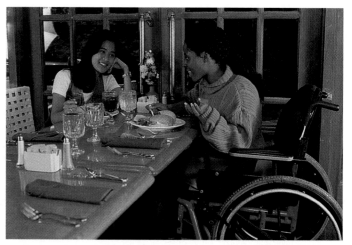

The motivation to improve quality of life within the framework of one's own unique capabilities is crucial to achieving health and wellness.

knowledge, influence values, and improve health decision making, health promotion goes well beyond the simple information campaign. By basing programs and services in communities, organizations, schools, and other places where most people spend their time, health promotion increases the likelihood of long-term success on the road to health and wellness.

Whether we use the term *health* or *wellness,* we are talking about a person's overall responses to the challenges of living. Occasional dips into the ice cream bucket and other dietary slips, failures to exercise every day, flare-ups of anger, and other deviations from optimal behavior should not be viewed as major failures. Actually, the ability to recognize that each of us is an imperfect being, attempting to adapt in an imperfect world, signals individual well-being.

We must also remember to be tolerant of others. Rather than be warriors against pleasure in our zeal to change the health behaviors of others, we need to be supportive, understanding, and nonjudgmental. *Health bashing*—intolerance or negative feelings, words, or actions aimed at people who fail to meet our expectations of health—may indicate our own deficiencies in the psychological, social, and/or spiritual dimensions of the health continuum.

Disease Prevention

Most health promotion initiatives include the term **disease prevention.** What does it really mean? Historically, the health literature describes three types of prevention: primary, secondary, and tertiary.

In a general sense, *prevention* means taking positive actions *now* to avoid becoming sick *later.* Getting immunized against diseases such as polio, deciding not to smoke cigarettes, and practicing safer sex constitute **primary prevention**—actions designed to reduce risk and avoid health problems before they start. **Secondary prevention** (also referred to as **intervention**) involves recognizing health risks or early problems and

Health promotion   Combined educational, organizational, policy, financial, and environmental supports to help people reduce negative health behaviors and promote positive change.

Risk behaviors   Behaviors that increase susceptibility to negative health outcomes.

Disease prevention   Actions or behaviors designed to keep people from getting sick.

Primary prevention   Actions designed to stop problems before they start.

Secondary prevention (intervention)   Intervention early in the development of a health problem.

New Standards Help Protect Info-Seeking Health Consumers

Interested in finding out about health-related topics on the Internet? It may surprise you to know that until very recently, every time you logged onto the net to seek health information, you may have been playing a risky game of Russian Roulette, with only a 50-50 chance of getting completely reliable and accurate information.

As of July 20, 2001, it has become much easier to determine whether the health-related websites you log onto provide reliable information. On this date, the American Accreditation Health Care Consumer organization (named ARAC from a previous accreditation name) took an active stance in protecting health information seekers. This organization, whose primary mission prior to this was to set quality standards for managed care companies, has come up with 50 criteria that health sites must meet to win its "seal of approval."*

Now, a rating scale and visible seal will tell you at a glance whether a site providing health information meets the rigorous standards for quality and accuracy that ARAC demands. In addition to policing the accuracy of health claims, this accreditation will evaluate health information and provide a forum for reporting misinformation, privacy violations, and other complaints.

Such an accreditation may cost in excess of $5000. The high cost increases the likelihood that a site bearing the "seal of approval" is sponsored by a stable, professional organization rather than by pseudoprofessionals operating their health networks out of home offices. Out of over 20,000 or more potential sites, fewer than 50 may seek this accreditation in the next year. The most likely candidates are sites that are sponsored by reputable, established professional organizations.

Although experts have recognized the potential threat from unmonitored information on the Internet for the last decade, efforts to police sites have not been able to garner the support or resources for the regular monitoring and enforcement that are needed in a rapidly changing health arena.

With over 100 million people accessing health information on the Internet each year, these risks have grown exponentially in the last few years, forcing professional groups to act quickly to help wary consumers get only the best information.

Numerous polls have indicated that consumers are skeptical of Internet-based information, yet they continue to access sites that lack credibility at alarming rates. Some populations, particularly those who lack formal health education or health-related knowledge, are among those who are most vulnerable. The accreditation listed above is one of the first major steps in bringing the most reliable sources of information into your home. If you have concerns about the accuracy of information or are wondering which sites might be the best for your particular needs, contact your local university health center and/or health education department, health care provider, or community-based support groups. Other reliable sources will be listed throughout this book.

*Source: Laura Landro, "Health Journal: Online Groups Step Up Attempts to Enforce Standards," Wall Street Journal, July 20, 2001, p. B1.

---

taking action (intervening) to stop the behavior before it leads to actual illness. Getting a young smoker to quit is an example of secondary prevention. The third type, **tertiary prevention,** involves treatment and/or rehabilitation after the person is already sick. Typically, it is offered by medical specialists.

In the United States, two of every three deaths and one of every three hospitalizations are linked to preventable lifestyle behaviors, such as tobacco use, sedentary lifestyle, alcohol consumption, and overeating. This means that primary and secondary prevention offer our best hope for reducing the **incidence** (number of new cases) and **prevalence** (number of existing cases) of disease and disability.

It is clear that we need to move from a mind-set of tertiary prevention to focus on earlier intervention designed to remove barriers and help individuals succeed in their behavior change strategies. Health educators in U.S. schools and communities offer an affordable and effective delivery of prevention and intervention programs. **Certified Health Education Specialists (CHES)** make up a trained cadre of public health workers with special credentials and competencies to plan, implement, and evaluate prevention programs that offer scientifically sound, behaviorally based methods to help

individuals and communities increase the likelihood of success. As a nation that historically spends little on prevention, however, such a shift has been and will continue to be difficult.

Achievements in Public Health

To those of us in the field of public health, the saying "We've come a long way, baby" accurately reflects the health achievements of the past 100 years. The Centers for Disease Control

---

Tertiary prevention Treatment and/or rehabilitation efforts.

Incidence The number of new cases.

Prevalence The number of existing cases.

Certified Health Education Specialists (CHES) Academically trained health educators who have passed a national competency examination for prevention and intervention programming.

and Prevention (CDC) have named the following as the ten greatest public health achievements of the twentieth century:[12]

1. *Vaccinations.* Vaccinations have eradicated smallpox, eliminated poliomyelitis, and significantly controlled a number of infectious diseases, including measles, rubella, tetanus, diphtheria, and *Haemophilus influenzae* Type B, which once claimed the lives of large numbers of people in the early 1900s, many before they had reached age 5.

2. *Motor vehicle safety.* Motor vehicle safety has improved as a result of engineering advances that have made both vehicles and highways safer and as a result of successful public policy efforts to change personal behavior. These personal behavior changes include the use of safety belts, child safety seats, and motorcycle helmets and the avoidance of drinking and driving.

3. *Workplace safety.* Work-related health risks common at the beginning of the century are now either under better control or completely eliminated. Since 1980, the rate of fatal occupational injuries has fallen by 40 percent.

4. *Control of infectious diseases.* Clean water and improved sanitation have greatly reduced the development and transmission of infectious diseases since 1900. In addition, antimicrobial therapy, such as the discovery of and treatment with antibiotics, has greatly reduced the risk of contracting such diseases as tuberculosis and sexually transmitted infections.

5. *Cardiovascular disease (CVD) and stroke deaths.* The incidence of CVD and stroke has declined as a result of efforts to educate the public on how to modify health risk factors, such as smoking and high blood pressure, coupled with earlier detection and better treatment.

6. *Safe and healthy foods.* Since 1900, technology for eradicating microbial contaminants from foods has increased dramatically. In addition, the identification of essential micronutrients and establishment of food-fortification programs have almost eliminated major nutritional deficiency diseases, such as rickets, goiter, and pellagra.

7. *Maternal and infant care.* Better hygiene and nutrition, wider availability of antibiotics, greater access to health care, and technological advances in medicine have greatly reduced the risks to infants and mothers. Since 1900, infant mortality has decreased by 90 percent, and maternal mortality has declined by 99 percent.

8. *Family planning.* Access to family planning and contraceptive services has altered social and economic roles of women. Family planning has provided health benefits that have helped reduce the number of infant, child, and maternal deaths; increased opportunities for preconceptional counseling and screening; and increased the use of barrier contraceptives to prevent unwanted pregnancies and transmission of sexually transmissible infections.

9. *Fluoridated drinking water.* Fluoridation of drinking water began in 1945 and in 1999 reached an estimated 144 million persons in the United States. Fluoridation safely and inexpensively prevents tooth decay, regardless of socioeconomic status or access to health care. It has played an important role in reducing tooth decay in children and tooth loss in adults.

10. *Recognition of tobacco as a health hazard.* Public antismoking campaigns have changed social norms to prevent people from initiation of tobacco use, promote cessation of use, and reduce exposure to environmental tobacco smoke. Since the 1964 Surgeon General's report on the health risks of smoking, millions of smoking-related health problems have been prevented, and millions of lives have been saved.

While we have indeed come a long way, the possibilities for health and well-being in the future defy the imagination. Living longer, living more disease-free years, and injecting more quality into the extra years of life will be major goals. The more we learn about the remarkable resilience of the human body and spirit, and the more technology stretches our imagination and enlarges our possibilities, the more likely that the twenty-first century will rival the twentieth for health-related breakthroughs.

> **What do you think?**
>
> *What do you consider the greatest achievements in public health in the twentieth century?* ✳ *What do you think would be the most important achievement that public health could make in the next 50 years?*

Gender Differences and Health Status

You don't have to be a health expert to know there are physiological differences between men and women. Although much of male and female anatomy is identical, major differences exist in susceptibility to disease and other health factors. Many diseases—osteoporosis, multiple sclerosis, and Alzheimer's disease, for example—are far more common in women than in men. Finally, although women live longer than men, they don't necessarily enjoy better quality of life.[13]

Much of the current interest in exploring women's health came after 1990, when a highly publicized government study raised concern about the uneven numbers of women included in clinical trial research conducted by the National Institutes of Health (NIH). In response, the NIH established the Office of Research on Women's Health (ORWH) in 1990 to oversee the representation of women in NIH studies. According to Vivian Pinn, ORWH's director, "For too long, medicine has viewed women as 'abnormal men' when considering health problems."[14]

Researchers have historically excluded women of childbearing age from clinical trials of many new drugs. One reason was concern about the possibility that a medication might harm a fetus; another was that women's menstrual cycles can influence the effects of a drug. Of course, men and women do vary physiologically, so the elimination of women from many studies meant that the results from these studies were not applied to women directly.

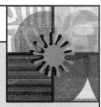

Consumer Beware: Health Information on the Internet

Looking for health-related information? Always consult your doctor first. However, to get additional information, there are innumerable resources right at your fingertips on the internet. But how do you know how reliable the information is? Which of the thousands of websites should you click onto first? Not all health websites are created equal.

Here are some hints to help you recognize those that are likely to be reliable.

– Websites sponsored by an official government agency, a college or university, or a hospital tend to have accurate, up-to-date information about a wide range of health topics. Government sites are easily identified by their .gov extensions (for example, the National Institute of Mental Health at http://www.nimh.nih.gov/); college and university sites typically have .edu extensions (Johns Hopkins University: http://www.jhu.ed/.) Hospitals often have an .org extension (Mayo Clinic: http://www.mayohealth.org/), although some have other extensions as well.

– Links provided within proven websites are often valuable resources.

– Many medical journal websites, such as The New England Journal of Medicine, http://www.nejm.org/; or the Journal of the American Medical Association (JAMA), http://www.ama-assn.org/, are good sources of current breakthroughs in research. (While some of these sites may require a fee for access, often you can locate basic information, such as a weekly table of contents, that can help you conduct a library search.) However, not all medical journals are of this caliber. If you have questions about a journal's reputation, ask your doctor or another qualified medical professional.

– In most cases, it is important that websites include fresh content; however, beware of information that is trendy or based on fads. This information is not always the most accurate or useful. Also, if a site contains encyclopedic information, such as definitions of diseases and other health-related issues, it is not necessary that they be updated as frequently as those sites containing current research.

– Use discretion and don't believe everything you read. If you notice grammatical or spelling errors, that should raise a red flag. If the site you're using is sponsored by a pharmaceutical company or a retail medical operation, consider whose best interests are being served.

As in everyday practice, quackery runs rampant on the internet. This is particularly true if you visit health usenet groups or bulletin boards. Just because some claim to be physcians or experts does not mean that they are telling the whole truth. In the same vein, if you are seeking information pertaining to a personal health issue, make sure you have checked your source's credentials. Privacy on the internet is a valuable and rare commodity that you want to preserve.

In addition to the many government and education-based sites, there are useful sites that are independently sponsored. The following are just a sample:

1. Adam: www.adam.com
2. HealthAnswers.com: www.healthanswers.com
3. Dr. Koop.com: www.drkoop.com
4. ThriveOnline: www.thriveonline.com
5. InteliHealth: www.intelihealth.com
6. HealthAtoZ.com: www.healthatoz.com
7. WebMD Health: http://my.webmd.com
8. America's Doctor: www.americasdoctor.com
9. Drug Infonet: www.druginfonet.com

Throughout this book, you will find some of these sites among the many that are provided in each chapter. These sites are related to each of the health areas presented so that you can further enhance your knowledge base. Use good judgment; be a health-wise consumer of information.

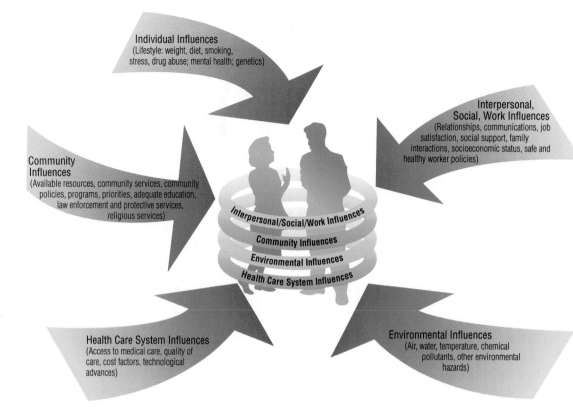

Figure 1.2
Factors That Influence Health Status

To address concerns about women's health, the government has specified that equal amounts of money and time must be spent on men's and women's health research.[15] The National Heart, Blood, and Lung Institute is conducting the **Women's Health Initiative (WHI).** This 15-year, $625 million study focuses on the leading causes of death and disease in more than 160,000 postmenopausal women. WHI researchers hope to find out how a healthful lifestyle and increased medical attention can help prevent women's cancers, heart disease, and osteoporosis.[16]

> **What do you think?**
> *Do you think there are true disparities between men's and women's health status?* * *What are some indicators or examples?* * *Can you think of programs, policies, or individual actions that would reduce such disparities?*

Women's Health Initiative (WHI)   National study of postmenopausal women, in conjunction with the NIH mandate for equal research priorities for women's health issues.

Improving Your Health

Factors Influencing Your Health Status

Table 1.1 summarizes the leading causes of death in the United States, by age. Note that Americans aged 15–24 are most likely to die from unintentional injuries, followed by homicide, legal intervention, and suicide. Unintentional injuries are also the major killer in the next age group, 25–44, followed by malignant neoplasms (cancer), and heart disease.

Individual behavior is a major determinant of good health, but heredity, access to health care, and the environment can also influence health status (Figure 1.2). When these factors are considered together and form the basis of a person's lifestyle choices, the net effect on health can be great.

Health Behaviors

Most experts believe that several key behaviors will help people live longer, such as

- Getting a good night's sleep (minimum of seven hours)
- Maintaining healthy eating habits
- Managing weight
- Participating in physical recreational activities
- Avoiding tobacco products

Table 1.1
Leading Causes of Death in the United States by Age (Years)

RANK	ALL AGES	1–4	5–14	15–24	25–44	45–65	65+
1	Diseases of heart	Unintentional injuries	Unintentional injuries	Unintentional injuries	Unintentional injuries	Malignant neoplasms	Diseases of heart
2	Malignant neoplasms	Congenital anomalies	Malignant neoplasms	Homicide and legal intervention	Malignant neoplasms	Diseases of heart	Malignant neoplasms
3	Cerebrovascular disease	Homicide and legal intervention	Homicide and legal intervention	Suicide	Diseases of heart	Unintentional injuries	Cerebrovascular diseases
4	Chronic obstructive disease	Malignant neoplasms	Congenital anomalies	Malignant neoplasms	Suicide	Cerebrovascular diseases	Chronic obstructive pulmonary diseases
5	Unintentional injuries	Diseases of heart	Diseases of heart	Diseases of heart	Human immunodeficiency virus infection	Diabetes mellitus	Pneumonia and influenza
6	Pneumonia and influenza	Pneumonia and influenza	Suicide	Congenital anomalies	Homicide and legal intervention	Chronic obstructive pulmonary diseases	Diabetes mellitus
7	Diabetes mellitus	Septicemia	Chronic obstructive pulmonary disease	Chronic obstructive pulmonary diseases	Chronic liver disease and cirrhosis	Chronic liver disease and cirrhosis	Unintentional injuries
8	Suicide	Conditions of perinatal period	Pneumonia and influenza	Pneumonia and influenza	Cerebrovascular diseases	Suicide	Nephritis, nephrotic syndrome, and nephrosis
9	Nephritis, nephrotic syndrome, and nephrosis	Cerebrovascular diseases	Benign neoplasms	Human immunodeficiency virus infection	Diabetes mellitus	Pneumonia and influenza	Alzheimer's disease
10	Chronic liver disease and cirrhosis	Benign neoplasms	Cerebrovascular diseases	Cerebrovascular diseases	Pneumonia and influenza	Human immunodeficiency virus infection	Septicemia

Source: S. Murphy, "Deaths: Final Data for 2000," National Vital Statistics Reports, vol. 48 (11) from the Centers for Disease Control and Prevention, (2001), National Center for Health Statistics, Hyattsville, MD. http://www.cdc.gov/nchs/data

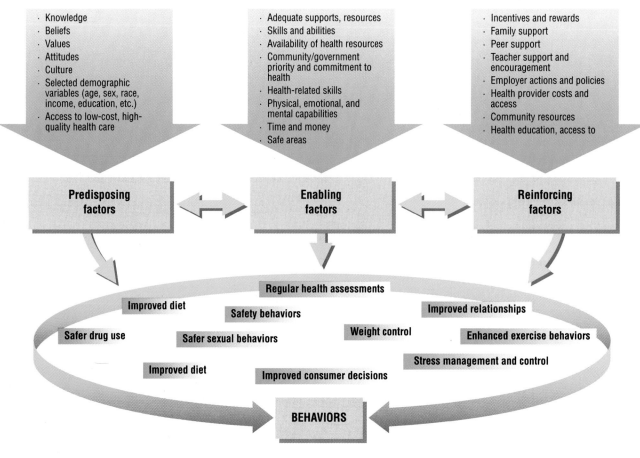

Figure 1.3
Factors That Influence Behavior-Change Decisions

- Practicing safer sex
- Limiting intake of alcohol
- Scheduling regular self-exams and medical checkups

Several other actions may not add "years to your life" but may significantly add "life to your years." They include the following:

- Controlling the real and imaginary stressors in life
- Forming and maintaining meaningful relationships with family and friends
- Making time for yourself
- Participating in at least one fun activity each day
- Respecting the environment and the people in it
- Considering alternatives when making decisions and assessing how actions affect others
- Valuing each day and making the best of opportunities
- Viewing mistakes as opportunities to learn and grow
- Being as kind to yourself as to others
- Understanding the health care system and using it wisely

Though it's easy to list things that one should do, change is not easy. All of us, no matter where we are on the health/wellness continuum, have to start somewhere. All people have faced personal and external challenges to their at-

tempts to change health behaviors. Some have not done so well, some have been extremely successful, and some have made only small changes that add up to significant improvements in how they feel and how they live.

Preparing for Behavior Change

Mark Twain said that "habit is habit, and not to be flung out the window by anyone, but coaxed downstairs a step at a time." The chances of successfully changing negative behavior improve when you make gradual changes that give you time to unlearn negative patterns and to substitute positive ones. To understand the process of behavior change, first identify specific behavior patterns and attempt to understand the reasons for them.

Factors Influencing Behavior Change

Figure 1.3 identifies major factors that influence behavior and behavior-change decisions. They can be divided into three general categories: predisposing, enabling, and reinforcing.

Predisposing Factors Our life experiences, knowledge, cultural and ethnic heritage, and current beliefs and values are all *predisposing factors* influencing behavior and behavior change. Factors that may predispose us to certain conditions include age, sex, race, income, family background, educational background, and access to health care. For example, if your parents smoked, you are 90 percent more likely to start smoking than someone whose parents didn't. If your peers smoke, you are 80 percent more likely to smoke than someone whose friends don't.

Enabling Factors An *enabling factor* is anything that makes a behavior-change decision more convenient or difficult. Enabling factors include your physical, emotional, and mental capabilities, your skills, and your access to resources. Positive enablers encourage you to carry through on your intentions. Negative enablers work against your intentions to change. For example, suppose you would like to join a local fitness center but discover that the closest one is four miles away and that the membership fee is $500. Those are negative enablers that may convince you to stay home. But suppose that your

---

SKILLS FOR BEHAVIOR CHANGE

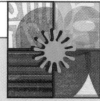

Staging for Change

On any given day, countless numbers of us get out of bed and resolve to begin to change a given behavior "today." Whether it be losing weight, drinking less, exercising more, being nicer to others, managing time better, or some other change in a negative behavior, we start out with high expectations. In a short time, however, a vast majority of people fail and are soon doing whatever it was they thought they shouldn't be doing.

Why do so many good intentions end up as failures? According to Dr. James Prochaska, psychologist and head of the Health Promotion. Partnership at the University of Rhode Island, and Dr. Carlos DiClimente, these failures occur because we are going about things in the wrong way. According to Prochaska and DiClimente, fewer than 20 percent of us are really prepared to take action, Yet, prevention specialists, doctors, and other professionals continue to force us to "Just Do It! and do it *now!*" After considerable research, Prochaska and DiClimente believe that behavior changes usually do not succeed if they start with the change itself. Instead, they believe that we must go through a series of "stages" to adequately prepare, or ready, ourselves for that eventual change. They insist that through proper reinforcement and help during each of the following stages, our chances of making and keeping those New Year's resolutions will be greatly enhanced.

1. *Precontemplation.* People in the precontemplation stage have no current intention of changing. They may have tried to change a behavior before and may have all but given up, or they may just be in denial and unaware of any problem. People in this stage don't have to worry about failure and have no intention of taking any actions.
   Strategies for Change: *Although a very touchy area, sometimes a few frank, yet kind words from friends may be enough to make the precontemplator take a closer look at him- or herself. This is not to say that you should become a "warrior against pleasure" or that you should feel justified in telling people what to do when they haven't asked for advice. Recommended readings or tactful suggestions, however, can be useful.*

2. *Contemplation.* In the contemplation stage, the person recognizes that he or she has a problem and begins to think about the need to change. Acknowledgment usually results from increased awareness, often due to feedback from family and friends or access to information. Despite this acknowledgment, people can languish in this stage for years, knowing that they have a problem but never finding the time or energy to make the change.
   Strategies for Change: *Often, contemplators need a little push to get them started. This may come in the*

form of helping them set up a change plan (e.g., an exercise plan), buying them a gift that helps with the plan (i.e., a low-fat cookbook), giving them articles about a particular problem, or inviting them to go with you to hear a speaker on a related topic. In this stage, people often need skill building or time to think about what they might want to do. Your assistance can help them move off the point of indecision.

3. *Preparation.* Most people in this stage are close to taking action. They've thought about several things they might do and may even have come up with a plan. Rather than thinking only about the reasons why they *can't* begin action, they have started to focus on what they can do to start action.
   Strategies for Change: *Successful change requires following some standard guidelines at this stage: set realistic goals (large and small), take small steps toward change, change only a couple of things at once, reward small milestones, and seek support from friends. Identify those factors that have enabled success or served as a barrier to success in the past, and change or modify those conditions where possible.*

4. *Action.* In the action stage, the individual begins to follow the action plan he or she has put together. People who have prepared for change, thought about alternatives, engaged social

Continued on page 18

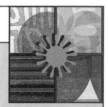

Staging for Change

support, and made a plan of action are more ready for action than those who have given it little thought. Unfortunately, too many people start behavior change here rather than going through the first three stages. Without a plan, without enlisting the help of others, or without a realistic goal, failure is likely. **Strategies for Change:** *Publicly stating the desire to change often helps ensure success. Encourage a friend making a change to share his or her plan with you. Whenever possible, offer to help, and try to remove potential obstacles. Social support and the buddy system often help motivate even the most reluctant person.*

5. *Maintenance.* Maintenance requires vigilance, attention to detail, and long-term commitment. Many people reach their goals, only to relax and slip back into the undesired behavior. In this stage, it is important to be aware of the potential for relapses and develop strategies for dealing with such challenges. Common causes of relapse include overconfidence, daily temptations, stress or emotional distractions, and self-deprecation for failure. **Strategies for Change:** *During maintenance, you must continue doing the same things that led to success in the first place. Find fun and creative ways to maintain the positive behav-*

iors. This is where a willing and caring support group can be vital. Knowing where to turn on your campus for help when you don't have a close support network also can be helpful.

6. *Termination.* In this stage, the behavior is so ingrained that the current level of vigilance may be unnecessary. The new behavior has become an essential part of daily living. Can you think of someone you know who has made a major behavior change that has now become an essential part of that person's life?

---

school's fitness center is two blocks away, stays open until midnight, and offers a special student membership. Those are positive enablers that will probably convince you to join the center. Identifying positive and negative enabling factors and devising alternative plans when the negative factors outweigh the positive are part of planning for behavior change.

Reinforcing Factors The presence or absence of support, encouragement, or discouragement from significant people in your life is a *reinforcing factor.* For example, suppose you decide to stop smoking and your family and friends continue smoking in your presence. You may be tempted to start smoking again because your smoking behavior was reinforced. Suppose, however, that you are overweight and you lose a few pounds and all your friends tell you how terrific you look. Their encouragement will reinforce your positive behavior, and you will be more likely to continue your weight-loss plan.

The manner in which you reward or punish yourself also plays a role. Accepting small failures and concentrating on your successes can foster further achievements. Telling yourself that you're worth the extra time and effort and giving yourself a pat on the back for small accomplishments are

often overlooked factors in positive behavior change. In contrast, berating yourself because you, for example, binged on ice cream or argued with a friend may create an internal environment in which failure becomes almost inevitable.

Motivation

Wanting to change is a prerequisite of the change process, but there is much more to the process than motivation. Motivation must be combined with common sense, commitment, and a realistic understanding of how best to move from point A to point B.[17] *Readiness* is the state of being that precedes behavior change. People who are ready to change possess the knowledge, attitudes, skills, and internal and external resources that make change a likely reality. To be ready for change, a person must take certain basic steps and make adjustments in thinking.

Beliefs and Attitudes

We often assume that when rational people realize what they are doing carries a risk, they will act to reduce that risk. But this is not necessarily true. Consider the number of health professionals who smoke, consume high-fat diets, and act in other unhealthy ways. They surely know better, but their "knowing" is disconnected from their "doing." Why is this so? Two strong influences on behavior are at work: beliefs and attitudes.

A **belief** is an appraisal of the relationship between some object, action, or idea (for example, smoking) and

Belief Appraisal of the relationship between some object, action, or idea and some attribute of that object, action, or idea.

some attribute of that object, action, or idea (for example, smoking is expensive, is dirty, and causes cancer—or, smoking is relaxing). An **attitude** is a relatively stable set of beliefs, feelings, and behavioral tendencies in relation to something or someone.

Psychologists studying the relationship between beliefs and health habits have determined that although beliefs can subtly influence behavior, they may not actually cause people to behave differently. In 1966, psychologist I. Rosenstock developed a classic theory, the **Health Belief Model (HBM),** to show when beliefs affect behavior change.[18] Although many other models attempt to explain the influence of beliefs on behaviors, the HBM remains one of the most widely accepted. It holds that several factors must support a belief before change is likely:

- *Perceived seriousness of the health problem.* How severe would the medical and social consequences be if the health problem were to develop or be left untreated? The more serious the perceived effects, the more likely that the person will take action.
- *Perceived susceptibility to the health problem.* Next, what is the likelihood of developing the health problem? People who perceive themselves at high risk are more likely to take preventive action.
- *Cues to action.* Those who are reminded or alerted about a potential health problem are more likely to take action.

Three other factors are linked to perceived risk for health problems: *demographic variables,* including age, gender, race, and ethnic background; *sociopsychological variables,* including personality traits, social class, and social pressure; and *structural variables,* including knowledge about or prior contact with the health problem.

The Health Belief Model is followed many times every day. Take, for example, smokers. Older smokers are likely to know other smokers who have developed serious heart or lung problems. They are thus more likely to perceive tobacco as a threat to their health than a teenager who has just begun smoking. The greater the perceived threat of health problems caused by smoking, the greater the chance a person will quit.

However, many chronic smokers know the risks yet continue to smoke. Why do they fail to take actions to avoid further harm? According to Rosenstock, some people do not believe that they will be affected by a severe problem—they act as though they believed they have some kind of immunity—and are unlikely to change their behavior. In some cases, they may think that even if they get cancer or have a heart attack, the health care system will cure them. They also may feel that the immediate pleasure outweighs the long-range cost.

Intentions to Change

Our attitudes reflect our emotional responses to situations and follow from our beliefs. According to the **Theory of Rea-** soned Action, our behaviors result from our intentions to perform actions. An intention is a product of our attitude toward an action and our beliefs about what others may want us to do.[19] A behavioral intention, then, is a written or stated commitment to perform an action.

In brief, the more consistent and powerful your attitudes about an action and the more you are influenced by others to take that action, the greater will be your stated intention to do so. The more you verbalize your commitment to change, the more likely you are to succeed.

What do you think?
*What is one major behavior that you believe you should change? * How serious a threat to your health is this behavior right now? * What might happen if you don't make the change? * What can you do right now to reduce your risk of developing a problem? * List the steps that you intend to take today and this week.*

Significant Others as Change Agents

Many people are highly influenced by the approval or disapproval (real or imagined) of close friends, loved ones, and the social and cultural groups to which they belong. Such influences can support healthy behavior, or they can interfere with even the best intentions.

Your Family   From the time of your birth, your parents have given you strong cues about which actions are socially acceptable and which are not. Brushing your teeth, bathing, wearing deodorant, and chewing food with your mouth closed are all behaviors that your family probably instilled in you long ago. Your family culture influenced your food choices, religious beliefs, political beliefs, and all your other values and actions. If you deviated from your family's norms, your mother or father probably let you know fairly quickly. Good family units share a dedication to the healthful development of all family members, unconditional trust, and a commitment to work out difficulties.

Attitude   Relatively stable set of beliefs, feelings, and behavioral tendencies in relation to something or someone.

Health Belief Model (HBM)   Model for explaining how beliefs may influence behaviors.

Theory of Reasoned Action   Model for explaining the importance of our intentions in determining behaviors.

When the loving family unit does not exist, when it does not provide for basic human needs, or when dysfunctional, irresponsible individuals try to build a family under the influence of drugs or alcohol, it becomes difficult for a child to learn positive health behaviors. Healthy behaviors get their start in healthy homes; unhealthy homes breed unhealthy habits. Healthy families provide the foundation for a clear and necessary understanding of what is right and wrong, what is positive and negative. Without this fundamental grounding, many young people have great difficulties.[20]

Your Social Bonds   Like family, personal environments also mold behaviors. If you deviated from the actions expected in your hometown, you probably suffered strange looks, ostracism by some high school cliques, and other negative social reactions. The more you value the opinions of other people, the more likely you are to change a behavior that offends them. If you couldn't care less what they think, you probably brush off their negative reactions or suggested changes. How often have you told yourself, "I don't care what so-and-so thinks. I'll do what I darn well please"? Although most of us have thought or said these words, often we care too much about what even the insignificant people in our lives think. In general, the lower your self-esteem and self-efficacy, the higher the chances that others will influence your actions.

Sometimes, the influence of others can be a powerful social support for positive behavior changes.[21] At other times, we are influenced to drink too much, party too hard, eat too much, or engage in some other negative action because we don't want to be left out or criticized. Learning to understand the subtle and not-so-subtle ways in which other people influence our actions is an important step toward changing our behaviors.

Choosing a Behavior-Change Strategy

Once you have analyzed all the factors that influence what you do, you must decide which behavior-change technique will work best for you. These techniques include shaping, visualization, modeling, controlling the situation, reinforcement, and changing self-talk.

Shaping   Using a series of small steps to get to a particular goal gradually.

Imagined rehearsal   Practicing, through mental imagery, to become better able to perform an event in actuality.

Modeling   Learning specific behaviors by watching others perform them.

Shaping

Regardless of how motivated you are, some behaviors are almost impossible to change immediately. To reach your goal, you may need to take a number of individual steps, each designed to change one small piece of the larger behavior. This process is known as **shaping.**

For example, suppose that you have not exercised for a while. You decide that you want to get into shape, and your goal is to jog three to four miles every other day. You realize that you'd face a near-death experience if you tried to run even just a few blocks in your current condition. So you decide to start slowly and build up to your desired fitness level gradually. During week 1, you will walk for one hour every other day at a slow, relaxed pace. During week 2, you will walk for the same amount of time but will speed up your pace and cover slightly more ground. During week 3, you will speed up even more and will try to go even farther. You will continue taking such steps until you reach your goal.

Whatever the desired behavior change, all shaping involves the following items:

- Starting slowly and trying not to cause undue stress during the early stages of the program
- Keeping the steps small and achievable
- Being flexible and ready to change if the original plan proves uncomfortable
- Refusing to skip steps or to move to the next step until the previous step has been mastered

Behaviors don't develop overnight, so they won't change overnight.

Visualization

Mental practice and rehearsal can help change unhealthy behaviors into healthy ones. Athletes and others use a technique known as **imagined rehearsal** to reach their goals. By visualizing their planned action ahead of time, they are better prepared when they put themselves to the test.

For example, suppose you want to ask someone out on a date. Imagine the setting (walking together to class) for the action. Then practice exactly what you're going to say ("Minh, there's a great concert this Sunday and I was wondering if") in your mind and out loud. Mentally anticipate different responses ("Oh, I'd love to, but I'm busy that evening") and what you will say in reaction ("How about if I call you sometime this week?"). Careful mental and verbal rehearsal—you could even try out your scenario on a friend—will greatly improve the likelihood of success.

Modeling

Modeling, or learning behaviors through careful observation of other people, is one of the most effective strategies for changing behavior. For example, suppose that you have trouble talking to people you don't know very well. One of the easiest ways to improve your communication skills is to select friends whose "gift of gab" you envy. Observe their social skills. Do they talk more or listen more? How do people respond to them? Why are they such good communicators? If you carefully observe behaviors you admire and isolate their components, you can model the steps of your behavior-change strategy on a proven success.

Controlling the Situation

Sometimes, the right setting or the right group of people will positively influence your behaviors. Many situations and occasions trigger certain actions. For example, in libraries, houses of worship, and museums, most people talk softly. Few people laugh at funerals. The term **situational inducement** refers to an attempt to influence a behavior by using situations and occasions to control it.

For example, you may be more apt to stop smoking if you work in a smoke-free office, a positive situational inducement. But a smoke-filled bar, a negative situational inducement, may tempt you to resume. By carefully considering which settings will help and which will hurt your effort to change, and by making a firm decision to seek the first and avoid the second, you will improve your chances for change.

Reinforcement

A **positive reinforcement** is a reward that is given to increase the likelihood that a behavior change will occur. Each of us is motivated by different reinforcers. Although a special T-shirt may be a positive reinforcer for young adults entering a race, it would not be for a 40-year-old runner who dislikes message-bearing T-shirts.

Most positive reinforcers can be classified under five headings: consumable, activity, manipulative, possessional, and social.

- *Consumable reinforcers* are delicious edibles, such as candy, cookies, or gourmet meals.
- *Activity reinforcers* are opportunities to do something enjoyable, such as to watch TV, go on a vacation, or go swimming.
- *Manipulative reinforcers* are incentives, such as getting a lower rent in exchange for mowing the lawn or the promise of a better grade for doing an extra-credit project.
- *Possessional reinforcers* are tangible rewards, such as a new TV or a sports car.
- *Social reinforcers* are signs of appreciation, approval, or love, such as loving looks, affectionate hugs, and praise.

When choosing reinforcers, determine what would motivate you to act in a particular way. Research has shown that people can be motivated to change their behaviors, such as not smoking during pregnancy or abstaining from cocaine, if they set themselves up on a *token economy* system, whereby they earn tokens or points that can be exchanged for meaningful rewards, such as financial incentives.[22] The difficulty often lies in determining *which* incentive will be most effective. Your reinforcers may initially come from others (extrinsic rewards), but as you see positive changes in yourself, you will begin to reward and reinforce yourself (intrinsic rewards). Keep in mind that reinforcers should immediately follow a behavior, but beware of overkill. If you reward yourself with a movie on the VCR every time you go jogging, this reinforcer will soon lose its power. It would be better to give yourself this reward after, say, a full week of adhering to your jogging program.

Changing Self-Talk

Self-talk, or the way you think and talk to yourself, can also play a role in modifying health-related behaviors. Here are some cognitive procedures for changing self-talk.

Rational—Emotive Therapy   This form of cognitive therapy or self-directed behavior change is based on the premise that there is a close connection between what people say to themselves and how they feel. According to psychologist Albert Ellis, most emotional problems and related behaviors stem from irrational statements that people make to themselves when events in their lives are different from what they would like them to be.[23]

For example, suppose that after doing poorly on an exam, you say to yourself, "I can't believe I flunked that easy exam. I'm so stupid." By changing this irrational, "catastrophic" self-talk into rational, positive statements about what is really going on, you can increase the likelihood that positive behaviors will occur. Positive self-talk might be phrased as follows: "I really didn't study enough for that exam, and I'm not surprised I didn't do very well. I'm certainly not stupid. I just need to prepare better for the next test." Such self-talk will help you to recover quickly from disappointment and take positive steps to correct the situation.

Meichenbaum's Self-Instructional Methods   Behavioral psychologist Donald Meichenbaum is perhaps best known for a process known as stress inoculation, which subjects clients to extreme stressors in a laboratory environment. Before a stressful event (e.g., going to the doctor), clients practice individual coping skills (e.g., deep breathing exercises) and self-instruction (e.g., "I'll feel better once I know what's

---

Situational inducement   Attempt to influence a behavior through situations and occasions that are structured to exert control over that behavior.

Positive reinforcement   Presenting something positive following a behavior that is being reinforced.

causing my pain"). Meichenbaum demonstrated that clients who practiced coping techniques and self-instruction were less likely to resort to negative behaviors in difficult situations. In Meichenbaum's behavioral therapies, clients are encouraged to give themselves "self-instructions" ("Slow down, don't rush") and "positive affirmations" ("My speech is going fine—I'm almost done!") instead of self-defeating thoughts ("I'm talking too fast—my speech is terrible") whenever a situation seems to be getting out of control.

Blocking/Thought Stopping   By purposefully blocking or stopping negative thoughts, a person can concentrate on taking positive steps toward behavior change. For example, suppose you are preoccupied with your ex-partner, who has recently deserted you for someone else. You consciously stop dwelling on the situation and force yourself to think about something more pleasant (e.g., dinner tomorrow with your best friend). By refusing to dwell on negative images and forcing yourself to focus elsewhere, you can save wasted energy, time, and emotional resources and move on to positive change.

Changing Your Behavior

Self-Assessment: Antecedents and Consequences

Behaviors, thoughts, and feelings always occur in a context—the situation. Situations can be divided into two components: the events that come before and after. *Antecedents* are the setting events for a behavior; they cue or stimulate a person to act in certain ways. Antecedents can be physical events, thoughts, emotions, or the actions of other people. *Consequences*—the results of behavior—affect whether a person will repeat that action.[24] Consequences can also consist of physical events, thoughts, emotions, or the actions of other people.

Suppose you are shy and must give a speech in front of a large class. The antecedents include walking into the class, feeling frightened, wondering whether you are capable of doing a good job, and being unable to remember a word of your speech. If the consequences are negative—if your classmates laugh and you get a low grade—your terror about speaking in public will be reinforced, and you will continue to dread this kind of event. In contrast, if you receive positive feedback from the class or instructor, you may actually learn to like speaking in public.

Learning to recognize the antecedents of a behavior and acting to modify them is one method of changing behavior. A diary noting your undesirable behaviors and identifying the settings in which they occur can be a useful tool. Figure 1.4 identifies several factors that can make behavior change more difficult.

Analyzing Personal Behavior

Successful behavior change requires determining what you want to change. All too often we berate ourselves by using generalities: "I'm lousy to my friends, I need to be a better person." Determining the specific behavior you would like to change—in contrast to the general problem—will allow you to set clear goals. What are you doing that makes you a lousy friend? Are you gossiping or lying about your friends? Have you been a "taker" rather than a "giver"? Or are you really a good friend most of the time?

Let's say the problem is gossiping. You can analyze this behavior by examining the following components:

- *Frequency.* How often are you gossiping—all the time, or only once in a while?
- *Duration.* How long have you been doing this?
- *Seriousness.* Is your gossiping just idle chatter, or are you really trying to injure the other person? What are the consequences for you? For your friend? For your relationship?
- *Basis for problem behavior.* Is your gossip based on facts, perceptions of facts, or deliberate embellishment of the truth?
- *Antecedents.* What kinds of situations trigger your gossiping? Do some settings or people bring it out in you more than others? What triggers your feelings of dislike or irritation toward your friends? Why are you talking behind their backs?

Decision Making: Choices for Change

Now it is time to make a decision that will lead to positive health outcomes. Choosing among alternatives isn't easy, particularly when friends, family, media, and pleasurable options tempt you. "Just saying no" is usually easier said than done. However, if you are trying to fit in, be liked, or satisfy other emotional needs, decision making will become even more difficult. That's why anticipating what might occur in a given setting and thinking through all possible safe alternatives is important as you implement behavior change.

For example, suppose you know that you are likely to be offered a drink when you go to a party. What kind of response could you make that would be okay in your social group? If someone is flirting with you and the conversation takes on a distinct sexual overtone, what might you do to prevent the situation from turning bad? Advance preparation will help you stick to your behavior plan.

Remember that things typically don't "just happen." By staying alert to potential problems, being aware of your alternatives, maintaining a good sense of your own values, and sticking to your beliefs under pressure, you can gain control over many situations in your life.

OBSTACLE	STRATEGY
Stress (intrinsic and extrinsic)	Identify potential sources of stress, and find constructive ways to lower stress level.
Social pressures to repeat old habits	Enlist the support of friends. Identify specifics of these pressures.
Not expecting mistakes, perfectionist, hypercritical	Accept that slips are inevitable, but maintain control. Acknowledge that humans are imperfect beings.
Self-blame for poor coping or a weak personality	Blame pressures from the environment or lack of skills, rather than innate weakness.
Lack of effort, lack of motivation	Assess effort and make sure it is adequate. Provide rewards for successes.
Faulty beliefs, low self-efficacy	Develop new skills, focus on successes, and plan ahead for difficult situations. Change self-talk.

Figure 1.4
Obstacles to Behavior Change. Psychologists offer a number of explanations for why you may fail in your efforts to change your behavior and strategies for overcoming these obstacles.
Source: From Self-Directed Behavior: Self-Modification for Personal Adjustment, by D. L. Watson and R. G. Tharp. Copyright 1997, 1993, 1989, 1985, 1981, 1977, 1972 Brooks/Cole Publishing Company, Pacific Grove, CA 93950, a division of Thomson Publishing Inc. By permission of the publisher.

Setting Realistic Goals

Changing behavior is not easy, but sometimes we make it even harder by setting unrealistic and unattainable goals. To start making positive changes, ask yourself these questions.

1. *What do I want?* What is your ultimate goal—to lose weight? Exercise more? Reduce stress? Have a lasting relationship? Whatever it is, you need a clear picture of the target outcome.
2. *Which change is the greatest priority at this time?* Often people decide to change several things all at once. Suppose that you are gaining unwanted weight. Rather than saying, "I need to eat less, start jogging, and really get in shape," you need to be specific about your current behavior. Are you eating too many sweets? Are you eating too many foods high in fat? Perhaps a realistic goal, therefore, would be, "I am going to try to eat less fat during dinner every day." Choose the behavior that constitutes your greatest problem, and tackle that first. You can always work on something else later. Take small steps, experiment with alternatives, and find the best way to meet your unique goals.
3. *Why is this important to me?* Think through why you want to change. Are you doing it because of your health? To look better? To win someone else's approval? Usually, do-

ing something because it's right for you rather than to win others' approval is a sound strategy. If you are doing it for someone else, what happens when that other person isn't around?
4. *What are the potential positive outcomes?* What do you hope to accomplish?

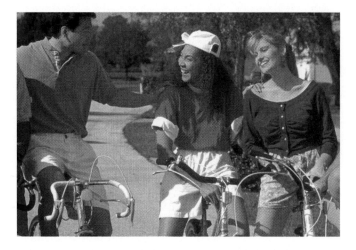

The support and encouragement of friends who have similar goals and interests will strengthen your commitment to develop and maintain positive health behaviors.

5. *What health-promoting programs and services can help me get started?* Nearly all campuses offer resources that can help you in your behavior change. You might buy a self-help book at the campus bookstore, speak to a counselor, or enroll in an aerobics class at the local fitness center. College communities typically offer a number of outreach opportunities designed to get you started in your efforts to change behaviors.

6. *Are there family or friends whose help I can enlist?* Social support is one of your most powerful allies. Getting a friend to exercise with you, asking your partner to help you stop smoking by quitting at the same time, and making a commitment with a friend to never let each other drive if you've had something to drink—these are all examples of how people can help each other make positive changes.

Taking Charge

Managing Behavior Change

Regardless of the model or the strategy employed, each of us has a unique road to follow. Every chapter in this book lists activities and choices that will enable you to develop healthy behaviors.

Checklist for Change

Making Personal Choices

✓ Are you ready to make this change? Are you in a healthy emotional state? Are you doing it for yourself or to please someone else?
Have you:

✓ Completed a personal health history to assess your risks from various sources?

✓ Developed an action plan with short- and long-term goals? Have you set priorities?

✓ Assessed your personal resources? Where can you go for support and advice?

✓ Planned alternative actions in case you run into obstacles or begin to sabotage yourself?

✓ Set up a list of reinforcers and supports that will keep you motivated along the way?

✓ Established a set of guidelines for success? Will you set small goals to achieve at selected intervals, or will you consider yourself successful only if you meet your ultimate goal?

Making Community Choices

✓ Have you taken time to become educated about issues and concerns affecting others in your community?

✓ Have you prioritized actions to take to help change community behaviors? Do you have a particular goal?

✓ Do you analyze what is happening in your school, community, state, and nation by reading about issues, actively discussing problems and possible solutions, and developing personal opinions?

✓ Do you listen carefully to what your elected officials say and take constructive action if you disagree with them?

✓ Do you vote for officials whose policies, rhetoric, and past histories indicate that they support improvements in health care for all people, the environment, and education?

✓ Do you, at least once every term, volunteer to help others who are less fortunate?

✓ Do you purchase products and services from companies that have proven records of supporting the health and well-being of others through their organizational practices?

Summary

❋ Health encompasses the whole dynamic process of fulfilling one's individual potential in the physical, social, emotional, spiritual, intellectual, and environmental dimensions of life. Wellness means achieving the highest level of health possible along several dimensions.

❋ Although the average American life expectancy has increased over the past century, the span of quality life still needs improvement. Programs such as *Healthy People 2000, Healthy People 2010,* and *AHRQ Guidelines* have established national objectives for increasing life expectancy and improving the quality of life for all Americans through health promotion and disease prevention.

* Gender continues to play a major role in health status and care. Women have longer lives but more medical problems than do men. To close the gender gap in health care, researchers have begun to include more women in medical research and training.

* In the 15- to 24-year-old age group, the leading causes of death are unintentional injuries, homicide, and suicide. In older age groups, heart disease, cancer, and stroke are major killers. Many of the risks associated with heart disease, stroke, and cancer can be reduced through lifestyle changes. Many of the risks associated with injuries, legal intervention, homicide, and suicide can be reduced through preventive measures.

* Several factors contribute to a person's health status, but not all of them are within the person's control. Beliefs and attitudes, intentions to change, support from significant others, and readiness to change are factors over which individuals have some degree of control. Reinforcing, predisposing, and enabling factors that influence health decisions include access to health care, genetic predisposition, and health policies that support positive choices.

* Applying behavior-change techniques, such as shaping, visualization, modeling, controlling the situation, reinforcement, and changing self-talk help people succeed in making behavior changes.

* Decision making has several key components. Each person must explore his or her own problems, the reasons for making change, and the expected outcomes. The next step is to plan a course of action best suited to the individual's needs.

Discussion Questions

1. How are the terms *health* and *wellness* similar? What, if any, are important distinctions between these terms? What is health promotion? Disease prevention?

2. How healthy are Americans today? How will health promotion and illness and accident prevention both increase life expectancy and improve quality of life right now? In the future?

3. What are some of the major differences in the way men and women are treated in the health care system? Why do you think these differences exist?

4. What are the leading causes of death across different ages and races? What are the leading causes of death for people aged 15 to 24? Why are these statistics so different? Explain why it is important to look at these statistics by age rather than just in total. What lifestyle changes can you make to lower your risks for contracting major diseases?

5. What is the Health Belief Model? What is the Theory of Reasoned Action? How may each of these models operate when a young woman decides to smoke her first cigarette? Her last cigarette?

6. Explain the predisposing, reinforcing, and enabling factors that might influence a young welfare mother as she decides whether to sell drugs to support her children.

7. Using the Stages of Change model found in the Skills for Behavior Change Box, discuss what you might do (in stages) to help a friend stop smoking. Why is it important that a person be ready to change before trying to change?

Application Exercise

Reread the What Do You Think? scenarios at the beginning of the chapter and answer the following questions.

1. From what you learned in this chapter, why are young people at high risk for accidents, homicide, and suicide? Why do these risks decline with age?

2. On your campus, or in your community, what programs, services, or policies are in place to reduce risk related to these problems?

3. Who is most likely to develop a health problem or sustain an injury—Matt, Kathy, or Ted? What steps might this student take to reduce such risks?

Accessing Your Health on the Internet

Visit the following Internet sites to explore further topics and issues related to personal health. To visit an organization's website, go to the Companion Website for *Health: The Basics, Fifth Edition* at www.aw.com/donatelle, click on the book image, and select "Accessing Your Health on the Internet" from the navigation menu on the left.

1. **National Center for Health Statistics.** Outstanding place to start for information about health status in the United States. Links to key documents such as *Health United States* (published new yearly), national survey information, and information on mortality by age, race, gender, geographic location, and other important data. Includes comprehensive information provided by the Centers for

Disease Control and Prevention (CDC) as well as easy links to at least ten of the major health resources currently being utilized for policy and decision making about health in the United States.

2. **CDC Wonder.** Oustanding reference for comprehensive information from the CDC, including special reports, guidelines, and access to national health data.

3. **National Health Information Center.** Excellent resource for consumer information about health.

4. **Web MD.** Reputable and comprehensive overview of various diseases and conditions. Written for the public in an easy-to-understand format with links to more in-depth information.

5. **Mayo Clinic.** Reputable resource for specific information about health topics, diseases, and treatment options. Easy to navigate and consumer friendly.

Further Reading

Robins, Alexander, and Abby Wilner. Quarterlife Crisis: The Unique Challenges of Life in Your 20s. J P Tarcher Paperbacks, 2001. Overview of challenges facing young adults in America today.

Olpin, M., and D. Gotthoffer. *Health on the Net 2001.* Boston: Allyn & Bacon, 2001.
This easy-to-use resource makes the vast potential of the Internet easily accessible to health students.

U.S. Department of Health and Human Services. *Healthy People 2010: National Health Promotion and Disease Prevention Objectives for the Year 2010.* Washington, DC: Government Printing Office, 1998.
This plan constitutes the Surgeon General's long-range goals for increasing life expectancy for all Americans by three years and improving access to health for all Americans, regardless of sex, race, socioeconomic status, and other variables.

U.S. Department of Health and Human Services. *Health United States: 2001.* Centers for Disease Control and Prevention. Washington, DC: Government Printing Office, 2001.
Provides an up-to-date overview of U.S. health statistics, risk factors, and trends.

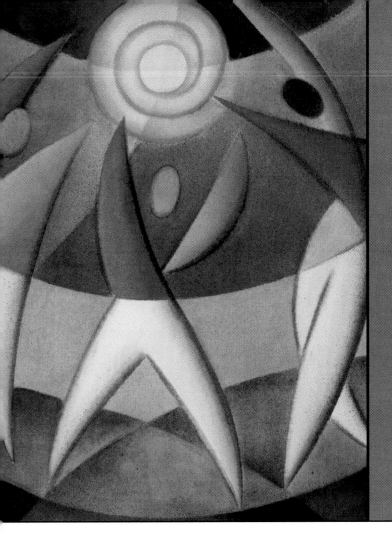

2

Psychosocial Health

*BEING MENTALLY, EMOTIONALLY,
SOCIALLY, AND SPIRITUALLY WELL*

objectives

* Define psychosocial health in terms of its mental, emotional, and social components, and identify the basic elements shared by psychosocially healthy people.

* Identify the internal and external factors influencing psychosocial health, and consider how each may affect you.

* Discuss the positive steps you can take to enhance psychosocial health.

* Discuss the dimension of spirituality and the role that it plays in health and wellness.

* Discuss the mind–body connection and how emotions (including optimism and happiness) influence health status.

* Identify and describe common psychosocial problems of adulthood, and explain their causes, methods of prevention, and available treatments.

* Illustrate the warning signs of suicide and actions that can be taken to help a suicidal individual.

* Identify the different types of health professionals and therapies.

Have there been days when you felt mentally and physically exhausted? Were you so tired that you found it hard to stay awake long enough to study or go out with friends? In contrast, have there been other days when you felt energized from the moment you woke up in the morning? Although you were busy all day, you may have felt too awake to even think about going to bed.

The example in the What Do You Think box illustrates the close link between psychosocial and physical health. Although often overlooked during the pursuit of a fit and firm body, a fit mind can be equally important in determining not only the number of years we live, but also the quality of those years. Like Amy, all of us go through times when life seems difficult. Whatever the cause for the "lows" in our lives, they have the power to sap energy, drain emotions, and break the spirit. Over the long haul, they can even shorten life expectancy.

However, human beings possess a resiliency that enables us to cope, adapt, and thrive, regardless of life's challenges. How we feel and think about ourselves, those around us, and our environment can tell us a lot about our psychosocial health and whether we are healthy emotionally, spiritually, and mentally. Increasingly, health professionals recognize that having a solid social network, being emotionally and mentally healthy, and acknowledging and developing spiritual capacity may put life into years, as well as add years to life.

Defining Psychosocial Health

Psychosocial health encompasses the mental, emotional, social, intellectual, and spiritual dimensions of health (Figure 2.1). It is the result of a complex interaction between a person's his-

tory and his or her conscious and unconscious thoughts about and interpretations of the past. Psychosocially healthy people are emotionally, mentally, socially, intellectually, and spiritually resilient. They respond to challenges and frustrations in appropriate ways most of the time, despite occasional slips. Most authorities identify several basic elements shared by psychosocially healthy people.[1]

- *They feel good about themselves.* Healthy people are not typically overwhelmed by fear, love, anger, jealousy, guilt, or worry. They know who they are, have a realistic sense of their capabilities, and respect themselves even though they realize they aren't perfect.
- *They feel comfortable with other people.* Psychosocially healthy individuals enjoy satisfying and lasting personal relationships and do not take advantage of others, nor do they allow others to take advantage of them. They can give love, consider others' interests, respect personal differences, and feel responsible for their fellow human beings.
- *They control tension and anxiety.* They recognize the underlying causes and symptoms of stress in their lives and

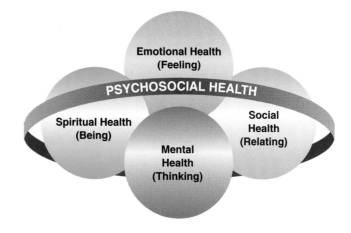

Figure 2.1
Psychosocial Health. Psychosocial health is a complex interaction of mental, emotional, social, and spiritual health.

Psychosocial health   The mental, emotional, social, and spiritual dimensions of health.

consciously struggle to avoid irrational thoughts, unnecessary aggression, hostility, excessive excuse making, and blaming others for their problems.

- *They are able to meet the demands of life.* They try to solve problems as they arise, accept responsibility, and plan ahead. They set realistic goals, think for themselves, and make independent decisions. Acknowledging that change is inevitable, they welcome new experiences. They use their natural abilities to control their environment whenever possible and fit themselves into the environment when necessary.
- *They curb hate and guilt* by acknowledging and combating tendencies to respond with hate, anger, thoughtlessness, selfishness, vengeful acts, or feelings of inadequacy. They do not try to knock others aside to get ahead but rather reach out to help others—even those they don't particularly care for.
- *They maintain a positive outlook.* Psychosocially healthy people approach each day with a presumption that things will go well. They block out most negative and cynical thoughts and give the good things in life star billing. They look to the future with enthusiasm rather than dread.
- *They enrich the lives of others* because they recognize that there are others whose needs are greater than their own.
- *They cherish the things that make them smile.* Reminders of good experiences brighten their day. Fun is an integral part of their lives. So is making time for themselves.
- *They value diversity.* Psychosocially healthy people do not feel threatened by people who are of a different race, gender, religion, sexual orientation, ethnicity, or political party. They appreciate creativity in others as well as in themselves.
- *They appreciate and respect nature.* They take the time to enjoy their surroundings and are conscious of their place in the universe.

Of course, few of us ever achieve perfection in these areas. Attaining psychosocial health and wellness involves many complex processes (Figure 2.2 on page 30). This chapter will help you understand not only what it means to be psychosocially well, but also why we may run into problems. In addition, learning how to assess your own health and to help yourself or seek help from others are important parts of psychosocial health (see Assess Yourself, page 31).

> **What do you think?**
> *Which psychosocial qualities do you value the most in your friends?* ✳ *Do you think that you are strong in these areas yourself?* ✳ *Explain your answer.*

Mental Health: The Thinking You

The term **mental health** is often used to describe the "thinking" part of psychosocial health. As a thinking being, you have the ability to reason, interpret, and remember events from a unique perspective; to sense, perceive, and evaluate what is happening; and to solve problems. In short, you are intellectually able to sort through the clutter of events, contradictory messages, and uncertainties of a situation and attach meaning, either positive or negative, to it. (People often refer to this subset of mental health as *intellectual health*). Your values, attitudes, and beliefs about your body, your family, your relationships, and life in general are usually—at least in part—a reflection of your mental health.

A mentally healthy person is likely to respond in a positive way even when things do not go as expected. For example, a mentally healthy student who receives a D on an exam may be disappointed but will try to assess why she did poorly. Did she study enough? Did she attend class and ask questions about the things she didn't understand? Even though the test result may be very important to her, she will find a constructive way to deal with her frustration. She may talk to the instructor, spend more time studying, or hire a tutor. In contrast, a mentally unhealthy person may respond in an irrational manner. She may believe that her instructor is out to get her or that other students cheated on the exam. She may allow her low grade to provoke a major crisis in her life. She may spend the next 24 hours getting wasted, decide to quit school, try to get back at her instructor, or even blame her roommate for preventing her from studying.

When a person's mental health begins to deteriorate, he or she may experience sharp declines in rational thinking ability and increasingly distorted perceptions. The person may become cynical and distrustful, experience volatile mood swings, or choose to be isolated from others. Extreme negative reactions may even threaten the life and health of others. People who show such extreme behavior are classified as having mental illnesses, discussed later in this chapter.

Emotional Health: The Feeling You

The term **emotional health** is often used interchangeably with *mental health*. Although the two are closely intertwined, emotional health more accurately refers to the "feeling," or subjective, side of psychosocial health. **Emotions** are intensified feelings or complex patterns of feelings that we experience on a minute-by-minute, day-to-day basis. Love, hate, frustration, anxiety, and joy are only a few of the many

Mental health   The "thinking" part of psychosocial health. Includes your values, attitudes, and beliefs.

Emotional health   The "feeling" part of psychosocial health. Includes your emotional reactions to life.

Emotions   Intensified feelings or complex patterns of feelings we constantly experience.

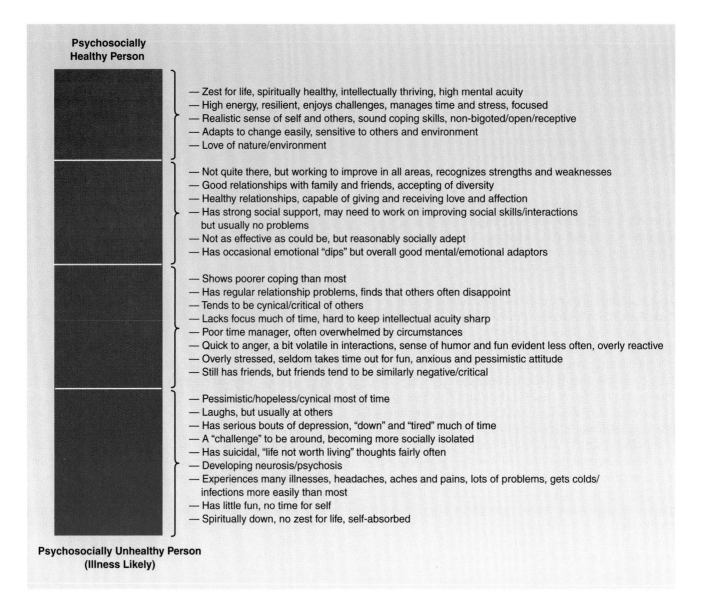

Psychosocially Healthy Person

— Zest for life, spiritually healthy, intellectually thriving, high mental acuity
— High energy, resilient, enjoys challenges, manages time and stress, focused
— Realistic sense of self and others, sound coping skills, non-bigoted/open/receptive
— Adapts to change easily, sensitive to others and environment
— Love of nature/environment

— Not quite there, but working to improve in all areas, recognizes strengths and weaknesses
— Good relationships with family and friends, accepting of diversity
— Healthy relationships, capable of giving and receiving love and affection
— Has strong social support, may need to work on improving social skills/interactions but usually no problems
— Not as effective as could be, but reasonably socially adept
— Has occasional emotional "dips" but overall good mental/emotional adaptors

— Shows poorer coping than most
— Has regular relationship problems, finds that others often disappoint
— Tends to be cynical/critical of others
— Lacks focus much of time, hard to keep intellectual acuity sharp
— Poor time manager, often overwhelmed by circumstances
— Quick to anger, a bit volatile in interactions, sense of humor and fun evident less often, overly reactive
— Overly stressed, seldom takes time out for fun, anxious and pessimistic attitude
— Still has friends, but friends tend to be similarly negative/critical

— Pessimistic/hopeless/cynical most of time
— Laughs, but usually at others
— Has serious bouts of depression, "down" and "tired" much of time
— A "challenge" to be around, becoming more socially isolated
— Has suicidal, "life not worth living" thoughts fairly often
— Developing neurosis/psychosis
— Experiences many illnesses, headaches, aches and pains, lots of problems, gets colds/ infections more easily than most
— Has little fun, no time for self
— Spiritually down, no zest for life, self-absorbed

Psychosocially Unhealthy Person
(Illness Likely)

Figure 2.2
Psychosocially Healthy Individuals Versus Psychosocially Unhealthy Individuals

emotions we feel. Typically, emotions are described as the interplay of four components: physiological arousal, feelings, cognitive (thought) processes, and behavioral reactions. Each time you are put in a stressful situation, you react physiologically while your mind tries to sort things out. You consciously or unconsciously react based on how rationally you interpret the situation.

Psychologist Richard Lazarus has indicated that there are four basic types of emotions: (1) emotions resulting from harm, loss, or threats; (2) emotions resulting from benefits; (3) borderline emotions, such as hope and compassion; and (4) more complex emotions, such as grief, disappointment, bewilderment, and curiosity.[2] Each of us may experience any of these feelings in any combination at any time. As rational beings, it is our responsibility to evaluate our individual emotional responses, the environment that is causing these responses, and the appropriateness of our actions.

Emotionally healthy people are usually able to respond in an appropriate manner to upsetting events. When they feel threatened, they are not likely to react in an extreme fashion, behave inconsistently, or adopt an offensive attack mode. Even when their feelings are trampled on or they suffer agonizing pain because of a lost love, they keep their emotions in check.

Emotionally unhealthy people are much more likely to let their feelings overpower them. They may be highly volatile and prone to unpredictable outbursts and inappropriate, sometimes frightening responses to events.

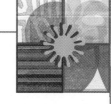

Assessing Your Psychosocial Health

Being psychosocially healthy requires both introspection and the willingness to work on areas that need improvement. Often it is difficult to assess one's own behaviors and actions. Ask someone who is close to you to take the same test and respond with their perceptions of you. Carefully assess areas where your responses differ from those of your friend or family member. Which areas might need some work? Which areas are in good shape?

1 = Never describes me   2 = Describes me infrequently   3 = Describes me fairly frequently
4 = Describes me most of the time   5 = Describes me all of the time

1. My actions and interactions indicate that I am confident in my abilities.	1	2	3	4	5
2. I am quick to blame others for things that go wrong in my life.	1	2	3	4	5
3. I am spontaneous and like to have fun with others.	1	2	3	4	5
4. I am able to give love and affection to others and show my feelings.	1	2	3	4	5
5. I am able to receive love and signs of affection from others without feeling uneasy.	1	2	3	4	5
6. I am generally positive and upbeat about things in my life.	1	2	3	4	5
7. I am cynical and tend to be critical of others.	1	2	3	4	5
8. I have a large group of people whom I consider to be good friends.	1	2	3	4	5
9. I make time for others in my life.	1	2	3	4	5
10. I take time each day for myself for quiet introspection, having fun, or just doing nothing.	1	2	3	4	5
11. I am compulsive and competitive in my actions.	1	2	3	4	5
12. I handle stress well and am seldom upset or stressed out by others.	1	2	3	4	5
13. I try to look for the good in everyone and every situation before finding fault.	1	2	3	4	5
14. I am comfortable meeting new people and interact well in social settings.	1	2	3	4	5
15. I would rather stay in and watch TV or read than go out with friends or interact with others.	1	2	3	4	5
16. I am flexible and can adapt to most situations, even if I don't like them.	1	2	3	4	5
17. Nature, the environment, and other living things are important aspects of my life.	1	2	3	4	5
18. I think before responding to my emotions.	1	2	3	4	5
19. I am selfish and tend to think of my own needs before those of others.	1	2	3	4	5
20. I am consciously trying to be a "better person."	1	2	3	4	5
21. I like to plan ahead and set realistic goals for myself and others.	1	2	3	4	5
22. I accept others for who they are.	1	2	3	4	5
23. I value diversity and respect others' rights, regardless of culture, race, sexual orientation, religion, or other differences.	1	2	3	4	5

Continued on page 32

24. I try to live each day as though it might be my last.	1	2	3	4	5
25. I have a great deal of energy and appreciate the little things in life.	1	2	3	4	5
26. I cope with stress in appropriate ways.	1	2	3	4	5
27. I get enough sleep each day and seldom feel tired.	1	2	3	4	5
28. I have healthy relationships with my family.	1	2	3	4	5
29. I am confident that I can do most things if I put my mind to them.	1	2	3	4	5
30. I respect others' opinions and believe that others should be free to express their opinions, even when they differ from my own.	1	2	3	4	5

Look at items 2, 7, 11, 15, and 19. Add up your score for these five items and divide by 5. Is your average for these items above or below 3? Did you score a 5 on any of these items? Do you need to work on any of these areas?

Now look at your scores for the remaining items. (There should be 25 items.) Total these scores and divide by 25. Is your average above or below 3? On which items did you score a 5? Obviously you're doing well in these areas. Now remove these items from this grouping of 25 (scores of 5), and add up your scores for the remaining items. Then divide your total by the number of items included. Now what is your average?

Do the same for the scores completed by your friend or family member. How do your scores compare? Which ones, if any, are different, and how do they differ? Which areas do you think you need to work on?

What actions can you take now to improve your ratings in these areas?

An ex-boyfriend who is so jealous of your new relationship that he begins to hit you and push you around is showing an extremely unhealthy and dangerous emotional reaction. Such violent responses have become a problem of epidemic proportions in the United States (see Chapter 4).

Emotional health also affects social health. Someone feeling hostile, withdrawn, or moody may become socially isolated. People in the midst of emotional turmoil may be grumpy, nasty, irritable, or overly quiet; they may cry easily or demonstrate other disturbing emotional responses. Because they are not much fun to be around, their friends may avoid them at the very time they are most in need of emotional support. Social isolation is just one of the many potential negative consequences of unstable emotional responses.

For students, a more immediate concern is the impact of emotional trauma or turmoil on academic performance. Have you ever tried to study for an exam after a fight with a close friend or family member? Emotional turmoil may seri-

ously affect your ability to think, reason, and act rationally. Many otherwise rational, mentally healthy people do ridiculous things when they are going through a major emotional upset. Mental functioning and emotional responses are intricately connected.

Social Health: Interactions with Others

Social health is the part of psychosocial health dealing with interactions with others and the ability to adapt to social situations. Socially healthy individuals have a wide range of interactions with family, friends, and acquaintances. They are able to listen, express themselves, form healthy relationships, act in socially acceptable and responsible ways, and find the best fit for themselves in society. Numerous studies have documented the importance of social life in achieving and maintaining health, and two aspects of social health have proven to be particularly important.[3]

- *Presence of strong social bonds.* **Social bonds,** or social linkages, reflect the general degree and nature of our interpersonal contacts and interactions. Social bonds serve six major functions, providing (1) intimacy, (2) feelings of belonging to or integration with a group, (3) opportunities

Social bonds Degree and nature of interpersonal contacts.

for giving or receiving nurturance, (4) reassurance of one's worth, (5) assistance and guidance, and (6) advice. People who are more "connected" to others manage stress more effectively and are much more resilient when bombarded by life's crises.

- *Presence of key social supports.* **Social supports** refer to relationships that bring positive benefits to the individual. Social supports can be either *expressive* (emotional support, encouragement) or *structural* (housing, money). Families provide both structural and expressive support to children. Adults need to develop their own social supports. Psychosocially healthy people create a network of friends and family with whom they can give and receive support.

Social health also reflects the way we react to others. In its most extreme forms, a lack of social health may be represented by aggressive acts of prejudice and bias toward other individuals or groups. **Prejudice** is a negative evaluation of an entire group of people that is typically based on unfavorable (and often wrong) ideas about the group. In its most obvious manifestations, prejudice is reflected in acts of discrimination, in overt acts of hate and bias, and in purposeful intent to harm individuals or groups.

> ### What do you think?
>
> *What do social health, mental health, and emotional health mean to you?* ✳ *What are your strengths and weaknesses in the area of psychosocial health?* ✳ *What can you do to enhance your strengths?* ✳ *How can you improve areas that are not so strong?*

Spiritual Health

Although mental health and emotional health are key factors in overall psychosocial functioning, it is possible to be mentally and emotionally healthy and still not achieve optimal well-being. What is missing? For many people, the difficult-to-describe element that gives zest to life is the spiritual dimension. For a complete discussion of spiritual health, see the section later in this chapter and in Chapter 3.

Factors Influencing Psychosocial Health

External Factors That Influence Psychosocial Health

Most of our mental, emotional, and social reactions to life are a direct outcome of our experiences and social and cultural expectations. We often interpret situations based on learned reactions to certain environmental and social stimuli. Our psychosocial health is based, in part, on how we perceive life experiences. While some experiences are under our control, others are not. External influences are those factors in life that we do not control, such as who raised us and where we live.

The Family Families have a significant influence on psychosocial development. Children raised in healthy, nurturing, happy families are more likely to become well-adjusted, productive adults. Children raised in **dysfunctional families**—which show characteristics such as violence, negative behaviors, distrust, anger, dietary deprivation, drug abuse, parental discord, or sexual, physical, or emotional abuse—may have a harder time adapting to life. In dysfunctional families, love, security, and unconditional trust are so lacking that children often become confused and psychologically bruised. Yet not all people raised in dysfunctional families become psychosocially unhealthy, and not all children from healthy environments become well adjusted. Obviously, more factors are involved in our "process of becoming" than just our family.

The Wider Environment Although isolated negative events may do little damage to psychosocial health, persistent stressors, uncertainties, and threats can cause significant problems. Children raised in environments where crime is rampant and daily safety is in question, for example, run an increased risk of psychosocial problems. Drugs, crime, violent acts, school failure, unemployment, and a host of other bad things can happen to good people. But it is believed that certain protective factors, such as having a positive role model in the midst of chaos, can help children from even the worst environments remain healthy and well adjusted.

Another important influence is access to health services and programs designed to enhance psychosocial health. Going to a support group or seeing a trained therapist is often a crucial first step in prevention and intervention efforts. Individuals from poor socioeconomic environments who cannot afford such services often find it difficult to secure help in improving their psychosocial health.

Social Supports and Social Bonds Although often overlooked, a stable, loving support network of family and friends is key to psychosocial health. Social supports and the social bonds that come from close relationships help us get through

Social supports Structural and functional aspects of social interactions.

Prejudice A negative evaluation of an entire group of people that is typically based on unfavorable and often wrong ideas about the group.

Dysfunctional families Families in which there is violence; physical, emotional, or sexual abuse; parental discord; or other negative family interactions.

even the most difficult times. Having those with whom we can talk, share thoughts, and practice good and bad behaviors without fear of losing their love is an essential part of growth.

> **What do you think?**
> *Over which external factors does an individual have the most control?* ✳ *Which factors had the greatest impact on making you who you are today?*

Internal Factors That Influence Psychosocial Health

Many internal factors also work to shape a person's development. These factors include hereditary traits, hormonal functioning, physical health (including neurological functioning), physical fitness level, and certain elements of mental and emotional health.

Self-Efficacy, Self-Esteem

During our formative years, successes and failures in school, athletics, friendships, intimate relationships, jobs, and every other aspect of life subtly shape our beliefs about our own personal worth and abilities. These beliefs in turn become internal influences on our psychosocial health. Psychologist Albert Bandura used the term **self-efficacy** to describe a person's belief about whether he or she can successfully engage in and execute a specific behavior. Prior success in academics, athletics, or social events will lead to expectations of success in the future. In general, the more self-efficacious a person is and the more positive his or her past experiences have been, the more likely this person will keep trying to execute a specific behavior successfully. Self-efficacious people are also more likely to feel a sense of **personal control** over situations, that their own internal resources allow them to control events. In contrast, someone with low self-efficacy may give up easily or never even try to change a behavior. Always being the last chosen to play basketball or long-term difficulty with making friends, for example, may make failure seem inevitable.

Self-efficacy Belief in one's own ability to perform a task successfully.

Personal control Belief that one's own internal resources can control a situation.

Self-esteem Sense of self-respect or self-confidence.

Learned helplessness Pattern of responding to situations by giving up because of repeated failure in the past.

Self-esteem refers to one's sense of self-respect or self-worth. It can be defined as one's evaluation of oneself and one's own personal worth as an individual. People with high self-esteem tend to feel good about themselves and have a positive outlook on life. People with low self-esteem often do not like themselves, constantly demean themselves, and doubt their ability to succeed.

Our self-esteem is a result of the relationships we have with our parents and family during our formative years, with our friends as we grow older, with our significant others as we form intimate relationships, and with our teachers, co-workers, and others throughout our lives. If we felt loved and valued as children, our self-esteem may allow us to believe that we are inherently "lovable individuals."

Learned Helplessness Versus Learned Optimism

Psychologist Martin Seligman has proposed that people who continually experience failure may develop a pattern of responding known as **learned helplessness,** in which they give up and fail to take any action to help themselves. Seligman ascribes this in part to society's tendency toward "victimology," blaming one's problems on other people and circumstances. Although viewing ourselves as victims may make us feel better temporarily, it does not address the underlying causes of a problem. Ultimately, it can erode self-efficacy and foster learned helplessness by making us feel that we cannot do anything to improve the situation.[4]

Countering this is Seligman's principle of *learned optimism.* Just as we learn to be helpless, so can we teach ourselves to be optimistic. His research provides growing evidence for the central place of mental health in overall positive development.[5]

In one study, university freshmen who had been identified as pessimistic on the basis of a questionnaire were randomly assigned to an experimental group or a control group. The experimental group attended a 16-hour workshop in which they practiced social and study skills and learned to dispute chronic negative thoughts. The control group did not participate. Eighteen months later, 15 percent of the control group members were experiencing severe anxiety, and 32 percent were suffering from moderate to severe depression. In contrast, only 7 percent of workshop participants suffered from anxiety and 22 percent from depression. Seligman concluded that even relatively brief interventions, such as this workshop, can produce measurable improvements in coping skills.[6]

Personality

Your personality is the unique mix of characteristics that distinguish you from others. Hereditary, environmental, cultural, and experiential factors influence how each person develops. Personality determines how we react to the challenges of life, interpret our feelings, and resolve conflicts.

Most of the recent schools of psychosocial theory promote the idea that we have the power not only to understand our behavior but also to actively change it and thus mold our own personalities. Although much has been written about the importance of a healthy personality, there is little consensus on what that concept really means. In general, however, people who possess the following traits often appear to be psychosocially healthy:[7]

- *Extroversion.* This refers to the ability to adapt to a social situation and demonstrate assertiveness as well as power or interpersonal involvement.
- *Agreeableness.* This refers to the ability to conform, be likable, and demonstrate friendly compliance as well as love.
- *Openness to experience.* This refers to the ability to demonstrate curiosity and independence (also referred to as *inquiring intellect*).
- *Emotional stability.* Someone who demonstrates emotional stability is able to maintain social control.
- *Conscientiousness.* Someone who is conscientious demonstrates self-control and is dependable. This person has a need to achieve.[8]

Our personalities are not static. Rather, they change as we move through the stages of our lives. Our temperaments also change as we grow: consider, for example, the extreme emotions experienced by many early adolescents. Most of us learn to control our emotions as we advance toward adulthood.

Enhancing Psychosocial Health

Attaining self-fulfillment is a lifelong, conscious process that involves building self-esteem, understanding and controlling emotions, and learning to solve problems and make decisions.

Developing and Maintaining Self-Esteem and Self-Efficacy

There are several ways to develop and maintain self-esteem and self-efficacy. These include finding a support group, completing required tasks, forming realistic expectations, making time for yourself, maintaining your physical health, and examining your problems and seeking help.

Find a Support Group   The best way to maintain self-esteem is through a support group—peers who share your values. The prime prerequisite for a support group is that it makes you feel good about yourself and forces you to take an honest look at your actions and choices. Although the idea of finding a support group seems to imply establishing a wholly new group, remember that old ties are often the strongest.

   Keeping in contact with old friends and important family members can provide a foundation of unconditional love that will help you through the many life transitions

ahead. Try to be a support for others, too. Join a discussion, political action, or recreational group. Write more postcards and "thinking of you" notes to people who matter. This will build both your own self-esteem and that of your friends.

Complete Required Tasks   A way to boost your self-efficacy is to complete required tasks well and develop a history of success. You are less likely to succeed in your studies if you leave term papers until the last minute or fail to ask about points that are confusing to you. Most college campuses provide study groups and learning centers that offer tips for managing time, understanding assignments, dealing with professors, and preparing for tests. Poor grades, or grades that do not meet expectations, are major contributors to emotional distress among college students.

Form Realistic Expectations   Set realistic expectations for yourself. If you expect perfect grades, a steady stream of Saturday-night dates and soap-opera romances, and the perfect job, you may be setting yourself up for failure. Assess your current resources and the direction in which you are heading. Set small, incremental goals that are possible for you to meet.

Make Time for You   Taking time to enjoy yourself is another way to boost your self-esteem and psychosocial health. Viewing each new activity as something to look forward to and an opportunity to have fun is an important part of keeping the excitement in your life. Wake up focusing on the fun things you have to look forward to each day, and try to make this anticipation a natural part of your day.

Maintain Physical Health   Regular exercise fosters a sense of well-being. Nourishing meals can help you avoid the weight gain that many college students experience. (See Chapter 9 for information on nutrition and Chapter 10 for more information on the role of exercise on health.)

Examine Problems and Seek Help   Knowing when to seek help from friends, support groups, family, or professionals is another important factor in boosting self-esteem. Sometimes you can handle life's problems alone; at other times, you need assistance. Recognizing your strengths and acting appropriately are keys to psychosocial health.

Sleep: The Great Restorer

Sleep serves at least two biological purposes in the body: *conservation* of energy, so that we are rested and ready to perform during high-performance daylight hours; and *restoration,* so that neurotransmitters that have been depleted during waking hours can be replenished. This process clears the brain of daily minutiae to prepare for a new day. Getting enough sleep is a key factor in optimal physical and psychosocial health.

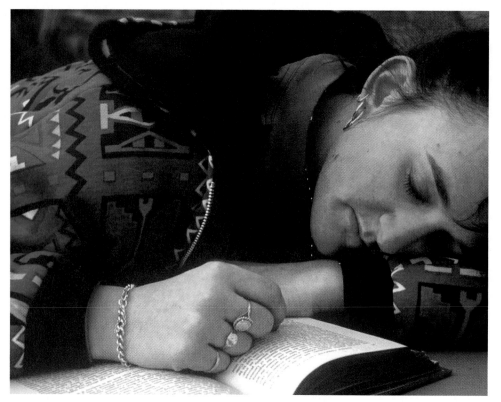

Without adequate sleep, a person may have a hard time facing the challenges of college life.

How much sleep do we need? This depends on many factors. There is a genetically based need for sleep that is different for each species. Sleep duration is also controlled by *circadian rhythms,* which are linked to the hormone *melatonin.* People may also control sleep patterns by staying up late, drinking coffee, getting lots of physical exercise, eating a heavy meal, or using alarm clocks. The most important period of sleep is known as the time of *rapid eye movement, or REM, sleep.* This is the period of deepest sleep, during which we dream. Getting enough REM sleep is essential to feeling rested and refreshed. If we miss this period of sleep, we are left feeling groggy and sleep deprived.

Many people turn to over-the-counter sleeping pills, barbiturates, or tranquilizers to get some sleep, which can potentially be harmful. The following methods for conquering insomnia are less risky:[9]

- Establish a consistent sleep schedule. Go to bed and get up at about the same time every day.
- Evaluate your sleep environment, and change anything that could be keeping you awake. If it's noise, wear earplugs. If it's light, try room-darkening shades.
- Exercise regularly. It's hard to feel drowsy if you have been sedentary all day. However, don't exercise right before bedtime; activity speeds up your metabolism and makes it harder to go to sleep.
- Limit caffeine and alcohol. Caffeine can linger in your body for up to 12 hours and cause insomnia. Although alcohol

may make you drowsy at first, it interferes with the normal sleep-wake cycle and can make you wake up early.
- Avoid eating a heavy meal, particularly at bedtime. Don't drink large amounts of liquid before bed.
- If you're unable to get to sleep in 30 minutes, get up and do something else for a while. Read, play solitaire, or try other relaxing activities, and return to bed when you feel drowsy.
- If you nap, do so only during the afternoon, when circadian rhythms make you especially sleepy. Don't let naps interfere with your normal sleep schedule.
- Establish a relaxing nighttime ritual that puts you in the mood to sleep. Take a warm shower, relax in a comfortable chair, don your favorite robe. Doing this consistently will cue your mind and body that it's time to wind down.

Spirituality: An Inner Quest for Well-Being

Most of us have heard from others or recognized in our own lives the importance of a spiritual dimension. This might range from a zest for nature to a great love for a deity. For millennia, philosophers and humanists have discussed spirituality, religious crusaders have promoted spirituality throughout the world. Today, researchers extol the virtues of spirituality for everything from saving interpersonal relationships to reducing stress.

But what, exactly, does **spirituality** mean? Most experts agree that spiritual health refers to a belief in some unifying force that gives purpose or meaning to life, or a sense of belonging to a scheme of being that is greater than the purely physical or personal dimensions of existence. For some, this unifying force is nature; for others, it is a feeling of connection to other people; for others still, the unifying force is a god or some other spiritual symbol. Dr. N. Lee Smith, internist and associate professor of medicine at the University of Utah, defines spiritual health in the following ways:[10]

- The quality of existence in which one is at peace with oneself and in good standing with the environment
- A sense of empowerment and personal control that includes feeling heard and valued and feeling in control over one's responses (but not necessarily in control of one's environment)
- A sense of connectedness to one's deepest self, to other people, and to all regarded as good
- A sense of meaning and purpose, which provides a sense of mission by finding meaning and wisdom in the here and now
- Enjoying the process of growth and having a vision of one's potential
- Having hope, which translates into positive expectations

On a day-to-day basis, many of us focus on acquiring material possessions and satisfying basic human needs. But there comes a point when we discover that material possessions do not automatically bring happiness or a sense of self-worth. This realization may be triggered by a crisis. A failed relationship, a terrible accident, the death of a close friend or family member, or other loss often prompts a search for meaning, for the answer to the proverbial question "Is that all there is?" Whatever the reason, this search brings new opportunities for understanding ourselves.

As we develop into spiritually healthy beings, we begin to recognize our identity as unique individuals. We reach a better appreciation of our strengths and shortcomings and our place in the universe. By developing an understanding of spirituality and how it is interwoven intricately into our existence, we embrace its power to improve health and our overall perspective on life. In turn, we may begin to notice more, feel more, and experience more of life. Perhaps most important, we gain an appreciation for the here-and-now, rather than living for aspirations that we may never achieve.

In its purest sense, spirituality addresses four main themes: interconnectedness, the practice of mindfulness, spirituality as a part of everyday life, and living in harmony with the community.

- *Interconnectedness.* This concept of **interconnectedness** refers to one's connectedness to self, to others, and to a larger meaning or purpose. Connecting with oneself involves exploring feelings, taking time to consider how you feel in a given situation, assessing your reactions to people and experiences, and taking mental notes when things or people cause you to lose equilibrium. It also involves considering your values and achieving congruence between what you consider important (your goals) and what you can do to achieve your goals without compromising your values. You may choose to connect with people in a physical, emotional, social, occupational, intellectual, or spiritual way.

- *Practice of mindfulness.* **Mindfulness** refers to the ability to be fully present in the moment. Mindfulness has been described as a way of nurturing greater awareness, clarity, and acceptance of present-moment reality or a form of inner "flow"—a holistic sensation you feel when you are totally involved in the moment.[11] According to mindfulness experts, you can achieve this inner flow through an almost infinite range of opportunities for enjoyment and pleasure, either through the use of physical and sensory skills ranging from athletics to music to yoga, or through the development of symbolic skills in areas such as poetry, philosophy, or mathematics.[12] The psychologist Abraham Maslow referred to these moments as peak experiences, during which a person feels integrated, synergistic, and at one with the world.

- *Spirituality as a part of daily life.* Spirituality is embodied in the ability to discover and articulate our own basic purpose in life; to learn how to experience love, joy, peace, and fulfillment; and to help ourselves and others achieve their full potential.[13] This ongoing process of growth fosters three convictions: faith, hope, and love. **Faith** is the belief that helps us realize our purpose in life; **hope** is the belief that allows us to look confidently and courageously to the future; and **love** involves accepting, affirming, and respecting self and others regardless of who they are.[14]

- *Living in harmony with our community.* Our values are an extension of our beliefs about the world and attitude toward life. They are formed over time through a series of life experiences, and they are reflected in our hopes,

Spirituality A form of well-being in which a person acknowledges the need for having, relating, being, and transcendence in the quest for meaning and purpose in life.

Interconnectedness A web of connections, including our relationship to ourselves, to others, and to a larger meaning or purpose in life.

Mindfulness Awareness and acceptance of the reality of the present moment.

Faith Belief that helps each person realize a unique purpose in life.

Hope Belief that establishes confidence and courage in facing the future.

Love Acceptance, affirmation, and respect for the self and others.

dreams, desires, goals, and ambitions.[15] Though most people have some idea of what is important to them, many spend life largely unaware of how their values impact themselves or those around them, until a life-altering event shakes up their usual perspective on life.

Spirituality: A Key to Health and Wellness   Although many experts affirm the importance of spirituality in achieving health and wellness, the specific impact of this dimension remains elusive. Some researchers describe the spiritual dimension as a factor of well-being, which is achieved when four basic kinds of needs are satisfied:[16]

1. The need for having
2. The need for relating
3. The need for being
4. The need for *transcendence*, or that sense of well-being that is experienced when a person finds purpose and meaning in life. Nonphysical in nature, transcendence can best be described as spiritual.

A Spiritual Resurgence   Over recent decades, studies have shown that most Americans want spirituality in their lives, although not necessarily in the form of religion. Many find spiritual fulfillment in music, poetry, literature, art, nature, and intimate relationships.[17] Researcher Wade Clark Roof, of the University of California at Santa Barbara, found that in the 1960s and 1970s, baby boomers abandoned organized religion in large numbers: 84 percent of Jews, 69 percent of mainline Protestants, 61 percent of conservative Protestants, and 67 percent of Catholics.[18] Many dropped out of formal religious practice not because they lost interest in spirituality, but because they felt organized religion was not meeting their needs.

However, today we are seeing a return to formal religious participation and a similar increase in concern for spiritual growth and development. National polls show that 9 out of 10 Americans believe in God and consider religion and/or spirituality to be important in their lives.[19] Many religious groups have spawned new philosophies that are more inclusive and often influenced by "New Age" ideas. An estimated 32 million baby boomers have turned to Eastern practices, New Age philosophies, twelve-step programs, Greek mythology, shamanistic practices, massage, yoga, and a host of other traditions and practices.[20]

For some, spirituality means a "quest for self and self-lessness"—a form of therapy and respite from a sometimes

Healing Through Faith and Spirituality

Dozens of studies have begun to examine the effects of religion and spirituality on mental health. Several of them provide interesting preliminary results:

• *Stress.* The Alameda County Study, which tracks nearly 7,000 Californians, showed that West Coast worshippers who participate in church-sponsored activities are markedly less stressed over finances, health, and other daily concerns than nonreligious types.
• *Blood pressure.* Elderly people in a Duke University study who attended religious services, prayed, or read the Bible regularly had lower blood pressure than their nonpracticing peers.
• *Recovery.* In another Duke University study, devout patients recovering from surgery spent an average of 11 days in the hospital, compared with nonreligious patients, who spent 25 days.
• *Mortality.* Research on 1,931 older adults indicates that those who attend religious services regularly have a lower mortality rate.
• *Immunity.* Research on 1,700 adults found that those who attend religious services were less likely to have elevated levels of interleukin-6, an immune substance prevalent in people with chronic diseases.
• *Lifestyle.* A recent review of several studies suggests that spirituality is linked with low suicide rates, less alcohol and drug abuse, less criminal behavior, fewer divorces, and higher marital satisfaction.
• *Depression.* Women with pious mothers are 60 percent less likely to be depressed over the course of 10 years than women whose mothers aren't so reverent, according to a Columbia University study. Daughters belonging to the same religious denomination as their mothers are even less likely (71 percent) to suffer the blues; sons are 84 percent less likely.
• A Duke University study of 577 men and women hospitalized for physical illness showed that the more patients used positive coping strategies (seeking spiritual support from friends and religious leaders, praying, meditating, and so on), the lower the level of their depressive symptoms and the higher their quality of life.

Sources: From D. N. Elkins, "Spirituality: It's What's Missing in Mental Health," September/October, 1999, *Psychology Today*, p. 48; *Journal of Gerontology: Psychological Sciences*, 1998.

challenging personal environment. This quest for a "life force," which helps people deeply experience the moments of their lives rather than just living through them, has received much scholarly and popular attention. Self-help books that focus on spirituality consistently top the bestseller lists. Television programs promote the virtues of a spiritual or natural existence. Writers and psychologists such as William James, Carl Jung, Gordon Allport, Erich Fromm, Viktor Frankl, Abraham Maslow, and Rollo May have made spirituality a major focus of their work.

Spiritual health courses have emerged in public health and medical school training. For example, the Harvard Medical School of Continuing Education offers a course called "Spirituality and Healing in Medicine," which brings together scholars and medical professionals from around the world to discuss the role of spirituality in treating illness and chronic pain. Self-help workshops focusing on spiritual elements of health are popular throughout the world.

The Mind–Body Connection

Can negative emotions make a person physically sick? Can positive feelings help us stay well? Researchers are exploring the interaction between emotions and health, especially in conditions of uncontrolled, persistent stress. According to one theory, the brain of an emotionally overwrought person sends signals to the adrenal glands, which respond by secreting cortisol and epinephrine (adrenaline), the hormones that activate the body's stress response. These chemicals are also known to suppress immune functioning, so a persistently overwrought person may undergo subtle immune changes. What remains to be shown is how these changes affect overall health, if they do at all.

Happiness: A Key to Well-Being

Although we can list the actions that we should perform to become physically healthy, such as eating the right foods, getting enough rest, exercising, and so on, it is less clear how to achieve that "feeling-good state" that researchers call **subjective well-being (SWB).** This refers to that uplifting feeling of inner peace and wonder that we call "happiness." Psychologists David Myers and Ed Deiner completed a major study of this thing called happiness and noted that people experience it in many different ways, based on age, culture, gender, and other factors.[21] However, in spite of the differences in the way it is experienced, SWB is defined by three central components:[22]

1. *Satisfaction with present life.* People who are high in SWB tend to like their work and are satisfied with their current personal relationships. They are sociable, outgoing, and willing to open up to others. They also like themselves and enjoy good health and self-esteem.
2. *Relative presence of positive emotions.* People with high SWB more frequently feel pleasant emotions, mainly

because they evaluate the world around them in a generally positive way. They have an optimistic outlook, and they expect success in what they undertake.
3. *Relative absence of negative emotions.* Individuals with a strong sense of subjective well-being experience fewer and less severe episodes of negative emotions, such as anxiety, depression, and anger.

Do you have to be happy all of the time to achieve overall subjective well-being? Of course not. Everyone experiences disappointments, unhappiness, and times when life seems unfair. However, people with SWB are typically resilient, are able to look on the positive side, get themselves back on track fairly quickly, and are less likely to fall into deep despair over setbacks. There are several myths about happiness: that it depends on age, gender, race, and socioeconomic status. Research and empirical evidence, however, have debunked these myths:[23]

- *There is no "happiest age."* Age is not a predictor of SWB. Most age groups exhibit similar levels of life satisfaction, although the things that bring joy often change with age.
- *Happiness has no "gender gap."* Women are more likely than men to suffer from anxiety and depression, and men are more at risk for alcoholism and personality disorders. Equal numbers of men and women report being fairly satisfied with life.
- *There are minimal racial differences in happiness.* For example, African Americans and European Americans report nearly the same levels of happiness, and African Americans are slightly less vulnerable to depression. Despite racism and discrimination, members of disadvantaged minority groups generally seem to "think optimistically" by making realistic self-comparisons and attributing problems less to themselves than to unfair circumstances.
- *Money does not buy happiness.* Wealthier societies report greater well-being. However, once the basic necessities of food, shelter, and safety are provided, there is a very weak correlation between income and happiness. Having no money is a cause of misery, but wealth itself does not guarantee happiness.

Fortunately, humans are remarkably resourceful creatures. We respond to great loss, such as the death of a loved one or a traumatic event, with an initial period of grief, mourning, and sometimes abject rage. Yet, with time and the support of loving family and friends, we can pick ourselves up, brush off the bad times, and manage to find satisfaction and peace. Typically, humans learn from suffering and emerge even stronger and more ready to deal with the next crisis. Most find some measure of happiness after the initial shock and

> **Subjective well-being (SWB)** That uplifting feeling of inner peace and wonder that we call "happiness."

pain of loss. Those who are otherwise healthy, in good physical condition, and part of a strong social support network can adapt and cope effectively.

Does Laughter Enhance Health?

Remember the last time you laughed so hard that you cried? Remember how relaxed you felt afterward? Scientists are just beginning to understand the role of humor in our lives and health. For example, laughter has been shown to have the following effects:

- Stressed-out people with a strong sense of humor become less depressed and anxious than those whose sense of humor is less well developed.
- Students who use humor as a coping mechanism report that it predisposes them to experiencing a positive mood.
- In a study of depressed and suicidal senior citizens, patients who recovered were the ones who demonstrated a sense of humor.
- Telling a joke, particularly one that involves a shared experience, increases our sense of belonging and social cohesion.

Laughter helps us in many ways. People like to be around people who are fun-loving and laugh easily. Learning to laugh puts more joy into everyday experiences and increases the likelihood that fun-loving people will keep company with us.

Psychologist Barbara Fredrickson argues that positive emotions such as joy, interest, and contentment serve valuable life functions. Joy is associated with playfulness and creativity. Interest encourages us to explore our world, enhancing knowledge and cognitive ability. Contentment allows us to savor and integrate experiences, an important step to achieving mindfulness and insight. By building our physical, social, and mental resources, these positive feelings empower us to cope more effectively with life's challenges. While the actual emotions may be transient, their effects can be permanent and provide lifelong enrichment.[24]

Laughter also seems to have positive physiological effects. A number of researchers, such as Lee Berk, M.D., and Stanley Tan, M.D., have noted that laughter sharpens our immune systems by activating T-cells and natural killer cells and increasing production of immunity-boosting interferon.[25] It also reduces levels of the stress hormone cortisol.

Major depressive disorder   Severe depression that entails chronic mood disorder, physical effects such as sleep disturbance and exhaustion, and mental effects such as the inability to concentrate.

Chronic mood disorder   Experience of persistent sadness, despair, and hopelessness.

In one experiment, Fredrickson monitored the cardiovascular responses of human subjects who suffered fear and anxiety induced by an unsettling film clip. Some of them then viewed a humorous film clip while others did not. Those who watched the humorous film returned more quickly to their baseline cardiovascular state, indicating that laughter may counteract some of the physical effects of negative emotions.[26]

In another study, 50 women with advanced breast cancer who were randomly assigned to a weekly support group lived an average of 18 months longer than 36 cancer patients not in the support group. The implication of this finding is that the women in the support group cheered each other on and that this allowed them to sleep and eat better, which promoted their survival.[27] Other researchers have found that a fighting spirit and the determination to survive are vital adjuncts to standard cancer therapy.[28]

A large body of evidence points to an association between the emotions and physical health, although we still have much to learn about this relationship. Does an emotional state trigger negative behaviors that lead to decreased immune functioning? Or do emotions directly affect health by stimulating the production of hormones that tax the immune system? In the meantime, however, it appears that happiness and an optimistic mind-set don't just feel good—they are also good for you.

When Psychosocial Health Deteriorates

Sometimes circumstances overwhelm us to such a degree that we need outside assistance to help us get back on track toward healthful living.

Depression: The Full-Scale Tumble

In a recent meeting of the American Psychological Association, the organization's president remarked, "Depression has been called the common cold of psychological disturbances, which underscores its prevalence, but trivializes its impact."[29] According to experts, major depression is, in fact, one of the most common psychiatric disorders in the United States, affecting over 15 million Americans. Many of them are misdiagnosed, underdiagnosed, and not receiving treatment, despite its availability.[30]

It is normal to feel blue or depressed in response to certain experiences, such as the death of a loved one, divorce, loss of a job, or an unhappy ending to a long-term relationship. However, people with **major depressive disorder** experience a form of **chronic mood disorder** that involves, on a day-to-day basis, extreme and persistent sadness, despair, and hopelessness. People with this disorder typically feel discouraged by life and circumstances and experience feelings of intense guilt and worthlessness. Usually they show some impairment of social and occupational

Table 2.1
Are You Depressed?

Sadness and despair are the main symptoms of depression. Other common signs include the following:

- Loss of motivation or interest in pleasurable activities
- Preoccupation with failures and inadequacies; concern over what others are thinking
- Difficulty concentrating; indecisiveness; memory lapses
- Loss of sex drive or interest in close interactions with others
- Fatigue and loss of energy; slow reactions
- Sleeping too much or too little; insomnia
- Feeling agitated, worthless, or hopeless
- Withdrawal from friends and families
- Diminished or increased appetite
- Recurring thoughts that life isn't worth living, thoughts of death or suicide
- Significant weight loss or weight gain

Some depressed people mask their symptoms with a forced, upbeat sense of humor or high energy levels. Communication may cease or seem frantic.

functioning, although their behavior is not necessarily bizarre. Approximately 15 percent of them eventually attempt suicide or succeed in committing suicide.[31]

According to the National Institutes of Mental Health (NIMH), women experience depression at nearly two times the rate of men. Between 8 and 11 percent of men experience depression, in contrast to between 19 and 23 percent of women. About 6 percent of women and 3 percent of men have experienced episodes severe enough to require hospitalization.[32]

There are a few exceptions to these findings, however. Among Jews, males are equally as likely as females to have major depressive episodes.[33] In recent years, there has also been a noteworthy increase in depression among children, the elderly, and adolescents, particularly adolescent girls, and perhaps in Native American and homosexual young people as well.[34] Writers, composers, and entertainers also seem to have higher than expected rates of major depression, and people experiencing chronic, unrelenting pain have the highest rates of any group.[35]

Depression can strike at any age, but the first episode usually occurs before age 40. Some people experience one bout of depression and never have problems again, but others suffer recurrences throughout their lives. Stressful life events are often catalysts for these recurrences.

Risks for Depression Major depressive disorders are caused by interaction between biology, learned behavioral responses, and cognitive factors. Chemical and genetic processes may predispose people to depression, and irrational ideas and beliefs can guide them to negative coping behaviors.[36] Some people, because of genetic history, environment, situational triggers and stressors, poor behavioral skills, and brain–body chemistry, may be particularly vulnerable.

Facts and Fallacies About Depression Although it is one of the fastest-growing problems in U.S. culture, depression remains one of the most misunderstood mental disorders (Table 2.1). Myths and misperceptions about the disease abound.[37] Some of these misperceptions are corrected below:

- *True depression is not a natural reaction to crisis and loss.* It is a pervasive and systemic biological problem. Symptoms may come and go, and their severity will fluctuate, but they do not simply go away. Crisis and loss can lead an already depressed person over the edge to suicide or other problems, but crisis and loss do not inevitably result in depression.
- *People will not snap out of depression by using a little willpower.* Telling a depressed person to "snap out of it" is like telling a diabetic to produce more insulin. Medical intervention in the form of antidepressant drugs and therapy is often necessary for recovery. Understanding the seriousness of the disease and supporting people in their attempts to recover are key elements.
- *Frequent crying is not a hallmark of depression.* Some people who are depressed bear their burdens in silence or may even be the life of the party. Some depressed individuals don't cry at all. Rather, biochemists theorize that crying may actually ward off depression by releasing chemicals that the body produces as a positive response to stress.
- *Depression is not "all in the mind."* Depression isn't a disease of weak-willed, powerless people. In fact, research suggests that depressive illnesses originate with an inherited chemical imbalance in the brain. In addition, some physiological conditions, such as thyroid disorders, multiple sclerosis, chronic fatigue syndrome, and certain cancers have depressive side effects. Certain medications also are known to prompt depressive-like symptoms.

- *It is not true that only in-depth psychotherapy can cure long-term clinical depression.* No single psychotherapy method works for all cases of depression.

Depression and Gender For reasons that are not well understood, two-thirds of all people suffering from depression are women. Researchers have proposed biological, psychological, and social explanations for this fact. Women appear to be at greater risk for depression during times when their hormone levels change significantly, such as the premenstrual phase of the menstrual cycle, following the birth of a child, and at onset of menopause. Men's hormone levels appear to remain more stable throughout life. Some researchers theorize that women are inherently more at risk for depression, yet evidence to support this theory is inconsistent or contrary.

Although adolescent and adult females have been found to experience depression at twice the rate of males, the college population seems to represent a notable exception, with equal rates experienced by males and females. Why? Several theories have been suggested:[38]

- The social institutions of the college campus provide more egalitarian roles for men and women.
- College women experience fewer negative events than do high school females. Men in college report more negative events than they experienced in high school.
- College women report smaller and more supportive social networks.

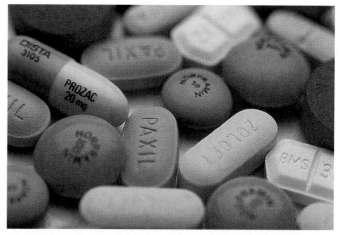

In addition to prescription antidepressant drugs, a number of related natural supplements are sold over the counter. One such supplement, melatonin, has grown in popularity in recent years.

Finally, researchers have observed gender differences in coping strategies, or the response to certain events or stimuli, and have proposed that women's strategies make them more vulnerable to depression. Presented with "a list of things people do when depressed," college students were asked to indicate how likely they were to engage in each behavior. Men were more likely to assert that "I avoid thinking of reasons why I am depressed," "I do something physical,"

REALITY CHECK

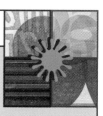

Depression Strikes Increasing Numbers of Young People

While statistics indicate a rising incidence of depression among all age groups, the most alarming aspect of these numbers is that they are probably gross "underestimations" of the true problem. Consider the following:

✓ Many of the drug and alcohol problems facing Americans have their roots in a hopeless, depressed psychological state in which victims turn to drugs to ease their suffering. In addition, many drugs cause victims to be depressed.

✓ More than 80 percent of people with depression can be treated successfully with medication, therapy, or a

combination of both; however, most people never seek treatment.

✓ Nearly 20 percent of Americans will seek psychological help from trained professionals during their lifetimes. Many of those who seek help will be suffering from depression-related problems.

✓ The risk of depression increases for those who have a parent or sibling who suffered from depression before age 30.

✓ Suicide is one of the leading causes of death in the United States, and between 35,000 to 40,000 depressed people in the United States kill themselves every year.

✓ Antidepressant medications are among the most prescribed drugs in the United States, with dramatic increases in the numbers of prescriptions filled and the length of time that patients are on these medications.

Sources: From U.S. Department of Health and Human Services, *U.S. Health,* (Washington, DC: Author, 1999); and M. Clements, "How Healthy Are We?" *Parade* magazine, September 7, 1997, pp. 4–7.

or "I play sports." Women were more likely to answer "I try to determine why I am depressed," "I talk to other people about my feelings," and "I cry to relieve the tension." In other words, the men tried to distract themselves from a depressed mood, whereas the women focused on it. If focusing on negative feelings intensifies these feelings, women's response style may predispose them to depression. This hypothesis has not been directly tested, but some supporting evidence suggests its validity.[39]

Treating Depression   The best treatment involves determining the person's type and degree of depression and its possible causes. Both psychotherapeutic and pharmacological modes of treatment are recommended for clinical (severe and prolonged) depression. Drugs often relieve the symptoms of depression, such as loss of sleep or appetite, while psychotherapy can be equally helpful by improving the ability to function (Table 2.2).[40]

In some cases, psychotherapy alone may be the most successful treatment. The two most common psychotherapeutic therapies for depression are cognitive and interpersonal therapy.

Cognitive therapy aims to help a patient look at life rationally and correct habitually pessimistic thought patterns. It focuses on the here-and-now rather than analyzing a patient's past. To pull a person out of depression, cognitive therapists usually need six to 18 months of weekly sessions that include reasoning and behavioral exercises. *Interpersonal therapy*, which is sometimes combined with cognitive therapy, also addresses the present but focuses on correcting chronic relationship problems. Interpersonal therapists focus on patients' relationships with their families and other people.

Antidepressant drugs relieve symptoms in nearly 80 percent of people with chronic depression. Several types of the medications known as *tricyclics* are available and work by preventing excessive absorption of mood-lifting neurotransmitters. Tricyclics can take six weeks to three months to become effective. Newer antidepressant drugs, called *tetracyclics*, work in one or two weeks.

In recent years, words like Zoloft and Prozac have become such a common part of our vocabulary that it doesn't seem at all unusual to know someone who is taking an antidepressant. This could lead one to think that antidepressants can be taken like aspirin. However, countless emergency room visits occur when people misuse antidepressants, try to quit by going "cold turkey," or suffer reactions to the drugs. The potency and dosage of each vary greatly. Antidepressants should be prescribed only after a thorough psychological and physiological examination.

Electroconvulsive therapy (ECT) is another treatment for depression. A patient given ECT is sedated under light general anesthesia, and electric current is applied to the patient's temples for five seconds at a time for 15 or 20 minutes. Between 10 and 20 percent of people with depression who do not respond to drug therapy are responsive to ECT. However, because it carries a risk of permanent memory loss, some therapists do not recommend ECT under any circumstances.

Anxiety Disorders: Facing Your Fears

One of several **anxiety disorders** is panic attack, a little-understood yet common psychological problem. Consider John Madden, former head coach of the Oakland Raiders and a true "man's man," who has outfitted his own bus and drives every weekend across the country to serve as commentator on NFL football games. What's the reason behind this exhausting driving schedule? Madden is terrified of getting on a plane.

Anxiety disorders are the number-one mental health problem in the United States, affecting over 19 million people aged 18–54 each year, or about 13 percent of all adults.[41] Some sources place the number as high as 25 percent. Anxiety is also a leading mental health problem among adolescents, affecting 13 million youngsters aged 9–17. Between 1997 and 1999, the number of "hits" on the website of the Anxiety Disorders Association of America soared from 500,000 to over 21.6 million.[42] Costs associated with an overly anxious populace are growing rapidly; conservative estimates cite nearly $50 billion a year spent in doctors' bills and workplace losses in America. According to a study by the World Health Organization, the odds of developing an anxiety disorder have doubled in the past four decades.[43] These numbers don't begin to address the human costs incurred when a person is too fearful to leave the house or talk to anyone outside the immediate family. Anxiety-related ailments include generalized anxiety disorders, panic disorder, specific phobias, and social phobias.

Generalized Anxiety Disorders   One common form of anxiety disorder, **generalized anxiety disorder (GAD),** is severe enough to significantly interfere with daily life. Generally, the person with this disorder is a consummate "worrier" who develops a debilitating level of anxiety. Often multiple sources of worry exist, and it is hard to pinpoint the root cause of the anxiety. A diagnosis of GAD depends on showing at least three of the following symptoms for more days than not during a period of six months.[44]

1. Restlessness or feeling keyed up or on edge
2. Being easily fatigued
3. Difficulty concentrating or mind going blank
4. Irritability
5. Muscle tension
6. Sleep disturbances (difficulty falling or staying asleep or restless sleep)

Anxiety disorders   Disorders characterized by persistent feelings of threat and anxiousness in coping with everyday problems.

Generalized anxiety disorder (GAD)   A constant sense of worry that may cause restlessness, difficulty in concentrating, and tension.

Table 2.2
Drug Treatments for Depression

ANTIDEPRESSANT CLASS	INDICATIONS/CONTRAINDICATIONS	SIDE EFFECTS
TRICYCLICS (TCAs) Desipramine (Norpramin) Nortriptyline (Pamelor) Imipramine (Trofranil) Amitriptyline (Elavil) Protriptyline (Vivactil) Doxepin (Sinequan)	Due to their sedating effects, TCAs are useful for patients with insomnia. They may pose a risk for individuals with cardiovascular disease, such as arrhythmias.	Most common: dry mouth, constipation. Others: weight gain, dizziness caused by a drop in blood pressure on sitting or standing up (orthostatic hypotension), changes in sexual desire, difficulty urinating, increased sweating, and sedation. TCAs can be lethal in overdose.
SELECTIVE SEROTONIN REUPTAKE INHIBITORS (SSRIs) Fluoxetine (Prozac) Sertraline (Zoloft) Paroxetine (Paxil) Fluvoxamine (Luvox) Serzone	SSRIs are generally the first-line choice because they have fewer side effects than other antidepressants, do not require blood monitoring, and are safe in overdose. Newer versions have fewer side effects.	Insomnia, agitation, sexual dysfunction, occasional nausea or heartburn, headache, occasional drowsiness, dizziness, tremor, diarrhea/constipation, and dry mouth (rare).
MONOAMINE OXIDASE INHIBITORS (MAOIs) Isocarboxazid (Marplan) Tranylcypromine (Parnate) Phenelzine (Nardil)	MAOIs can cause severe and sudden rise in blood pressure if ingested with certain drugs (e.g., over-the-counter cold preparations, diet pills, and amphetamines) or foods containing tyramine (e.g., red wines, aged cheeses). They interact with epinephrine in some topical anesthetics and are not advised with other antidepressants.	Agitation, insomnia, sexual dysfunction, disturbed appetite, faintness (like orthostatic hypotension). Weight gain is most prominent with MAOIs.
BUPROPION (WELLBUTRIN)	This drug doesn't interact significantly with other drugs. At high doses it can cause seizures in some people, most commonly those who have seizure disorders, anorexia, or bulimia. It has been used experimentally to counteract sexual side effects of SSRIs.	Agitation, insomnia, sedation, blurred vision, dizziness, headache/migraine, dry mouth, tremor, appetite loss, weight loss, excessive sweating, rapid heartbeat, constipation, rashes.
TRAZODONE (DESYREL)	Trazodone is often used with another antidepressant to alleviate insomnia induced by the initial drug.	Drowsiness, faintness, nausea, and vomiting.
MAPROTILINE (LUDIOMIL)	This drug is used to treat agitation and anxiety associated with depression but is not advised for people with seizure disorders. It is somewhat risky for patients with cardiovascular disease.	Similar to those of TCAs.
SEROTONIN AND NOREPINEPHRINE REUPTAKE INHIBITORS (SNRIs) Venlafaxine (Effexor)	SNRIs work something like a combination of an SSRI and a TCA and are useful for patients who don't respond to other antidepressants.	Similar to those of SSRIs.
NEFAZODONE (SERZONE)	This drug shouldn't be taken with the nonsedating antihistamines terfenadine (Seldane) and astemizone (Hismanal).	Headache, dry mouth, nausea, drowsiness, faintness, constipation.

Source: Table of antidepressant drugs in "Antidepressants" excerpted by permission from the December 1995 issue of Harvard Women's Health Watch, *Vol. 3, No. 4, p. 3. © 1995, President and Fellows of Harvard College. Nichols, Mark. "The Quest for a New Cure: New Drugs and Therapies Join the Battle against Depression."* Maclean's, *December 1, 1997, V. 110, No. 48, pp. 60–63.*

Often GAD runs in families and is readily treatable with benzodiazepines such as Librium, Valium, and Xanax, which calm the person for short periods. More effective long-term treatments are achieved through individual therapy.

Panic Disorder   **Panic attacks** are typically described as sudden bursts of disabling terror. The panic may be "free-floating anxiety" that has no connection with the person's present experience. During a panic attack, at least four of the following symptoms develop abruptly and reach a peak within 10 minutes:[45]

1. Palpitations, pounding of the heart, or accelerated heart rate
2. Sweating
3. Trembling or shaking
4. Sensations of shortness of breath, smothering, or choking
5. Chest pain or discomfort
6. Nausea or abdominal distress
7. Feeling dizzy, unsteady, lightheaded, or faint
8. Derealization (feeling of unreality) or depersonalization (being detached from oneself)
9. Fear of losing control or going crazy
10. Fear of dying
11. Paresthesias (numbness or tingling sensations)
12. Chills or hot flashes

Specific Phobias   In contrast with panic disorders, **phobias,** or phobic disorders, involve a persistent and irrational fear of a specific object, activity, or situation, often out of proportion to the circumstances. About 13 percent of Americans suffer from phobias, such as fear of spiders, snakes, public speaking, and so on. Social phobias are perhaps the most common phobic response.[46]

Social Phobias   A **social phobia** is an anxiety disorder characterized by the persistent fear and avoidance of social situations. Essentially, the person dreads these situations for fear of being humiliated, embarrassed, or even looked at.[47] These disorders vary in scope. Some cause difficulty only in specific situations, such as getting up in front of the class to give a report. In more extreme cases, a person avoids all contact with others.

Seasonal Affective Disorder

An estimated 6 percent of Americans suffer from **seasonal affective disorder (SAD),** a type of depression, and an additional 14 percent experience a milder form of the disorder known as the winter blues. SAD strikes during the winter months and is associated with reduced exposure to sunlight. People with SAD suffer from irritability, apathy, carbohydrate craving and weight gain, increases in sleep time, and general sadness. Researchers believe that SAD is caused by a malfunction in the hypothalamus, the gland responsible for regulating responses to external stimuli. Stress may also play a role.

Certain factors seem to put people at risk for SAD. Women are four times more likely to suffer from it than men. Although SAD can occur at any age, people aged 20–40 appear to be most vulnerable. Certain families appear to be at risk. And residents of northern states, where there are fewer hours of sunlight during the winter, are more at risk than those living in the South. An estimated 10 percent of the population in Maine, Minnesota, and Wisconsin experience SAD, compared to fewer than 2 percent of those in Florida and New Mexico.

Therapies for SAD are simple but effective. The most beneficial is light therapy, which exposes patients to lamps that simulate sunlight. Eighty percent of patients experience relief from their symptoms within four days of treatment. Other treatments for SAD include diet change (eating more complex carbohydrates), increased exercise, stress management techniques, sleep restriction (limiting the number of hours slept in a 24-hour period), psychotherapy, and antidepressants.

Schizophrenia

Perhaps the most frightening of all mental disorders is **schizophrenia,** which affects about 1 percent of the U.S. population. Schizophrenia is characterized by alterations of the senses (including auditory and visual hallucinations); the inability to sort out incoming stimuli and make appropriate responses; an altered sense of self; and radical changes in emotions, movements, and behaviors. Victims of this disease often cannot function in society.

For decades, scientists believed that schizophrenia was an environmentally provoked form of madness. They blamed abnormal family interactions or early childhood traumas. Since the mid-1980s, however, when magnetic resonance imaging (MRI) and positron emission tomography (PET) have allowed us to study brain function more closely, scientists

Panic attack   Severe anxiety attack in which a particular situation, often for unknown reasons, causes terror.

Phobia   A deep and persistent fear of a specific object, activity, or situation that results in a compelling desire to avoid the source of the fear.

Social phobia   A phobia characterized by fear and avoidance of social situations.

Seasonal affective disorder (SAD)   A type of depression that occurs in the winter months, when sunlight levels are low.

Schizophrenia   A mental illness with biological origins that is characterized by irrational behavior, severe alterations of the senses (hallucinations), and, often, an inability to function in society.

have recognized that schizophrenia is a biological disease of the brain. The brain damage occurs early in life, possibly as early as the second trimester of fetal development. However, symptoms most commonly appear in late adolescence.

Schizophrenia is treatable but not curable at present. Treatments usually include some combination of hospitalization, medication, and supportive psychotherapy. Supportive psychotherapy, as opposed to psychoanalysis, can help the patient acquire skills for living in society.

Even though environmental theories of the causes of schizophrenia have been discarded in favor of biological theories, a stigma remains attached to the disease. Families of people with schizophrenia often experience anger and guilt associated with misunderstandings about the causes of the disease. They often need help in the form of information, family counseling, and advice on how to meet the schizophrenic person's needs for shelter, medical care, vocational training, and social interaction.

Gender Issues in Psychosocial Health

Gender bias often gets in the way of correct diagnosis of psychosocial disorders. In one study, for instance, 175 mental health professionals, of both genders, were asked to diagnose a patient based upon a summarized case history. Some of the professionals were told that the patient was male, others that the patient was female. The gender of the patient made a substantial difference in the diagnosis (though the gender of the clinician did not). When subjects thought the patient was female, they were more likely to diagnose hysterical personality, a "women's disorder." When they believed the patient to be male, the more likely diagnosis was antisocial personality, a "male disorder."

A major controversy is the inclusion of a "provisional" diagnosis for premenstrual syndrome (PMS) in the American Psychiatric Association's *Diagnostic and Statistical Manual of Mental Disorders* (now in its fourth edition, known as DSM-IV). The provisional inclusion, in an appendix to DSM-IV, signals that PMS merits further study and may be included as an approved diagnosis in future editions of the DSM. In other words, PMS could be considered a mental disorder in the future.

PMS is characterized by depression, irritability, and other symptoms of increased stress typically occurring just prior to menstruation and lasting for a day or two. A more severe case of PMS is known as *premenstrual dysphoric disorder*, or PMDD. Whereas PMS is somewhat disruptive and uncomfortable, it does not interfere with daily function; PMDD does. To be diagnosed with PMDD, a woman must have at least five symptoms of PMS for a week to 10 days, with at least one symptom being serious enough to interfere with her ability to function at work or at home. In these more severe cases, antidepressants may be prescribed. The point of contention lies in whether administering this treatment indicates that PMDD is viewed as a mental disorder rather than a physical problem.[48] Is it legitimate to attach a label indicating dysfunction and disorder to symptoms experienced only once or twice a month? Further controversy stems from the possible use (or misuse) of the diagnostic label to justify exclusion of women from certain desirable jobs.

Suicide: Giving Up on Life

There are over 35,000 reported suicides each year in the United States. Experts estimate that there may actually be closer to 100,000 cases. The disparity is due to the difficulty in determining many causes of suspicious deaths. More lives are lost to suicide than to any other single cause except cardiovascular disease and cancer. Suicide often results from poor coping skills, lack of social support, lack of self-esteem, and the inability to see one's way out of a bad situation.

College students are more likely than the general population to attempt suicide; suicide is the third leading cause of death in people between the ages of 15 and 24. In fact, this age group now accounts for nearly 20 percent of all suicides.[49] The pressures, joys, disappointments, challenges, and changes of the college environment are believed to be in part responsible for these rates. However, young adults who choose not to go to college but who are searching for direction in careers, relationships, and other life goals are also at risk.

Risk factors for suicide include a family history of suicide, previous suicide attempts, excessive drug and alcohol use, prolonged depression, financial difficulties, serious illness in the suicide contemplator or in his or her loved ones, and loss of a loved one through death or rejection. Societal pressures often serve as a catalyst.

In most cases, suicide does not occur unpredictably. In fact, between 75 and 80 percent of people who commit suicide give a warning of their intentions.

Warning Signs of Suicide

Common signs of possible suicide include the following:[50]

- Recent loss and a seeming inability to let go of grief
- Change in personality—sadness, withdrawal, irritability, anxiety, tiredness, indecisiveness, apathy
- Change in behavior—inability to concentrate, loss of interest in classes
- Diminished sexual interest—impotence, menstrual abnormalities
- Expressions of self-hatred
- Change in sleep patterns
- Change in eating habits
- A direct statement about committing suicide, such as, "I might as well end it all"
- An indirect statement, such as, "You won't have to worry about me anymore"
- "Final preparations," such as writing a will, repairing poor relationships with family or friends, giving away prized possessions, or writing revealing letters
- A preoccupation with themes of death

Suicide: A Neglected Problem Among Diverse Populations

One of the most underrated public health problems facing Americans today, suicide accounts for more than 35,000 preventable deaths each year, nearly 10,000 more than deaths from homicide. It touches all ages, races, and social groups and is on the rise in many segments of the population.

- Recent reports from the Centers for Disease Control showed that the rate of suicide among African American teens aged 15–19 more than doubled between 1980 and 1995.
- For every successful suicide, another 17 are attempted.

- Elderly men use the most violent means of suicide and are the most likely to be successful.
- After age 75, suicide rates are three times the national average, and after age 80, six times the national average.
- Males outnumber females five to one in completed suicides, whereas females are two times more likely to attempt suicide, often by using less lethal means such as drugs or alcohol. Native Americans have a higher suicide rate than whites of all ages.
- Teen suicides often occur in clusters, particularly when friends or prominent national figures, such as rock stars, commit suicide.
- Rates of suicide are considerably higher in western states, followed by the South, Midwest, and Northeast.
- People who have never been married are twice as likely to commit suicide as

currently married people. The highest rates of all occur among the divorced or widowed.
- Suicide rates are lower in rural areas than in cities.
- Suicide rates are highest in German-speaking countries, Switzerland, Scandinavia, Eastern Europe, and Japan, and lowest in Greece, Italy, and Spain.

Sources: From S. Stapleton, "The Surgeon General Calls for Suicide Prevention," 1998, *American Medical News,* 41, p. 9; and "Suicide Among Black Youth, 1980–1995," *Journal of the American Medical Association,* 279, p. 1431.

- A sudden and unexplained demonstration of happiness following a period of depression
- Marked changes in personal appearance
- Excessive risk taking and an "I don't care what happens to me" attitude

Taking Action to Prevent Suicide

Most people who attempt suicide really want to live but see suicide as the only way out of an intolerable situation. Crisis counselors and suicide hotlines may help temporarily, but the best way to prevent suicide is to get rid of conditions that may precipitate attempts, including alcoholism, drug abuse, loneliness, isolation, and access to guns.

If someone you know threatens suicide or displays any warning signs, take the following actions:

- Monitor the warning signals. Try to keep an eye on the person involved, or see that there is someone around the person as much as possible.
- Take any threats seriously. Don't just brush them off.
- Let the person know how much you care about him or her. State that you are there if he or she needs help.
- Listen. Try not to discredit or be shocked by what the person says. Empathize, sympathize, and keep the person talking. Talk about stressors and listen to the responses.
- Ask directly, "Are you thinking of hurting or killing yourself?"

- Do not belittle the person's feelings or say that he or she doesn't really mean it or couldn't succeed at suicide. To some people, these comments offer the challenge of proving you wrong.
- Help the person think about alternatives. Be ready to offer choices. Offer to go for help with the person. Call your local suicide hotline and use all available community and campus resources. Recommend a counselor or other person to talk to.
- Remember that your relationships with others involve responsibilities. If you need to stay with the person, take the person to a health care facility, or provide support, give of yourself and your time.
- Tell your friend's spouse, partner, parents, brothers and sisters, or counselor. Do not keep your suspicions to yourself. Don't let a suicidal friend talk you into keeping your discussions confidential. If your friend succeeds in a suicide attempt, you will have to live with the consequences.

What do you think?

If your roommate showed some of the warning signs of suicide, what action would you take? ✳ Whom would you contact first? ✳ Where on campus might your friend get help? ✳ What if someone in class whom you hardly know gave some of the warning signs? ✳ What would you then do?

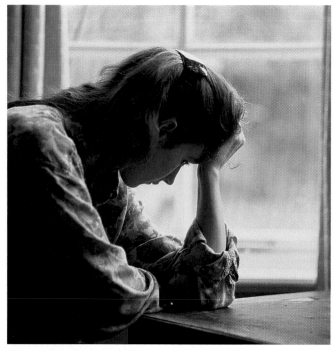

When experiencing problems such as depression or anxiety, it is unwise to try to "go it alone." A qualified, caring therapist can help.

Seeking Professional Help

Whereas a physical ailment will readily send most of us to the nearest health professional, seeking professional help for psychosocial problems is too often viewed as an admission of personal failure. However, increasing numbers of Americans are turning to mental health professionals, and nearly one in five seeks such help. Researchers cite breakdown in support systems, high societal expectations of the individual, and dysfunctional families as the three major reasons why more people are asking for assistance than ever before.

You should consider seeking help in any of the following circumstances:

- You think you need help.
- You experience wild mood swings.
- A problem is interfering with your daily life.
- Your fears or feelings of guilt frequently distract your attention.
- You begin to withdraw from others.
- You have hallucinations.

Psychiatrist A licensed physician who specializes in treating mental and emotional disorders.

Psychologist A person with a Ph.D. degree and training in psychology.

- You feel that life is not worth living.
- You feel inadequate or worthless.
- Your emotional responses are inappropriate to various situations.
- Your daily life seems to be nothing but repeated crises.
- You feel you can't "get your act together."
- You are considering suicide.
- You turn to drugs or alcohol to escape from your problems.
- You feel out of control.

Getting Evaluated for Treatment

If you are considering treatment for a psychosocial problem, schedule a complete evaluation first. Consult a credentialed health professional for a thorough examination, which should include three parts:

- A physical checkup, which will rule out thyroid disorders, viral infections, and anemia—all of which can result in depressive-like symptoms—and a neurological check of coordination, reflexes, and balance, to rule out brain disorders
- A psychiatric history, which will attempt to trace the course of the apparent disorder, genetic or family factors, and any past treatments
- A mental status examination, which will assess thoughts, speaking processes, and memory, as well as an in-depth interview with tests for other psychiatric symptoms[51]

Once physical factors have been ruled out, you may decide to consult a professional who specializes in psychosocial health.

Mental Health Professionals

Several types of mental health professionals, or providers, are available to help you. The most important criterion is not how many degrees this person has, but whether you feel you can work together.

Psychiatrist A **psychiatrist** is a medical doctor. After obtaining an M.D. degree, a psychiatrist spends up to 12 years studying psychosocial health and disease. As a licensed physician, a psychiatrist can prescribe medications for various mental or emotional problems and may have admitting privileges at a local hospital. Some psychiatrists are affiliated with hospitals, while others are in private practice.

Psychologist A **psychologist** usually has a Ph.D. degree in counseling or clinical psychology. In addition, many states require licensure. Psychologists are trained in various types of therapy, including behavior and insight therapy. Most can conduct both individual and group counseling sessions. Psychologists may also be trained in certain specialties, such as family counseling or sexual counseling.

Psychoanalyst A **psychoanalyst** is a psychiatrist or psychologist having special training in psychoanalysis. Psychoanalysis is a type of therapy that helps patients remember early traumas that have blocked personal growth. Facing these traumas helps them resolve conflicts and begin to lead more productive lives.

Clinical/Psychiatric Social Worker A **social worker** has at least a master's degree in social work (M.S.W.) and two years of experience in a clinical setting. Many states require an examination for accreditation. Some social workers work in clinical settings, whereas others have private practices.

Counselor A **counselor** often has a master's degree in counseling, psychology, educational psychology, or related human service. Professional societies recommend at least two years of graduate course work or supervised practice as a minimal requirement. Many counselors are trained to do individual and group therapy. They often specialize in one type of counseling, such as family, marital, relationship, children, drug, divorce, behavioral, or personal counseling.

Psychiatric Nurse Specialist Although all registered nurses can work in psychiatric settings, some continue their education and specialize in psychiatric practice. The psychiatric nurse specialist can be certified by the American Nursing Association in adult, child, or adolescent psychiatric nursing.

Many different types of counseling exist, ranging from individual therapy, which involves one-on-one work between therapist and client, to group therapy, in which two or more clients meet with a therapist to discuss problems. Table 2.3 identifies traditional forms of psychotherapy.

What to Expect in Therapy

The first trip to a therapist can be extremely difficult. Most of us have misconceptions about what therapy is and about what it can do. That first visit is a verbal and mental sizing up between you and the therapist. You may not accomplish much in that first hour. If you decide that this professional is not for you, you will at least have learned how to present your problem and what qualities you need in a therapist.

1. Before meeting, briefly explain your needs. Ask what the fee is. Arrive on time. Wear comfortable clothing. Expect to spend about an hour during your first visit.

Psychoanalyst A psychiatrist or psychologist having special training in psychoanalysis.

Social worker A person with an M.S.W. degree and clinical training.

Counselor A person having a variety of academic and experiential training who deals with the treatment of emotional problems.

2. The therapist will want to take down your history and details about the problems that have brought you to therapy. Answer as honestly as possible. Many will ask how you feel about aspects of your life. Do not be embarrassed to acknowledge your feelings.
3. Therapists are not mind readers. They cannot tell what you are thinking. It is therefore critical to the success of your treatment that you trust this person enough to be open and honest.
4. Do not expect the therapist to tell you what to do or how to behave. The responsibility for improved behavior lies with you.
5. Find out if you can set your own therapeutic goals and timetables. Also, find out whether, later in therapy, your therapist will allow you to determine what is and is not helping you.
6. If after your first visit (or even after several visits), you feel you cannot work with this person, you must say so.

Taking Charge 2 ² 2

Managing Your Psychosocial Health

Psychosocial health is a complex concept. Finding the best way to help yourself achieve optimal psychosocial health requires careful introspection and planned action. Remembering the following points and acting on them whenever possible will help you along the way.

Checklist for Change

✓ Consider life a constant process of discovery.

✓ Accept yourself as the best that you are able to be right now.

✓ Remember that nobody is perfect.

✓ Remember that the most difficult times in life occur during transitions and can be opportunities for growth even when they are painful.

✓ Be open to other perspectives.

✓ Recognize the sources of your own anxiety, and act to reduce them.

✓ Ask for help when you need it; discuss your problems with others.

✓ Try to find joy and happiness in both the little and big things in life.

✓ Nurture your friendships.

✓ Become sensitive to and aware of your own body's signals—take care of yourself.

✓ Find a meaning for your life and work toward achieving your goals.

✓ Develop strategies to get through problem situations.

✓ Remain open to emotional experiences—give yourself to today rather than always reserving yourself for tomorrow.

✓ Even when you fail, be proud of yourself for trying.

✓ Keep your sense of humor— learn to laugh at yourself.

✓ Never quit trying to grow, to experience, to love, and to live life to its fullest.

Summary

❋ Psychosocial health is a complex phenomenon involving mental, emotional, social, and spiritual health.

❋ Many factors influence psychosocial health, including life experiences, family, the environment, other people, self-esteem, self-efficacy, and personality. Some of these are modifiable; others are not.

❋ Developing self-esteem and self-efficacy and getting enough sleep are key to enhancing psychosocial health.

❋ Many people believe spirituality is important to wellness. Though the exact reasons have not been established, many studies show a connection.

❋ Happiness is a key factor in determining overall reaction to life's challenges. The mind–body connection is an important link in overall health and well-being.

❋ Indicators of deteriorating psychosocial health include depression. Identifying depression is the first step in treating this disorder.

❋ Common psychosocial problems include anxiety disorders, panic attacks, phobias, seasonal affective disorder, and schizophrenia.

❋ Suicide is a result of negative psychosocial reactions to life. People intending to commit suicide often give warning signs of their intentions. Such people can often be helped.

✳ Mental health professionals include psychiatrists, psychoanalysts, psychologists, clinical/psychiatric social workers, counselors, and psychiatric nurse specialists. Many different kinds of therapy methods exist, including group and individual therapy. It is wise to interview a therapist carefully before beginning treatment.

Discussion Questions

1. What is psychosocial health? What indicates that you either are or aren't psychosocially healthy? Why might the college environment provide a real challenge to your psychosocial health?
2. Discuss the factors that influence your overall level of psychosocial health. What factors can you change? Which ones may be more difficult to change?
3. What steps could you take today to improve your psychosocial health? Which steps require long-term effort?
4. What are four main themes of spirituality, and how are they expressed in daily life?
5. Why is laughter therapeutic? How can humor help you better achieve wellness?
6. What factors appear to contribute to psychosocial difficulties and illnesses? Which of the common psychosocial illnesses is likely to affect people in your age group?
7. What are the warning signs of suicide? Of depression? Why is depression so pervasive among young Americans today? Why are some groups more vulnerable to suicide and depression than are others? What would you do if you heard a friend in the cafeteria say to no one in particular that he was going to "do the world a favor and end it all"?
8. Discuss the different types of health professionals and therapies. If you felt depressed about breaking off a long-term relationship, which professional and therapy do you think would be most beneficial? Explain your answer. What services are provided by your student health center? What fees are charged to students?
9. What psychosocial areas do you need to work on? Which are most important? Why? What actions can you take today?

Application Exercise

Reread the What Do You Think? scenario at the beginning of the chapter and answer the following questions.

1. What factors may have contributed to Amy's behavior? Why might her friends be hesitant about reaching out to help her?
2. What services on your campus would be available to help students improve their psychosocial health? What community services are available to nonstudents who have limited incomes?
3. What could you do to help fellow students or friends who are having problems in this area?

Accessing Your Health on the Internet   http

Visit the following Internet sites to explore further topics and issues related to personal health. To visit an organization's website, go to the Companion Website for *Health: The Basics, Fifth Edition* at www.aw.com/donatelle, click on the book image, and select "Accessing Your Health on the Internet" from the navigation menu on the left.

1. **National Institute of Mental Health (NIMH):** Overview of mental health information, new research, and so on relating to mental health.
2. **Mental Health Net.** Provides information for mental health practitioners as well as those whom they serve. Includes many mental health links.
3. **American Psychological Association.** Includes APA newsletters, links to other sites, information on books, journals, employment, and public, practical, and educational materials.

Further Reading

Dalai Lama and H. C. Cutler. *The Art of Happiness: A Handbook for Living.* New York: Riverhead, 1998.
Explores the reasons why so many people are unhappy and offers strategies for becoming happy. Through a series of interviews, the authors explore questions of meaning, motives, and the interconnectedness of life.

Koening, H. G. *The Healing Power of Faith: Science Explores Medicine's Last Great Frontier.* New York: Simon and Schuster, 1999.
Layperson's overview of the role of faith and spirituality in health. Offers insights in past research and future areas worth studying.

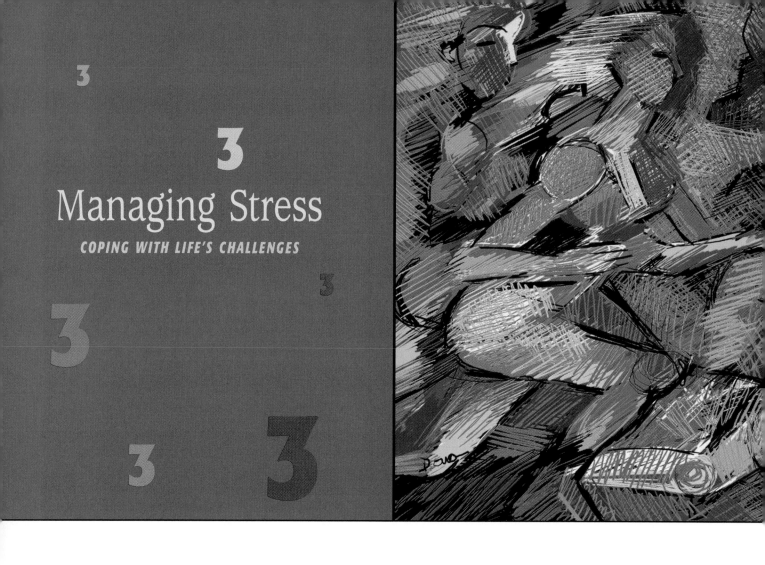

3
Managing Stress
COPING WITH LIFE'S CHALLENGES

objectives

* Define stress, and examine the potential impact of stress on health, relationships, and success in college.

* Explain the three phases of the general adaptation syndrome, and describe what happens physiologically when people experience a real or perceived threat.

* Examine the health risks that may occur with chronic stress.

* Discuss psychosocial, environmental, and self-imposed sources of stress. Examine ways in which you might reduce risks from these stressors or inoculate yourself against stressful situations.

* Examine the special stressors that affect college students and strategies for reducing risk.

* Explore techniques for coping with unavoidable stress, reducing exposure to stress, and making optimum use of positive stressors to promote growth and enrich life experiences.

Loud music. Relationship problems. Too much to do. Not enough time. The excitement of a new relationship. Financial worries. Stress! You can't get away from it; there's no place to hide. Seemingly, stress is an inevitable part of modern life. Whether it seems frightening or invigorating, we all experience its effect.

Often, stress is insidious, and we don't even notice things that affect us. As we sleep it encroaches on our psyche through noise or incessant worries over things that need to be done. While we work at the computer, stress may interfere in the form of noise from next door, strain on our eyes, and tension in our backs. The exact toll stress exacts from us during a lifetime of stress overload is unknown, but it is much more than an annoyance. Rather, it is a significant health hazard that can rob the body of needed nutrients, damage the cardiovascular system, raise blood pressure, and dampen the immune system's defenses, leaving us vulnerable to infections and a host of diseases. In addition, it can drain our emotional reserves, contribute to depression, anxiety, and irritability, and cause social interactions to be punctuated with hostility and anger. Stress is a major concern in the United States, and it appears to be getting worse: One-third of U.S. workers report an increase in job-related stress over the past year. Although much has been written about stress, we are only beginning to understand the multifaceted nature of the stress response and its tremendous potential for harm or benefit.

What Is Stress?

Often, we think of stress as an externally imposed factor that threatens or makes a demand on our minds and bodies. But for most of us, stress usually results from an internal state of emotional tension that occurs in response to the various demands of living. Most current definitions state that **stress** is the mental and physical response of our bodies to the changes and challenges in our lives. Inherent in these definitions is the idea that we sometimes take ourselves and our lives too seriously: that we should loosen up, worry less, and gain greater control over our minds as well as our bodies.

A **stressor** is any physical, social, or psychological event or condition that causes the body to adjust to a specific situation. Stressors may be tangible, such as an angry parent or a disgruntled roommate, or intangible, such as the mixed emotions associated with meeting your significant other's parents for the first time. **Adjustment** is the attempt to cope with a given situation. **Strain** is the wear and tear the body and mind sustain during the adjustment process.

Stress and strain are associated with most daily activities. Generally, positive stress, or stress that presents the opportunity for personal growth and satisfaction, is called **eustress.** Getting married, starting school, beginning a career,

Stress   Mental and physical responses to change.

Stressor   A physical, social, or psychological event or condition that requires an adjustment.

Adjustment   The attempt to cope with a given situation.

Strain   The wear-and-tear sustained by the body and mind in adjusting to or resisting a stressor.

Eustress   Stress that presents opportunities for personal growth.

developing new friendships, and learning a new physical skill all give rise to eustress. **Distress,** or negative stress, is caused by those events that result in debilitative stress and strain. Examples include financial problems, the death of a loved one, academic difficulties, and the breakup of a relationship.

In many cases, we cannot prevent distress: like eustress, it is a part of life. However, we can train ourselves to recognize the events that cause distress and to anticipate the reactions we have to them. We can learn to practice coping skills and to develop techniques to manage stress once it does occur.

The Body's Response to Stress

Whenever we're surprised by a sudden stressor, such as someone swerving into our lane of traffic, the adrenal glands jump into action. These two almond-sized glands sitting atop the kidneys secrete adrenaline and other hormones into the bloodstream. As a result, the heart speeds up, breathing rate increases, blood pressure elevates, and the flow of blood to the muscles increases with a rapid release of blood sugars into the bloodstream. This sudden burst of energy and strength is believed to provide the extra edge that has helped generations of humans survive during adversity. Known as the **fight-or-flight response,** this physiological reaction is believed to be one of our most basic, innate survival instincts. It is a point at which our bodies go on the alert either to fight or to escape.

The General Adaptation Syndrome (GAS)

What has just been described in very general terms is a complicated physiological response to stress in which our bodies move from **homeostasis,** a level of functioning in which systems operate smoothly and maintain equilibrium, to one of crisis, in which the body attempts to return to homeostasis. This adjustment is referred to as an **adaptive**

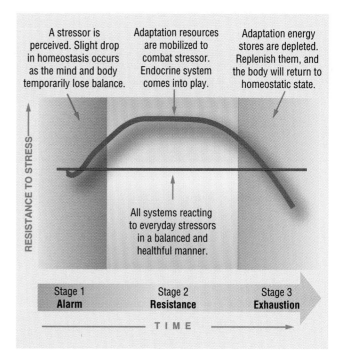

Figure 3.1 The General Adaptation Syndrome

response. First characterized by Hans Selye in 1936, this internal fight to restore balance is known as the **general adaptation syndrome (GAS)** (Figure 3.1). It has three distinct phases: alarm, resistance, and exhaustion.[1]

Alarm Phase When the body is exposed to a stressor, whether real or perceived, the fight-or-flight response kicks into gear. Stress hormones flow into the body, and the body prepares to do battle with whatever is causing the upset. The subconscious perceptions and appraisal of the stressor stimulate the areas in the brain responsible for emotions. Emotional stimulation, in turn, starts the physical reactions that we associate with stress (Figure 3.2). This entire process takes only a few seconds.

Suppose that you are walking to your car after a latenight class on a dimly lighted campus. As you pass a particularly dark area, you hear someone cough behind you and sense that this person is fairly close. You walk faster, only to hear the quickened footsteps of the other person. Your senses become increasingly alert, your breathing quickens, your heart races, and you begin to perspire. The stranger is getting closer and closer. In desperation you stop, clutching your book bag in your hands, determined to use force if necessary to protect yourself. You turn around quickly and let out a blood-curdling yell. To your surprise, the only person you see is Mrs. Fletcher, a woman in your class, who has been trying to stay close to you out of her own anxiety about walking alone in the dark. She screams and jumps back off the street, only to trip and fall. You look at her in startled embarrassment, help her to her feet, and nervously laugh about your reaction. You have just experienced the alarm and resistance phases of GAS.

Distress   Stress that can have a negative effect on health.

Fight-or-flight response   Physiological arousal response in which the body prepares to combat a real or perceived threat.

Homeostasis   A balanced physical state in which all the body's systems function smoothly.

Adaptive response   Form of adjustment in which the body attempts to restore homeostasis.

General adaptation syndrome (GAS)   The pattern followed in the physiological response to stress, consisting of the alarm, resistance, and exhaustion phases.

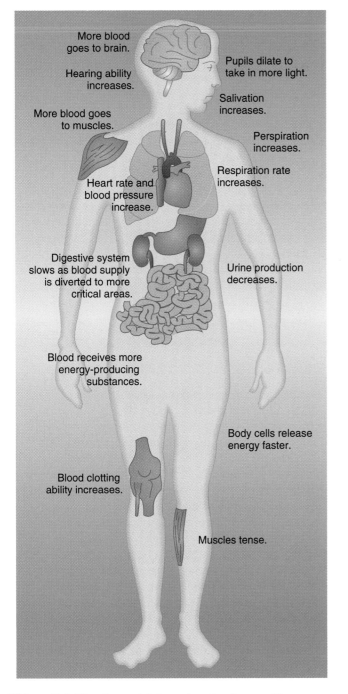

More blood goes to brain.

Hearing ability increases.

Pupils dilate to take in more light.

Salivation increases.

More blood goes to muscles.

Perspiration increases.

Respiration rate increases.

Heart rate and blood pressure increase.

Digestive system slows as blood supply is diverted to more critical areas.

Urine production decreases.

Blood receives more energy-producing substances.

Body cells release energy faster.

Blood clotting ability increases.

Muscles tense.

Figure 3.2 The General Adaptation Syndrome: Alarm Phase

When the mind perceives a stressor (either real or imaginary), such as a potential attacker, the *cerebral cortex,* the region of the brain that interprets the nature of an event, is called to attention. If the cerebral cortex perceives a threat, it triggers an **autonomic nervous system (ANS)** response that prepares the body for action. The ANS is the portion of the central nervous system that regulates bodily functions that we do not normally consciously control, such as the beating of the heart, breathing, and glandular

function. When we are stressed, the activity rate of all these bodily functions increases dramatically to give us the physical strength to protect ourselves or to mobilize internal forces.

The ANS has two branches: the sympathetic nervous system and parasympathetic nervous system. The **sympathetic nervous system** energizes the body for either fight or flight by signaling the release of several stress hormones that speed the heart rate, increase the breathing rate, and trigger many other stress responses. The **parasympathetic nervous system** functions to slow all the systems stimulated by the stress response. Thus, the parasympathetic branch of the ANS serves as a system of checks and balances on the sympathetic branch. In a healthy person, these two branches work together in a balance that controls the negative effects of stress. However, long-term stress can strain this balance. As stress reactions become the dominant forces in a person's body, chronic physical problems can occur.

The responses of the sympathetic nervous system to stress involve a complex series of biochemical exchanges between different parts of the body. The **hypothalamus,** a section of the brain, functions as the control center of the sympathetic nervous system and determines the overall reaction to stressors. When the hypothalamus perceives that extra energy is needed to fight a stressor, it stimulates the adrenal glands, located near the top of the kidneys, to release the hormone **epinephrine,** also called adrenaline. Epinephrine causes more blood to be pumped with each beat of the heart, dilates the bronchioles (air sacs in the lungs) to increase oxygen intake, increases the breathing rate, stimulates the liver to release more glucose (which fuels muscular exertion), and dilates the pupils to improve visual sensitivity. The body is then poised to act immediately.

As epinephrine secretion increases, blood is diverted away from the digestive system, possibly causing nausea and cramping if the distress occurs shortly after a meal, and drying of nasal and salivary tissues, producing dry mouth.

Autonomic nervous system (ANS) The portion of the central nervous system that regulates bodily functions that a person does not normally consciously control.

Sympathetic nervous system Branch of the autonomic nervous system responsible for stress arousal.

Parasympathetic nervous system Part of the autonomic nervous system responsible for slowing systems stimulated by the stress response.

Hypothalamus A section of the brain that controls the sympathetic nervous system and directs the stress response.

Epinephrine Also called adrenaline, a hormone that stimulates body systems in response to stress.

The alarm phase also provides for longer-term reaction to stress. The hypothalamus triggers the pituitary gland, which in turn releases another powerful hormone, **adrenocorticotrophic hormone (ACTH).** ACTH signals the adrenal glands to release **cortisol,** a hormone that makes stored nutrients more readily available to meet energy demands. Finally, other parts of the brain and body release endorphins, the body's naturally occurring opiates, which relieve pain that may be caused by a stressor.

Resistance Phase The resistance phase of the GAS begins almost immediately after the alarm phase starts. In this stage, the body has reacted to the stressor and adjusted in a way that allows the system to return to homeostasis. As the sympathetic nervous system energizes the body via the hormonal action of epinephrine, norepinephrine, cortisol, and other hormones, the parasympathetic nervous system helps control these energy levels and return the body to a normal level of functioning.

Exhaustion Phase In the exhaustion phase of the GAS, the physical and emotional energy used to fight a stressor has been depleted. The toll stress takes on the body depends on the type of stress or the period of time spent under stress. Short-term stress probably would not deplete all of a person's energy reserves, but chronic stress experienced over a period of time can create continuous states of alarm and resistance, resulting in total depletion of energy and susceptibility to illness. The key to warding off the effects of stress lies in what many researchers refer to as *adaptation energy stores,* the physical and mental foundations of our ability to cope with stress.

There are two levels of adaptation energy stores: deep and superficial. We apparently have little control over deep stores; their size appears to be preset by heredity. Superficial adaptation energy stores, however, are renewable. They present the first line of defense against stress; they are tapped into initially as the body fights stress. Only when superficial stores are exhausted does the body tap into the deep energy stores. As our adaptation energy stores are depleted, we tire more quickly and require more rest. Without this replenishing sleep, the alarm and resistance phases eventually will limit our ability to rebound properly.

> **Adrenocorticotrophic hormone (ACTH)** A pituitary hormone that stimulates the adrenal glands to secrete cortisol.
>
> **Cortisol** Hormone released by the adrenal glands that makes stored nutrients more readily available to meet energy demands.
>
> **Immunocompetence** The ability of the immune system to respond to assaults.

As the body adjusts to chronic unresolved stress, the adrenal glands continue to release cortisol, which remains in the bloodstream for longer periods of time due to slower metabolic responsiveness. Over time, without relief, cortisol can reduce **immunocompetence,** or the ability of the immune system to respond to various onslaughts. Blood pressure can remain dangerously elevated, and our body systems become unable to respond with the same vigor they once did. The net effect? Greater chance of minor illnesses at one end of the continuum; greater risk of life-threatening disease at the other end.

Stress management, therefore, depends on the ability to replenish superficial stores and conserve deep stores. Besides getting adequate amounts of rest, adaptation energy stores can be replenished by aerobic exercise, finding a balance between work and relaxation, practicing good nutritional habits, setting realistic goals, and maintaining supportive relationships.

Stress and Your Health

Although much has been written about the negative effects of stress, researchers have only recently begun to untangle the complex web of physical and emotional interactions that actually cause the body to break down over time. Stress is often described as a "disease of prolonged arousal" that leads to other negative health effects. Nearly all systems of the body become potential targets for this onslaught, and the long-term effects may be devastating.

Much of the initial impetus for studying the health effects of stress came from indirect observations. Cardiologists in the Framingham Heart Study (a large, longitudinal study of CVD risks) and other research projects noted that highly stressed individuals seemed to experience significantly greater risks for cardiovascular disease (CVD) and hypertension.[2] Monkeys exposed to high levels of unpredictable stressors in studies showed significantly increased levels of disease and mortality.[3] In a landmark study, M. D. Jeremko observed that chronic stress activation can result in headaches, asthma, hypertension, ulcers, lower back pain, and other medical conditions, a finding substantiated by a meta-analysis of over 100 similar studies.[4] Moreover, a Harvard study concluded that mental health was the most important predictor of physical health.[5] While the battle over the legitimacy of these observations continues to be waged in research labs across the country, the theory that chronic stress increases susceptibility to certain ailments has gained credibility.

Stress and CVD Risks

Since Friedman and Rosenman's classic study of Type A and Type B personalities and heart disease from the late 1960s and early 1970s (discussed later in this chapter), researchers have tried to definitively link personality, emotions, and a host of other variables to heart disease.[6] It is generally assumed that too much stress contributes to several adverse physiological changes:

- Increased plaque buildup in the arteries due to elevations in cholesterol level
- Hardening of the arteries
- Alterations in heart rhythms
- Increased blood pressure
- Difficulties in cardiovascular system responsiveness due to all of the above

For more information about CVD risks, see also Chapter 12.

Stress and Impaired Immunity

A new area of scientific investigation known as **psychoneuroimmunology (PNI)** analyzes the intricate relationship between the mind's response to stress and the ability of the immune system to function effectively. An article in the *Journal of the American Medical Association (JAMA)* reviews the research linking stress to adverse health consequences.[7] Among the findings: Too much stress, over a long period, can negatively regulate various aspects of the cellular immune response. In particular, stress disrupts bidirectional communication networks between the nervous, endocrine, and immune systems. When these networks fail, messenger systems that regulate hormones, blood cell formation, and a host of other health-regulating systems begin to falter or send faulty information.[8]

During prolonged stress, elevated levels of adrenal hormones destroy or reduce the ability of the white blood cells, known as natural killer T-cells, to aid the immune response. When killer T-cells are suppressed and other regulating systems aren't working correctly, illness may occur. Several key studies link stress with infectious diseases:

- Mice that are forced to live in crowded cages prior to and after infection with tuberculosis have much poorer outcomes than mice in less crowded situations. Social disruption in mice also seems to trigger outbreaks of herpes viruses.[9]
- Caregivers of Alzheimer's patients who were vaccinated against the flu still had a much greater chance of getting the flu or becoming ill than non-caregivers who received the same vaccine.[10]
- People with self-reported high stress levels were much more likely to develop upper respiratory infections than those who reported lower levels of stress.[11]
- Certain changes in lifestyle may increase resistance to infectious diseases. These changes include broadening one's social involvement (e.g., joining social or spiritual groups, having a confidant, spending time with supportive friends) and maintaining healthful practices, such as proper diet, exercise, and sleep.[12]

- Students' disease-fighting mechanisms are weaker during high-stress times, such as exam weeks and on days when they are upset. In one experiment, a stressful event increased the severity of symptoms in a group of volunteers who were knowingly infected with a cold virus. In another, 47 percent of subjects living high-stress lives developed colds after a virus was dropped into their noses, but only 27 percent of those living relatively stress-free lives caught these colds.[13]

Although strong indicators support the hypothesis of a relationship between high stress and increased risk for disease, we are only beginning to understand this link. Some research indicates that such a relationship does not exist and that other factors, such as genetics and environmental stimuli, may be involved. However, in spite of questions, studies supporting this relationship outnumber those that don't.[14]

Stress and the Mind

Stress may be one of the single greatest contributors to mental disability and emotional dysfunction in the United States. Whether it be from lost work productivity, difficulties in relationships, abuse of drugs and other substances, displaced anger and aggressive behavior, or a host of other problems, stress overload does much more than cause the heart rate to soar. Evidence suggests a strong relationship between stress and the potential for negative mental health reactions. Consider the following:[15]

- Numerous researchers have demonstrated that provoking stressors, interacting with low self-esteem and/or maladaptive coping styles, predict depression and anxiety.
- Depression and drug abuse are highly correlated with excessive exposure to stress.
- Among college students, low self-esteem or depression and concerns about stress and health were identified as unresolved problems for 35 percent and 20 percent of the respondents, respectively.
- Mature coping styles predict happiness, occupational and social success, enjoyment, and absence of addictions.
- Persons with high nervous tension have increased risk for mental illness, suicide, and coronary heart disease.
- A recent national study of Americans ages 15 to 54 found that almost half will suffer a mental and addictive disorder during their lifetime. Many of these disorders are believed to be stress related.
- Mental illness is on the increase in almost all segments of U.S. society.

> **Psychoneuroimmunology (PNI)** Science of the interaction between the mind and the immune system.

Sources of Stress

Both eustress and distress have many sources. These sources include psychosocial factors, environmental stressors, and self-imposed stress.

Psychosocial Sources of Stress

Psychosocial stress refers to the factors in our daily lives that cause stress (see the Assess Yourself box below). Interactions with others, the subtle and not-so-subtle expectations we and

---

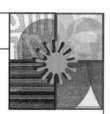

ASSESS YOURSELF

How Stressed Are You?

Each of us reacts differently to life's little challenges. Faced with a long line at the bank, most of us will get heated up for a few seconds before we shrug and move on. But for others—the one in five of us whom researchers call "Hot Reactors"—such incidents are an assault on good health. That's why rating your stress requires you both to tally your life's stressors (Part One) and to figure out whether you are particularly susceptible to stress (Part Two).

PART ONE: THE STRESS IN YOUR LIFE

How often are the following stressful situations a part of your daily life?

   1 = Never   2 = Rarely   3 = Sometimes   4 = Often   5 = All the time

I work long hours.	1	2	3	4	5
There are signs that my job isn't secure.	1	2	3	4	5
Doing a good job goes unnoticed.	1	2	3	4	5
It takes all my energy just to make it through the day.	1	2	3	4	5
There are severe arguments at home.	1	2	3	4	5
A family member is seriously ill.	1	2	3	4	5
I'm having problems with child care.	1	2	3	4	5
I don't have enough time for fun.	1	2	3	4	5
I'm on a diet.	1	2	3	4	5
My family and friends count on me to solve their problems.	1	2	3	4	5
I'm expected to keep up a certain standard of living.	1	2	3	4	5
My neighborhood is crowded or dangerous.	1	2	3	4	5
My home is a mess.	1	2	3	4	5
I can't pay my bills on time.	1	2	3	4	5
I'm not saving money.	1	2	3	4	5

Your Total Score _____

Below 38: You have a Lower-Stress Life.

38 & Above: You have a High-Stress Life.

PART TWO: YOUR STRESS SUSCEPTIBILITY

Try to imagine how you would react in these hypothetical situations.

   You've been waiting 20 minutes for a table in a crowded restaurant, and the host seats a party that arrived after you. You feel your anger rise as your face gets hot and your heart beats faster.   True or False

---

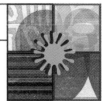

Your sister calls out of the blue and starts to tell you how much you mean to her. Uncomfortable, you change the subject without expressing what you feel.   True or False

You come home to find the kitchen looking like a disaster area and your spouse lounging in front of the TV. You tense up and can't seem to shake your anger.   True or False

Faced with a public speaking event, you get keyed up and lose sleep for a day or more, worrying about how you'll do.   True or False

On Thursday your repair shop promises to fix your car in time for a weekend trip. As the hours go by, you become increasingly worried that something will go wrong and your trip will be ruined.   True or False

Two or Fewer True: You're a Cool Reactor, someone who tends to roll with the punches when a situation is out of your control.

Three or More True: Sorry, you're a Hot Reactor, someone who responds to mildly stressful situations with a fight-or-flight adrenaline rush that drives up blood pressure and can lead to heart rhythm disturbances, accelerated clotting, and damaged blood vessel linings. Some hot reactors can seem cool as a cucumber on the outside, but inside their bodies are silently killing them.

WHAT YOUR SCORES MEAN

Combine the results from Parts One and Two to get your total stress rating.

Lower-Stress Life   Cool Reactor
Whatever your problems, stress isn't one of them. Even when stressful events do occur—and they will—your health probably won't suffer.

Lower-Stress Life   Hot Reactor
You're not under stress—at least for now. Though you tend to overreact to problems, you've wisely managed your life to avoid the big stressors. Before you honk at the guy who cuts you off in rush hour traffic, remember that getting angry can destroy thousands of heart muscle cells within minutes.

High-Stress Life   Cool Reactor
You're under stress, but only you know if it's hurting. Even if you normally thrive with a full plate of challenges, now you might be biting off more than you can chew. Note any increase in headaches, backaches, or insomnia; that's your body telling you to lighten your load. If your job is the main source of stress, think about reducing your hours. If that's not possible, find a way to make your job more enjoyable, and stress will become manageable.

High-Stress Life   Hot Reactor
You're in the danger zone. Make an extra effort to exercise, get enough sleep, and keep your family and friends close. Unfortunately, even being physically fit does little to protect you if your body is in perpetual stress mode. To survive, you may need to make major changes—walking away from a life-destroying job or relationship, perhaps—as well as to develop a whole new approach to life's hourly obstacles. Such effort will be rewarded, too. In one experiment, 77 percent of hot reactors were able to cool down—lower their blood pressure and cholesterol levels—by training themselves to stay calm.

Source: Reprinted by permission of Time Inc. Health from "How Stressed Are You?" *Health,* October 1994, 47. Researched by Lora Elise Ma. © 1994.

Chronic Stressors for College Students

Here are several chronic stressors that college students often experience. Each has the potential to cause serious health problems, particularly if experienced on a fairly regular basis (e.g., at least two or three times per week for the past month).

1. Roommate conflict
2. Homesickness
3. Friend conflict
4. Writing major papers
5. Dieting
6. Money/financial problems
7. Long-distance relationship
8. Juggling school and job
9. Time management difficulties
10. Noisy dorm or apartment
11. No car or car not working
12. Being underweight
13. Uncertainty over whether one has chosen the right major
14. Missing distant friends
15. Family illness
16. Loneliness
17. Job pressures
18. Lack of privacy
19. Friends with problems
20. Parental problems/family problems
21. Not enough sex/intimacy
22. Being behind in schoolwork
23. Problem with lover
24. Not enough exercise
25. Conflict with parents
26. Worries about academic performance
27. Being overweight
28. Feeling that one doesn't fit in; no friends
29. Difficult living/housing situations
30. Tuition bills/book costs
31. Health problems/not feeling well
32. Difficult class or instructor
33. Uncertainty regarding job future
34. Not enough sleep
35. Problem with drugs/alcohol

Source: Adapted from L. Towbes and L. Cohen, "Chronic Stress in the Lives of College Students: Scale Development and Prospective Predictions of Distress." *Journal of Youth and Adolescence* 25, no. 2 (1996): 202–203. By permission of Plenum Publishing Corporation.

others have of ourselves, and the social conditions we live in force us to readjust continually. Sources of psychosocial stress include change, hassles, pressure, inconsistent goals and behaviors, conflict, overload, and burnout.

Change Anytime change occurs in your normal daily routine, whether good or bad, you will experience stress. The more changes you experience and the more adjustments you must make, the greater the stress effects may be. In 1967, Drs. Thomas Holmes and Richard Rahe analyzed the social readjustments experienced by over 5,000 patients, noting which events seemed to occur just prior to disease onset.[16] They determined that certain events (both positive and negative) were predictive of increased risk for illness. They called their scale for predicting stress overload and the likelihood of illness the Social Readjustment Rating Scale (SRRS).[17] The SRRS has since served as the model for scales for certain groups, including college-aged students, as shown in the accompanying box, Chronic Stressors for College Students. Although many other factors must be considered, in general, the more of these stressors you experience, the more you need to change your behaviors or situation before problems occur.

What do you think?

*Think about the changes that you have made during the past couple of years. Which of these changes would you regard as positive? * Which as negative? * How did you react to these changes initially? * Did your reactions change later? * What are the biggest and most important changes that students must make as they enter colleges and universities? * What things help them prepare for and cope with unexpected changes?*

Hassles While Holmes and Rahe have focused on major stressors, psychologists such as Richard Lazarus have focused on petty annoyances and frustrations, collectively referred to as hassles.[18] Minor hassles—losing your keys, slipping and falling in front of everyone as you walk to your seat in a new class, finding that you went through a whole afternoon with a big chunk of spinach stuck in your front teeth—seem unimportant, but their cumulative effects may be harmful in the long run.

Pressure Pressure occurs when we feel forced to speed up, intensify, or shift the direction of our behavior to meet a higher standard of performance.[19] Pressures can be based on our personal goals and expectations, concern about what others think, or on outside influences. Among the most significant outside influences are society's demands that we compete and be all that we can be. The forces that push us to compete for the best grades, nicest cars, most attractive significant others, and highest-paying jobs create significant pressure to be the personification of American success.

Inconsistency between Goals and Behaviors For many of us, the negative effects of stress are magnified when there is a disparity between our goals (what we value or hope to obtain in life) and our behaviors (actions that may or may not lead to these goals). For instance, you may want good grades, and your family may expect them. But if you party and procrastinate throughout the term, your behaviors are inconsistent with your goals, and significant stress in the form of guilt, last-minute frenzy before exams, and disappointing grades may result. By contrast, if you dig in and work and remain committed to getting good grades, this may eliminate much of your negative stress. Thwarted goals can lead to frustration, and frustration has been shown to be a significant disrupter of homeostasis.

Determining whether behaviors are consistent with goals is an essential component of maintaining balance in life.

Conflict   Conflict occurs when we are forced to make difficult decisions concerning two or more competing motives, behaviors, or impulses or when we are forced to face incompatible demands, opportunities, needs, or goals.[20] What if your best friends all choose to smoke marijuana and you don't want to smoke but fear rejection? Conflict often occurs as our values are tested. College students who are away from home for the first time often face conflict between parental values and their own set of developing beliefs.

Overload   Overload, a state of being overburdened, results from excessive time pressure, too much responsibility, high expectations of yourself and those around you, and lack of support. Have you ever felt you had so many responsibilities that you couldn't possibly begin to fulfill them all? Have you longed for a weekend when you could just take time out with friends and not feel guilty? These feelings are symptoms of overload. Students suffering from overload may experience anxiety about tests, poor self-concept, a desire to drop classes or drop out of school, and other problems. In severe cases where they are unable to see any solutions to their problems, students may suffer from depression or turn to substance abuse.

Burnout   People who regularly suffer from overload, frustration, and disappointment may eventually experience burnout, a state of physical and mental exhaustion caused by excessive stress. People involved in the "helping professions," such as teaching, social work, drug counseling, nursing, and psychology, experience high levels of burnout, as do people who work in high-pressure, dangerous jobs, such as police officers and air-traffic controllers.

Other Forms of Psychosocial Stress   Other forms of psychosocial stress include problems with overcrowding, discrimination, and socioeconomic difficulties, such as unemployment and poverty. People of different ages or ethnic backgrounds may face disproportionately heavy impact from these sources of stress.

> **What do you think?**
> *What are your greatest sources of stress right now? ☀ On a scale of 1–10, with 10 being the highest level of stress, how stressed are you? ☀ Have you noticed any symptoms of stress? ☀ Can you eliminate or reduce your stress? ☀ How?*

Environmental Stress

Environmental stress results from events occurring in the physical environment. Environmental stressors include natural disasters, such as floods and hurricanes, and human-made disasters, such as chemical spills and explosions. As with other stressors, our bodies respond to environmental stressors with the general adaptation syndrome. Often as damaging as one-time disasters are **background distressors,** such as noise, air, and water pollution, although we may be unaware of them and their effects may not become apparent for decades. People who cannot escape background distressors may exist in a constant resistance phase, which can contribute to the development of stress-related disorders.

Self-Imposed Stress

Self-Concept and Stress   The **cognitive stress system** is the psychological system that governs our responses to stressors.[21] The cognitive stress system helps us recognize stressors; evaluate them on the basis of self-concept, past experiences, and emotions; and make decisions regarding how to cope with them.

Sensory organs serve as input channels for information reaching the brain. From that point on, attention to the problem, memory, reasoning processes, and problem solving are organized in various parts of the brain. This occurs before we act on the stressor. Because learning and memory involve the changing of various proteins in brain neurons, the emotions experienced during the stress response also "tickle" the memory storage neurons and contribute to responses. Behaviorally, we will respond to the stressor in ways consistent with our memories of similar situations.

Self-esteem is closely related to the emotions engendered by past experiences. Low self-esteem can lead to helpless anger. People suffering helpless anger have usually learned that they are wrong to feel anger, so instead of expressing it in healthy ways they turn it inward. They may "swallow" their rage in food, alcohol, or other drugs, or they may act in other self-destructive ways. One national priority of the former Secretary of Health and Human Services of the United States, Donna Shalala, is a program called "Girl Power," designed to improve the self-esteem of young women between the ages of 9 and 14, a time when low self-esteem is thought to trigger a host of negative health behaviors.

Research indicates that self-esteem significantly affects various disease processes. People with low self-esteem create a self-imposed stressor that can depress the immune system

---

Overload   A condition in which a person feels overly pressured by demands.

Burnout   Physical and mental exhaustion caused by excessive stress.

Background distressors   Environmental stressors of which people are often unaware.

Cognitive stress system   The psychological system that governs emotional responses to stress.

and increase the symptoms of diseases such as acquired immune deficiency syndrome (AIDS), herpes, multiple sclerosis, and Epstein-Barr syndrome.

Personality Types and Hardiness   A person's personality may contribute to the kind and degree of self-imposed stress he or she experiences. The coronary disease–prone personality was first described in 1974 by physicians Meyer Friedman and Ray Rosenman.[22] They identified two stress-related personality types: Type A and Type B. Type A personalities are hard-driving, competitive, anxious, time-driven, impatient, quick-tempered, and perfectionistic. Type B personalities are relaxed and noncompetitive. According to Rosenman and Friedman, people with Type A characteristics are more prone to heart attacks than their Type B counterparts.

Researchers today believe that more needs to be discovered about personality types before we can say that all Type A individuals have greater risks for heart disease. For one reason, most people are not one personality type all the time. For another reason, many other unexplained variables must be explored, such as why some Type A people seem to thrive in stress-filled environments. Now labeled Type C personalities, these individuals appear to succeed more often than Type B personalities and enjoy good overall health even while displaying Type A patterns of behavior.

Critics argue that these attempts to base ill health on personal behavioral patterns are crude. For example, researchers at Duke University contend that the Type A personality may be more complex than previously described. They have identified a "toxic core" in some Type A personalities. People who have this toxic core are angry, distrustful of others, and have above-average levels of cynicism. People who are angry and hostile often have below-average levels of social support and other increased risks for ill health. It may be this toxic core rather than the hard-driving nature of the Type A personality that makes people more vulnerable to self-imposed stress.[23]

According to psychologist Susanne Kobasa, **psychological hardiness** may negate self-imposed stress associated with Type A behavior. Psychologically hardy people are characterized by *control, commitment,* and *challenge.*[24] People with a sense of control are able to accept responsibility for their behaviors and change behaviors that they discover to be debilitating. People with a sense of commitment have good self-esteem and understand their purpose in life. People with a sense of challenge see changes in life as stimulating opportunities for personal growth.

Because some Type A behavior is "learned," it can be modified. Some Type A people are able to slow down and become more tolerant, patient, and better humored. Unfortunately, many people do not decide to modify their Type A

Psychological hardiness   A personality trait characterized by control, commitment, and challenge.

---

habits until after they become ill or suffer a heart attack. To prevent heart and circulatory disorders resulting from stress, the person needs to recognize and change dangerous behaviors before damage is done.

Self-Efficacy and Control   Whether people cope successfully with stressful situations often depends on their level of self-efficacy, or their belief in their skills and performance abilities.[25] If people have been successful in mastering similar problems in the past, they will be more likely to believe in their own effectiveness. Similarly, people who have repeatedly tried and failed may lack confidence in their abilities to deal with life's problems. In some cases, this insecurity may prevent them from trying to cope.

In addition, people who believe they lack control in a situation may become easily frustrated and give up. Those who feel they have no personal control tend to have an *external locus of control* and a low level of self-efficacy. People who are confident their behavior will influence the outcome tend to have an *internal locus of control*. Individuals who feel that they have limited control over their lives often have higher levels of stress.

Stress and the College Student

College students experience numerous stressors, including changes related to being away from home for the first time, pressure to make friends in a new and sometimes intimidating setting, the feeling of anonymity imposed by large classes, and test-taking anxiety.

College students may be especially vulnerable because they are in a period of transition, facing several key developmental tasks: (1) achieving emotional independence from family; (2) choosing and preparing for a career; (3) preparing for a relationship, commitment, and/or family life; and (4) developing an ethical system. These tasks require that the college student develop new social roles and modify old ones. Such changes can result in role strain, a major aspect of chronic stress.

In a large study of chronic stressors, male and female college students differed significantly in the things they perceived to be significant stressors.[26] Women indicated that among their most frequent stressors were (1) trying to diet, (2) being overweight, (3) having an overload of school work, and (4) gaining weight. Men, in contrast, tended to list the following items as major stressors: (1) being underweight, (2) problems relating to commuting to school, (3) not having someone to date, (4) not enough sex, (5) being behind in schoolwork, (6) not having enough friends, and (7) concerns about drug or alcohol use.[27]

Most colleges offer stress management workshops through health centers or student counseling departments. You should not ignore the symptoms of stress overload. If you experience one or more of the stressors listed in the box on page 60, act promptly to reduce their impact.

College can be a stressfull time for students, whether they are young people choosing a career path or older adults returning to school to change directions later in life.

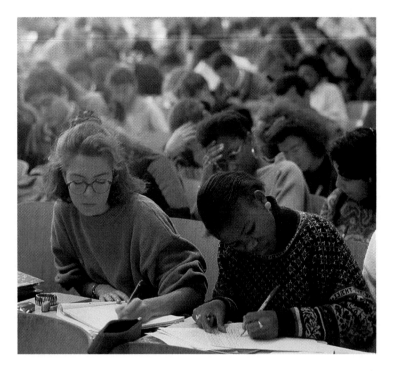

Stress Management

Stress can be challenging or debilitating, depending upon how you view it. In addition to creating stressful situations, college gives you the opportunity to evaluate and change how you manage stress. The most effective way to avoid problems is to learn a number of skills known collectively as *stress management*.

Building Skills to Reduce Stress

Dealing with stress involves assessing all aspects of a stressor, examining your response and how you can change it, and learning to cope with the stressor. Often we cannot change the requirements at our college, assignments in class, or unexpected stressors. Inevitably, we will be stuck in classes that bore us and for which we find no application in real life. We feel powerless when a loved one has died. Although the facts cannot be changed, our reactions to these distressors can be changed.

Assessing Your Stressors   After recognizing a stressor, evaluate it. Can you alter the circumstances to reduce the amount of distress you are experiencing, or must you change your behavior and reactions to reduce stress levels? For example, if five term papers for five different courses are due during the semester, your professors are unlikely to drop such requirements. You can, however, change your behavior by beginning the papers early and spacing them over time to avoid last-minute stress.

Changing Your Responses   Changing your responses requires practice and emotional control. If your roommate is habitually messy and this causes you stress, you can choose among several responses. You can express your anger by yelling; you can pick up the mess and leave a nasty note; or you can defuse the situation with humor. The first reaction that comes to mind is not always the best. Before you react, stop. Take the time you need to find an appropriate response. Ask yourself, "What is to be gained from my response?"

Many people change their responses to potentially stressful events through *cognitive coping strategies*. These strategies help them prepare for stressors through gradual exposure to increasingly higher stress levels.

Learning to Cope   Everyone copes with stress in different ways. Some people drink or take drugs; others seek help from counselors; and still others try to forget about it or engage in positive activities, such as exercise. **Stress inoculation**, one of the newer techniques, helps people prepare for stressful events ahead of time. For example, suppose you are petrified over speaking in front of a class. Practicing in front of friends or in front of a video camera are strategies that may inoculate and prevent your freezing up on the day of the

Stress inoculation   Newer stress management technique in which a person consciously tries to prepare ahead of time for potential stressors.

Taming Technostress

Cell phones that constantly ring; VCRs that you can't program; e-mail lists that grow on your desktop like an out-of-control fungus; laptop computers that somehow end up in your bags when you go on vacation; electronic organizers that beep during dinner or at the movies; voice message systems that don't allow you to talk to a live person; busy signals as you try to get on the Internet; and slow, slow, slow downloading of information. Can you almost feel your heart rate speeding up just thinking about these situations?

Millions of people today may be victims of a stressor unknown to previous generations. Known as *technostress,* this problem is defined as "personal stress generated by reliance on technological devices, . . . a panicky feeling when they fail, and a state of near-constant stimulation, or being perpetually 'plugged in.'" Technostress may interact with other sources of tension to create a synergistic, never-ending form of stimulation that keeps your stress response reverberating all day.

Part of the problem, ironically, is that technology enables us to be so productive. Because it encourages polyphasic activity, or "multi-tasking," people are forced to juggle multiple thoughts and actions at the same time, such as driving and talking on cell phones or checking hand-held devices for appointments. There is clear evidence that such multiple activity events contribute to auto accidents and other harmful consequences. What is less clear is what happens to someone who never takes downtime and is always plugged in.

What are the symptoms of technology overload? Although increased heart rate and blood pressure and other fight-or-flight symptoms are common responses to stress, so, too, are the inability to concentrate, irritability, and memory disturbances. Over time, many people with technostress may lose the ability to relax and find they feel nervous and anxious when they are supposed to be having fun. Headaches, stomach and digestive problems, skin irritations, more colds than usual, difficulty in wound healing, lack of sleep, ulcers, and a host of other problems may result.

TIPS FOR FIGHTING TECHNOSTRESS

- *Exercise.* Get away from any form of technology. Quiet walks or runs away from the blare of music and the sound of machines (typical in fitness centers) are best. Try to find a place that has few people and little noise—that usually means outdoors.
- *Become aware of what you are doing.* Log the time you spend on e-mail, voicemail, and so on. Set up a schedule to limit your use of technology. For example, limit all e-mail responses to two to three lines. Answer e-mails for no more than a half hour per day. Set up strict rules for when you log on, and make sure you don't log in other times. Prioritize your responses, and delete unnecessary intrusions into your life.
- *Give yourself more time for everything you do.* If you are surfing the web for resources for a term paper, start early rather than the night before the paper is due.
- *Set "time out" periods.* During these times, don't answer the phone, listen to the stereo, turn on the computer, or turn on the TV.
- *Take regular breaks.* Even when working, get up, walk around, stretch, do deep breathing, or get a glass of water, every hour or so. Look away from the screen and focus on something else.
- *Resist the urge to buy the newest and fastest technology.* Such purchases not only cause financial stress but also add to stress levels during setups.
- *Do not take laptops, hand-held devices, or other technological gadgets on vacation.* If you must take a cell phone for emergencies, use it only in true emergencies. Stay off the phone when driving.
- *Back up materials on your computer at regular intervals.* Writing a term paper only to lose it during a power outage can send you into hyperstress very quickly.

Source: From L. Rosen and M. Weil, *TechnoStress: Coping with Technology@ Work@Home@Play* (New York: Wiley, 1997).

---

presentation. Some health experts compare stress inoculation to a vaccine given to protect against a disease. Regardless of how you cope with a situation, your conscious effort to deal with it is an important step in stress management.

Downshifting   More and more people recognize that today's lifestyle is hectic and pressure-packed, and much of their stress comes from trying to keep up. Many also question whether "having it all" is worth it. In recent years, a number of top executives have said "enough" and have voluntarily left high-paying jobs to lead a simpler life. Although you may argue that it is easy to lead a simple life with a large bank account, the truth is that people of all walks of life are taking a step back and simplifying their lives. They are following a trend known as **downshifting.** Moving from a large urban area to the country or to small towns, buying a smaller house, exchanging the expensive SUV for a run-of-the-mill four-door sedan, and a host of other changes in lifestyle typify this move. Some dedicated downshifters have given up television, microwaves, phones, and even computers.

Downshifting   Conscious attempt to simplify life in an effort to reduce the stresses and strains of modern living.

Post Traumatic Stress: The Aftermath of Terror

For many of us, the vivid images of the planes hitting the Twin Towers of the World Trade Center on September 11, 2001, will be etched in our memory for the rest of our lives. Anger, horror, frustration, and a host of other emotions surrounding the terrorist attacks bring tears, stomach upset, and other bodily ills to those of us who sat helplessly watching the events surrounding the attack. As horrible as the events were for those who sat watching, the real trauma for those who lost loved ones, co-workers, and friends in the attack may have only begun. *Post traumatic stress disorder (PTSD)* is an acute stress disorder with extreme anxiety and behavioral disturbances that develops within the first hours or days after a traumatic event. Typically, persons suffering from PTSD have been soldiers returning from the atrocities of war, particularly those who saw friends and people they loved killed or mangled or who experienced terrible suffering and pain themselves. Many of these soldiers have continued to suffer from these experiences for decades after the events.

Other extreme traumatic events that can provoke PTSD have included rape or other severe physical assault, near-death experiences in accidents, witnessing a murder or death, street crime, being caught in a natural disaster, or being a victim of random terrorist attacks, such as the Oklahoma City bombing in the mid 1990s. Typically, symptoms of PTSD include the following:

- *Dissociation,* or perceived detachment of the mind from the emotional state or even the body. In dissociation, the person may have a sense of the world as a dreamlike or unreal place and have poor memory of the events, a form of *dissociative amnesia.*
- *Acute anxiety* or nervousness, in which the person is hyperaroused, may cry easily or experience mood swings, or may have flashbacks, nightmares, or recurrent thoughts or visual images. The person may feel as though the event were happening again and again and feel a vague uneasiness. Some people may experience intense physiological reactions, such as shaking or nausea, when something reminds them of the events. In some cases, a person may have difficulty returning to the area where the trauma occurred. For example, persons experiencing PTSD related to the Pentagon and World Trade Center attacks may be unable to work in tall buildings, have difficulty getting on a plane or traveling by air, or have acute fear when they hear planes flying overhead.
- *Persistent stress symptoms.* Sufferers may have two or more of these symptoms:

  ⇒ Difficulty falling or staying asleep
  ⇒ Irritability or outbursts of anger or other emotions
  ⇒ Difficulty concentrating
  ⇒ Hypervigilance
  ⇒ Exaggerated startle response

If these symptoms last more than one month, a post traumatic stress disorder may be diagnosed, either as an *acute form* (less than three months' duration) or a *chronic form* (duration longer than three months). In some cases, PTSD may appear months after the attack and be labeled as a *delayed onset* form of the ailment. Symptoms disappear within six months in the majority of people.[*]

Although exact figures for this illness may never be known, The National Institutes of Health indicate that as many as 5–8 percent of the American public may have chronic forms of post traumatic stress. It is almost twice as prevalent among women than among men. Victims of rape and survivors of torture and concentration camps have historically been among those most likely to have problems.[†]

Therapies designed to help trauma victims recover from victimization have become increasingly effective as our knowledge about this disorder has increased. Schools, communities, and workplaces now routinely bring in crisis experts immediately after an event to help survivors talk through their feelings and gain support from others during times of need. Having a supportive family, employer, and friends as well as access to professional counseling services is an important part of the recovery process. New generations of antianxiety drugs have also been developed to help individuals who have difficulties. Sleep aids and other options for symptom relief are also available to ease short-term symptoms.

[*] From Posttraumatic Stress Disorder Society, http://www.mentalhealth.com/dis1/p21-an06.html, September 1, 2001.
[†] From *Mental Health: A Report to the Surgeon General,* http://www.surgeongeneral.gov/library/mentalhealth/chapter4/sec2.html.

This trend toward simplicity was promoted by Henry David Thoreau in the nineteenth century, but for years it has been seen as an eccentric battle against machines or part of a back-to-nature movement. In recent years, however, the idea has become more mainstream. In one study, nearly 32 percent of those surveyed indicated that they would give up their current lifestyles for a return to simpler times.[28] According to researchers at Trends Institute, as many as 25 percent of all Americans will scale back their lives to some degree in the next 10 years. In fact, consultants who once coached clients on getting ahead now run programs that teach them how to be satisfied with less.

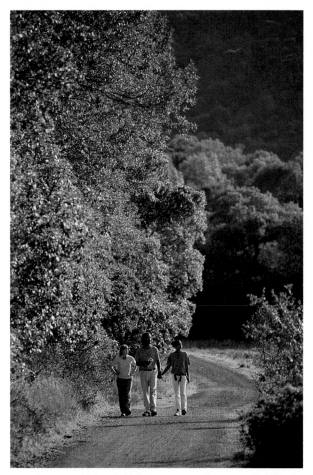

Finding time to take a walk in nature is an excellent stress reducer.

Self-help books, newsletters, and networking groups all pitch the simpler life.

Downshifting involves a fundamental alteration in values and honest introspection about what is important in life. When you consider any form of downshift or perhaps even start your career this way, it's important to move slowly and consider the following:

- *Determine your ultimate goal.* What is most important to you, and what will you need to reach that goal? What can you do without? Where do you want to live?
- *Make a short-term and long-term plan for simplifying your life.* Set up your plan in doable steps, and work slowly toward each step. Begin saying no to requests for your time, and determine which people you feel it is important to spend time with.
- *Complete a financial inventory.* How much money will you need to do the things you want to do? Will you rent or buy a home? What kind of car could you get by with? Pay off credit cards and eliminate existing debt, or consider debt consolidation. Get used to paying with cash. If you don't have the cash, don't buy.
- *Plan for health care costs.* Make sure that you budget for health insurance and basic preventive health services. This should be a top priority.

- *Select the right career.* Look for work that you enjoy and that isn't necessarily driven by salary. Can you be happy taking a lower-paying job that is less stressful and allows you the opportunity to have a life?
- *Consider options for saving money.* Downshifting doesn't mean you renounce money; it means you choose not to let money dictate your life. It's still important to save. If you're just getting started, you need to prepare for emergencies and for future plans. Avoid compulsive buying, and consider living with others to share the costs.
- *Clear out/clean out.* A cluttered life can be distressing. Take an inventory of material items, and get rid of things you haven't worn or used in the last year. Donate items to charity groups. Clean as you go, and get rid of the frills.

Managing Emotional Responses

Have you ever gotten all worked up about something only to find that your perceptions were totally wrong? We often get upset, not by realities, but by our faulty perceptions. For example, suppose you found out that everyone except you is invited to a party. You might easily begin to wonder why you were excluded. Does someone dislike you? Have you offended someone? Such thoughts are typical. However, the reality of the situation may have absolutely nothing to do with your being liked or disliked. Perhaps you were sent an invitation and it didn't get to you.

Stress management requires that you examine your *self-talk* and your emotional responses to interactions with others. With any emotional response to a stressor, you are responsible for the emotion and the behaviors elicited by the emotion. Learning to tell the difference between normal emotions and those based on irrational beliefs can help you either stop the emotion or express it in a healthy and appropriate way.

Fighting the Anger Urge Although much has been said about how hotheaded, short-fused people are at risk for health problems, recent research provides even more compelling reasons for "chilling out." A study of nearly 13,000 people found that anger, even in the absence of high blood pressure, can increase a person's risk of heart attack by more than 2.5 times. Stress hormones released during anger may constrict blood vessels in the heart or actually promote clot formation, which can cause a heart attack.

Anger results when our wants, desires, and dreams differ from what we actually "get" in life. People who spend all their emotional energy in a quest for justice or grow frustrated over events that seem impossible to change can become driven by anger. Because anger triggers the fight-or-flight reaction, these people operate with the stress response turned on long after it should have dissipated.

Angry individuals typically display cynicism, a brooding, hypercritical view of their world. Like angry people, cynical individuals keep fight-or-flight reactions reverberating through their bodies indefinitely. Often labeled as "hostile," these chronically stressed folks frequently have weakened

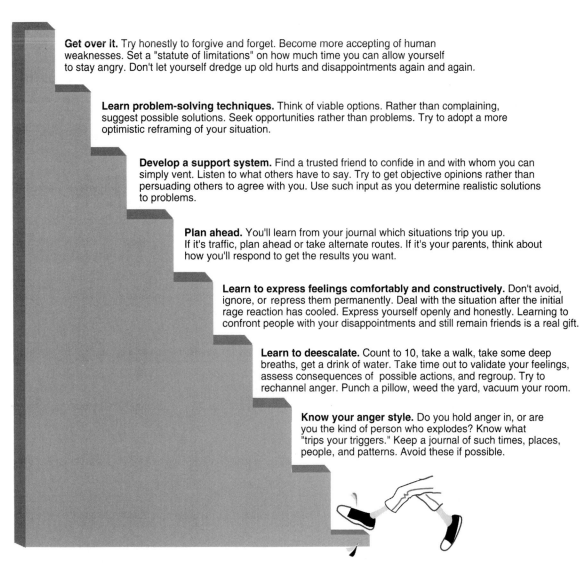

Get over it. Try honestly to forgive and forget. Become more accepting of human weaknesses. Set a "statute of limitations" on how much time you can allow yourself to stay angry. Don't let yourself dredge up old hurts and disappointments again and again.

Learn problem-solving techniques. Think of viable options. Rather than complaining, suggest possible solutions. Seek opportunities rather than problems. Try to adopt a more optimistic reframing of your situation.

Develop a support system. Find a trusted friend to confide in and with whom you can simply vent. Listen to what others have to say. Try to get objective opinions rather than persuading others to agree with you. Use such input as you determine realistic solutions to problems.

Plan ahead. You'll learn from your journal which situations trip you up. If it's traffic, plan ahead or take alternate routes. If it's your parents, think about how you'll respond to get the results you want.

Learn to express feelings comfortably and constructively. Don't avoid, ignore, or repress them permanently. Deal with the situation after the initial rage reaction has cooled. Express yourself openly and honestly. Learning to confront people with your disappointments and still remain friends is a real gift.

Learn to deescalate. Count to 10, take a walk, take some deep breaths, get a drink of water. Take time out to validate your feelings, assess consequences of possible actions, and regroup. Try to rechannel anger. Punch a pillow, weed the yard, vacuum your room.

Know your anger style. Do you hold anger in, or are you the kind of person who explodes? Know what "trips your triggers." Keep a journal of such times, places, people, and patterns. Avoid these if possible.

Figure 3.3 Steps in Anger Control
Source: Adapted from Brian L. Seaward. 1999. Managing Stress, Jones and Bartlett. p. 97–99.

immune responses and increased risk of disease. Counseling designed to determine the underlying cause of anger and deal with related issues can be effective. See Figure 3.3 for strategies to control and redirect anger.

What do you think?

Do you know people who display the angry and cynical personality traits discussed here? ☀ *How do others react to them?* ☀ *How do you feel when you are around them?* ☀ *Do you regard yourself as a "glass half empty" or a "glass half full"?* ☀ *What factors have been most important in molding your own anger/hostility profile?* ☀ *What actions would you recommend for someone trying to be more positive, less hostile, and less critical of others?*

Taking Mental Action

Stress management calls for mental action in two areas. First, positive self-esteem, which can help you cope with stressful situations, comes from learned habits. Successful stress management involves mentally developing and practicing self-esteem skills.

Second, because you can't always anticipate what the next stressor will be, you need to develop the mental skills necessary to manage your reactions to stresses after the stresses have occurred. The ability to think about and react quickly to stress comes with time, practice, experience with a variety of stressful situations, and patience.

Changing the Way You Think Once you realize that some of your thoughts may be irrational or overreactive, make a conscious effort to adjust your thinking. Reframe or change the way you've been thinking and focus on more positive patterns. Here are some specific actions you can take to develop these mental skills:

- *Worry constructively.* Don't waste time and energy worrying about things you can't change or events that may never happen.
- *Look at life as being fluid.* If you accept that change is a natural part of living and growing, the jolt of changes may become less stressful.
- *Consider alternatives.* Remember that there is seldom only one appropriate action. Anticipating options will help you plan for change and adjust more rapidly.
- *Moderate your expectations.* Aim high, but be realistic about your circumstances and motivation.
- *Weed out trivia.* Age-old advice offered by cardiologist Robert Eliot provided two rules for coping with life's challenges that continue to resonate today: (1) "Don't sweat the small stuff," and (2) Remember that "it's all small stuff."[29]
- *Don't rush into action.* Think before you act.

Taking Physical Action

Physical activities can complement the emotional and mental strategies of stress management.

Exercise Exercise reduces stress by raising levels of endorphins—mood-elevating, pain-killing hormones—in the bloodstream. As a result, exercise increases energy, reduces hostility, and improves mental alertness.

Most of us have relieved stress by engaging in aggressive physical activity: chopping wood when we are angry is one example. Exercise performed as an immediate response can help alleviate stress symptoms. However, a regular exercise program yields even more substantial benefits. Try to engage in at least 25 minutes of aerobic exercise three or four times a week. But even simply walking up stairs, parking farther away from your destination, or standing rather than sitting helps to conserve and replenish your adaptive energy stores. Although it may not improve your aerobic capacity, a quiet walk alone or with friends can refresh your mind and calm your stress response. Plan walking breaks with friends. Stretch after prolonged periods of study at your desk. A short period of physical exercise may provide the break you really need. For more information on the beneficial effects of exercise, see Chapter 11.

Relaxation Like exercise, relaxation can help you cope with stressful feelings, preserve adaptation energy stores, dissipate excess hormones associated with GAS, and refocus your energies. Practice relaxation daily until it becomes a habit. You will probably find that you enjoy it.

Once you have learned simple relaxation techniques, you can use them at any time—during a tough exam or stressful confrontation, for example. If you're facing a tough exam, you may choose to relax before it or at intervals during it. You can also use relaxation techniques when you face stressful confrontations or assignments. As your body relaxes, your heart rate slows, your blood pressure and metabolic rate decrease, and many other body-calming effects occur, allowing you to channel energy appropriately.

Eating Right Is food really a de-stressor? Whether foods can calm us and nourish our psyches is a controversial question. Much of what has been published about hyperactivity and its relation to the consumption of candy and other sweets has been shown to be scientifically invalid. High-potency vitamin and mineral supplements, which are touted as boosting resistance against stress-related ailments, are nothing more than gimmicks. But it is clear that eating a balanced, healthful diet will help provide the stamina you need to get through problems and will stress-proof you in ways that are not fully understood. It is also known that undereating, overeating, and eating the wrong kinds of foods can create distress in the body. For more information about the benefits of sound nutrition, see Chapter 9.

Managing Time

Time. Everybody needs more of it, especially students trying to balance the demands of classes, social life, earning money for school, and family obligations. Include the following time management tips in your stress management program:

- *Take on only one thing at a time.* Don't try to pay bills, clean the bathroom, wash clothes, and write your term paper all at once. Stay focused.
- *Clean off your desk.* According to Jeffrey Mayer, author of *Winning the Fight Between You and Your Desk,* most of us spend many stressful minutes each day looking for things that are lost on our desks or in our homes. Go through the things on your desk, toss the unnecessary papers, and put into folders the papers for tasks that you must do.
- *Find a clean, comfortable place to work.* Go somewhere where you won't be distracted.
- *Never handle papers more than once.* When bills and other papers come in, take care of them immediately. Write a check, and hold it for mailing. Get rid of the envelopes. Read your mail, and file it or toss it. If you haven't looked at something in over a year, toss it.
- *Prioritize your tasks.* Make a daily "to do" list, and try to stick to it. Categorize the things you must do today, the things that you have to do but not immediately, and the things that it would be nice to do. Prioritize the "must do now" and "have to do later" items, and put deadlines next to each. Only consider the "nice to do" items if you finish the others or if the "nice to do" list includes something fun for you. Give yourself a reward as you finish each task.
- *Don't be afraid to say no.* All too often we do things out of fear of what someone may think. Set your school and personal priorities. Please yourself as often as you can.
- *Avoid interruptions.* When you've got a project that requires your total concentration, schedule uninterrupted

time. Unplug the phone, or let your answering machine get it. Close your door, and post a *Do Not Disturb* sign. Go to a quiet room in the library or student union where no one will find you.

- *Reward yourself for being efficient.* Whenever you finish a task earlier than you had planned, take some time for yourself. Have a cup of coffee or hot chocolate. Go for a walk. Start reading something you've wanted to read but haven't had time for. Differentiate between rest breaks and work breaks. Work breaks simply mean switching tasks for awhile. Rest breaks give you time to yourself. Make sure that your rest breaks help you recharge and re-fresh your energy levels.

- *Become aware of your own time patterns.* Keep a time journal for one week. For many of us, minutes and hours drift by without our even noticing them. Chart your daily schedule, hour by hour, for one week. Note the time that was wasted and the time spent in productive work or restorative pleasure. Assess how you could be more pro-ductive and make more time for yourself.

- *Use time to your advantage.* If you're a morning person, schedule activities to coincide with the time when you're at your best. Study and write papers in the morning, and take breaks when you start to slow down. Take a short nap when you need it.

- *Break overwhelming tasks into small pieces, and allocate a certain amount of time to each.* If you are floundering in a task, move on and come back to it when you're refreshed.

- *Remember that time is precious.* Many people learn to value their time only when they face a terminal illness. Try to value each day. Time spent not enjoying life is a tremendous waste of potential.

Alternative Stress Management Techniques

Popular "stress fighters" include hypnosis, massage thera-pies, meditation, and biofeedback.

Hypnosis   Hypnosis is a process that requires a person to focus on one thought, object, or voice, thereby freeing the right hemisphere of the brain to become more active. The person then becomes unusually responsive to suggestions. Whether self-induced or induced by someone else, hypnosis can reduce certain types of stress.

Massage Therapy   If you have ever had someone massage your stiff neck or aching feet, you know that massage is an excellent way to relax. Massage techniques vary from vigor-ous Swedish massage to the gentler acupressure and Esalen massage. Before selecting a massage therapist, check his or her credentials carefully. The therapist should have training from a reputable program that teaches scientific principles for anatomic manipulation and be certified through the American Massage Therapy Association (AMTA).

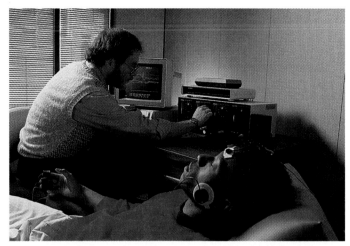

Biofeedback is an excellent way to train your body to cope with stressors.

Meditation   Meditation generally focuses on deep breath-ing, allowing tension to leave the body with each exhalation. It allows you to get away, to wipe all thoughts out of your mind, and turn inward. Practiced by Eastern religions for centuries, meditation is believed to be an important form of personal renewal and introspection. As a stress management tool, it can calm the body and quiet the mind, creating a sense of peace. There are several common forms of medita-tion. Most involve sitting quietly for 15 to 20 minutes, focus-ing on a particular word or symbol, controlling breathing, and getting in touch with the inner self.

Biofeedback   Biofeedback involves self-monitoring by ma-chine of physical responses to stress and attempts to control these responses. The machine records perspiration, heart rate, respiration, blood pressure, surface body temperature, muscle tension, and other stress responses. Then, by trial and error, the person using biofeedback techniques learns to lower his or her stress responses through conscious effort. Eventually, the person develops the ability to lower his or her stress responses at will, without using the machines.

Making the Most of Support Groups

Support groups are an important part of stress manage-ment. Friends, family members, and coworkers can provide emotional and physical support. Although the ideal support

Hypnosis   A process that allows people to become unusually responsive to suggestion.

Meditation   A relaxation technique that involves deep breathing and concentration.

Biofeedback   A technique involving machine self-monitoring of physical responses to stress.

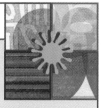

Social Connections and Social Support as a Stress Buffer

Although a number of "buffers" may inoculate individuals from the negative health effects of stress, social support may play a more important role than all others. Consider the following points, derived from several studies assessing the role of social support and social connections in dealing with stress.

✓ Being well integrated socially reduces all age-adjusted mortality by a factor of 2, about as much as having low versus high serum cholesterol levels, or being a nonsmoker versus a smoker. Furthermore, the nature of one's position in the social hierarchy has health consequences, including relatively higher status within the same social class.

✓ People are statistically more likely to die right after, rather than before, their birthdays and important holidays. These events include social interactions.

✓ Randomized trials have provided evidence that psychosocial support is associated with longer survival for patients with breast cancer, malignant melanoma, and lymphoma.

✓ Studies looking at the relationship between widowhood (regarded as a high stressor) and depression have found repeatedly that the death of a spouse is more strongly associated with depression among men than women.

What could be the possible reasons for the final item on the list? Though some argue that men depend more on women for daily activities of living, studies have shown that widowed men tend to cut off or reduce ties with surviving parents and adult children after such an event, presumably as they begin to search for a new partner. Women, in contrast, maintain and, in fact, increase their social connections during this time, which may serve as a stress buffer.

Sources: From S. Levine, D. M. Lyons, and A. F. Schatzberg, "Psychobiological Consequences of Social Relationships," *The Annals of the New York Academy of Science* 89, no. 7(1999): 210–218; M. G. Marmot, R. Fuhrer, S. L. Ettner, N. F. Marks, L. L. Bumpass, and C. D. Ryff, "Contributions of Psychosocial Factors to Socioeconomic Difference in Health," *Milbank Quarterly* 76 (1998): 403–448; D. P. Phillips, T. E. Ruth, and L. M. Wagner, "Psychology and Survival," *Lancet* 342 (1993): 1142–1145; D. Ornish et al., "Intensive Lifestyle Changes for Reversal of Coronary Heart Disease," *Journal of the American Medical Association,* 280 (1998): 2001–2007; and D. Spiegel, "Healing Words: Emotional Expression and Disease Outcome," *Journal of the American Medical Association* (1999).

group differs for each of us, you should have one or two close friends in whom you are able to confide and neighbors with whom you can trade favors. Try to participate in community activities at least once a week. A healthy committed relationship can also provide vital support.

If you do not have a close support group, find out where to turn when the pressures of life seem overwhelming. Family members are often a steady base of support on which you can rely. But if friends or family are unavailable, most colleges and universities have counseling services available at no cost for short-term crises. Clergy, instructors, and dorm supervisors may also be excellent resources. If university services are unavailable or if you are concerned about confidentiality, most communities offer low-cost counseling through mental health clinics.

Developing Your Spiritual Side: Mindfulness

In discussions of spirituality, the concept of mindfulness often emerges. As a meditative technique, mindfulness—fully experiencing and accepting the present moment—can aid relaxation, reduce emotional or physical pain, and help individuals connect more effectively with others, with their inner selves, and with nature. Practicing mindfulness can include strategies and activities that contribute to overall health and wellness. In fact, mindfulness and wellness are interconnected and can be developed concurrently, reinforcing each other.

The Physical Dimension: Moving in Nature

Far too many of us go for a walk or start working out while stewing about relationships, jobs, classes, or finances, and we end up maintaining stress levels that exercise should eliminate. Although exercising in a gym or other workout facility increases physical fitness, the optimum way to nourish and strengthen the body and build endurance and peace of mind is to interact with the natural environment. Activities such as walking, jogging, biking, and swimming all foster this interaction, providing sensory experiences (feeling, smelling, touching, listening, and hearing) as well as exercises to strengthen muscles and the cardiovascular system. By focusing on the sounds of birdsong or the crunch of your shoes on freshly fallen snow, you can free yourself of worry or anxious thoughts. Appreciating and absorbing the beauty of nature allow us to unwind emotionally even as our bodies are at work.

The Emotional Dimension: Dealing with Negative Feelings

Each person has positive and negative emotions that govern moods and behaviors throughout the day. We often take joy, happiness, and contentment for granted because we tend not to notice the *absence* of stress and distress. However, we typically are aware of negative emotions, such as jealousy, hatred, and anger, because they tend to deplete our energy reserves and cause us problems in interacting with others. To improve our emotional health and access our spiritual side, we must take notice of the situations that trigger negative emotions, such as anger. (See Fighting the Anger Urge, page 66.) What provokes the anger? What is our physiological response to it? What body parts seem to hold most of the anger? Does the body become hard or soft, pliable or rigid? How is body temperature related to anger? Does the body perspire more, feel hot and constrained in clothing? Where does the mind focus when angry—on another person or object? On ourselves and our pain? What do we say to ourselves when we are angry?

By stopping in the midst of anger and concentrating on physical reactions, we may begin to realize the full extent of the damage we inflict on ourselves when we allow negativity to get the best of us. This realization might bring a person to conclude, "I don't like allowing this kind of hit on my body. I've got to get a handle on this before I hurt myself or someone else." We might ask ourselves, Is it worth it? By practicing thought-stopping, blocking negative thoughts, and focusing on positive emotions via self-talk and other methods of diversion, we may help ourselves through a potentially negative experience.

The Social Dimension: Interacting, Listening, and Communicating

Developing the spiritual side is not only an isolated, internal process. It is also a social process that can enhance relationships with others. The ability to give and take, speak and listen, forgive and move on are all integral to spiritual development.

Today, life is busier than ever. While we constantly juggle responsibilities, it is easy to get so caught up in the stresses of our own lives that we find it difficult to give to others. Here again, we need to stop and think about how being too self-enmeshed can affect relationships and the ability to communicate with others. Communication is a two-way process, in which listening is every bit as important as speaking. Learning to *listen actively* is a potent asset. Active listeners take note of content, intent, and feelings being expressed. They listen to all levels of the communication. Sensitivity and honesty are also essential to the give-and-take of communication. Asking specific questions, rephrasing the speaker's ideas, and focusing genuine attention on the speaker can enhance its effectiveness. Through such active participation, we gain a greater insight into the other person, who in turn will more likely be encouraged to share more in the flow of the conversation. Sharing becomes more intimate and relationships more connected when people feel that others care for them and are genuinely interested in their well-being. Both parties benefit from such an interchange.

The Intellectual Dimension: Sharpening Intuition

One often underdeveloped aspect of spiritual health is taking the time to carefully assess events in life, their causes, and one's own involvement in them. This often involves putting aside our feeling dimension for a moment in order to reflect, read, and gain insight. Sometimes this process leads to startling new insights—"Ah-ha! . . . Now I get it; this all makes sense!" Such moments mean so much, but few people include this mental activity in daily rituals. Examining the past, how we've gotten to where we are in the present, and what actions might have changed the course of events is a critical element of spiritual growth. Using our minds for objective reasoning will develop the intellectual dimension of spiritual health.

Managing Stress

Stress is not something that you can run from or wish into nonexistence. To control stress, you must meet it head on and use as many resources as you can to ensure that your coping skills are fine-tuned and ready to help you. In planning your personal strategy for successfully managing stress, following a few simple guidelines can help you enjoy more guilt-free time and become more productive.

✓ *Plan life, not time.* Evaluate all your activities, even the most trivial, to determine whether they contribute to your life. If they don't, eliminate them.

✓ *Decelerate.* When rushed, ask yourself if you really need to be. What's the worst that could happen if you slow down? Tell yourself at least once a day that failure seldom results from doing a job slowly or too well.

✓ *Learn to delegate and share.* Don't be afraid to ask others to help or to share the work load and responsibilities.

✓ *Learn to say no.* Decide what you can do, you must do, and you want to do, and delegate the rest to someone else either permanently or until you complete your priority tasks. Before you take on a new responsibility, finish or drop an old one.

✓ *Schedule time alone.* Find time each day for quiet thinking, reading, exercising, or other enjoyable activities.

Checklist For Change

Assessing Your Life Stressors

✓ Have you assessed the major stressors in your life? Are they people, events, or specific activities?

✓ Do you often worry about things that never happen? Are you often anxious about nothing?

✓ Have you thought about what you could change to reduce your stress levels?

✓ Do you have a network of friends and family members who can help you reduce your stress levels? Do you know where to get professional advice about reducing them?

✓ Have you thought about what changes you'd like to work on first? Have you developed a plan of action? When do you want to start?

Assessing Community Stressors

✓ Have you considered what in your environment may cause stress for you and the people around you?

✓ Could these stressors be changed? If so, how? Why would changing them make a difference?

✓ What on your campus or in your living situation causes undue stress for you or your friends? What could you do to change these stressors?

✓ What advice might you give to your school administrators to help them reduce unnecessary stress among students?

Summary

❋ Stress is an inevitable part of our lives. Eustress refers to stress associated with positive events, distress to negative events.

❋ The alarm, resistance, and exhaustion phases of the general adaptation syndrome (GAS) involve physiological responses to both real and imagined stressors and cause a complex cascade of hormones to rush through the body. Prolonged arousal due to stress may be detrimental to health.

❋ Undue stress for extended periods of time can compromise the immune system and result in serious health consequences. Psychoneuroimmunology is the science that analyzes the relationship between the mind's reaction to stress and the function of the immune system. While increasing evidence links disease susceptibility to stress, much of this research remains controversial. Stress has been linked to numerous health problems, including CVD, cancer, and increased susceptibility to infectious diseases.

❋ Multiple factors contribute to stress and to the stress response. Psychosocial factors include change, hassles, pressure, inconsistent goals and behaviors, conflict, overload, and burnout. Other factors are environmental stressors and self-imposed stress.

❋ College can be especially stressful. Recognizing the signs of stress is the first step toward better health. Learning to reduce test anxiety and cope with multiple stressors is also important.

❋ Managing stress begins with learning coping mechanisms such as assessing stressors and changing responses. Finding out what works best for you—probably some combination of managing emotional responses, taking mental or physical action, downshifting, learning time management, or using alternative stress management techniques—will help you cope with stress.

* Developing the spiritual side involves practicing mindfulness and its many dimensions. These include the physical dimension (moving in nature); the emotional dimension (identifying and controlling negative emotions and feelings); the social dimension (interacting, listening, and communicating); and the intellectual dimension (sharpening intuition).

Discussion Questions

1. Compare and contrast distress and eustress. Are both types of stress potentially harmful?
2. Describe the alarm, resistance, and exhaustion phases of the general adaptation syndrome and the body's physiological response to stress. Does stress lead to more irritability or emotionality, or does emotionality lead to stress? Provide examples.
3. What are some of the health risks that result from chronic stress? How does the study of PNI link stress and illness?
4. What major factors seem to influence the nature and extent of a person's susceptibility to stress? Explain how social support, self-esteem, and personality may make a person more or less susceptible to stress.
5. Why are some students more susceptible to stress than others are? What services are available on your campus to help you deal with excessive stress?
6. What can college students do to inoculate themselves against negative effects of stress? What actions can you take to manage your stressors? How can you help others to manage their stressors more effectively?
7. How does anger affect the body? Discuss the steps you can take to fight your own anger urge and help your friends control theirs.

Application Exercise

Reread the What Do You Think? scenarios at the beginning of the chapter, and answer the following questions:

1. What could the students in the chapter opener have done to inoculate themselves against their negative reactions to stressful events? What services on campus could they have used to help them through their troubles?
2. What factors make stress potentially greater for students whose background or age differs from that of the "typical" student on a particular campus?
3. What direct and indirect health effects of stress may these students experience? What symptoms of stress should particularly concern them?
4. What strategies should these students follow to reduce the stress they are experiencing? As a friend, what action could you take to reduce their stress levels?

Accessing Your Health on the Internet http

Visit the following Internet sites to explore further topics and issues related to personal health. To visit an organization's website, go to the Companion Website for *Health: The Basics, Fifth Edition* at www.aw.com/donatelle, click on the book image, and select "Accessing Your Health on the Internet" from the navigation menu on the left.

1. *Center for Anxiety and Stress Treatment.* Provides resources and services regarding a broad range of stress-related topics.
2. **Hampden-Sydney College.** Links to helpful tips for dealing with stressful issues commonly experienced by college students.
3. *Mind Tools.* Focuses on all aspects of stress and stress management.

Further Reading

Coffey, R. *Unspeakable Truths and Happy Endings*. Veritas Programming, 1998. Web: http://www.sover.net/ ~ schwcof/ email.html. Author phone: (802)387-4356. *Outstanding resource focusing on survivors of trauma/stress and recovery from human cruelty. Reports on survivors of war, rape, sexual assault, street crime, terrorism, and domestic violence; encompasses all major stressors in contemporary life.*

Health and Stress: Newsletter of the American Institute of Stress. *Excellent monthly resource on stress. Reports on latest developments in all areas of stress research. Each issue contains a listing of meetings of interest and a book review. Web: http://www.stress.org/news.htm.*

Rice, P. L. *Stress and Health.* Monterey, CA: Brooks/Cole, 1998. *An overview of current perspectives on stress and the influence of personal control and behavior on health. Discusses stress management as a factor in controlling pain, anxiety, and depression. An excellent resource for health professionals.*

Seaward, B. *Managing Stress,* 3E. Jones & Bartlett, 2002. *Spirituality and stress expert provides complete overview of stress and health effects.*

Weil, A. *Ask Dr. Weil.* New York: Random House, 1998. *A New Age author who provides an overview of mind–body health and alternative strategies for coping with life's challenges.*

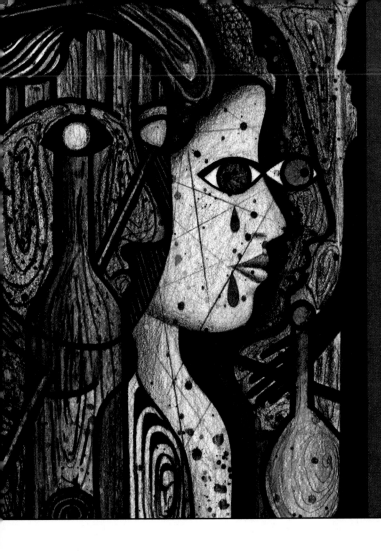

4

Violence and Abuse

CREATING HEALTHY ENVIRONMENTS

objectives

* Differentiate between intentional and unintentional injuries, and discuss societal and personal factors that contribute to violence in American society.

* Identify factors that contribute to homicide, domestic violence, sexual victimization, and other intentional acts of violence.

* Identify strategies to prevent intentional injuries and reduce their risk of occurrence.

* Identify types of crime that are common on college campuses, and explain ways in which the campus community, law enforcement officials, and individuals can prevent crime.

* Discuss the impact of unintentional injuries on American society, and explain actions that might contribute to personal risk of injuries of all types.

"Across the land, waves of violence seem to crest and break, terrorizing Americans in cities and suburbs, in prairie towns and mountain hollows."

"To millions of Americans few things are more pervasive, more frightening, more real today than violent crime. . . . The fear of being victimized by criminal attack has touched us all in some way."

"Among urban children ages 10–14, homicides are up 150 percent, robberies are up 192 percent, assaults are up 290 percent."

You might think these are statements from today's newspapers or television news. But they're not. The first quotation comes from President Herbert Hoover's 1929 inauguration speech, the second from the 1860 Senate report on crime, and the third from a 1967 report on children's violence.[1] Clearly, violence and our concern over its rising rates are not new concepts.

The term **violence** is used to indicate a set of behaviors that produce injuries, regardless of whether they are **intentional injuries** (committed with intent to harm) or **unintentional injuries** (committed without intent to harm, often accidentally). Any definition of *violence* implicitly includes the use of force, regardless of the intent, but as you'll see, some forms of violence are also extremely subtle. In this chapter, we focus on the various types of intentional and unintentional violence, the underlying causes of or contributors to these problems, strategies to reduce risk of encountering violence, and possible methods for preventing violence. Although certain indicators of violence, such as murders and deadly assaults, seem to be on the decline, other forms of violence, such as rape and hate crimes, are on the increase. Even more important is that for all we know about the incidence and prevalence of violence, a great deal remains unknown. Just how many people suffer in silence, failing to report violent acts because of fear of repercussions or accepting violence as "the way it is," remains unknown.

Violence in the United States

Even though violence has long been a major concern in American society, it wasn't until 1985 that the U.S. Public Health Service formally identified violence as a leading public health problem that was contributing to significant death and disability rates. The Centers for Disease Control and Prevention (CDC) created an entire section devoted to the prevention of violence, listing violence as a form of chronic disease that is pervasive at all levels of American society. Children, women, African American males, and the elderly were listed as vulnerable populations at high risk.

Violence   A set of behaviors that produce injuries, as well as the outcomes of these behaviors (the injuries themselves).

Intentional injuries   Injuries done on purpose with intent to harm.

Unintentional injuries   Injuries done without intent to harm.

Recent numbers indicate that we have made dramatic improvements in certain areas. Since 1991, FBI statistics show that overall crime and certain types of violent crime have actually decreased each year. In addition, a Department of Justice report on crime and safety on college campuses suggested that colleges and universities were relatively safe in the 1990s and numerous security measures have been enacted on campuses to insure safety in the next decade.[2] However, although a person's chances of being murdered or violently assaulted may have declined, the odds of being a victim of crime in general are on the increase. College campuses continue to report assaults, rapes, and other problems; however, students who are victimized often have more avenues for support and assistance than previous generations.

Unfortunately, violence affects everyone, directly or indirectly. Although the direct victims of violence and those close to them obviously suffer the most, others suffer in various ways because of the climate of fear that violence generates. Women are afraid to walk the streets at night. The elderly are often afraid to go out even in the daytime. Since the terrorist attack in 2001 on the World Trade Center in New York, some people are becoming afraid to fly, to work in tall buildings, or live in heavily populated areas. Tourists are afraid of being brutalized in many of our nation's cities. We hear of children dodging bullets while playing in city neighborhoods. Even people who live in "safe" areas often become victims of violence within their own homes or at the hands of family members.

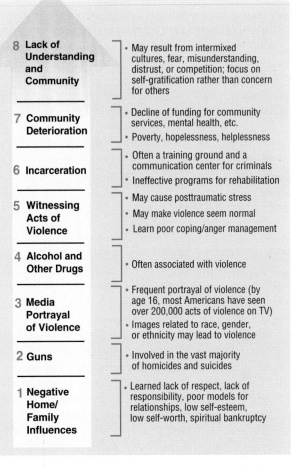

Figure 4.1
Correlations to Violence

Societal Causes of Violence

Several social, cultural, and individual factors increase the likelihood of violent acts (Figure 4.1). Commonly listed factors include the following[3]:

- *Poverty.* Low socioeconomic status and poor living conditions can create an environment of hopelessness, leaving one feeling trapped and seeing violence as the only way to obtain what is needed or wanted.
- *Unemployment.* It is a well-documented fact that when the economy goes sour, violent crime, suicide, assault, and other crimes increase.
- *Parental influence.* Violence is cyclical. Children raised in environments in which shouting, slapping, hitting, and other forms of violence are commonplace are more apt to "act out" these behaviors as adults. Horrifying reports in recent years have made this pattern impossible to ignore.
- *Cultural beliefs.* Cultures that objectify women and empower men to be tough and aggressive tend to have higher rates of violence in the home.
- *The media.* A daily dose of murder and mayhem can take a toll on even resistant minds.
- *Discrimination/oppression.* Whenever one group is oppressed by another, seeds of discontent are sown, and hate crimes arise.

- *Religious differences.* Religious persecution has been a part of the human experience since earliest times.
- *Breakdowns in the criminal justice system.* Overcrowded prisons, lenient sentences, early releases from prison, and trial errors subtly encourage violence in a number of ways.
- *Stress.* People who suffer from inordinate amounts of stress or are in crisis are more apt to be highly reactive, striking out at others or acting irrationally.

In addition to these broad, societally based factors, many personal factors also can lead to violence.

> **What do you think?**
> *Why do you think there is so much violent behavior in the United States?* ✳ *What actions can you take personally to prevent violence from occurring?*
> ✳ *What actions could be taken to reduce risk on your campus?* ✳ *In your community?*

Personal Precipitators of Violence

If you are like most people, you probably acted out your anger much more readily as a child than you do today. However, even the worst-behaved children usually grow up. As we mature, we learn to control outbursts of anger and approach conflict rationally, not aggressively.

Yet others go through life acting out their aggressive tendencies in much the same ways they did as children or their families did. Why do two children from the same neighborhood, or even from the same family, go in different directions when it comes to violence? There are several antecedents or predictors of future aggressive behavior.

Anger Anger is a spontaneous, usually temporary, biological feeling or emotional state of displeasure that occurs most frequently during times of personal frustration. Because life is stressful, anger becomes a part of daily life experiences. Anger can range from slight irritation to rage, a violent and extreme form of anger.[4] When it is acted out at home or on the road, the consequences can be deadly. (See the accompanying box, Skills for Behavior Change.)

What makes some people flare at the slightest provocation? Often, people who anger quickly are individuals who have a low tolerance for frustration, believing that they should not have to put up with inconvenience or petty annoyances. The cause may be genetic or physiological; there is evidence that some people are born unstable, touchy, or easily angered.[5] Another cause of anger is sociocultural. Because many people are taught not to express anger in public, many do not know how to handle it when it reaches a level that cannot be hidden. Family background may be the most important factor. Typically, anger-prone people come from families that are disruptive, chaotic, and unskilled in emotional expression.[6] In fact, the single largest predictor of future violence is past violence.[7]

Aggressive behavior is often a key aspect of violent interactions. **Primary aggression** is goal-directed, hostile self-assertion that is destructive in nature. **Reactive aggression** is more often part of an emotional reaction brought about by frustrating life experiences. Whether aggression is reactive or primary in nature, it is most likely to flare in times of acute stress, during relationship difficulties or loss, or when a person is so frustrated that the only recourse is to strike out at others.

Primary aggression   Goal-directed, hostile self-assertion, destructive in character.

Reactive aggression   Emotional reaction brought about by frustrating life experiences.

What do you think?

What are some examples of primary aggression? ❊ *Reactive aggression?* ❊ *Can both of these aggressive patterns result in the same degree of harm?* ❊ *Do you think our laws are more lenient when violent acts result from reactive aggression?* ❊ *Why?*

Substance Abuse Although much has been written about a link between substance abuse and violence, we have yet to show that substance abuse actually causes violence. In fact, many violent acts are carefully planned actions that involve no alcohol or drug abuse. In some situations, however, psychoactive substances appear to be a form of "ignition" for violence:

- Consumption of alcohol—by perpetrators of the crime, the victim of the crime, or both—immediately preceded over half of all violent crimes, including murder.[8]
- Chronic drinkers are more likely than others to have histories of violent behavior.[9]
- Criminals using illegal drugs commit robberies and assaults more frequently than nonusing criminals and do so especially during periods of heavy drug use.[10]
- In domestic assault cases, more than 86 percent of the assailants and 42 percent of victims reported using alcohol at the time of the attack. Nearly 15 percent of victims and assailants reported using cocaine at the time of the attack.[11]
- Ninety-two percent of assailants and 42 percent of victims reported having used alcohol or other drugs on the day of the assault.[12]
- Mentally ill patients who fail to adhere to prescription drug regimens and abuse alcohol and/or other drugs are significantly more likely to be involved in a serious violent act in the community.[13]
- Substance abuse markedly increases the risk of both homicide and suicide. Being in trouble at work because of drinking, being hospitalized for a drinking problem, using illicit drugs, and being arrested for using illicit drugs all placed subjects at risk for violent death by homicide. The combination of depression and use of alcohol or other drugs increased homicide and suicide rates threefold.[14]

Intentional Injuries

Anytime someone sets out to harm other people or their property, the incident may be referred to as one of intentional violence. Such incidents often result in intentional

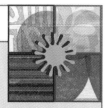

Road Rage!

We pulled out into traffic and immediately were serenaded by the sound of a blaring horn from a car speeding by in the next lane. Apparently we had pulled out in front of the car, causing the driver to swerve quickly to the left lane to avoid hitting us. We felt bad and were thankful that nothing serious had happened; however, the other driver wasn't so quick to forgive. For several miles she maneuvered in an effort to cause us to pull over, or slowed down in the neighboring lane in order to pull alongside our car. I wanted nothing to do with this and slowed down as well to avoid having to face her. Finally, she pulled over as she approached a right-hand turn, and as we went by, she stuck her head out the window and screamed venomous slurs our way. I'll never forget the expression on the woman's face as we went by. It was filled with such hatred and anger, such rage.
—From the author's files

Rage indeed. While drunk driving remains a critical problem, the facts about aggressive driving are surely as ominous. According to the National Highway Transportation Safety Association, 41,907 people died on the highways last year. An estimated two-thirds of these fatalities were caused at least in part by aggressive driving behavior.

Why is road rage becoming more common? One reason is sheer overcrowding. In the last decade, the number of cars has increased by more than 11 percent, and the number of miles driven has risen by 35 percent; however, the number of new road miles has increased by only 1 percent. That means more cars in the same amount of space, and the problem is magnified in urban areas. Also, people have less time and more things to do. When people try to fit more activities into the day, stress levels rise. Stress creates anxiety, which leads to short tempers and road rage.

ARE YOU IMMUNE TO ROAD RAGE?

You may think you are the last person who would drive aggressively, but you might be surprised. Have you ever tailgated a slow driver, honked long and hard at another car, or sped up to keep another driver from passing? If you recognize yourself in any of these situations, watch out!

AVOID THE "RAGE" (YOURS AND OTHER DRIVERS')

Whether you are getting angry at other drivers, or another driver is visibly upset with you, there are things you can do to avoid major confrontations:

- Avoid eye contact!
- If you need to use your horn, do it sparingly.
- Get out of the way. Even if the other guy is speeding, it's safest to not make a point by staying in your lane.
- If someone is following you after an on-the-road encounter, drive to a public place or the nearest police station.
- Report any aggressive driving incidents to the police department immediately. You may be able to prevent further occurrences by the same driver.
- Above all, always use your seat belt! Seat belt use saves 9,500 lives annually.

Source: Reprinted with permission of Allstate Insurance Co. "Don't Be Blinded by Road Rage," Allstate Insurance website, http://www.allstate.com/safety/auto/rage.html

---

injuries, which come in many forms. Whether the situation entails a simple outburst of anger or a fatal attack with a weapon, the resulting intentional injuries cause pain and suffering at the very least, and death and disability at the worst.

Gratuitous Violence

Often it is the most shocking or gratuitous crimes that gain the greatest attention, such as stories of innocent victims of drive-by shootings or young students who turn their internal rage outward on family, classmates, and teachers.

Assault/Homicide **Homicide,** death that results from intent to injure or kill, accounts for nearly 17,000 premature deaths in the United States.[15] These numbers are down slightly from 1997 but still represent a significant contributor to life lost in certain segments of the population. Although homicide was the fourteenth leading cause of death in the United States among all age groups in 1999, it was the second leading cause of death for persons aged 15 to 24. It also exacted a heavy toll among other groups, such as African American males and young Hispanic Americans, both male and female (Table 4.1 describes rates of violent deaths.)

For every violent death, violence also leads to at least 100 nonfatal injuries. In 1999, an estimated 28,874 firearm-related deaths occurred, including large numbers of homicides and suicides.[16] For every person shot and killed specifically by

Homicide Death that results from intent to injure or kill.

CAUSE OF DEATH	ALL AGES	AGES 15–24	AGES 25–34	AGES 35–44
All injury deaths	52.6	59.7*	56.0	55.6
Intentional self-harm	10.7	10.3	13.5	14.4
Accidents (unintentional injury)	35.9	36.2*	31.3	34.0
Assaults (homicide)	6.2	13.2*	11.2	7.2
Number of deaths/motor vehicles	42,401	10,128*	6,778	4,972
Number of deaths/accidental	821	251*	143	136

Highest rate/number age group.

Source: National Center for Health Statistics, Center for Disease Control and Prevention, *Health U.S., 2001.* 1999 Preliminary Data, Sept 21, 2001. FASTATS: http://www.cdc.gov/nehswww/FASTATS/Homicide.html.

a firearm, almost three others were treated annually for nonfatal shootings, many of them children under age 10.[17]

For the average American, the lifetime probability of being murdered is 1 in 153. For white women, the risk is 1 in 450; for Afican American men, it is 1 in 28. For a black man in the 20- to 22-year age group, the risk is 1 in 3. Combined across races, males represent 77 percent of all murder and nonnegligent manslaughter victims. African American males are 1.14 times more likely than white males to be murder victims; white females are 1.5 times more likely than African American females to be victims.[18] Over half of all homicides occur among people who know one another. In two-thirds of these cases, the perpetrator and the victim are friends or acquaintances; in one-third, they belong to the same family.[19]

Living in certain regions of the country, particularly poverty-stricken, inner city areas, also seems to increase one's risk for homicide. Statistics on homicides from other areas of the world provide an interesting comparison of international homicide risk.

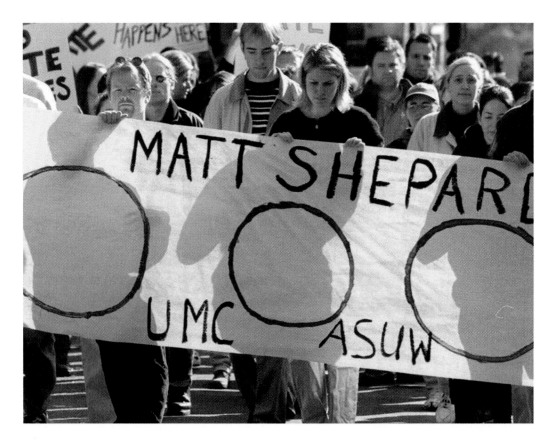

The grisly 1998 murders of Matthew Shepard and James Byrd served as grim reminders of the power and senselessness of hatred.

Bias and Hate Crimes   Even as the population of the United States becomes more diverse, intolerance of those differences continues to smolder. In 1998, nearly 10,000 hate crimes were reported in the United States, with over 1,000 of these being sex-bias crimes.[20]

Hate crimes vary along two dimensions: (1) the way they are carried out and (2) their effects on victims. Vicious gossip, nasty comments, and devilish pranks may not make campus headlines, but they can hurt nonetheless. Recent studies have identified three additional characteristics of hate crimes:[21]

- Excessively brutal
- Perpetrated at random on total strangers
- Perpetrated by multiple offenders

In addition, the perpetrators tend to be motivated by thrill, defensive feelings, or a mission to hate-mongering.

The murder in Wyoming of Matthew Shepard, a young gay student, served as another reminder of the emotions that can lie simmering beneath the surface. The incident shocked the nation on a number of levels, but not because it was a hate crime against a gay person. The attack was shocking because of its gruesome nature and because of where it took place: in a college community, an environment often seen as a bastion of liberalism and tolerance. But academic settings are not immune to hatred and bias. According to a report in the *Chronicle of Higher Education,* nearly one-third of our nation's campuses have reported incidents of hate crimes. Another study of four campuses found that victimization rates varied widely, from 12 percent of Jewish students to as high as 60 percent of Hispanic students. White students were victimized at rates ranging from 5 to 15 percent.[22] The sad truth is, however, that many minor assaults go unreported, so these statistics may reveal only part of the picture.

The tendency toward violent acts on campus might best be defined as campus **ethnoviolence,** a term that reflects relationships among groups in the larger society. Ethnoviolence is based on prejudice and discrimination. Although ethnoviolence often is directed randomly at persons affiliated with a particular group, the group itself is specifically targeted apart from other people, and that differentiation is usually ethnic in nature. Typically, the perpetrators agree that "the group is an acceptable target." For example, in a largely Christian community, Jews and Muslims may be considered acceptable targets.[23] Students bring with them attitudes and beliefs from past family and life experiences.

Prejudice and discrimination are always at the base of ethnoviolence. **Prejudice** is a set of negative attitudes toward a group of people. To say that a person is prejudiced against some group is to say that the person holds a set of beliefs about the group, has an emotional reaction to the group, and is motivated to behave in a certain way toward the group. **Discrimination** constitutes actions that deny equal treatment or opportunities to a group of people, often based on prejudice and bias.

Gang Violence   The growing influence of street gangs has had a harmful impact on health in our country. Whole neighborhoods feel the effects of drug abuse, gang shootings, beatings, thefts, and carjackings; people live in fear of being caught in the middle between gangs at war. As a result, these neighborhoods are, in a very real sense, held hostage by gang members. Once thought to be a phenomenon that occurred only in inner-city areas, gang violence now also occurs in both rural and suburban communities, particularly in the southeast, southwest, and western regions of the country.

Why do young people join gangs? Although the reasons are complex, gangs seem to meet many of their needs. Gangs provide a sense of belonging to a "family" that gives young people self-worth, companionship, security, and excitement. In other cases, gangs provide economic security through criminal activity, drug sales, or prostitution. Once young people become involved in the gang subculture, it is difficult for them to leave. Threats of violence or fear of not making it on their own dissuade even those who are most seriously trying to get out.

Who is at risk for gang membership? Membership varies considerably from region to region. The age range of gang members is typically 12 to 22 years. Risk factors include low self-esteem, academic problems, low socioeconomic status, alienation from family and society, a history of family violence, and living in gang-controlled neighborhoods.

Terrorism: Increased Risks from Multiple Sources

It wasn't so long ago that Americans considered acts of terrorism to be limited to isolated events that happened in distant cities, seldom amounting to more than a blip on the evening news. The bombing of the Oklahoma City Federal Building in 1995 garnered national attention on terrorism for a brief moment in time. Most of us, however, went about our daily business after the event, acknowledging that it was an act of a madman and sympathizing with victims. However, it wasn't until the September 11, 2001 World Trade Center and Pentagon attacks that Americans got a huge wake-up call about the vulnerability of our nation to domestic and international threats. The terms *terrorist attack, bioterrorism,* and *biological weapons* catapulted us into the new millennium with

---

Ethnoviolence   Violence directed randomly at persons affiliated with a particular group.

Prejudice   A set of negative attitudes and beliefs or an emotional reaction or way of thinking about a group of people.

Discrimination   Actions that deny equal treatment or opportunities to a group, often based on bias and prejudice.

Bioterrorism: Pandora's Box

For many, the threat of any kind of viable attack on the United States was incomprehensible until the World Trade Center and Pentagon attacks on September 11, 2001. As shocking as those attacks were, they may pale in comparison to the unleashing of a Pandora's box of insidious biological killers, which could threaten the health and well-being of the global population. Before the terrorist attacks in New York and Washington, D.C., many people had never heard of diseases such as Anthrax, but within a few days of the cataclysm, Americans watched as endless newscasts discussed the potential horrors of biological warfare.

As chilling as the threats of such attacks might be, the real potential for bioterrorism is actually much more far-reaching than any of us might have imagined. Included are a wide range of threats from both biological diseases and chemical agents, as indicated below. A complete overview of each of these as well as national initiatives for preventing bioterrorist attacks is available on the Centers for Disease Control (CDC) web site http://www.bt.cdc.gov/.

BIOLOGICAL AGENTS/DISEASES:

Class A diseases are pathogens that are rarely seen in the United States and pose a risk to national security because they (a) can be easily disseminated or transmitted person-to-person; (b) cause high mortality, with potential for major public health impact; (c) might cause public panic and social disruption; and (d) require special action for public health preparedness. The class A threats that are of greatest concern are highlighted below; a complete overview of others may be located at the above CDC web site.

- Bacillus Anthracis (**anthrax**): An acute infectious disease caused by a bacterium. This bacterium typically occurs in hoofed animals but can also infect humans. Three major forms of anthrax may occur: inhalation anthrax, cutaneous (skin) anthrax, and intestinal anthrax, all with symptoms that usually occur within 7 days after infection. Initial symptoms of inhalation anthrax resemble a common cold, followed by respiratory symptoms and shock, which is often fatal. The intestinal form of anthrax results in initial signs of nausea, vomiting, loss of appetite, and fever, followed by abdominal pain, bloody vomit, and severe diarrhea. It is believed that direct person-to-person spread of anthrax is very rare; thus, immunization and treatment of contacts is not recommended. If exposed, antibiotics are effective treatments in the early stages. Vaccination is also effective.

- Clostridium Botulinum toxin (**botulism**): Botulism is an acute muscle-paralyzing disease caused by a toxin that the bacteria produces. There are three major forms of botulism. Food-borne, the most common strain, leads to illness within hours of ingestion. Infant botulism occurs in infants who harbor the organism in their intestines. Wound botulism occurs when cuts are infected with the botulism organism and its toxins. Fortunately, botulism is not spread from person to person. Symptoms include double vision, blurred vision, slurred speech, difficulty swallowing, and muscle weakness that descends through the body and eventually causes paralysis of breath, and death. Antitoxins given to persons infected are effective if given early in the progression of the disease.

- Yersinia Pestis (**plague**): Plague is an infectious disease of animals and humans that is found in many parts of the world and is caused by a bacterium

an emotional reaction unlike any ever seen. America had lost its innocence and its spirit of invincibility. An undercurrent of fear and anxiety about potential threats from faceless strangers shook many of us in ways that we had never even considered.

What Is Terrorism?   According to the FBI, terrorism is the use of unlawful force or violence against persons or property to intimidate or coerce a government, the civilian population, or any segment thereof, in furtherance of political or social objectives. Typically, terrorism is of two major types: *Domestic terrorism,* which involves groups or individuals whose terrorist activities are directed at elements of our government or population without foreign direction, and *International terrorism,* which involves groups or individuals whose terrorist activities are foreign-based, transcend national boundaries, and are directed by countries or groups outside the United States.

Clearly, terrorist activities may have immediate impact in terms of loss of lives and resources. However, the September 11th attacks played out in such a way that there were far-reaching effects on the U.S. economy, airlines, and transportation systems. Perhaps most damaging in the aftermath of the attacks was the fear, anxiety, and altered behavior of countless Americans. How many people will fear working in skyscrapers for years to come? How many will fear getting on a plane, crossing bridges, or getting on the subway? How many will worry excessively about germs and potential threats from biological weapons? (See the accompanying Health in a Diverse World box.) Will worry about terrorist attacks disrupt our lives, cause us excessive stress or anxiety, or prompt us to harbor concerns or distrust others as we travel, interact with others, and live our lives?

As the media spurs our anxieties about germ, chemical, and nuclear warfare, and the multitude of ways that terrorists can breech our defenses, is it any wonder that an carried by rodents and their fleas. The plague organism infects the lungs. Fever, headache, weakness, and a watery, blood-laden cough is often present. Pneumonia progresses quickly, and over a course of 2–4 days, may cause septic shock. Without treatment, plague may cause death. Person to person contact with transfer of respiratory droplets spreads the disease. A vaccine has not been developed, but several antibiotics are effective if given early.

- Variola major **(smallpox):** Although smallpox was eliminated from the world in 1977, stockpiling of the virus that causes this disease has occurred in many regions of the world. The disease is spread from person to person by infected saliva droplets and is most contagious during the first week of illness. Initial symptoms include high fever, fatigue, and head- and backaches. A characteristic rash with flat red lesions that evolve into pustules most prominent on the face, arms, and legs follows in 2–3 days. Lesions crust early in the second week. Scabs develop, separate, and fall off after about 3–4 weeks. The majority of patients with smallpox recover, but death occurs in up to 30 percent of cases. Although most Americans were vaccinated prior to 1972, it is uncertain whether any lasting immunity was conferred from these shots. Although vaccines are effective, the current supply is limited. Treatment for smallpox focuses on relief of symptoms. New antiviral agents are being tested.

Francisella Tularensis (tularemia)
Viral Hemorrhagic Fever

Category B diseases
Coxiella burnetti (Q fever)
Brucella Species (Brucellosis)
Burkholderia Mallei (Glanders)
Ricin Toxin from Ricinus Communis (Caster beans)
Epsilon Toxin of Clostridium Perfringens
Staphylococcus enterotoxin B

Category C diseases
Nipah virus
Hantavirus
Tickborne hemorrhagic fever
Tickborne encephalitis viruses
Yellow fever
Multidrug-resistant tuberculosis

CHEMICAL AGENTS:

Blister/Vesicants:
    Distilled Mustard (HD)

    Lewisite (L)
    Various forms of nitrogen mustard and Lewisite combinations
Blood
    Arsine
    Cyanogen
    Hydrogen chloride
    Hydrogen cynanide
Choking/Lung/Pulmonary Damaging
    Chorine
    Diphosgene
    Nitrogen oxide
    Zinc oxide
    Others (see CDC list for complete overview)
Incapacitating
    Agent 15
    BZ
    Canniboids
    Fentanyls
    LSD
    Phenothiazines
Nerve
    Cyclohexyl sarin
    Sarin
    Others (See complete CDC listing.)
Riot control/tear
    See listing
Vomiting agents
    See listing

already stressed American public is demonstrating increasing concern? Is there anything that we can do to reduce our risk of terrorist attack? Be assured that the U.S. Department of Health and Human Services Centers for Disease Control and Prevention (CDC) has a wide range of ongoing programs and services designed to help Americans respond to terrorist threats and prepare for attacks. Information on programs and services is available on the CDC web site and is updated regularly. The FBI and other government agencies have also prepared a sweeping set of procedures and guidelines for ensuring citizen safety. The following lists things that you can do to help reduce risks of terrorist attacks:

- *Be aware of your own reactions to stress, anxiety, and fear.* Try to assess how much of your fear is justifiable for a given situation and how much of it is a product of media sensationalism. Practice stress reduction techniques, try to determine the source of your stressors, and react as prudently as possible.

- *Be more conscious of your surroundings.* If you note suspicious activities or irregularities, report them to a person in authority. Being a passive observer and not speaking up when warranted may put you and others at risk.

- *Stay informed.* Try to stay on top of the news and understand the underlying roots of violent activity. Persistent poverty and situations in which there is an imbalance of power and control and/or extreme and pervasive religious or political fanaticism may provide ample fodder for violent acts. Consider when a self-righteous contempt for others may lead to persecution and violation of human rights. Be skeptical about acts perpetrated in the name of some cause, and intervene if possible to diffuse violence.

- *Seek understanding.* Whenever two opposing groups mentally stop engaging with each other and/or when communication breaks down, possible hate, bigotry, and anger may occur. Knowing about other's customs, cultures, and beliefs, and keeping a line of communication open is a good first step in avoiding separation.

- *Seek information.* When political parties fight for power in election years, know your candidates. What are their underlying beliefs regarding national defense, spending for consumer protection, policies on immigration, human rights violations, diversity issues, hate crimes, gun control, and so forth? Are they more aligned with one ideology than another? What is their stance on government interference and control, punishment of offenders, and other key issues?
- *Know what to do in cases of disaster or emergency situations.* Who would you call? How would you access local and regional assistance? Do you have necessary provisions to keep safe in an emergency? Food? Water? First Aid? What happens when your electricity is off, your phone and communication systems are off line, and your access to health care is limited?

Domestic Violence

Domestic violence refers to the use of force to control and maintain power over another person in the home environment. It can involve emotional abuse, verbal abuse, threats of physical harm, and actual physical violence ranging from slapping and shoving to beatings, rape, and homicide.

Women as Victims   Whereas young men are more apt to become victims of violence from strangers, women are much more likely to become victims of violent acts perpetrated by spouses, lovers, ex-spouses, and ex-lovers. In 1999, more than 6 million women were victims of assault. In fact, six of every ten women in the United States will be assaulted at some time in their lives by someone they know.[24] Every year, approximately 12 percent of married women are the

victims of physical aggression perpetrated by their husbands, according to a national survey.[25] This aggression often includes pushing, slapping, and shoving, but it can also take more severe forms.

Each year about 4 percent of married women are beaten, threatened, or actually injured by knives or guns.[26] Acts of aggression by a husband or boyfriend are one of the most common causes of death for young women, and roughly 2,200 women in the United States are killed each year by their partners or ex-partners.[27] Over a recent 10-year period, according to the National Crime Survey, on average more than 2 million assaults on women occurred each year. More than two-thirds of these assaults were committed by someone the woman knew.[28]

The following U.S. statistics indicate the seriousness of this long-hidden problem:[29]

- The most vulnerable women are African American and Hispanic, live in large cities far from their families, and are young and unmarried.
- Every 15 seconds, someone batters a woman.
- Only 1 in every 250 such assaults is reported to the police.
- More than one-third of female victims of domestic violence are severely abused on a regular basis.
- About five women are killed every day in domestic violence incidents.
- Three of every four women who are murdered are killed by their husbands.
- Domestic violence is the single greatest cause of injury to women, surpassing rape, mugging, and auto accidents combined.
- About 25 to 45 percent of all women who are battered sustain such attacks during pregnancy.
- One-quarter of suicide attempts by women occur as a result of domestic violence.

How many times have you heard of a woman who is repeatedly beaten by her partner and wondered, "Why doesn't she just leave him?" There are many reasons why some women find it difficult to break their ties with their abusers. Many women, particularly those with small children, are financially dependent on their partners. Others fear retaliation against themselves or their children. Some women hope that the situation will change with time (it rarely does), and others stay because their cultural or religious beliefs forbid divorce. Finally, some women still love the abusive partner and are concerned about what will happen to him if they leave.[30]

Psychologist Lenore Walker developed a theory known as the "cycle of violence" to explain how women can get caught in a downward spiral without knowing what is happening to them.[31] The cycle has three phases:

1. *Tension building.* In this phase, minor battering occurs, and the woman may become more nurturant, more pleasing, and more intent on anticipating the spouse's needs in order to forestall another violent scene. She assumes guilt for doing something to provoke him and tries hard to avoid doing it again.

Domestic violence   The use of force to control and maintain power over another person in the home environment, including both actual harm and the threat of harm.

2. *Acute battering.* At this stage, pleasing her man doesn't help, and she can no longer control or predict the abuse. Usually, the spouse is trying to "teach her a lesson," and when he feels he has inflicted enough pain, he'll stop. When the acute attack is over, he may respond with shock and denial about his own behavior. Both batterer and victim may soft-pedal the seriousness of the attacks.

3. *Remorse/reconciliation.* During this "honeymoon" period, the batterer may be kind, loving, and apologetic, swearing he will never act violently again. He may "behave" for several weeks or months, and the woman may come to question whether she overreacted to past abuse.

When the tension that precipitated past abuse resurfaces, the man loses control and beats the woman again. Unless some form of intervention breaks this downward cycle of abuse, consisting of contrition, further abuse, denial, and contrition, it will repeat itself again and again—perhaps ending only in the woman's or, rarely, the man's death.

It is very hard for most women who get caught in this cycle of violence (which may include forced sexual relations and psychological and economic abuse as well as beatings) to summon up the resolution to extricate themselves. Most need effective outside intervention.

Men as Victims   Are men also victims of domestic violence? Some women do abuse and even kill their partners. Approximately 12 percent of men reported that their wives had engaged in physically aggressive behaviors against them in the past year—nearly the same percentage of reported claims as for women. The difference between male and female batterers is twofold. First, although the frequency of physical aggression may be similar, the impact is drastically different: women are typically injured in domestic incidents two to three times more often than men.[32] These injuries tend to be more severe and have resulted in significantly more deaths. Women do engage in moderate aggression, such as pushing and shoving, at rates almost equal to those of men, but severe aggression that is likely to land the victim in the hospital is almost always male-against-female. Second, a woman who is physically abused by a man is generally intimidated by him: she fears that he will use his power and control over her in some fashion. Men, however, generally report that they do not live in fear of their wives.

Causes of Domestic Violence   There is no single explanation for why people tend to be abusive in relationships. Although alcohol abuse is often associated with such violence, marital dissatisfaction seems to also be a predictor.[33] Numerous studies also point to differences in the communication patterns between abusive and nonabusive relationships.[34] While some argue that the hormone testosterone causes male aggression, studies have failed to show a strong association between physical abuse in relationships and this hormone.[35] Many experts believe that men who engage in severe violence are more likely than other men to suffer from personality disorders.[36]

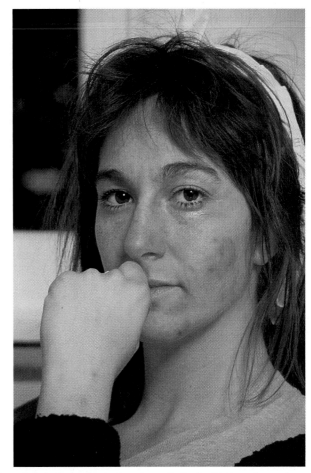

Despite obvious physical and psychological injury, it can be difficult for a woman to leave an abusive partner.

Regardless of the cause, it is the dynamics that *both* people bring to a relationship that will result in violence and allow it to continue. Community support and counseling services can help determine underlying problems and allow the victim and the batterer to break the cycle. The accompanying Assess Yourself box may help you determine whether you are a victim of abuse.

Child Abuse   Children raised in families in which domestic violence and/or sexual abuse occur are at great risk for damage to personal health and well-being. The effects of such violent acts are powerful and long-lasting. **Child abuse** refers to the systematic harm of a child by a caregiver, generally a parent.[37] The abuse may be sexual, psychological, physical, or any combination of these. Although exact figures are lacking, many experts believe that over 2 million cases of child abuse occur every year in the United States, involving severe injury, permanent disability, or death.

Child abuse   The systematic harming of a child by a caregiver, typically a parent.

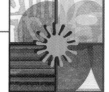

Are You a Victim of Abuse?

Although we often think of abuse as physical, much of the abuse that takes place in intimate relationships is more psychological in nature. If you feel constantly put down or controlled by your partner, ask yourself the following questions.

1 = Never	2 = Sometimes	3 = Usually	4 = Always

	1	2	3	4
1. Are you blamed by your partner whenever things go wrong?	1	2	3	4
2. Does your partner yell at you, curse you, or call you names?	1	2	3	4
3. Is your partner a "nasty" drunk or drug user?	1	2	3	4
4. Does your partner control your money?	1	2	3	4
5. Are you discouraged from enjoying outside friendships?	1	2	3	4
6. Is your free time restricted by your partner?	1	2	3	4
7. Do you "cover," or make excuses for, your partner's behavior?	1	2	3	4
8. Do you do more than your fair share of work around the house?	1	2	3	4
9. Are you forced into having unwanted sex after you've said no?	1	2	3	4
10. Do you feel you must ask permission to do things?	1	2	3	4
11. Are you sometimes "punished" for "misbehaving," either overtly or more subtly?	1	2	3	4
12. Was your mother or your partner's mother abused, or was your partner abused in the past?	1	2	3	4
13. If you express opinions opposed to those of your partner, does it cause a scene?	1	2	3	4
14. Are you afraid of your partner?	1	2	3	4
15. Does your partner repeatedly point out things that are wrong with you?	1	2	3	4

SCORING

If you answered "usually" or "always" to

1 or 2 items   Take notice. Work together to improve troubled areas in the relationship.
3 or 4 items   Seriously examine the relationship. Seek joint counseling from a qualified professional.
5 to 7 items   Abuse is definitely a problem. Counseling is necessary (joint counseling may be appropriate).
8 to 15 items   Crisis intervention is needed. Joint therapy is not appropriate.

Child abusers exist in all gender, social, ethnic, religious, and racial groups, but they tend to share certain characteristics: a history of abuse as a child, a poor self-image, feelings of isolation, extreme frustration with life, higher stress or anxiety levels than normal, a tendency to abuse drugs and/or alcohol, and unrealistic expectations of the child. It is estimated that one-half to three-quarters of men who batter their female partners also batter children. In fact, spouse abuse is the single most identifiable risk factor for predicting child abuse. Children with handicaps or other "differences" are more likely to be abused.

Child Sexual Abuse   **Sexual abuse of children** by adults or older children includes sexually suggestive conversations; inappropriate kissing; touching; petting; oral, anal, or vaginal intercourse; and other kinds of sexual interaction. The most frequent abusers are a child's parents or companions or spouses of the child's parents. Next most frequent are grandfathers and siblings. Girls are more commonly abused than boys, although young boys are also frequent victims, usually of male family members. Between 20 and 30 percent of all adult women report having had an unwanted childhood sexual encounter with an adult male, usually a father, uncle, brother, or grandfather. It is a myth that male deviance or mental illness accounts for most of these incidents: "Stories of retrospective incest patients typically involved perpetrators who are 'Everyman'—attorneys, mental health practitioners, businessmen, farmers, teachers, doctors, and clergy."[38]

Most sexual abuse occurs in the child's home. The risk is higher in the following situations:[39]

1. The child lives without one of his or her biological parents.
2. The mother is unavailable because she is either disabled, ill, or working outside the home.
3. The parents' marriage is unhappy.
4. The child has a poor relationship with his or her parents or is subjected to extremely punitive discipline.
5. The child lives with a stepfather.

Consider only two points about the impact of child abuse in later life: 99 percent of the inmates in the maximum security prison at San Quentin were either abused or raised in abusive households; and 300,000 children between the ages of 8 and 15 are living on the nation's streets, willing to prostitute themselves to survive rather than return to the abusive households they ran away from.[40]

Although most people who were abused as children do not end up as convicts or prostitutes, many do bear spiritual, psychological, and/or physical scars. Clinical psychologist Marjorie Whittaker has found that "of all forms of violence, incest and childhood sexual abuse are considered among the most 'toxic' because of their violations of trust, the confusion of affection and coercion, the splitting of family alignments, and serious psychological and physical consequences."[41]

Not all child violence is physical. Health can be severely affected by psychological violence—assaults on personality, character, competence, independence, or general dignity as a human being. The negative consequences of this kind of victimization can be harder to discern and therefore harder to combat. They include depression, low self-esteem, and a pervasive fear of doing something that will offend the abuser.

> ### What do you think?
> *What factors in society lead to child abuse and neglect?* ✳ *What are common characteristics of children's abusers?* ✳ *Why are family members often the perpetrators of child abuse and child sexual abuse?* ✳ *What actions can be taken to prevent such behaviors?*

Sexual Victimization

As with all forms of violence, men and women alike are susceptible to sexual victimization. However, sexual violence against women is of epidemic proportions. Therefore, much of our focus here is on women as victims. Sexual battering is the single greatest cause of injury to women in the United States, occurring more frequently than car accidents, muggings, and rapes combined.[42] Physical battering and emotional abuse often leave psychological as well as physical scars. One-quarter to one-third of high school and college students report involvement in dating violence, either as perpetrators, victims, or both.[43]

Sexual Assault and Rape **Sexual assault** is any act in which one person is sexually intimate with another person without that other person's consent. This may range from simple touching to forceful penetration and may include such acts as ignoring indications that intimacy is not wanted, threatening force or other negative consequences, and actually using force.

Rape is the most extreme form of sexual assault and is defined as "penetration without the victim's consent."[44] Whether committed by an acquaintance, a date, or a stranger, rape is a criminal activity that usually has serious emotional, psychological, social, and physical consequences for the victim. Most victims are young females; 29 percent are under 11 years of age, 32 percent are between the ages of 11 and 17, and 22 percent are between the ages of 18 and 24.[45] Rape is thought to be the most underreported of all violent crimes in the United States. Estimates of the number of rapes and other sexual assaults on women range from 310,000 to 700,000 every year.[46]

Incidents of rape generally fall into one of two types—aggravated or simple. An **aggravated rape** involves multiple attackers, strangers, weapons, or physical beatings. A **simple rape** is perpetrated by one person, whom the victim knows,

---

Sexual abuse of children Sexual interaction between a child and an adult or older child; includes, but is not limited to, sexually suggestive conversations, inappropriate kissing, touching, petting, and oral, anal, or vaginal intercourse.

Sexual assault Any act in which one person is sexually intimate with another person without that other person's consent.

Rape Sexual penetration without the victim's consent.

Aggravated rape Rape that involves multiple attackers, strangers, weapons, or a physical beating.

Simple rape Rape by one person known to the victim that does not involve a physical beating or use of a weapon.

and does not involve a physical beating or use of a weapon. Most incidents are classified as simple rapes. One report suggests that 82 percent of female rape victims have been victimized by acquaintances (53 percent), current or former boyfriends (16 percent), current or former spouses (10 percent), or other relatives (3 percent). With almost half of all rape charges dismissed before the cases reach trial and a perceived lack of male understanding of how rape affects women, it's easy to understand why experts feel that so-called simple rape is seriously underreported and ignored.

Acquaintance or Date Rape   Although the terms *date rape, friendship rape,* and *acquaintance rape* have become standard terminology, they are typically misused. Not all rapes occur on dates, not all the relationships are friendships, and sometimes the term *acquaintance* is used all too loosely. Many acquaintance rapes occur as the result of incidental contact at a party or when groups of people congregate at one person's house. These are crimes of opportunity, not necessarily the result of a prearranged date. This is an important distinction because the term *date* may suggest some type of reciprocal interaction arranged in advance. Whereas most date or acquaintance rapes happen to women aged 15 to 21 years, the 18-year-old new college student is the most likely victim.[47]

In a study of 6,000 college students from 32 different universities, researchers uncovered the following data:[48]

- More than 50 percent of the college women surveyed had endured some form of sexual abuse.
- More than 25 percent had been the victims of rape or attempted rape.
- Eighty-four percent of the assault victims knew their assailants.
- Fifty-seven percent of the assaults occurred on dates.
- Forty-one percent of the women raped were virgins at the time of the assault.
- Seventy-three percent of the assailants and 55 percent of the victims had used alcohol or drugs prior to the assault.
- Forty-two percent of the victims indicated that they had sex with the offender again (it is unknown whether the subsequent sex was voluntary).
- Twenty-five percent of the men admitted to some degree of aggressive sexual behavior.
- Men were most likely to commit sexual assaults during their senior year in high school or first year in college.

Sexual Harassment   If we think of violence as including verbal abuse and the threat of coercion, then sexual harassment is a form of violence. Under Title VII of the Civil Rights

Act, **sexual harassment** is defined as "unwelcomed sexual advances, requests for sexual favors, and other verbal or physical contact of a sexual nature." Despite what might appear to be a clear definition, sexual harassment is often difficult to identify. Although many people would say that sexual harassment is anything the offended person *believes* is harassment, others will say that this definition is too nebulous.

The issue of sexual harassment was brought to the collective consciousness of society in the early 1990s, when Anita Hill charged Supreme Court justice nominee Clarence Thomas with sexual harassment in a previous employment environment. The alleged harassment was partly in the form of sexually offensive humor, not all directed at the victim. What had long been dismissed as harmless behavior became a cause for concern in business, academia, and government. More recently, the Paula Jones and Monica Lewinsky scandals have kept sexual harassment issues in the news and have focused attention on additional aspects, such as improper touching, improper suggestions, and inappropriate uses of power. Most colleges and universities now offer courses on identifying and preventing sexual harassment, and most companies have established sexual harassment policies and procedures for dealing with it.

Most companies now have sexual harassment policies in place, as well as procedures for dealing with it. If you feel you are being harassed, the most important thing you can do is be assertive:

- *Tell the harasser to stop.* Be clear and direct about what is bothering you and why you are upset.
- *Document the harassment.* Keep a record of every incident, including a description of the harassment, when and where it happened. Having a record of exactly what occurred (and when and where) will be helpful in making your case.
- *Complain to a higher authority.* Talk to your manager about what happened.
- *Remember that you have not done anything wrong.* You will likely feel awful after being harassed (especially if you have to complain to superiors). However, you should feel proud that you are not keeping silent.

Social Contributors to Sexual Assault   According to many experts, certain common assumptions in our society prevent both the perpetrator and the wider public from recognizing the true nature of sexual assault.[49] These assumptions include the following:[50]

- *Minimization.* It is often assumed that sexual assault of women is rare because official crime statistics, including the Uniform Crime Reports of the FBI, show very few rapes per thousand population. However, rape is the most underreported of all serious crimes. Researchers have found that nearly 25 percent of women in the United States have been raped.
- *Trivialization.* Incredibly enough, sexual assault of women is still often viewed as a jocular matter. During a gubernatorial election in Texas a few years back, one of the

---

Sexual harassment   Any form of unwanted sexual attention.

---

candidates reportedly compared a bad patch of weather to rape: "If there's nothing you can do about it, just lie back and enjoy it." (He lost the election—to a woman.)

- *Blaming the victim.* Many discussions of sexual violence against women display a sometimes unconscious assumption that the woman did something to provoke the attack —that she dressed revealingly or flirted outrageously, for example.
- *"Boys will be boys."* According to this assumption, men just can't control themselves once they become aroused.

Over the years, psychologists and others have proposed several theories to explain why many males sexually victimize women. In one of the first major studies to explore this issue, almost two-thirds of the male respondents had engaged in intercourse unwanted by the woman, primarily because of male peer pressure.[51] By all indicators, these trends continue today. Peer pressure is certainly a strong factor, but a growing body of research suggests that sexual assault is encouraged by the socialization processes that males experience daily.[52]

- *Male socialization.* Throughout our lives, we are exposed to social norms that "objectify" women—make them appear as objects that can be used. Media portrayals of half-dressed and undressed women in seductive poses promoting products, for instance, contribute to sex-role stereotyping. These portrayals often show males as aggressors and females as targets. In addition, men are exposed from an early age to anti-female jokes and vulgar and obscene terms for women. These reinforce the idea that females are lesser beings who may be pushed around with impunity.[53] Males are also discouraged from acting in ways that society views as feminine. They are told to act tough and unemotional; to strive for power, status, and control; and to be aggressive and take risks.
- *Male attitudes.* Several studies have confirmed a greater tolerance of rape among men who accept the myth that rape is something women secretly desire, who believe in adversarial relationships between men and women, who condone violence against women, or who hold traditional attitudes toward sex roles. Such men are more apt to

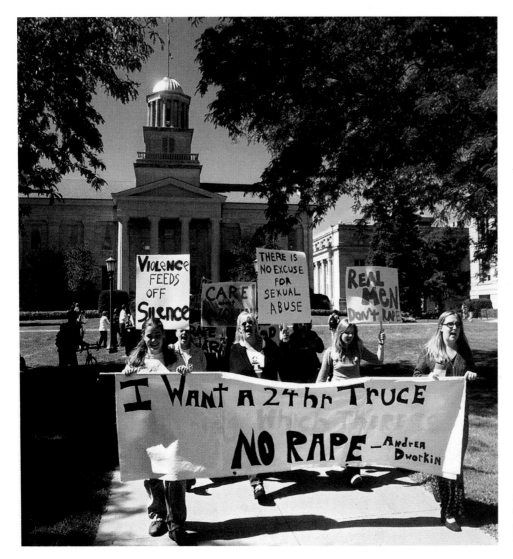

College students can organize vigils, marches, and educational programs to raise awareness about violence against women.

blame the victim and more likely to commit rape themselves if they think they will get away with it.[54]

- *Male sexual history and hostility.* Most rapists are not abnormal or psychologically disturbed. Rather, they tend to be people whose childhoods involved early, multiple sexual experiences (both forced and voluntary) and who feel hostility toward women.[55]

- *Male misperceptions.* Men who are convinced that women really want sex even if they say they don't are more likely to perpetrate sexual assaults. They more readily misinterpret a woman's words and behavior and act on their misperceptions—only to be surprised later when the woman claims that she has been assaulted.[56]

- *Situational factors.* Several factors increase the likelihood of sexual assault. Dates in which the male makes all the decisions, pays, drives, and in general controls what happens are more likely to end in sexual aggression. Alcohol and drug use increase the risk and severity of sexual assault. Length of relationship is another important situational factor: the more long-standing the relationship, the greater the chance of aggression. Finally, males who belong to a close-knit social group involving intense interaction are more prone to engage in a peer-pleasing assault.

What do you think?

What factors make men likely to commit sexual assault or rape? ✳ *What measures might be effective in preventing such behaviors?*

Crime on Campus: A Safe Haven?

Though the majority of crimes on campus still consist of nonviolent crimes—larceny, vandalism, and setting off fire alarms illegally—the rate of violent crime is increasing. Traditionally, most campus crimes were handled internally. This procedure has changed as more states have passed legislation requiring that colleges and universities warn their students about crime and danger both on campus property and in off-campus housing that they recommend.[57] In 1992, Congress passed the Campus Sexual Assault Victim's Bill of Rights, known as the Ramstad Act. The act gives victims the right to call in off-campus authorities to investigate serious campus crimes. In addition, universities must set up educational programs and notify students of available counseling.

Sexual Assault on Campus   Most studies of sexual assault among college students indicate that 25 percent to 60 percent of college men have engaged in some form of sexually coercive behavior.[58] This is consistent with the 27 percent of college women who have reported experiencing rape or attempted rape since they were 14 years old, and the 54 percent who claim to have been sexually victimized (forced to endure unwanted petting, kisses, and other advances).[59]

In Your Car

- Always keep your doors and windows locked.
- Purchase cars with an alarm system and remote entry.
- Don't stop for vehicles in distress; call for help.
- If your car breaks down, lock the doors and wait for help from the police.
- If you think someone is following you, do not drive to your home; drive to a busy place and attract attention.
- Stick to well-traveled routes.
- Keep your car in good running order and always filled with gas.
- On long trips, don't make it obvious you're traveling alone.
- Do not sleep in your car along interstate highways.
- Carry a cell phone with programmed emergency numbers.

On the Street

- Walk or jog at a steady pace.
- Walk or jog with others.
- At night, avoid dark parking lots, wooded areas, and any place that offers an assailant good cover.
- Listen for footsteps and voices.
- Be aware of cars that keep driving around in your area.
- Vary your running or walking routes.
- Carry pepper spray or other deterrents, or walk or jog with a dog… the bigger, the better!
- Carry change to make a phone call.
- Tell others where you are going, your route, and when you'll return.

Figure 4.2
Preventing Personal Assaults

In one survey, only 39 percent of the men sampled denied coercive involvement, 28 percent admitted to having used a coercive method at least once, and 15 percent admitted that they had forced a woman to have intercourse at least once.[60] And according to a large, nationally representative sample of college and university students, 25 percent of the male respondents had been involved in some form of sexual assault since age 14.[61] Since this early national study, many smaller studies have reported similar statistics.

As among the general public, the incidence of sexual assault on campuses is believed to be seriously underreported. In a recent report, one major university familiar to the author claimed there were no rapes on campus. But based on national averages, it seems highly unlikely that no forcible sexual encounters would occur in a setting where nearly 16,000 students date, drink, and socialize every week. The fact is that coercive sex or date rape is seldom reported to campus police, and when a rape victim seeks help at the campus health center, the center is not compelled to report the crime. In one study, 20 percent of female respondents at a midwestern university said they had been raped by someone they knew, but only 8 percent of them had reported it to the police. At another midwestern university, 20 percent of 247 women interviewed said they had experienced date rape, but few had reported it.[62] Needless to say, other sexual violations, such as obscene phone calls, stalking, sexual molestation that does not result in penetration, exhibitionism, voyeurism, and attempted rape, go equally unreported.[63]

Reducing Risks

After a violent act is committed against someone we know, we acknowledge the horror of the event, express sympathy, and go on with our lives. But the person who has been brutalized may take months or years to recover. It is far better to prevent a violent act than to recover from it.

Self-Defense Against Rape

Rape can occur no matter what preventive actions you take, but commonsense self-defense tactics can lower the risk. Self-defense is a process that includes learning increased awareness, self-defense techniques, reasonable precautions, and the self-confidence and judgment needed to determine appropriate responses to different situations.[64] Figure 4.2 identifies practical tips for preventing personal assaults.

Taking Control Most rapes by assailants unknown to the victim are planned in advance. They are frequently preceded by a casual, friendly conversation. Although many women have said that they started to feel uneasy during such a conversation, they denied the possibility of an attack to themselves until it was too late. Listen to your feelings, and trust your intuition. Be assertive and direct to someone who is getting out of line or threatening—this may convince the would-be rapist to back off. Stifle your tendency to be "nice," and don't fear making a scene. Let him know that you mean what you say and are prepared to defend yourself:

- *Speak in a strong voice, using firm language.* Use statements like "Leave me alone" rather than questions like "Will you please leave me alone?" Avoid apologies and excuses.
- *Maintain eye contact with the would-be attacker.*
- *Make sure your tone of voice conveys that you mean what you say.*
- *Stand up straight, act confident, and remain alert.* Walk as though you owned the sidewalk.

Many rapists use certain ploys to initiate their attacks. Among the most common are the following:

- *Request for help.* This allows him to get close—to enter your house to use the phone, for instance.
- *Offer of help.* This can also help him gain entrance to your home: "Let me help you carry that package."
- *Guilt trip.* "Gee, no one is friendly nowadays . . . I can't believe you won't talk with me for just a little while."
- *Purposeful accident.* He may bump into the back of your car, and then assault you when you get out to see the damage. Don't stop unless you have to in these situations, and if you do stop, stay in your car with the doors locked.
- *Authority.* Many women fall for the old "policeman at the door" ruse. If anyone comes to your door dressed in uniform, ask him to show his ID before you unlock the door. You can also call the police department to confirm his ID.

To prevent an attack, remember the following points:

- *Always be vigilant.* Rapes occur in even the safest cities and towns. Don't be fooled by a sleepy-little-town atmosphere.
- *Use campus escort services whenever possible.*
- *Be assertive in demanding a well-lighted campus.*
- *Don't use the same routes all the time.* Think about your movement patterns, and vary them.
- *Don't leave a bar alone with a friendly stranger.* Stay with your friends, and let the friendly stranger come along. Don't give your address to anyone you don't know.
- *Let friends and family know where you are going, what route you'll take, and when to expect your return.*
- *Stay close to others.* Avoid shortcuts through dark or unlighted paths. Don't be the last one to leave the lab or library late at night.
- *Keep your windows and doors locked.* Don't open the door to strangers.

If you are attacked, act immediately. Don't worry about causing a scene. Draw attention to yourself and your assailant. Scream "Fire" loudly. Research has shown that passersby are much more likely to help if they hear the word *fire* rather than just a scream. Your attacker may also be caught off balance by the action.

What To Do If a Rape Occurs

If you are a rape victim, report the attack. This gives you a sense of control. Follow these steps:

- Call 911 (if available).
- Do not bathe, shower, douche, clean up, or touch anything the attacker may have touched.
- Do not throw away or launder the clothes you were wearing. They will be needed as evidence.
- Bring a clean change of clothes to the clinic or hospital.
- Contact the rape assistance hotline in your area, and ask for advice on therapists or counseling if you need additional help or advice.

If a friend is raped, here's how you can help:

- Believe her, and don't ask questions that may appear to implicate her in the assault.
- Recognize that rape is a violent act and that the victim was not looking for this to happen.
- Encourage her to see a doctor immediately, because she may have medical needs but feel too embarrassed to seek help on her own.
- Encourage her to report the crime.
- Be understanding, and let her know you will be there for her.
- Recognize that this is an emotional recovery and that it may take six months to a year for her to bounce back.
- Encourage her to seek counseling.

A Campuswide Response to Violence

Increasingly, college campuses have become microcosms of the greater society, complete with the risks, hazards, and dangers people face in the world. Many college administrators have been proactive in establishing violence prevention policies, programs, and services.[65]

Changing Roles   To increase student protection, campus law enforcement has changed over the years, both in numbers and in their authority to prosecute student offenders. Campus police are responsible for emergency responses to situations that threaten safety, human resources, the general campus environment, traffic and bicycle safety, and other dangers. Campus police have the power to enforce laws with students in the same way they are handled in the general community. In fact, many campuses now hire state troopers or local law enforcement officers to deal with campus issues rather than maintain a separate police staff.

Many of these law enforcement groups follow a *community policing* model in which officers have specific responsibilities for certain areas of campus, departments, or events. By narrowing the scope of each officer's territory, officers get to know people in the area and are better able to anticipate and prevent risks. This differs from earlier safety policies, in which campus security typically swooped down only in times of trouble.

Prevention Efforts   Many colleges and universities now include crime prevention and safety specialists in their law enforcement agencies. These specialists work to improve university policies and procedures to reduce risk to students and others on campus. They commonly recommend the following activities:

- A rape awareness and education program for members of the campus community
- A crime prevention orientation program for new faculty and staff as well as students
- Specialized safety workshops for particular groups, such as commuters, international students, athletes, and students with disabilities

- Printed and electronic educational messages about personal safety
- A notification process to distribute information about special hazards
- Alcohol and drug programs dealing with policy, awareness, education, and enforcement
- A "grounds safety" program, including measures such as removing shrubs from dark areas and providing good lighting throughout the campus
- A system of emergency call boxes or telephones across campus
- Escort services for students who must be out after dark
- Motorist assistance programs for persons with car trouble
- Antitheft programs, including regular patrols of parking lots and other areas
- Victim advocacy programs, such as rape or abuse counseling

The Role of Student Affairs   Although there may be some overlap with law enforcement activities, student affairs offices need to play a vital role in all on-campus programs, both to prevent trouble and resolve problems that do occur. Student groups should monitor progress, identify potential threats, and advocate for improvements in any areas found to be deficient. A student affairs office can play a key role in making sure that mental health services, student assistance programs, and other services are high quality, are easily accessible, and meet student needs. A human services or student affairs office should seek to involve the wider student body and ensure that all are acutely aware of its services. If these programs are not visible or proactive in ensuring campus safety, their roles and responsibilities should be carefully assessed. Student leaders can play a major role in shaping such services and advocating for the campus population.

Community Strategies for Preventing Violence

Because the causes of homicide and assaultive violence are complex, community strategies for prevention must be multidimensional. Successful strategies include the following:[66]

- Developing and implementing educational programs to teach people communication, conflict resolution, and coping skills
- Working with individuals to help them develop self-esteem and respect for others
- Rewarding youngsters for good behavior and never spanking a child when angry (Children need to know that anger is sometimes acceptable, but violence never is. Use family meetings to resolve conflicts.)
- Establishing and enforcing policies that forbid discrimination on the basis of gender, religious affiliation, race, sexual orientation, marital status, and age

- Increasing and enriching educational programs for family planning
- Increasing efforts by health care and social service programs to identify victims of violence
- Improving treatment and support for victims
- Treating the psychological as well as the physical consequences of violence

Unintentional Injuries

As stated previously, unintentional injuries occur without planning or intention to harm. Examples of unintentional injuries include car accidents, falls, water accidents, accidental gunshots, recreational accidents, and workplace accidents. None of these injuries happen on purpose, yet they may result in pain, suffering, and possibly even death. Most efforts to prevent unintentional injuries focus on changing something about the *person,* the *environment,* or the *circumstances* (policies, procedures) that put people in harm's way.

Residential Safety

Injuries within the home typically occur in the form of falls, burns, or intrusions by others. Some populations, such as the elderly, are particularly vulnerable to household injuries. However, the elderly are not the only victims; each year, hundreds of children suffer severe burns or die from accidental fires, falls, and other home-based injuries. To reduce risk of such injuries, consider the following:

Fall-Proofing Your Home

- Eliminate clutter, particularly objects you may stumble over in the dark. Leave nothing lying around on the floor.
- Make sure all rugs are securely fastened to the floor and don't slide when stepped on. Inexpensive rubberized mats or strips will hold rugs in place.
- Train your pets to stay out from under your feet. Many an unsuspecting person has ended up on the floor while trying to avoid a pet.
- Make sure handrails are secure and within easy reach. All stairs should have slip-proof treads.
- Install slip-proof mats or decals in showers and tubs. Adding handrails and places to grab for stability in tubs and showers is a good idea.

Avoiding Burns

- Extinguish all cigarettes in ashtrays before you go to bed. Don't smoke and drink before bed. In fact, don't smoke in bed at any time! Don't throw spent matches in the trash with paper and other combustibles. Soak matches in water before discarding.

- Set all lamps away from drapes, linens, and paper, particularly halogen lights or specialty lamps that can get extremely hot.
- Keep all hotpads and kitchen cloths away from stove burners. When not using a cloth, set it on a counter far from the stove.
- Keep candles under control and away from combustibles. Although it may seem romantic to go to sleep by candlelight, it is highly risky. Don't do it.
- Whenever possible, purchase stoves and ovens with controls in front so you can avoid reaching over hot pans to change burner temperature.
- Use caution when lighting barbecue grills and other home-based fires. Never spray combustible fluids directly onto the fire.
- Check chimneys and fireplaces regularly for buildup of flammable soot.
- Service furnaces annually, and be sure to change the filters.
- Avoid overloading electrical circuits with appliances and cords. Older buildings are at particular risk for fire from such overloads.
- Program phones with emergency numbers for speed dialing, and keep these numbers in clear sight near phones as well.
- Replace batteries in fire alarms periodically, and test them regularly to make sure the batteries are working.
- Have the proper fire extinguishers ready in case of fire.

Preventing Unwanted Intruders

- Close blinds and drapes whenever you are away and in the evening when you are home. Remove large bushes and obstructions from around your windows and doors so that anyone lurking outside will be visible.
- Install dead bolts on all doors and locks on windows. Put a peephole in the main entryway to your home, and do not let anyone in without checking.
- If you have a screen door, lock it. If an unfamiliar visitor comes to the door, this door can serve as a barrier.
- If possible, install a low-cost home alarm system.
- Rent apartments that require a security code or clearance to gain entry.
- Avoid apartments that are easily accessible, such as first-floor units with large patio doors.
- Don't give information about your home or schedule to telephone solicitors. Try to vary the times of day that you come home for lunch, or make quick stops to check on things.
- Don't let repairmen in without identification. Ask your landlord to let you know about such visits well in advance. Even so, have someone else with you when repairmen are there working. Just because a person is licensed to fix refrigerators does not mean he can be trusted.
- Avoid dark parking structures, laundry rooms, and the like. Try to use these areas only when others are around.
- Use initials for first names on mailboxes and in phone listings. Keep your address out of phone books.

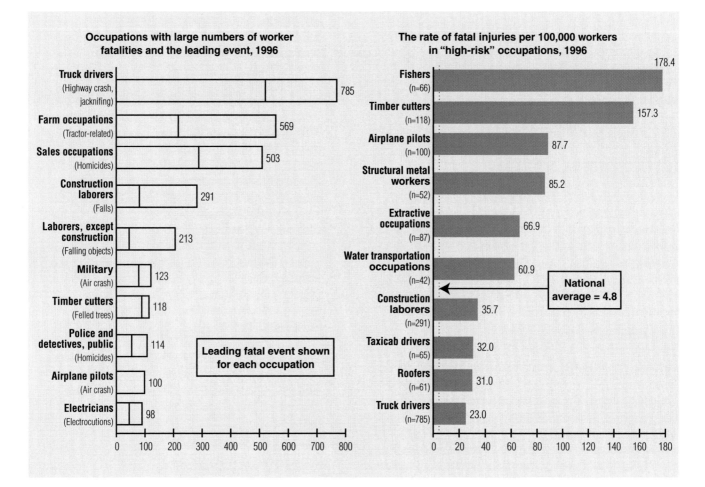

Figure 4.3

Occupations with Large Numbers of Fatalities Are Not Always Those with the Highest Risk, 1996
Source: Guy A. Toscano, *1996 Census of Fatal Occupational Injuries,* Bureau of Labor Statistics, U.S. Department of Labor. Presentation at National Safety Council Congress, October 29, 1997. Website: www.bls.gov/oshhome.htm.

- Keep a cell phone near your bed and program it to 911. Unlike what you see on TV, many intruders do not cut phone lines. More commonly, they simply pick up the receiver in another room as they walk through, thereby disabling a bedroom phone.
- Get to know your neighbors. Organize a neighborhood watch.
- Be careful of "doggy doors." Some thieves let their smallest associate crawl through and unlock the door.
- Be careful of skylights and other areas that open up from the outside. Keep them locked and bolted.
- When you plan to be away, put the lights in different rooms on timers set to come on and go off at different times. Stop your mail and newspaper.

Although no amount of security will prevent all threats of intrusion, following these precautions and actively searching for well-maintained housing in low-crime areas are good steps toward preventing break-ins. If a break-in does occur, keep in mind that, usually, intruders are searching for items to sell and enter with theft in mind. If you encounter an intruder, it is far better to give up your money than to fight.

> **What do you think?**
> *Do a "spot check" of your home. What areas might pose a risk for home accidents or forced entry?*
> ✱ *Do you have a fire extinguisher in your house?*
> ✱ *Do you know the phone number of the local fire department or police department?* ✱ *What would you do if the house caught on fire and you needed to escape immediately?*

Workplace Safety

American adults spend most of their waking hours on the job. Whereas most job situations are pleasant and productive, others pose physical and emotional hazards. Stress, burnout, hostile or abusive interactions with others, discrimination, power struggles, sexual harassment, and a host of other threats are possible whenever people are cloistered together for prolonged periods of time. The nature of the job itself, the corporate culture, and the policies and procedures that characterize certain professions can add to stressful workplace problems.

Fatal Injuries   Certain industries are inherently more hazardous than others (Figure 4.3). Outdoor occupations show the highest fatality and injury rates. Although workplaces have begun to institute serious programs, policies, and services designed to reduce risks, the following statistics indicate a continuing problem:[67]

- In 1999, job-related fatalities reached their highest levels since record keeping began.
- Highway crashes were the leading cause of on-the-job fatalities and accounted for 23 percent of fatal work injury totals in 1999. Most involved truck drivers.
- Twenty percent of worker fatalities resulted from other types of transportation-related incidents, such as tractors and forklifts overturning in fields or warehouses, workers being struck by vehicles, aircraft and railway crashes, and water vessels capsizing.
- Workplace homicides have declined in recent years but continued as the second leading cause of death. Disputes involving co-workers and former co-workers and shootings during the course of robbery led the list.
- Falls, being struck by objects, and electrocutions were the next leading causes of worker fatality.
- On average, about 17 workers were fatally injured each day in 1999. Hundreds more were permanently or temporarily disabled.

- Most fatally injured workers under 16 years of age were killed while doing farm work.

Nonfatal Work Injuries   Although work-related deaths capture more media attention, injury and disability are also serious problems in the workplace. Chronic, debilitating pain and other injuries can cause great economic strain on organizations as a result of workers' compensation claims and days lost from work. Injuries that cause the greatest number of lost work days include carpal tunnel syndrome, hernia, amputation of a limb, fractures, sprains and strains (often of the back), cuts or lacerations, and chemical burns.[68] For example, nearly half of all workers with carpal tunnel syndrome missed 30 days or more of work in 1999. Because so many work injuries are due to repetitive motion, overexertion, or inappropriate motion, they are largely preventable through training and techniques designed to reduce employees' risks.

What do you think?

What can be done to prevent fatal injuries? ✳ Nonfatal injuries? ✳ Are students on your campus at risk from any of the problems discussed? ✳ Are injury prevention strategies in place on your campus? ✳ Who is in charge of student safety? ✳ Do you think more has to be done? ✳ If so, what are your thoughts?

Taking Charge

Managing Campus Safety

Most campuses have initiated programs, services, and policies designed to protect students from potential threats against personal health and safety. Setting limits on where you go, at what time, and with whom are themes of this chapter. What limits do you set when you're out with friends, either casual or intimate ones? Answering the following questions may help you assess your personal behavior and determine your college administrators' degree of interest in and commitment to a violence-free setting.

Checklist for Change

Making Personal Choices

✓ Do you decide before going on a date to limit your sexual behavior?

✓ Do you travel in groups whenever possible?

✓ Do you avoid being out alone at night?

✓ Do you avoid high-crime areas?

✓ Do you take the precautions necessary to reduce your risk of injury from violence?

Making Community Choices

✓ Does your health center offer workshops on the prevention of rape and other sexual offenses?

✓ Does your campus offer courses focused on understanding human diversity?

✓ Does your campus offer workshops or information for students to help them avoid situations that put them at risk for violent interactions?

Taking Charge

4 4 4

✓ Does your campus offer confidential counseling or assistance to victims of sexual assault?

✓ Does your campus offer workshops or educational sessions dealing with suicide?

✓ Does your campus offer information, workshops, or other services dealing with partner and domestic violence?

✓ Does your campus have strict substance abuse policies?

✓ Are rides and escort services available after hours to prevent rapes and assaults? Has your university increased the role of campus security to improve student safety?

✓ Is your campus well lighted and open in the evenings?

✓ Are campus health educators, counselors, and other professionals trained to spot victimization in clients and recommend appropriate services?

✓ Does your campus have a code of conduct that mandates swift and prudent punishment for alcohol and other drug abuse and acts of campus violence?

Summary

* Intentional injuries result from actions committed with intent to harm. Unintentional injuries are the result of actions involving no intent to harm. Violence is at epidemic levels in the United States. Many factors lead people to be violent. Among them are anger, substance abuse, and root causes of oppression, mental health, and economic difficulties.

* Violence affects everyone in society—from the direct victims, to those who live in fear, to those who pay higher taxes and insurance premiums. Over half of homicides are committed by people, who knew their victims. Bias and hate crimes divide people, and gang violence continues to grow. Violence on campus may be increasing, but

victims' rights have also increased as a result of major legislation.

* Preventing violent acts begins with avoiding situations in which harm may occur. Reducing risks involves action not only on the part of the individual, but also through the community, school, and workplace. Many crimes of general society are now commonplace at universities and colleges, including personal assaults, harassment, hate crimes, and even murder.

* Unintentional injuries frequently occur in homes and worksites and can produce serious consequences, including death.

Discussion Questions

1. What major types of crimes are committed in the United States? What is the difference between primary and reactive aggression?
2. What major factors lead to violent acts?
3. Who tends to be susceptible to the appeal of gang membership?
4. Compare spousal abuse against men and against women. What are the differences? What are the similarities? What are the causes of domestic violence?
5. What conditions put a child at risk for abuse? What can be done to prevent or decrease the amount of child abuse?

6. What is sexual harassment, and what factors contribute to it in the workplace?
7. What factors increase risk for sexual assault?
8. What are the most effective violence prevention strategies on your campus?
9. What steps can you take to lower your risk of injury from unintentional violence?

Application Exercise

Reread the What Do You Think? scenarios at the beginning of the chapter, and answer the following questions:

1. What do you think are the major reasons why violent incidents occur? What actions could we take as a society to reduce violence?

2. Do you believe that violence is really much worse than it was back in the "good old days"? Or are we just more aware of it because of increased media coverage?
3. How safe is your campus? What policies, procedures, or safeguards are in place to protect you? What other actions could be taken?

Accessing Your Health  on the Internet

Visit the following Internet sites to explore further topics and issues related to personal health. To visit an organization's website, go to the Companion Website for *Health: The Basics, Fifth Edition* at www.aw.com/donatelle, click on the book image, and select "Accessing Your Health on the Internet" from the navigation menu on the left.

1. ***National Institute for Occupational Safety and Health (NIOSH.)*** Excellent reference for national statistics on injury and violence, both in the community and in the workplace.

2. ***Workplace Solutions.*** Provides information that helps promote well-being by helping people understand the nature of interpersonal conflict, stress, and violence at work.

3. ***Crimes on College Campuses.*** Comprehensive source of information and statistics of colleges and universities across America.

Further Reading

Hoffman, A., J. Schuh, and R. Fenske, *Violence on Campus.* Gaithersburg, MD: Aspen, 1998.
Overview of violence on campus, unique factors that lead to violence and abuse on college campuses, and current programs and policies designed to reduce risk.

U.S. Department of Health and Human Services. *Inventory of Federal Data Systems for Injury, Surveillance, Research and Prevention Activities.* Washington, DC: Government Printing Office, 2001.
Excellent reference for data, reporting mechanisms, and instruments used in assessing U.S. violence statistics.

U.S. Department of Labor. "News." Bureau of Labor Statistics.
Major source of up-to-date information about workplace injuries and illnesses. Internet site:
http://stats.bls.gov/OSH Home.htm

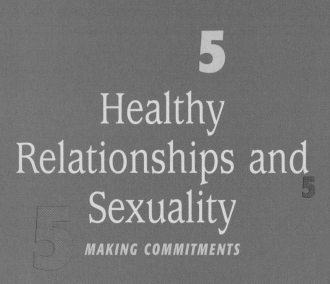

5

Healthy Relationships and Sexuality

MAKING COMMITMENTS

objectives

* Discuss ways to improve communication skills and interpersonal interactions.

* Explain the characteristics of intimate relationships, the purposes they serve, types of intimacy, and how effective relationships develop and are maintained.

* Discuss any differences between men and women in communication styles.

* Discuss the importance of commitment, honesty, and mutual respect in relationships.

* Discuss factors that affect life decisions, such as whether to remain single and whether to have children or not. Examine childrearing practices in the United States.

* Discuss the warning signs of relationship decline and

where to get help with relationship problems.

* Define sexual identity, and discuss the role of gender identity.

* Identify major features and functions of reproductive anatomy and physiology.

* Classify sexual dysfunctions, and describe major disorders.

Bob and Kathy have been sexually active since they met during their freshman year two years ago. During the first year, they dated other people, and each knows the other probably was not monogamous sexually. Although they enjoy each other's company, including the sex, they both recognize that they probably will go separate ways after graduation. One night, when they were talking about their sex life, Bob asked Kathy about her dating history. He wanted to know how many other people she'd been involved with sexually and whether she considered their relationship to be "normal."

Does Bob have a right to know about Kathy's past? ❋ *Does she have a right to keep it private?* ❋ *Why do people typically ask about past sexual partners?* ❋ *Which of these reasons, if any, do you believe are legitimate?* ❋ *How does our society define* normal? ❋ *What sexual behaviors do you consider normal?*

Kate, a 26-year-old senior at a large southern university, hopes to become a hospital administrator. She is attractive and accomplished, and several people have asked to date her. But she has clearly indicated that she is *not* interested in a love relationship, wishes to remain single, and also does not want to have children. In spite of her wishes, her family and friends continually try to "fix her up" with someone, which she finds frustrating. Her parents also pressure her about having grandchildren.

What difficulties might someone face who wishes to remain single in our society? ❋ *How do you react when you hear that someone chooses to remain single and/or avoid having children?* ❋ *Can a healthy person choose to avoid all intimate relationships?* ❋ *Why or why not?* ❋ *If you were Kate's friend, how might you help her be who she wants to be?*

Humans are "social animals"—we have a basic need to belong and to feel loved, appreciated, and wanted.[1] We can't live without relating to others in some way. In fact, a study done by researchers at the Harvard School of Public Health shows that the ability to relate well with people throughout your life can have almost as much impact on your health as exercise and good nutrition.[2]

All relationships involve a degree of risk. However, only by taking these risks can we grow and truly experience all that life has to offer. By looking at our intimate and non-intimate relationships, components of sexual identity, gender roles, and sexual orientation, we will come to better understand who we are.

Communicating: A Key to Good Relationships

From the moment of birth, we struggle to be understood. We flail our arms, cry, scream, smile, frown, belch, and make a number of sounds and gestures to attract attention, get a reaction from someone we care about, or have someone understand what we want or need from them.

Years later as we enter adulthood, each of us has perfected a unique way of "talking" to others with a series of gestures, words, expressions, and body positions. In fact, no two of us communicate in the exact same way or have the same need for "connecting" with others. Some of us are outgoing and quick to express our emotions and thoughts. Others of us are quiet and withdrawn and are reluctant to talk about our feelings and emotions with others.

In fact, males and females have their own styles of communication. Countless pop psychologists have written about the great differences that exist between the sexes in their basic interactions and communication needs. Entire series of books in the *Men Are from Mars, Women Are from Venus* genre suggest that although there are similarities between the sexes, differences in conversational styles between men and women make communication confusing and difficult.[3] In her highly regarded book *You Just Don't Understand: Women and Men in Conversation,* psychologist Deborah Taennen coins the term **genderlect** to characterize very real differences in word choices, interruption patterns, questioning patterns, language interpretations and misinterpretations, and vocal inflections based on gender.[4] Tannen is not alone

Genderlect The "dialect," or individual speech pattern and communication style, of each gender.

in her research. In fact, communication patterns between women and men have been studied for generations, and a consensus opinion is that women are more expressive, more relationship oriented, and more concerned with creating and maintaining intimacy; men tend to be more instrumental, task oriented, and concerned with gathering information or with establishing and maintaining social status or power.[5]

Different cultures not only have different languages and dialects, but also have different ways of expressing themselves and use body language in different ways to communicate information.[6] Some cultures gesture wildly; others maintain a closed and rigid means of speaking. Some cultures are offended by apparent "fixed and dilated" staring; others welcome a steady look in the eyes.

Although it is well established that people differ in the way they communicate, it doesn't mean that one sex, culture, or group is better, worse, wrong, right, or should be a model for the others. What it means is that individuals have to be willing to accept and acknowledge differences and work to ensure that they make every effort to keep communication lines open and fluid. Appearing interested, actively engaged in the interaction, and open and willing to exchange ideas and thoughts is something that we typically learn with practice and hard work.

Communicating How You Feel

Do you find it easy to convey how much you care about friends and family members with hugs, verbal expressions of appreciation and love, and other gestures of feelings? If you are comfortable telling friends and family you love them and that they mean a lot to you, and if you find it easy to express these feelings, chances are that you will also be able to tell them when you are feeling bad, when you are disappointed, or when you are angry or frustrated. However, it's important to realize that some people were not raised in affectionate families, that they do not readily discuss feelings or emotions, and that sometimes these individuals may struggle to find the "right words" for expressing what they feel in a given situation.

When two people begin a relationship, they bring their past communication styles along with them.[7] How often have you heard someone say, "We just can't communicate," or, "You're sending mixed messages?" These exchanges occur regularly as people start relationships or work through ongoing communication problems in an existing relationship. Because communication is a process, our every action, word, facial expression, gesture, or body posture becomes a part of our shared history and part of the evolving impression we make on others. If we are snippy and angry in our responses, others will be reluctant to interact with us. If we bring "baggage" from past bad interactions to new relationships, we may be cynical and distrustful and be guarded in our exchanges with others. If we are positive and happy and share openly with others, they may be more likely to engage in open communication styles.

Improving Communication/ Improving Relationships

Because people have such different ways of communicating, there is no one recipe for how to communicate best in a given situation. At times, silence may be the best means of communication. However, there are things that each of us can do to become better communicators and to encourage and assist others in their attempts to interact with us.

Learning to Share/Self-Disclose Learning when to share, how much to share, and who you can trust in sharing information is never an easy task. We've all experienced frustrations and disappointments by sharing too much when we probably should have stopped earlier; whenever you self-disclose, you take a risk. Sharing personal feelings and thoughts makes you vulnerable. However, if you have taken time to really think about what you believe in, if you have analyzed your feelings and the meanings that certain things have for you, it is often easier to self-disclose because you know that you have relayed information that you believe is important and honest. Also, it is wise to move cautiously in self-disclosing. Get to know a person better before you "tell all." Remember that you can't take back things that you have relayed, so you should consider why you are sharing and what the consequences of sharing might be. If a person seems too inquisitive or seems to be pushing you to share information that you'd rather not share, ask them why it is important to them. Remember, too, that disclosing information about past sexual partners, drug histories, and so forth, is now often done as part of responsible sexual behavior. Although you may feel uncomfortable in asking about sexual history, you have a responsibility to disclose information and receive information that might put a prospective partner at risk.

Learning to Listen All of us have tried to talk with someone who won't let us get a word in edgewise. We listen to them to be polite or to avoid conflict. How did it make you feel? Frustrated? Angry? Wanting to run? The unfortunate thing is that these nonstop talkers often don't have a clue that they are driving people away. They may see themselves as charming and entertaining, and it is hard to steer them to listen more and talk less. However, for comfortable interactions to occur, a gentle prod about listening more and talking less may be in order. Nearly everyone could benefit from working on their listening and speaking skills. Below are a few key pointers:

- *Focus on the speaker.* Maintain eye contact, nod, ask questions, and use body language to let the speaker know you are listening.
- *Avoid interruptions.* Let the speaker finish a thought before you cut in.
- *Avoid focusing on speaker quirks.* Sometimes we get so picky about a speaker's habits that they consume all our attention.

Standing Up for Yourself

You know that sinking feeling. Someone asks you to do something, and your stomach lurches. You don't want to go along, but you can't come up with a good excuse. It's hard to say no. How often are you caught in the "I can't say no" trap? Read the following situations and assess your response according to the following 5-point scale:

1 = never, 2 = very seldom, 3 = sometimes, 4 = frequently, 5 = always.

1. Friends ask you to ride home with them after they've all been drinking. You know you shouldn't go, but you think one of them is cute, and you don't want to seem like a prude. You take the ride.	1	2	3	4	5
2. Someone says something really nasty about someone you like. You jump to the defense of the person being criticized, even though you are in the minority opinion.	1	2	3	4	5
3. You feel strongly about a political issue, but it is the opposite of the opinion your parents hold. You remain silent rather than getting into an argument.	1	2	3	4	5
4. You start out by saying no to something but get talked into doing it after a short time.	1	2	3	4	5
5. You're stressed out, with too much to do and too little time, but you can't seem to say no when someone asks for a favor.	1	2	3	4	5
6. Someone is critical of something you do. You quickly defend your actions by explaining why you did what you did.	1	2	3	4	5
7. You would describe yourself as assertive and tend to quickly let others know your thoughts about certain issues.	1	2	3	4	5
8. Your decisions can be easily swayed by a strong argument from someone else pushing you in the opposite direction.	1	2	3	4	5

Think about your responses to each statement. Do your responses indicate an assertive communication style in which you stand up for your feelings or beliefs? What factors cause you to hold back when you should probably speak up? How can you work to improve your communication behaviors in this area?

- *Demonstrate understanding.* Try to avoid constant philoso-phizing or moralizing to the person who is pouring his heart out.
- *Avoid challenging the speaker or becoming defensive.* Listen objectively, and try to get a sense of what the person is really saying or feeling.
- *Try using "I" messages* when you do choose to respond, particularly in potentially volatile situations.
- *Avoid generalities.* Be specific in what you are telling a person you want from them, and tune in when they respond.

Although there are no foolproof communicating strategies, it is important to speak honestly, respectfully, and to pay attention to how your listener is responding to what you're saying. Sometimes the real message lies not in what is actually being said, but in the nonverbal message of what is *not* said. Rolling your eyes in reaction to the speaker's comments, looking at your watch, pointing your finger, or other such actions can send signals that ignite responses that you were not looking for. Getting a handle on these behaviors and learning to interact more effectively with friends, family members, and lovers can make a huge difference in the quality of your relationships.

Characteristics of Intimate Relationships

We can define **intimate relationships** in terms of four characteristics: *behavioral interdependence, need fulfillment, emotional attachment,* and *emotional availability.* Each of these characteristics may be related to interactions with family, close friends, and romantic partners.[8]

Behavioral interdependence refers to the mutual impact that people have on each other as their lives and daily activities intertwine. What one person does influences what the other person wants to do and can do. Behavioral interdependence may become stronger over time to the point that each person would find a great void if the other person were gone.

Intimate relationships also fulfill psychological needs and so are a means of *need fulfillment.* Through relationships with the others, we fulfill our needs for the following:

Intimate relationships Relationships with family members, friends, and romantic partners, characterized by closeness and understanding.

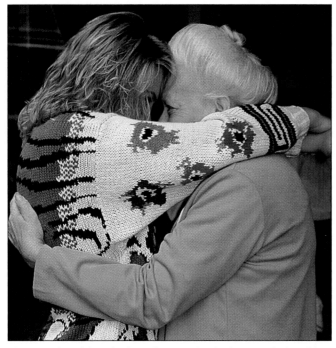

The emotional bonds that characterize intimate relationships often span the generations and help individuals gain insight and understanding into each other's worlds.

- Approval and a sense of purpose in life—requiring the assurance that what we say and do counts
- Intimacy—requiring someone with whom we can share our feelings freely
- Social integration—requiring someone with whom we can share our worries and concerns
- Being nurturant—requiring someone whom we can take care of
- Assistance—requiring someone to help us in times of need
- Reassurance or affirmation of our own worth—requiring someone who will tell us that we matter

In rewarding, intimate relationships, partners and friends meet each other's needs. They disclose feelings, share confidences, and provide support and reassurance.

In addition to behavioral interdependence and need fulfillment, intimate relationships involve strong bonds of *emotional attachment,* or feelings of love and attachment. Often, when we hear the word *intimacy,* we immediately think of a sexual relationship. Although sex can play an important role in emotional attachment, a relationship can be very intimate and not be sexual. Two people can be emotionally inti-

Family of origin   People present in the household during a child's first years of life—usually parents and siblings.

Nuclear family   Parents (usually married, but not necessarily) and their offspring.

mate (share feelings) or spiritually intimate (share spiritual beliefs and meanings), or be intimate friends. The intimacy level experienced by any two people cannot easily be judged by those outside the relationship.

Emotional availability, the ability to give to and receive from others emotionally without fear of being hurt or rejected, is the fourth characteristic of intimate relationships. At times, all of us may limit our emotional availability—for example, after a painful breakup we may decide not to jump into another relationship immediately. Holding back can offer time for introspection and healing as well as considering the "lessons learned." However, because of intense trauma, some people find it difficult ever to be fully available emotionally. This limits their ability to experience and enjoy intimate relationships.

Forming Intimate Relationships

In the early years of life, families provide the most significant relationships. Gradually, the circle widens to include friends, co-workers, and acquaintances. Ultimately, most of us develop romantic or sexual relationships with significant others. Each of these relationships plays a significant role in psychological, social, spiritual, and physical health.

Families: The Ties That Bind

The United Nations defines seven basic types of families, including single-parent families, communal families (unrelated people living together for ideological, economic, or other reasons), extended families, and others. But most Americans think of family in terms of the "family of origin" or the "nuclear family." The **family of origin** includes the people present in the household during a child's first years of life—usually parents and siblings. However, the family of origin may also include stepparents, grandparents, aunts and uncles, partners, and friends. The family of origin has a tremendous impact on the child's psychological and social development. The **nuclear family** consists of parents (usually married, but not necessarily) and their offspring.

The modern American family looks quite different from families of previous generations. Over half of today's moms work outside the home, and large numbers of children are cared for by single parents, grandparents, relatives, stepparents, friends, nannies, day care centers, and other caregivers. No particular family structure is inherently good or bad. Families that promote the most positive health outcomes for all members appear to be those that offer a sense of security, safety, love, and the opportunity for members to grow through positive interactions.

If parents are not afraid to share feelings, affection, or love with each other and their offspring, their children are likely to become emotionally connected adults. If the home environment provides stability and seems safe, it is likely that the children will learn to express feelings and develop intimacy skills. Sibling interactions provide a way to learn and practice interpersonal skills. When the family itself is healthy, people can practice positive behaviors and learn the rights and wrongs of negative behaviors in a safe and non-judgmental environment. However, if the family is psychologically or physically unhealthy, it may pose significant barriers to later relationships, as we discuss later in the section on dysfunctional families.

Establishing Friendships

A Friend is one who knows you as you are
understands where you've been
accepts who you've become
and still gently invites you to grow.

—*Author Unknown*

Good friends—they can make a boring day fun, a cold day warm, or a gut-wrenching worry disappear. They can make us feel that we matter and that we have the strength to get through just about anything. They can also make us angry, disappoint us, or seriously jolt our own comfortable ideas about right and wrong. No friendship is perfect, and most friendships need careful attention if they are to remain stable over time. Psychologists believe that people are attracted to and form relationships with people who give them positive reinforcement and that they dislike those who punish them. The basic idea is simple: you like the people who like you. Another factor that affects the development of a friendship is a real or perceived similarity in attitudes, opinions, and background.[9] In addition, true friends have a sense of *equity* that allows them to share confidences, contribute fairly and equally to maintaining the friendship, and consistently try to give as much as they get back from the interactions.[10]

Though we all know that friends enrich our lives, most people don't realize that real health benefits result from strong social bonds. Social support has been shown to boost the immune system, improve the quality and possibly the length of life, and even reduce the risks of heart disease.[11]

Although most of us have a fairly clear idea of the distinction between a friend and a lover, this difference is not always easy to verbalize. Some people believe that the major difference is that no intimate physical involvement exists between friends. Others have suggested that intimacy levels are much lower between friends than between lovers. But as we have stated, people can be intimate with each other without being sexually involved. Also, many people have sex with others more as friends than as true lovers and partners. Confused? You are probably not alone. Surprisingly, little research has been done to clarify these terms. Psychologists Jeffrey Turner and Laurna Rubinson have described the characteristics that make a good friendship:[12]

- *Enjoyment.* Friends enjoy each other's company most of the time, although temporary states of anger, disappointment, or mutual annoyance may occur.
- *Acceptance.* Friends accept each other as they are, without trying to change or make the other into a different person.

- *Trust.* Friends share mutual trust. Each assumes that the other will act in his or her friend's best interest.
- *Respect.* Friends respect each other in the sense that each assumes that the other exercises good judgment in making life choices.
- *Mutual assistance.* Friends are inclined to assist and support one another. Specifically, they can count on each other in times of need, trouble, or personal distress.
- *Confiding.* Friends share experiences and feelings with each other that they don't share with other people.
- *Understanding.* Friends have a sense of what is important to each and why each behaves as he or she does. Friends are not puzzled or mystified by each other's actions.
- *Spontaneity.* Friends feel free to be themselves in the relationship, without being required to play a role, to wear a mask, or to inhibit revelation of personal traits.

Significant Others, Partners, Couples

Most people choose at some point to enter into an intimate sexual relationship with another person. Numerous studies have analyzed the ways in which couples form significant partnering relationships. Most couples fit into one of four categories of significant sexual or committed relationships: married heterosexual couples, cohabiting heterosexual couples, lesbian couples, and gay male couples. These groups are discussed in greater detail later in this chapter.

Love relationships in each of these four groups typically include all the characteristics of friendship as well as other characteristics related to passion and caring:[13]

- *Fascination.* Lovers tend to pay attention to the other person even when they should be involved in other activities. They are preoccupied with the other and want to think about, look at, talk to, or merely be with the other.
- *Exclusiveness.* Lovers have a special relationship that usually precludes having the same relationship with a third party. The love relationship takes priority over all others.
- *Sexual desire.* Lovers want physical intimacy with the partner, desiring to touch, hold, and engage in sexual activities with the other.
- *Giving the utmost.* Lovers care enough to give the utmost when the other is in need, sometimes to the point of extreme sacrifice.
- *Being a champion or advocate.* Lovers actively champion each other's interests and attempt to ensure that the other succeeds.

> **What do you think?**
>
> *What is the difference between a friend and someone you'd select as a partner—only sex?* ✴ *Can you have a good relationship with a partner and not have sex?* ✴ *Can you have sex with a friend and be just friends?* ✴ *What issues are at stake in both instances?*

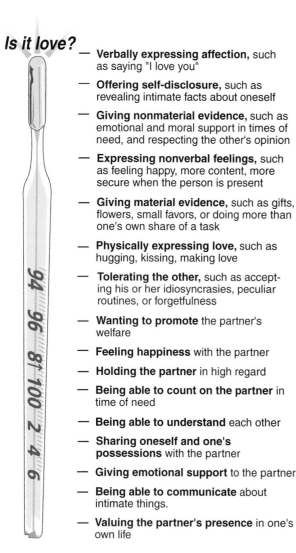

Is it love?

- **Verbally expressing affection,** such as saying "I love you"
- **Offering self-disclosure,** such as revealing intimate facts about oneself
- **Giving nonmaterial evidence,** such as emotional and moral support in times of need, and respecting the other's opinion
- **Expressing nonverbal feelings,** such as feeling happy, more content, more secure when the person is present
- **Giving material evidence,** such as gifts, flowers, small favors, or doing more than one's own share of a task
- **Physically expressing love,** such as hugging, kissing, making love
- **Tolerating the other,** such as accepting his or her idiosyncrasies, peculiar routines, or forgetfulness
- **Wanting to promote** the partner's welfare
- **Feeling happiness** with the partner
- **Holding the partner** in high regard
- **Being able to count on the partner** in time of need
- **Being able to understand** each other
- **Sharing oneself and one's possessions** with the partner
- **Giving emotional support** to the partner
- **Being able to communicate** about intimate things.
- **Valuing the partner's presence** in one's own life

Figure 5.1
Common Experiences of Love

Source: B. Strong, C. DeVault, and B. Sayad, *Human Sexuality* (Mountain View, CA: Mayfield Publishing Co., 1999), pp. 207–209.

This Thing Called Love

What is love? Finding a definition of love may be more difficult than listing characteristics of a loving relationship. The term *love* has more entries in *Bartlett's Familiar Quotations* than any other word except *man*.[14] This four-letter word has been written about and engraved on walls; it has been the theme of countless novels, movies, and plays. There is no one definition of *love,* and the word may mean different things to people, depending on cultural values, age, gender, and situation. Yet we all know what it is when it strikes (Figure 5.1).

Many social scientists maintain that love may be of two kinds: *companionate* and *passionate*. Companionate love is a secure, trusting attachment, similar to what we may feel for family members or close friends. In companionate love, two people are attracted, have much in common, care about each other's well-being, and express reciprocal liking and respect. Passionate love, in contrast, is a state of high

arousal, filled with the ecstasy of being loved by the partner and the agony of being rejected.[15] The person experiencing passionate love tends to be preoccupied with his or her partner and to perceive the love object as being perfect.[16] According to Hatfield and Walster, passionate love will not occur unless three conditions are met.[17] First, the person must live in a culture in which the concept of "falling in love" is idealized. Second, a "suitable" love object must be present. If the person has been taught by parents, movies, books, and peers to seek partners having certain levels of attractiveness or belonging to certain racial or social economic groups or having certain socioeconomic status, and if no such partner is available, the person may find it difficult to allow himself or herself to become involved. Finally, for passionate love to occur, there must be some type of physiological arousal that occurs when a person is in the presence of the beloved. Often this arousal takes the form of sexual excitement.

In his article "The Triangular Theory of Love," researcher Robert Sternberg attempts to clarify further what love is by isolating three key ingredients:[18]

- *Intimacy:* the emotional component, which involves feelings of closeness
- *Passion:* the motivational component, which reflects romantic, sexual attraction
- *Decision/commitment:* the cognitive component, which includes the decisions you make about being in love and the degree of commitment to your partner

According to Sternberg's model, the higher the levels of intimacy, passion, and commitment, the more likely a person is to be involved in a healthy, positive love relationship.

According to anthropologist Helen Fisher (and others), attraction and falling in love follow a fairly predictable pattern based on (1) *imprinting,* in which our evolutionary patterns, genetic predispositions, and past experiences trigger romantic reaction; (2) *attraction,* in which neurochemicals produce feelings of euphoria and elation; (3) *attachment,* in which endorphins—natural opiates—cause lovers to feel peaceful, secure, and calm; and (4) *production of a cuddle chemical,* in which the brain secretes the chemical *oxytocin,* thereby stimulating sensations during lovemaking and eliciting feelings of satisfaction and attachment.[19]

Lovers who claim that they are swept away by passion may not, therefore, be far from the truth.

> *A meeting of the eyes, a touch of the hands or a whiff of scent may set off a flood that starts in the brain and races along the nerves and through the blood. The familiar results— flushed skin, sweaty palms, heavy breathing—are identical to those experienced when under stress. Why? Because the love-smitten person is secreting chemical substances such as dopamine, norepinephrine, and phenylethylamine (PEA) that are chemical cousins of amphetamines.[20]*

Although attraction may in fact be a "natural high," with PEA levels soaring, this hit of passion loses effectiveness over time as the body builds up a tolerance. Needing a continual fix of passion, many people may become attraction junkies, seeking the intoxication of love much as the drug user seeks a chemical high.[21]

Fisher speculates that PEA levels drop significantly over a three- to four-year period, leading to the "four-year itch" that shows up in the peaking fourth-year divorce rates present in over 60 cultures. Romances that last beyond the four-year decline of PEA are influenced by another set of chemicals, known as endorphins, which are soothing substances that give lovers a sense of security, peace, and calm.[22]

Oxytocin is also being studied for its role in the love formula. Produced by the brain, it sensitizes nerves and stimulates muscle contractions, the production of breast milk, and the desire for physical closeness between mother and infant. Scientists speculate that oxytocin may encourage similar cuddling between men and women. Oxytocin levels have also been shown to increase dramatically during orgasm for both men and women.[23]

In addition to such possible chemical influences, past experiences significantly affect our attractions for others. Our parents' modeling of traits we believe are desirable or undesirable may play a role in drawing us to people with similar traits. Many researchers have investigated the possible link between males seeking their own mothers and females seeking their fathers in partners. To date, research on chemical attractions and parent-seeking tendencies is inconclusive and should be viewed only as preliminary. Much more research is needed to confirm these provocative theories.

Gender Issues in Relationships

When it comes to relationships, are men really from Mars and women from Venus? If they are not planets apart, how far apart are they, and what are the implications of the disparities?

Differences in Communication Styles

Psychologist Deborah Tannen has described several basic differences in conversational styles between men and women that can make communication between genders challenging.[24] Recent research validates much of Tannen's work and indicates that women are more expressive, relationship oriented, and concerned with creating and maintaining intimacy; men tend to be more instrumental, task oriented, and concerned with gathering information or with establishing and maintaining social status or power.[25] Unlike women, men tend to believe that they are not supposed to show emotions and are brought up to believe that "being strong" is often more important than having close friendships. As a result, according to research, only one male in ten has a close male friend to whom he divulges his innermost thoughts.[26]

Although men are often perceived as less emotional than women, the question remains whether they really feel less or just express their feelings differently. In one study,

when men and women were shown scenes of people in distress, the men exhibited little outward emotion, whereas the women communicated feelings of concern and distress. However, physiological measures of emotional arousal (such as heart rate and blood pressure) indicated that the male subjects were actually as affected emotionally as the female subjects. In other studies, men and women responded very differently to the same test.[27]

Understanding gender differences in communication patterns, rather than casting blame at each other, is an important step toward bettering communication between men and women. Don't expect members of the other sex to change their style of communication. Instead, learn to interpret messages while explaining your own unique way of communicating. Both men and women want to be heard and understood in their relationships. Understanding the different ways in which we use language will help us all achieve this goal.

Picking Partners

Just as males and females may find different ways to express emotions themselves, the process of partner selection also shows distinctly different patterns. For both males and females, more than just chemical and psychological processes influence the choice of partners. One of these factors is *proximity,* or being in the same place at the same time. The more you see a person in your hometown, at social gatherings, or at work, the more likely that an interaction will occur. Thus, if you live in New York, you'll probably end up with another New Yorker. If you live in northern Wisconsin, you'll probably end up with another Wisconsinite.

You also pick a partner based on *similarities* (attitudes, values, intellect, interests); the old adage that "opposites attract" usually isn't true. If your potential partner expresses interest or liking, you may react with mutual regard known as *reciprocity.* The more you express interest, the safer it is for someone else to return the regard, and the cycle spirals onward. (See the accompanying box, Reality Check.)

Another factor that apparently plays a significant role in selecting a partner is *physical attraction.* Whether such attraction is caused by a chemical reaction or a socially learned behavior, males and females appear to have different attraction criteria. Men tend to select their mates primarily on the basis of youth and physical attractiveness. Although physical attractiveness is an important criterion for women in mate selection, they tend to place higher emphasis on partners who are somewhat older, have good financial prospects, and are dependable and industrious.

> **What do you think?**
> *What factors do you consider the most important in a potential partner?* ✳ *Which are absolute musts?* ✳ *What differences exist between what you believe to be important in a relationship and what your parents considered important?*

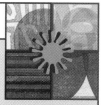

Computer Dating: Issues for the Communication Age

Ten years ago, the thought of meeting a perfect stranger in cyberspace or sharing intimate life details with a faceless stranger who has a "screen name" rather than a real name would have been virtually unthinkable. Today, such "chancy" meetings may lead to excitement, intrigue, or "happy-ever-after" encounters. In increasingly large numbers, however, they also lead to disappointments as the computer persona is found to be a rather ordinary, dull person in real life. Occasionally, as recent newspaper headlines point out, chance computer relationships can lead to victimization and death. In one such instance, a woman had been communicating daily with her "computer friend" for several months. When her friend began to use increasingly vivid and kinky sexual references and seemed to know more about her than she wished, she became uncomfortable and tried to "cool" the interaction. She was relentlessly "stalked" via her home and work computer, and it became evident that her computer stalker knew her address and much about her personal life. Eventually, she was found dead, the result of a vicious attack by the person she knew only via computer.

Though this incident is a dramatic example of computer interactions gone wrong, it is important to remember that there are many inherent risks in engaging in communications with people unknown to you in any traditional sense. Remembering these key points of computerized communication may save you many hours of worry and frustration.

✓ Never give your real name or vital information (e.g., credit card numbers) to a computer chat partner. Use a screen name only, and avoid giving information that may help chat partners home in on you personally.

✓ If your conversations become suggestive or otherwise threatening and weird, terminate the session. Report such violations to your Internet service provider.

✓ Never arrange to meet a stranger at your home or his or her home. Pick a safe meeting place, and bring a friend. Do not give specific identifying information until you know much more about the person. Keep job location and employment information out of the conversation, except in generic terms.

✓ Ask yourself why you are seeking intimacy from strangers on the computer, rather than taking time to interact with others in your social group, particularly if the computer seems to be taking up a disproportionate amount of your time. If your hours online are excessive, you may need to talk to a counselor or friend about the nature and extent of this problem.

Overcoming Barriers to Intimacy

Obstacles to intimacy include lack of personal identity, emotional immaturity, and a poorly developed sense of responsibility. The fear of being hurt, low self-esteem, mishandled hostility, chronic "busyness" (and its attendant lack of emotional presence), a tendency to "parentify" loved ones, and a conflict of role expectations may be equally detrimental. In addition, individual insecurities and difficulties in recognizing and expressing emotional needs can lead to an intimacy barrier. These barriers to intimacy may have many causes, including a dysfunctional family background and jealousy.

Dysfunctional family A family in which the interaction between family members inhibits rather than enhances psychological growth.

Dysfunctional Families

As noted earlier, the ability to sustain genuine intimacy is largely developed in the family of origin. If you were to examine even the most pristine family under a microscope, you would likely find some problems. No group of people can interact perfectly all the time, but this does not necessarily make them dysfunctional. In a truly **dysfunctional family,** interaction between family members inhibits psychological growth, self-love, emotional expression, and individual development. Negative interactions are the norm rather than the exception.

Children raised in dysfunctional settings tend to face tremendous obstacles to growing up healthy. Coming to terms with past hurts may take years. However, with careful planning and introspection, support from loved ones, and counseling when needed, children from even the worst homes have proved to be remarkably resilient. Many are able to forget the past and to focus on the future, developing into healthy, well-adjusted adults. But some have problems throughout their lives.[28] For example, adults who grew up with alcoholic parents may have serious problems creating and maintaining intimate relationships. The family messages that these children receive are typically contradictory, as the family usually tries to hide the presence of alcohol abuse in the home.

Many adult children of alcoholics (ACOAs) claim that they become involved in unhealthy relationships and have difficulty trusting others, communicating with partners, and defining a healthy relationship.[29] Research supporting this theory is conflicted, and many questions remain concerning how past experiences affect relationships for ACOAs.

Another tragically large group of people struggling with intimacy problems originating in the family of origin are survivors of childhood emotional, physical, or sexual abuse (see Chapter 4). It is important to note that dysfunctional families are found in every social, ethnic, religious, economic, and racial group.

Jealousy in Relationships

"Jealousy is like a San Andreas fault running beneath the smooth surface of an intimate relationship. Most of the time, its eruptive potential lies hidden. But when it begins to rumble, the destruction can be enormous."[30] **Jealousy** has been described as an aversive reaction evoked by a real or imagined relationship involving one's partner and a third person.

Contrary to what many of us may believe, jealousy is not a sign of intense devotion to the person who is its target. Instead, jealousy is often a sign of underlying problems that may prove to be a significant barrier to a healthy intimate relationship. Causes of jealousy typically include the following:

- *Overdependence on the relationship.* People who have few social ties and who rely exclusively on their significant others tend to be fearful of losing them.
- *High value on sexual exclusivity.* People who believe that sexual exclusiveness is a crucial indicator of a love relationship are more likely to become jealous.
- *Severity of the threat.* People may feel uneasy if a person with a fantastic body, stunning good looks, and a great personality appears interested in their partners. But they may brush off the threat if they appraise their rival "unworthy" in terms of appearance or other characteristics.
- *Low self-esteem.* People who feel good about themselves are less likely to feel unworthy and to fear that someone else is going to snatch their partners away from them. The underlying question that torments people with low self-esteem is "Why would anyone want me?"
- *Fear of losing control.* Some people need to feel in control of the situation. Feeling that they may be losing the attachment of or control over a partner can cause jealousy.

In both sexes, jealousy is related to the expectation that it would be difficult to find another relationship if the current one should end. For men, jealousy is positively correlated with self-evaluative dependency, the degree to which the man's self-esteem is affected by his partner's judgments. Though a certain amount of jealousy can be expected in any

loving relationship, it doesn't have to threaten a relationship as long as partners communicate openly about it.[31]

What do you think?

"Jealousy is not a barometer by which the depth of love can be read. It merely records the depth of the lover's insecurity" (anthropologist Margaret Mead, 1901–1978). ✴ *Do you agree or disagree with this statement?* ✴ *What other factors may play a role in jealousy?*

Committed Relationships

Commitment in a relationship means that there is an intent to act over time in a way that perpetuates the well-being of the other person, oneself, and the relationship. Polls show that the majority of Americans—as many as 96 percent—strive to develop a committed relationship. These relationships can take several forms, including marriage, cohabitation, and gay and lesbian partnerships.

Marriage

In many societies around the world, traditional committed relationships take the form of marriage. In the United States, marriage means entering into a legal agreement that includes shared financial plans, property, and responsibility for raising children. Many Americans also view marriage as a religious sacrament that emphasizes certain rights and obligations for each spouse.

Close to 90 percent of all Americans marry at least once. U.S. Census Bureau data shows that we are marrying later than ever before. In 1970, the median age for first marriage was 22.5 years for men and 20.6 years for women; by 1998, this had risen to 26.7 years for men and 25.0 years for women.[32] This trend appears to be continuing.

Many Americans believe that marriage involves **monogamy,** or exclusive sexual involvement with one partner. In fact, the lifetime pattern for many Americans appears to be **serial monogamy,** which means that a person has a monogamous sexual relationship with one partner before moving on to another monogamous relationship. However,

Jealousy An aversive reaction evoked by a real or imagined relationship involving a person's partner and a third person.

Monogamy Exclusive sexual involvement with one partner.

Serial monogamy A series of monogamous sexual relationships.

Differences in Marital and Dating Relationships: The Male/Female Perspective

Although there are many indicators that men and women adapt or cope with their relationship stressors in vastly different ways, certain relationship behaviors appear to be more beneficial for one gender than for the other. Consider the following:

- Research has shown that marriage is more beneficial for men than for women and that on marital dissolution, men suffer more distress than do women. Married women generally suffer from more depression and are at risk for more stressors and resultant negative health effects, whereas married men tend to be healthier and live longer, illness-free lives.

- In a study of nonmarried college students in long-distance dating relationships, vast differences appeared in adjustment to physical separation and breakup. Breakups increased men's distress but decreased women's. Women adjusted better than men to both physical separation and breakup. Frequency of contact prior to separation did not show a consistent pattern of effects on adjustment. Men, but not women, adjusted better to the breakup if they had initiated it. The most distressed subjects were men whose partners initiated the breakup, most likely because they were less prepared for it. Many of the sex differences found for dating relationships paralleled those found in marriage.

- In a study of sexual concerns and problems in relationships, 71 percent of men and 85 percent of women reported one or more sexual concerns in their sexual relationship. The two most common sexual concerns the men expressed were, "I like to do things my partner does not," and "I am not interested in sex." The two most common sexual concerns women expressed were, "I am not interested in sex," and "I am unable to relax." Interestingly, when men and women were asked to indicate what problems they believed that their sexual partners had, both sexes said, "reaching orgasm too quickly," and "trouble getting excited." None of the nearly 100 long-term couples interviewed had sought any kind of counseling for their sexual troubles.

Sources: V. Helgeson, "Long-Distance Romantic Relationships: Sex Differences in Adjustment and Breakup," *Personality and Social Psychology Bulletin* 20 (1996): 254–266; S. MacNeil and S. Byers, "The Relationship between Sexual Problems, Communication, and Sexual Satisfaction," *Canadian Journal of Human Sexuality* 6 (1997): 277–284; T. W. Smith, "The Emerging 21st-Century American Family," *GSS Social Change Report* 41, 2001 Chicago, NORC.

---

some people prefer to have an **open relationship,** or open marriage, in which the partners agree that there may be sexual involvement for each person outside their relationship.

Humans are not naturally monogamous; most of us are capable of being sexually and/or emotionally involved with more than one person at a time. Sexual infidelity is an extremely common factor in divorces and breakups. So why do we continue to get married?

Certainly marriage is socially sanctioned and highly celebrated in our culture, so there are numerous incentives for couples to formalize their relationship with a wedding ceremony. A healthy marriage provides emotional support by combining the benefits of friendship and a loving committed relationship. A happy marriage also provides stability for both the couple and for those involved in the couple's life.

Considerable research indicates that married people live longer, feel happier, remain mentally alert longer, engage in less risky behavior, take better care of themselves, engage in sex more often, have higher incomes and better health insurance, and suffer fewer physical and mental health problems.[33] Even people who divorce seem to miss being married; nearly 80 percent of them remarry.

Although a successful marriage can bring much satisfaction, traditional marriage does not work for everyone. Some research suggests that today's women who choose marriage may not be as happy as their mothers were.[34] This may reflect increasing pressure on women to perform multiple roles, such as taking care of a family while working outside the home. Other studies suggest that the happiness of never-married men has increased. Traditional marriage is not the only path to a successful committed relationship.

Open relationship   A relationship in which partners agree that sexual involvement can occur outside the relationship.

Cohabitation   Living together without being married.

Cohabitation

Cohabitation is defined as two unmarried people with an intimate connection who live together in the same household. For a variety of reasons, increasing numbers of Americans are choosing cohabitation. These relationships can be very stable and happy, with a high level of commitment between the partners. In some states, cohabitation that lasts a designated number of years (usually seven) legally constitutes a **common-law marriage** for purposes of real estate and other financial obligations.

Cohabitation can offer many of the same benefits that marriage does: love, sex, companionship, and the ongoing opportunity to know a partner better over time. In addition to enjoying emotional and physical benefits, some people may cohabit for practical reasons, such as the opportunity to share bills and housing costs. Although many cohabitors are young, some older adults choose this lifestyle because they would lose income, such as Social Security or a late spouse's pension, if they were to marry.

Successful cohabitations can also offer benefits not found in marriage. Partners may feel greater autonomy and independence than they might find in a traditional arrangement. Furthermore, if they decide to separate, they do not experience the legal problems and expense of a divorce.

Although cohabitation has its advantages, it also has some drawbacks. Perhaps the greatest disadvantage is the lack of societal validation for the relationship. Many cohabitors must deal with pressures from parents and friends, difficulties in obtaining insurance and tax benefits, and legal issues over property. In 1996, Congress reaffirmed tax advantages for married couples and effectively blocked cohabiting heterosexual and homosexual couples from these benefits through the Defense of Marriage Bill. Today, controversy continues over whether traditional marriage should remain the only means of eligibility for tax deductions, health insurance, and other benefits. In general, there appears to be a trend toward recognizing the validity of unmarried relationships. The state of Vermont, for example, has passed a law that allows partners to form "civil unions."[35] Also, some companies now offer insurance benefits to employees' unmarried partners.

Gay and Lesbian Partnerships

Most adults want intimate, committed relationships, whether they are gay or straight, men or women. Lesbians and gay men seek the same things in primary relationships that heterosexual partners do: friendship, communication, validation, companionship, and a sense of stability.

The 2000 U.S. Census revealed a significant increase in the number of same-sex partner households across the country—more than three times the total reported in the 1990 Census. The states with the most reported same-sex households are California, New York, Florida, Illinois, and Georgia. According to Lee Badgett, research director of the Institute for Gay and Lesbian Strategic Studies, the actual number of households is probably much higher. Many gay and lesbian partners hesitate to report their relationship because of concerns about discrimination.[36]

Studies of lesbian couples indicate high levels of attachment and satisfaction and a tendency toward monogamous, long-term relationships. Gay men, too, tend to form commit-

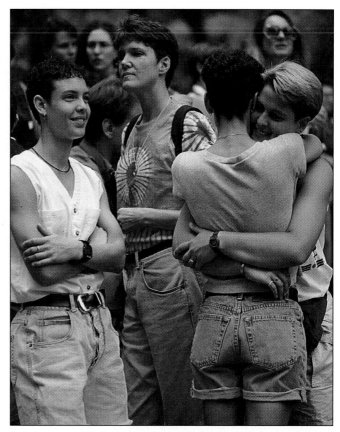

The process of "coming out" and making one's sexual orientation known takes a great deal of courage for gays and lesbians. Many express a sense of relief after having done so.

ted, long-term relationships, especially as they age, much like their heterosexual counterparts.

Challenges to successful lesbian and gay male relationships often stem from discrimination and from difficulties dealing with social, legal, and religious doctrines. For lesbian and gay couples, obtaining the same level of "marriage benefits," such as tax deductions, power-of-attorney, and other rights, continues to be a challenge. However, commitment ceremonies and marriage ceremonies are becoming more frequent in some U.S. cities and in several countries. As mentioned above, Vermont now recognizes same-sex civil unions.[37]

Staying Single

Increasing numbers of adults—of all ages—are electing to remain single. In 1970, 18.9 percent of adult men and 13.7 percent of adult women had decided that marriage wasn't for them. By the year 2000, the proportion of adult Americans

Common-law marriage   Cohabitation lasting a designated period of time (usually seven years) that is considered legally binding in some states.

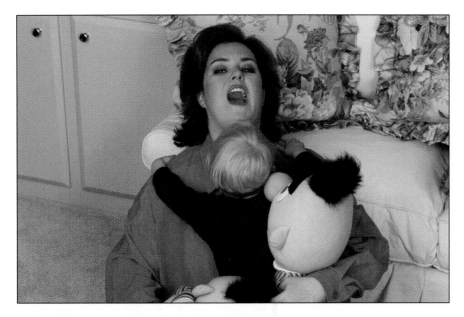

Whether as a result of a divorce, death, or not finding a suitable partner, many single men and women have opted to become parents on their own. Talk show host Rosie O'Donnell adopted children when she was on her own.

who were single by choice or by chance (sometimes after failed marriages) had increased significantly, to more than 37 percent of men and over 41 percent of women.[38] Other changes are reflected in the following facts:

- Over 10 percent of all people say they would never marry.
- People marrying today have more than a 50 percent chance of divorcing.
- As more women enjoy financial independence, they are less likely to remarry after divorce.
- Increasing numbers of widows and widowers are opting not to remarry.

Today, large numbers of people prefer to remain single. Singles clubs, social outings arranged by communities and religious groups, extended family environments, and a large number of social services support the single lifestyle. Many singles live rich, rewarding lives and maintain a large network of close friends and families. Although sexual intimacy may or may not be present, the intimacy achieved through other interactions with loved ones is a key aspect of the single lifestyle.

Some research indicates that single people live shorter lives, are more unhappy, and are more likely to experience financial and health problems than their married peers. However, other studies refute these conclusions. Few research studies to date have controlled for other confounding variables, such as environmental conditions, past histories, and other factors that may carry more weight than the married or single state.

> ### What do you think?
>
> *Although there are advantages and disadvantages in marriage, many people feel that marriage is a desirable option. Are there any advantages in remaining single?* ✳ *What are potential disadvantages?* ✳ *Are there any societal or organizational supports for the single lifestyle?*

Success in Relationships

Most people's definition of success in a relationship tends to be based on whether a couple stays together over the years. Learning to communicate, respecting each other, and sharing a genuine fondness are crucial to relationship success. Many social scientists agree that the happiest committed relationships are flexible enough to allow the partners to grow throughout their lives.

Partnering Scripts

Parents often believe that their children will achieve happiness by living much as they have. Accordingly, most children are reared with a very strong script for what is expected of them as adults. Each group in society has its own partnering script that prescribes standards regarding sex, age, social class, race, religion, physical attributes, and personality types. By adolescence, people generally know exactly what type of person they are expected to befriend or date. By which partnering script were you raised? Just picture whom you could or couldn't bring home to meet your family.

Society provides constant reinforcement for traditional couples, but it may withhold this reinforcement from couples of the same sex, mixed race, mixed religion, or mixed age. People who have not chosen an "appropriate" partner are subject to a great deal of external stress. In addition to denying recognition to such couples, friends and family often blame the "inappropriateness" of the couple if the relationship fails. Nonetheless, many nontraditional relationships survive and flourish. For example, the number of interracial marriages has quadrupled since the late 1960s, and the number of same-sex partner households has grown from 145,130 to almost half a million over the past ten years.[39] Recognizing that this stress is external to the relationship can help alleviate criticism and distancing between the partners.

Being Self-Nurturant

It is often stated that you must love yourself before you can love someone else. What does this mean? Learning how you function emotionally and how to nurture yourself through all life's situations is a lifelong task. You should certainly not postpone intimate connections with others until you have achieved this state. However, a certain level of individual maturity helps in maintaining a committed relationship. For example, divorce rates are much higher for couples under age 30 than for older couples.

Two concepts that are especially important to a good relationship are accountability and self-nurturance. **Accountability** means that both partners in a relationship see themselves as responsible for their own decisions and actions. They don't hold the other person responsible for positive or negative experiences.

Self-nurturance goes hand in hand with accountability. In order to make good choices in life, a person needs to balance many physical and emotional needs, including sleeping, eating, exercising, working, relaxing, and socializing. When the balance is disrupted, as it will inevitably be, self-nurturing people are patient with themselves and try to put things back on course. It is a lifelong process to learn to live in a balanced and healthy way. Two people who are on a path of accountability and self-nurturance together have a much better chance of maintaining a satisfying relationship.

Having Children . . . or Not?

When a couple decides to raise children, their relationship changes. Resources of time, energy, and money are split many ways, and the partners no longer have each other's undivided attention. Babies and young children do not time their requests for food, sleep, and care to the convenience of adults. Therefore, individuals or couples whose own basic needs for security, love, and purpose are already met make better parents. Any stresses that already exist in a relationship will be further accentuated when parenting is added to the list of responsibilities. Having a child does not save a bad relationship—in fact, it only seems to compound the problems that already exist. A child cannot and should not be expected to provide the parents with self-esteem and security.

Changing patterns in family life affect the way children are raised. In modern society, it is not always clear which partner will adjust his or her work schedule to provide the primary care of children. Nearly half a million children each year become part of a blended family when their parents remarry; remarriage creates a new family of stepparents and stepsiblings. In addition, an increasing number of individuals are choosing to have children in a family structure other than a heterosexual marriage. Single women can choose adoption or alternative (formerly called "artificial") insemination as a way to create a family. Single men can choose to adopt or can obtain the services of a surrogate mother. According to the 2000 census, over 9 percent of all U.S. households were headed by a man or woman raising a child alone, reflecting a growing trend in America and in the international community.[40] Regardless of the structure of the family, certain factors remain important to the well-being of the unit: consistency, communication, affection, and mutual respect. See Table 5.1 for emerging trends in childrearing.

Some people become parents without a lot of forethought. Some children are born into a relationship that was supposed to last and didn't. This does not mean it is too late to do a good job of parenting. Children are amazingly resilient and forgiving if parents show respect and communicate about household activities that affect their lives. Even children who grew up in a household of conflict can feel loved and respected if the parents treat them fairly. This means that parents must take responsibility for their own conflicts and make it clear to children that they are not the reason for the conflict.

Today, families that want to achieve their dream of living in a nice home in suburbia may discover that two incomes are needed. That's why more than 80 percent of all mothers with children under the age of 5 work outside the home. Day care, extended family and friends, grandparents, neighbors, and nannies "mind the kids." Some employers offer family leave arrangements that allow parents more latitude in taking time from work.

> ### What do you think?
> *What are the essential characteristics of a healthy family environment? ✳ Why is having such an environment important to the future development of children? ✳ Do you think that day-care centers, extended family units, and full-time baby-sitters can equally provide a positive environment for personal growth? ✳ Why or why not?*

When Relationships Falter

Breakdowns in relationships usually begin with a change in communication, however subtle. Either partner may stop listening, ceasing to be emotionally present for the other. In turn, the other feels ignored, unappreciated, or unwanted. Unresolved conflicts increase, and unresolved anger can cause problems in sexual relations.

When a couple who previously enjoyed spending time alone together find themselves continually in the company of others, spending time apart, or preferring to stay home

Accountability   Accepting responsibility for personal decisions, choices, and actions.

Self-nurturance   Developing individual potential through a balanced and realistic appreciation of self-worth and ability.

Table 5.1
The Emerging Twenty-First-Century American Family

	Percentage of Children in Various Types of Families				
	ONE SINGLE PARENT	**TWO PARENT, CONTINUING**	**TWO PARENT, REMARRIED**	**TWO ADULTS, EX-MARRIED**	**ADULTS, NEVER MARRIED**
1972	4.7	73.0	9.9	3.8	8.6
1978	10.2	65.3	13.6	4.0	6.9
1982	14.3	59.3	13.7	5.2	7.3
1988	18.6	54.7	13.0	5.0	8.7
1990	14.9	56.1	17.9	5.1	6.0
1994	18.4	52.8	14.7	7.1	7.0
1998	18.2	51.7	12.3	8.6	9.2

Note: Single parent = only one adult in household; *two parents, continuing* = married couple, never divorced; *two parents, remarried* = married couple, at least one remarried (unknown whether children came before or after remarriage); *two adults, ex-married* = two or more adults, previously but not currently married; *adults, never married* = two or more adults, never married (this category also includes some other family structures). *Source: General Social Survey News,* Number 13, August 1999. Published by the National Opinion Research Center.

alone, it may be a sign that the relationship is in trouble. Of course, the need for individual privacy is not a cause for worry—it's essential to health. If, however, a partner decides to change the amount and quality of time spent together without the input or understanding of the other, it may be a sign of hidden problems.

College students, particularly those who are socially isolated and far from family and hometown friends, may be particularly vulnerable to staying in unhealthy relationships. They may become emotionally dependent on a partner for everything from eating meals to recreational and study time, and mutual obligations such as shared rental arrangements, transportation, and child care can make it tough to leave.

It's also easy to mistake unwanted sexual advances for physical attraction or love. Without a network of friends and supporters to talk with, to obtain validation for feelings or to share concerns, a student may feel stuck in a relationship that is headed nowhere.

Honesty and verbal affection are usually positive aspects of a relationship. In a troubled relationship, however, they can be used to cover up irresponsible or hurtful behavior. "At least I was honest" is not an acceptable substitute for acting in a trustworthy way. The words "But I really do love you" should not be used as a license to be inconsiderate or rude.

Most communities have trained therapists who specialize in relationship difficulties, and most student health centers offer these services at reduced fees for students. If you are unaware of such services, ask your instructor for suggestions.

When and Why Relationships End

Based on recent statistics, it has been predicted that 20 percent of those who marry today will divorce within five years; one-third may divorce within ten years; and 40 percent will divorce before their fifteenth anniversary. Ultimately, half of all marriages will end in divorce.[41] While these numbers may seem alarming, the actual number of failed relationships is probably much higher. Many people never go through a legal divorce process and therefore are not counted in these statistics. Cohabitors and unmarried partners who raise children, own homes together, and exhibit all the outward appearances of marriage without the license are also not included.

Why do relationships end? There are many reasons, including illness, financial concerns, and career problems. Other breakups arise from unmet expectations. Many people enter a relationship with certain expectations about how they and their partner will behave. Failure to communicate these expectations to a partner can lead to resentment and disappointment. Differences in sexual needs may also contribute to the demise of a relationship.

Under stress, communication and cooperation between partners can break down. One of the greatest predictors of divorce appears to be husband dissatisfaction in the first five years of marriage.

Coping with Loneliness

When a relationship ends, it is normal to experience painful emotions of anger, guilt, rejection, and unworthiness. No matter how miserable the relationship was, feelings of failure are common. Counselors estimate that it takes at least a year and often longer to recover from the loss of a major relationship, whether by death or separation.

Although it may be painful, reflecting on the past relationship can help prevent similar mistakes in the future. Concentrating on the negative aspects of an ex-partner is a natural tendency, but it is equally important to remember what you loved in the other person and what is lovable about you. When we accept the risk and challenge of close relationships, we accept one of the greatest gifts life has to offer.

With time, support from others, and community or professional help, most people do recover and establish rewarding new relationships.

Building Better Relationships

Most relationships start with great optimism and true love. So why do so many run into trouble? "We just don't know how to handle the negative feelings that are the unavoidable by-product of the differences between two people, the very differences that attract them to each other in the first place. Think of it as the friction any two bodies would generate rubbing against each other countless times each day," says Howard Markman, Ph.D., professor of psychology at the University of Denver.[42] According to Markman, most unhappy couples don't need therapy; they need education in how relationships work and the special skills that make them work well. Markman and others promote **psychoeducation,** the teaching of crucial psychological skills—giving people knowledge so they can help themselves. Psychoeducation courses aren't therapy per se, but they typically have a therapeutic effect on couples.

Elements of Healthy Relationships

Relationships that are satisfying and stable share certain characteristics. A key ingredient is **trust,** the degree of confidence partners feel in a relationship. Without trust, intimacy will not develop, and the relationship could fail. Trust includes three fundamental elements:

- *Predictability* means that you can predict your partner's behavior, based on the knowledge that your partner acts in consistently positive ways.
- *Dependability* means that you can rely on your partner to give support in all situations, particularly those in which you feel threatened with hurt or rejection.
- *Faith* means that you feel absolutely certain about your partner's intentions and behavior.

Trust can develop even when it is initially lacking. This requires opening yourself to others, which carries the risk of hurt or rejection.

Other characteristics of happy relationships include the following:

- Partners interpret each other's behavior in the context of their own relationship, without overreacting to behaviors that remind them of past relationships.
- Partners who like each other and find each other interesting are happier than those who don't. Although most relationships have their share of ups and downs, members of successful couples are able to talk, listen, and touch each other in an atmosphere of caring.
- Sexual intimacy is a major component of healthy relationships, but sex is not a major reason for the existence of

the relationship. Some couples admit to sexual dissatisfaction but find the relationship more important than sexual satisfaction. Many couples report that as communication and trust increase, the sexual relationship also improves.
- Another important quality is a shared and cherished history, including private jokes, special places where key events have occurred, nicknames, rituals, emotions, and significant shared time and activities.

Your Sexual Identity

Sexual identity, the recognition of oneself as a sexual being, is determined by a complex interaction of genetic, physiological, environmental, and social factors. The beginning of sexual identity occurs at conception with the combining of chromosomes that determine sex. It is the biological father who determines whether a baby will be a boy or a girl. All eggs (ova) carry an X sex chromosome; sperm may carry either an X or a Y chromosome. If a sperm carrying an X chromosome fertilizes an egg, the resulting combination of sex chromosomes (XX) provides the blueprint to produce a female. If a sperm carrying a Y chromosome fertilizes an egg, the XY combination produces a male.

The genetic instructions included in the sex chromosomes lead to the differential development of male and female gonads at about the eighth week of fetal life. Once the male **gonads** (testes) and the female gonads (ovaries) are developed, they play a key role in all future sexual development because the gonads are responsible for the production of sex hormones. The primary sex hormones produced by females are estrogen and progesterone. In males, the sex hormone of primary importance is testosterone. The release of testosterone in a maturing fetus signals the development of a penis and other male genitals. If no testosterone is produced, female genitals form.

At the time of **puberty,** sex hormones again play major roles in development. Hormones released by the **pituitary gland,** called gonadotropins, stimulate the gonads (testes

---

Psychoeducation   The teaching of crucial psychological skills, giving people knowledge so they can help themselves.

Trust   The degree of confidence partners feel in a relationship.

Sexual identity   Recognition of oneself as a sexual being; a composite of biological sex, gender identity, gender roles, and sexual orientation.

Gonads   The reproductive organs in a male (testes) or female (ovaries).

Puberty   The period of sexual maturation.

Pituitary gland   The endocrine gland controlling the release of hormones from the gonads.

and ovaries) to make appropriate sex hormones. The increase of estrogen production in females and testosterone production in males leads to the development of **secondary sex characteristics.** Male secondary sex characteristics include deepening of the voice, development of facial and body hair, and growth of the skeleton and musculature. Female secondary sex characteristics include growth of the breasts, widening of the hips, and the development of pubic and underarm hair.

Thus far, we have described sexual identity only in terms of a person's sex. Sex simply refers to the biological condition of being male or female based on physiological and hormonal differences. **Gender,** in contrast, refers to the psychosocial condition of being masculine or feminine as defined by the society in which one lives. Each of us expresses our maleness or femaleness to others on a daily basis by the **gender roles** we play. **Gender identity** refers to the personal sense or awareness of being masculine or feminine, a male or a female. It may sometimes be difficult to express one's true sexual identity because of the bounds established by gender-role stereotypes. **Gender-role stereotypes** are generalizations about how males and females should express themselves and the characteristics each possesses. Our traditional sex roles are an example of gender-role stereotyping.

On the one hand, men are thought to be independent, aggressive, better in math and science, logical, and always in control of their emotions. Women, on the other hand, have traditionally been expected to be passive, nurturing, intuitive, sensitive, and emotional. **Androgyny** is the combination of traditional masculine and feminine traits in a single person. Androgynous people do not always follow traditional sex roles but rather try to act appropriately based on the given situation.

The process by which a society transmits behavioral expectations to its individual members is called **socialization.** Gender roles are shaped, or socialized, by parents, peers, schools, textbooks, advertisements, and many forms of media, including television, music, and movies. Think about the current television shows you watch. Do the characters play out traditional gender roles?

By now you can see that defining sexual identity is not a simple matter. It is a lifelong process of growing and learning. Your sexual identity is made up of the unique combination of your sex, gender identity, chosen gender roles, sexual orientation, and personal experiences. No other person on this earth is exactly like you, and it is up to you to take every opportunity to get to know and like yourself so that you may enjoy your life to the fullest.

> **What do you think?**
> *How often do you challenge existing gender-role stereotypes? ✳ What is the outcome? ✳ Do you think men and women have the same degree of freedom in gender-role expression?*

Secondary sex characteristics Characteristics associated with sex but not directly related to reproduction, such as vocal pitch, degree of body hair, and location of fat deposits.

Gender The psychological condition of being feminine or masculine as defined by the society in which one lives.

Gender roles Expression of maleness or femaleness in everyday life.

Gender identity Personal sense or awareness of being masculine or feminine, a male or a female.

Gender-role stereotypes Generalizations concerning how males and females should express themselves and the characteristics each possesses.

Androgyny Combination of traditional masculine and feminine traits in a single person.

Socialization Process by which a society communicates behavioral expectations to its individual members.

External female genitals The mons pubis, labia majora and minora, clitoris, urethral and vaginal openings, and the vestibule of the vagina and its glands.

Vulva The female's external genitalia.

Mons pubis Fatty tissue covering the pubic bone in females; in physically mature women, the mons is covered with coarse hair.

Reproductive Anatomy and Physiology

An understanding of the functions of the male and female reproductive systems will help you derive pleasure and satisfaction from your sexual relationships, be sensitive to your partner's wants and needs, and make responsible choices regarding your own sexual health.

Female Reproductive Anatomy and Physiology

The female reproductive system includes two major groups of structures, the external genitals (Figure 5.2) and the internal genitals. The **external female genitals** include all structures that are outwardly visible and are referred to as the vulva. Specifically, the **vulva,** or external genitalia, includes the mons pubis, the labia minora and majora, the clitoris, the urethral and vaginal openings, and the vestibule of the vagina. The **mons pubis** is a pad of fatty tissue covering the pubic bone. The mons serves to protect the pubic bone, and

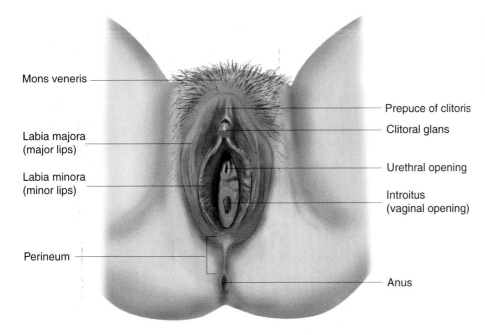

Figure 5.2
External Female Genital Structures

Source: From R. D. McAnulty and M. M. Burnette, *Human Sexuality: Making Healthy Decisions* (Boston: Allyn and Bacon, 2001).

Mons veneris

Labia majora
(major lips)

Labia minora
(minor lips)

Perineum

Prepuce of clitoris

Clitoral glans

Urethral opening

Introitus
(vaginal opening)

Anus

after puberty it becomes covered with coarse hair. The **labia minora** are folds of mucous membrane, and the **labia majora** are folds of skin and erectile tissue that enclose the urethral and vaginal openings. The labia minora are found just inside the labia majora.

The **clitoris** is the female sexual organ whose only known function is sexual pleasure. It is located at the upper end of the labia minora and beneath the mons pubis. Directly below the clitoris is the urethral opening through which urine leaves the body. Below the **urethral opening** is the vaginal opening, or opening to the vagina. In some women, the vaginal opening is covered by a thin membrane called the **hymen.** It is a myth that an intact hymen is proof of virginity. The **perineum** is the area between the vulva and the anus. Although not technically part of the external genitalia, the tissue in this area has many nerve endings and is sensitive to touch; it can play a part in sexual excitement.

The **internal female genitals** of the reproductive system include the vagina, uterus, fallopian tubes, and ovaries. The **vagina** is a tubular organ that serves as a passageway from the uterus to the outside of a female's body. This passageway allows menstrual flow to exit from the uterus during a female's monthly cycle and serves as the birth canal during childbirth. The vagina also receives the penis during intercourse. The **uterus,** also known as the **womb,** is a hollow, muscular, pear-shaped organ. Hormones acting on the inner lining of the uterus, called the **endometrium,** either prepare the uterus for implantation and development of a fertilized egg or signal that no fertilization has taken place, in which case the endometrium deteriorates and becomes menstrual flow.

The lower end of the uterus, the **cervix,** extends down into the vagina. The **ovaries** are almond-sized structures suspended on either side of the uterus. The ovaries produce the hormones estrogen and progesterone and are also the reser-

voir for immature eggs. All the eggs a female will ever have are present in the ovaries at birth. Eggs mature and are released from the ovaries in response to hormone levels. Extending from the upper end of the uterus are two thin,

Labia minora   "Inner lips," or folds of tissue just inside the labia majora.

Labia majora   "Outer lips," or folds of tissue covering the female sexual organs.

Clitoris   A pea-sized nodule of tissue located at the top of the labia minora.

Urethral opening   The opening through which urine is expelled.

Hymen   Thin tissue covering the vaginal opening.

Perineum   Tissue extending from the vulva to the anus.

Internal female genitals   The vagina, uterus, fallopian tubes, and ovaries.

Vagina   The passage in females leading from the vulva to the uterus.

Uterus (womb)   Hollow, pear-shaped muscular organ whose function is to contain the developing fetus.

Endometrium   Soft, spongy matter that makes up the uterine lining.

Cervix   Lower end of the uterus, which opens into the vagina.

Ovaries   Almond-sized organs that house developing eggs and produce hormones.

flexible tubes called the **fallopian tubes.** The fallopian tubes are where sperm and egg meet and fertilization takes place. Following fertilization, the fallopian tubes serve as the passageway to the uterus, where the fertilized egg becomes implanted and development continues.

The Onset of Puberty and the Menstrual Cycle With the onset of puberty, the female reproductive system matures, and the development of secondary sex characteristics transforms young girls into young women. The first sign of puberty is the development of breast buds, which occurs around age 11. Under the direction of the endocrine system, the pituitary gland, the **hypothalamus,** and the ovaries all secrete hormones that act as chemical messengers among them. Working in a feedback system, hormonal levels in the bloodstream act as the trigger mechanism for release of more or different hormones.

At around the age of $9\frac{1}{2}$ to $11\frac{1}{2}$ in females, the hypothalamus receives the message to begin secreting **gonadotropin-releasing hormone (GnRH).** The release of GnRH in turn signals the pituitary gland to release hormones called gonadotropins. Two gonadotropins, **follicle-stimulating hormone (FSH)** and **luteinizing hormone (LH),** signal the ovaries to start producing **estrogens** and **progesterone.** In-

Fallopian tubes   Tubes that extend from the ovaries to the uterus.

Hypothalamus   An area of the brain located near the pituitary gland. The hypothalamus works in conjunction with the pituitary gland to control reproductive functions.

Gonadotropin-releasing hormone (GnRH)   Hormone that signals the pituitary gland to release gonadotropins.

Follicle-stimulating hormone (FSH)   Hormone that signals the ovaries to prepare to release eggs and to begin producing estrogens.

Luteinizing hormone (LH)   Hormone that signals the ovaries to release an egg and to begin producing progesterone.

Estrogens   Hormones that control the menstrual cycle.

Progesterone   Hormone secreted by the ovaries; helps keep the endometrium developing in order to nourish a fertilized egg; also helps maintain pregnancy.

Menarche   The first menstrual period.

Ovarian follicles (egg sacs)   Areas within the ovary in which individual eggs develop.

Ovulation   The point of the menstrual cycle at which a mature egg ruptures through the ovarian wall.

Human chorionic gonadotropin (HCG)   Hormone that calls for increased levels of estrogen and progesterone secretion if fertilization has taken place.

creased estrogen levels assist in the development of female secondary sex characteristics. In addition, estrogens regulate the reproductive cycle. The normal age range for the onset of the first menstrual period, termed the **menarche,** is 9 to 17 years, with the average age being $11\frac{1}{2}$ to $13\frac{1}{2}$ years. Body fat heavily influences the onset of puberty, and increasing rates of obesity in children may account for the fact that girls here and in other countries seem to be reaching puberty much earlier than they used to.[43] Very thin girls, such as young athletes, tend to start menstruating later.

The average menstrual cycle is 28 days long and consists of two phases: the *menstrual/proliferative* (also known as the follicular) phase, and the *secretory* or *luteal* phase. During the proliferative phase, the pituitary gland releases FSH and LH. The FSH acts on the ovaries to stimulate the maturation process of several **ovarian follicles (egg sacs).** These follicles secrete estrogens, and in response to this estrogen stimulation, the lining of the uterus, the endometrium, begins to grow and develop. The inner walls of the uterus become coated with a thick, spongy lining composed of blood and mucus. In the event of fertilization, this endometrial tissue will become a nesting place for the developing embryo. The increased estrogen level also signals the pituitary to slow down FSH production but increase LH secretion. Of the several follicles developing in the ovaries, only one each month normally reaches complete maturity. Under the influence of LH, this one ovarian follicle rapidly matures, and about the fourteenth day of the proliferative phase, it releases an ovum into the fallopian tube—a process referred to as **ovulation.** Just prior to ovulation, the mature egg's follicle begins to increase secretion of progesterone, the first function of which is to spur the addition of further nutrients to the developing endometrium.

After ovulation, the secretory phase begins. The ovarian follicle is converted into the *corpus luteum,* or yellow body, which continues to secrete estrogen and progesterone but in decreasing amounts. In addition, FSH also falls back to preproliferative levels. Essentially, the woman's body is "waiting" to see whether fertilization will occur. During this time, LH declines and progesterone levels begin to rise, causing additional tissue growth in the endometrium.

If fertilization takes place, cells surrounding the developing embryo release a hormone called **human chorionic gonadotropin (HCG).** HCG increases estrogen and progesterone secretion, which maintains the endometrium while signaling the pituitary gland not to start a new menstrual cycle.

When fertilization does not occur, the egg gradually disintegrates within approximately 72 hours. The corpus luteum gradually becomes nonfunctional, causing levels of progesterone and estrogen to decline. As hormonal levels decline, the endometrial lining of the uterus loses its nourishment, dies, and is sloughed off as menstrual flow.

Some issues associated with menstruation that you may be interested in reading about are premenstrual syndrome (PMS), toxic shock syndrome (TSS), and dysmenorrhea, or painful menstruation.

Ritual Genital Mutilation

Despite hundreds of years of tradition, Hajia Zuwera Kassindja would not let it happen to her 17-year-old daughter, Fauziya. Hajia's own sister had died from it. So Hajia gave her daughter her inheritance from her deceased husband, which amounted to only $3,500 but left Hajia a pauper. Fauziya used the money to buy a phony passport and flee from the African country of Togo to the United States.

Upon arrival in the United States, Fauziya requested asylum from persecution. However, she was put into prison for more than a year. But then, in 1996, the Board of Immigration Appeals finally agreed that Fauziya was fleeing persecution, and she was allowed to remain in the United States. She now lives and studies near Washington, D.C. From what had Hajia's sister died? From what was Fauziya escaping? Ritual genital mutilation.

Cultures in some parts of Africa and the Middle East ritually mutilate or remove the entire clitoris or, in some cases, just the clitoral hood. Removal of the clitoris, or clitoridectomy, is a rite of initiation into womanhood in many of these predominantly Islamic cultures. It is often performed as a puberty ritual in late childhood or early adolescence (not at birth, like male circumcision).

The clitoris gives rise to feelings of sexual pleasure in women. Its removal or mutilation represents an attempt to ensure the girl's chastity, because it is assumed that uncircumcised girls are consumed with sexual desires. Cairo physician Said M. Thabit says, "With circumcision we remove the external parts, so when a girl wears tight nylon underclothes she will not have any stimulation." Some groups in rural Egypt and in the northern Sudan, however, perform clitoridectomies primarily because it is a social custom that has been passed down from ancient times. Some perceive it as part of their faith in Islam. However, neither Islam nor any other religion requires it. Ironically, many young women do not grasp that they are victims. They assume that clitoridectomy is part of being female.

Clitoridectomies are performed under unsanitary conditions without benefit of anesthesia. Medical complications are common, including infections, bleeding, tissue scarring, painful menstruation, and obstructed labor. The procedure is psychologically traumatizing. An even more radical form of clitoridectomy, called infibulation or pharaonic circumcision, is practiced widely in the Sudan. Pharaonic circumcision involves complete removal of the clitoris along with the labia minora and the inner layers of the labia majora. After removal of the skin tissue, the raw edges of the labia majora are sewn together. Only a tiny opening is left to allow passage of urine and menstrual discharge. The sewing together of the vulva may be intended to ensure girls' chastity until marriage. Medical complications are common, including menstrual and urinary problems, and even death. After marriage, the opening is enlarged to permit intercourse. Enlargement is a gradual process that is often made difficult by scar tissue from the circumcision. Hemorrhaging and tearing of surrounding tissues are common consequences. It may take three months or longer before the opening is large enough to allow penile penetration. Mutilation of the labia is now illegal in the Sudan, although the law continues to allow removal of the clitoris. Some African countries have outlawed clitoridectomies, although such laws are rarely enforced.

Millions of women in Africa and the Middle East—130 million by some estimates (World Health Organization [WHO], 1997)—have undergone ritual genital mutilation. Clitoridectomies remain common or even universal in nearly 30 countries in Africa, in many countries in the Middle East, and in parts of Malaysia, Yemen, Oman, Indonesia, and the India-Pakistan subcontinent. Thousands of African immigrant girls living in European countries and the United States have also been mutilated.

Do not confuse male circumcision with the maiming inflicted on girls. Former representative Patricia Schroeder of Colorado depicts the male equivalent of female genital mutilation as cutting off the penis. The *New York Times* columnist A. M. Rosenthal (1995) calls female genital mutilation the most widespread existing violation of human rights in the world. The Pulitzer Prize–winning African American novelist Alice Walker has condemned it in her novel *Possessing the Secret of Joy* (1992). She called for its abolition in her book and movie *Warrior Marks*.

In 1996, the United States outlawed ritual genital mutilation within its borders. The government also directed U.S. representatives to world financial institutions to deny aid to countries that have not established educational programs to bring an end to the practice. Yet calls from Westerners to ban the practice in parts of Africa and the Middle East have sparked controversy on grounds of "cultural condescension"—that people in one culture cannot dictate the cultural traditions of another (Women's Health—Female Genital Mutilation, 1997). Yet for Alice Walker, "torture is not culture." As the debate continues, some 2 million African girls continue to undergo ritual genital mutilations each year (WHO, 1997).

Sources: Adapted from A. R. Rathus, J. S. Nevid, and L. Fichner-Rathus, *Essentials of Human Sexuality* (Boston: Allyn and Bacon, 1998), pp. 30–31; "Women's Health—Female Genital Mutilation: Common, Controversial, and Bad for Women's Health," *Population Briefs* 3, 2 (1997); World Health Organization, "Fact Sheet 153: Female Genital Mutilation" (New York: The Population Council, 1997), www.who.ch/inf-fs/en/fact153.html. See also http://www.who.int/inf-fs/en/fact241.html (World Health Organization website on genital mutilation); and http://www.fgm.org (Female Genital Mutilation [FGM] Information Page).

Menopause Just as menarche signals the beginning of a female's reproductive years, **menopause**—the permanent cessation of menstruation—signals the end. Generally occurring between the ages of 40 and 60, and at age 51 on average, menopause results in decreased estrogen levels, which may produce troublesome symptoms in some women. Decreased vaginal lubrication, hot flashes, headaches, dizziness, and joint pains have all been associated with the onset of menopause. It has long been reported that taking hormones such as estrogen through **estrogen replacement therapy (ERT)** or hormone replacement therapy (HRT) containing estrogen and progesterone could relieve women's menopausal symptoms, such as bloating and hot flashes, as well as reduce risks of heart disease and osteoporosis. Several studies in 2000 and 2001 have raised questions about possible reduction of the risk of cardiovascular disease (CVD) through HRT. Other studies have continued to support HRT for osteoporosis benefits and reductions in menopausal symptoms. However, looming questions about increased risks of gall bladder disease, blood clotting, and breast cancer remain unanswered.[44] All women need to discuss the risks and benefits of HRT with their health care provider and come to an informed decision. Finding a doctor who specializes in women's health and who carefully studies and keeps up to date with the latest research findings is crucial. Certainly

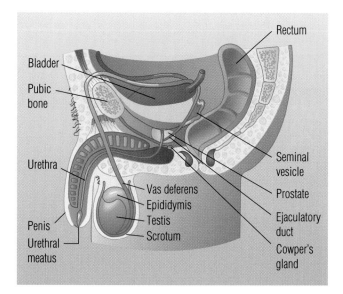

Figure 5.3
Side View of the Male Reproductive Organs

Source: From Jeffrey S. Turner and Laurna Rubinson, *Contemporary Human Sexuality,* ©1993, 64. Reprinted by permission of Prentice-Hall, Englewood Cliffs, NJ.

What do you think?

Why is it so important that we understand the function of our sexual anatomy? ✳ *Do men need to understand how the menstrual cycle works? Why?* ✳ *Some people are not comfortable using the proper terms for parts of the sexual anatomy. Why do you think this is so?*

---

lifestyle changes, such as regular exercise and a diet low in fat and adequate in calcium, can also help protect post-menopausal women from heart disease and osteoporosis.

Male Reproductive Anatomy and Physiology

The structures of the male reproductive system may be divided into external and internal genitals (Figure 5.3). The penis and the scrotum make up the **external male genitals.** The **internal male genitals** include the testes, epididymides, vasa deferentia, and urethra, and three other structures—the seminal vesicles, the prostate gland, and the Cowper's glands—that secrete components which, with sperm, make up semen. These three structures are sometimes referred to as the **accessory glands.**

The **penis** serves as the organ that deposits sperm in the vagina during intercourse. The urethra, which passes through the center of the penis, acts as the passageway for both semen and urine to exit the body. During sexual arousal, the spongy tissue in the penis becomes filled with blood, making the organ stiff, or erect. Further sexual excitement leads to **ejaculation,** a series of rapid spasmodic contractions that propel semen out of the penis.

Situated behind the penis and also outside the body is a sac called the **scrotum.** The scrotum serves to protect the testes and also helps control the temperature within the testes, which is vital to proper sperm production. The **testes** (singular: *testis*) are egg-shaped structures in which sperm are manufactured. The testes also contain cells that manufacture

---

Menopause The permanent cessation of menstruation.

Estrogen replacement therapy (ERT) Use of synthetic or animal estrogens to compensate for decreases in estrogens in a woman's body.

External male genitals The penis and scrotum.

Internal male genitals The testes, epididymides, vasa deferentia, ejaculatory ducts, urethra, and accessory glands.

Accessory glands The seminal vesicles, prostate gland, and Cowper's glands.

Penis Male sexual organ that releases sperm into the vagina.

Ejaculation The propulsion of semen from the penis.

Scrotum Sac of tissue that encloses the testes.

Testes Two organs, located in the scrotum, that manufacture sperm and produce hormones.

Circumcision: Risk versus Benefit

Circumcision involves the surgical removal of the foreskin, a fold of skin covering the end of the penis. Most circumcisions in the United States have traditionally been performed for religious or cultural reasons or for reasons of hygiene. In uncircumcised males, the foreskin, which is fully attached to the glans at birth, naturally separates from the glans anywhere from weeks to several years after birth. Once it can be retracted, the glans underneath the foreskin should be cleaned regularly. Some studies have suggested that uncircumcised males may be at slightly greater risk for penile cancer and some sexually transmitted infections, including syphilis, gonorrhea, and HIV. Poor hygiene, that is, failing to clean the area between the foreskin and glans, is suspected as the cause of all of these risks. However, other, apparently stronger, data suggest that uncircumcised men are no more likely to contract STIs than circumcised men are, and an equal number of deaths result from circumcision as from penile cancer.

Overall, research does not support the practice of circumcision for health reasons. In 1999, the American Academy of Pediatrics concluded that because no data suggest that circumcision benefits the health of the child, circumcision is not a medically necessary procedure. Parents who choose to circumcise should do so for religious, aesthetic, or other personal reasons, not because of concern for their son's health. New parents must decide whether their male infant will be circumcised. What decision do you think you would make for your son? Give your reasons.

Sources: American Academy of Pediatrics, "Care of the Uncircumcised Penis," 2001 (see www.aap.org/family/uncirc.htm); American Academy of Pediatrics Task Force on Circumcision, "Circumcision Policy Statement," *Pediatrics* 103 (1999): 686–693; E. O. Laumann, C. M. Masi, and E. W. Zuckerman, "Circumcision in the United States: Prevalence, Prophylactic Effects, and Sexual Practices," *Journal of the American Medical Association* 277 (1997): 1052–1057; H. Shingleton and C. W. Heath, "Letter to Dr. Perter Rappo, American Academy of Pediatrics from the American Cancer Society," 1996 (see www.nocirc.org/position/acs.html).

---

testosterone, the hormone responsible for the development of male secondary sex characteristics.

The development of sperm is referred to as **spermatogenesis.** Like the maturation of eggs in the female, this process is governed by the pituitary gland. Follicle-stimulating hormone (FSH) is secreted into the bloodstream to stimulate the testes to manufacture sperm. Immature sperm are released into a comma-shaped structure on the back of the testis called the **epididymis** (plural: *epididymides*), where they ripen and reach full maturity.

The epididymis contains coiled tubules that gradually "unwind" and straighten out to become the **vas deferens.** The two vasa deferentia, as they are called in the plural, make up the tubular transportation system whose sole function is to store and move sperm. Along the way, the **seminal vesicles** provide sperm with nutrients and other fluids that compose **semen.**

The vasa deferentia eventually connect each epididymis to the ejaculatory ducts, which pass through the prostate gland and empty into the urethra. The **prostate gland** contributes more fluids to the semen, including chemicals to aid the sperm in fertilizing an ovum, and neutralize the acidic environment of the vagina to make it more conducive to sperm motility (ability to move) and potency (potential for fertilizing an ovum).

Just below the prostate gland are two pea-shaped nodules called the **Cowper's glands.** The Cowper's glands secrete a fluid that lubricates the urethra and neutralizes any acid that may remain in the urethra after urination. Urine and semen do not come into contact with each other. During ejaculation of semen, a small valve closes off the tube to the urinary bladder.

Testosterone   The male sex hormone manufactured in the testes.

Spermatogenesis   The development of sperm.

Epididymis   A comma-shaped structure atop the testis where sperm mature.

Vas deferens   A tube that transports sperm toward the penis.

Seminal vesicles   Storage areas for sperm where nutrient fluids are added to them.

Semen   Fluid containing sperm and nutrient fluids that increase sperm viability and neutralize vaginal acid.

Prostate gland   Gland that secretes nutrients and neutralizing fluids into the semen.

Cowper's glands   Glands that secrete a fluid which lubricates the urethra and neutralizes any acid remaining in the urethra after urination.

Human Sexual Response

Human psychological traits greatly influence sexual response and sexual desire. Thus, we may find relationships with one partner vastly different from those we might experience with other partners.

Sexual response is a physiological process that generally follows a pattern. Laboratory research has delineated four stages within the response cycle, and researchers agree that each individual has a personal response pattern that may or may not conform to these phases. Both males' and females' sexual responses are somewhat arbitrarily divided into four stages: excitement/arousal, plateau, orgasm, and resolution. Regardless of the type of sexual activity (stimulation by a partner or self-stimulation), the response stages are the same.

During the first stage, *excitement/arousal,* male and female genital responses are caused by **vasocongestion,** or increased blood flow in the genital region. Increased blood flow to these organs causes them to swell. The vagina begins to lubricate in preparation for penile penetration, and the penis becomes partially erect. Both sexes may exhibit a "sex flush," or light blush all over their bodies. Excitement/arousal can be generated by touching other parts of the body, by kissing, through fantasy, by viewing films or videos, or by reading erotic literature.

During the *plateau phase,* the initial responses intensify. Voluntary and involuntary muscle tensions increase. The female's nipples and the male's penis become erect. A few drops of fluid, which may contain sperm, are secreted from the penis at this time. This fluid is termed *pre-ejaculatory fluid.*

During the *orgasmic phase,* vasocongestion and muscle tensions reach their peak, and rhythmic contractions occur through the genital regions. In females, these contractions are centered in the uterus, outer vagina, and anal sphincter. In males, the contractions occur in two stages. First, contractions within the prostate gland begin propelling semen through the urethra. In the second stage, the muscles of the pelvic floor, urethra, and anal sphincter contract. Semen usually, but not always, is ejaculated from the penis. In both sexes, spasms in other major muscle groups also occur, particularly in the buttocks and abdomen. Feet and hands may also contract, and facial features often contort.

Muscle tension and congested blood subside in the *resolution phase,* as the genital organs return to their pre-arousal states. Both sexes usually experience deep feelings of well-being and profound relaxation. Following orgasm and resolution, many females can become aroused again and experience additional orgasms. However, some men experience a *refractory period,* during which their systems are incapable of subsequent arousal. This refractory period may last from a few minutes to several hours. The length of the refractory period increases with age.

Men and women experience the same stages in the sexual response cycle; however, the length of time spent in any one stage varies. Thus, one partner may be in the plateau phase while the other is in the excitement or orgasmic phase. Such variations in response rates are entirely normal. Some couples believe that simultaneous orgasm is desirable for sexual satisfaction. Although simultaneous orgasm is pleasant, so are orgasms achieved at different times.

Sexual pleasure and satisfaction are also possible without orgasm or even intercourse. Expressing sexual feelings for another person involves many pleasurable activities, of which intercourse and orgasm may be only a part.

Expressing Your Sexuality

Finding healthy ways to express your sexuality is an important part of developing sexual maturity. Many avenues of sexual expression are available.

Sexual Orientation

Sexual orientation refers to a person's enduring emotional, romantic, sexual, or affectionate attraction to other persons. You may be primarily attracted to members of the other sex **(heterosexual),** your same sex **(homosexual),** or both sexes **(bisexual).** Homosexuality refers to emotional and sexual attachment to persons of the same sex. Many homosexuals prefer the terms *gay* and *lesbian* to describe their sexual orientations, as these terms go beyond the exclusively sexual connotation of the term *homosexual.* The term *gay* applies to both men and women, but *lesbian* refers only to women.

Bisexuality refers to emotional attachment and sexual attraction to members of both sexes. Bisexuals may face great social stigma because they are often ostracized by both homosexuals and heterosexuals. Little research has been done on this segment of the population, and many bisexuals remain hidden or closeted.

Throughout history, scientists and laypersons alike have debated the mental health status of gays and lesbians. In 1973, the American Psychiatric Association's board of trustees unanimously voted that homosexuality was not a

---

Vasocongestion   The engorgement of the genital organs with blood.

Sexual orientation   A person's enduring emotional, romantic, sexual, or affectionate attraction to other persons.

Heterosexual   Experiencing primary attraction to and preference for sexual activity with people of the other sex.

Homosexual   Experiencing primary attraction to and preference for sexual activity with people of the same sex.

Bisexual   Experiencing attraction to and preference for sexual activity with people of both sexes.

mental illness or psychiatric disorder. This position was affirmed by the American Psychological Association and the Sexuality Information and Education Council of the United States (SIECUS). Recently, the issue of homosexuality as a treatable "disease" has been resurrected. Therapies labeled as conversion or reparative therapies are being promoted in national newspapers and television ads. Mental health professionals have found these ads so troubling that the American Psychological Association passed a resolution reaffirming that homosexuality is *not* a disease in need of a "cure."[45]

Most researchers today agree that sexual orientation is best understood using a multifactorial model, which incorporates biological, psychological, and socioenvironmental factors.[46] Biological explanations focus on research into genetics, hormones (perinatal and postpubertal), and differences in brain anatomy, while psychological and socioenvironmental explanations examine parent–child interactions, sex roles, and early sexual and interpersonal interactions. Collectively, this growing body of research suggests that the origins of homosexuality, like heterosexuality, are complex. To diminish the complexity of sexual orientation to "a choice" is a clear misrepresentation of current research. Homosexuals do not "choose" their sexual orientation any more than heterosexuals do.

Irrational fear or hatred of homosexuality creates anti-gay prejudice and is expressed as **homophobia.** Homophobic behaviors range from avoiding hugging same-sex friends to name-calling and physical attacks. Herek and colleagues surveyed 2,259 gay and lesbian people and found that one in five women and one in four men had been victimized in the preceding five years because of their sexual orientation.[47]

> ### What do you think?
> *Why is sexual orientation so controversial in our society?* ❋ *Do you think homophobic behavior is increasing or decreasing? Explain your answer.* ❋ *What can you do to help prevent hate crimes?*

Sexual Behavior: What Is "Normal"?

Most of us want to fit in and be identified as normal, but how do we know which sexual behaviors are considered normal? What or whose criteria should we use? These are not easy questions.

Every society sets standards and attempts to regulate sexual behavior. Boundaries arise that distinguish good from bad, acceptable from unacceptable, and result in criteria used to establish what is viewed as normal or abnormal. Common sociocultural standards for sexual behavior in Western culture today include the following:

- *The heterosexual standard.* Sexual attraction should be limited to members of the other sex.
- *The coital standard.* Penile/vaginal intercourse (coitus) is viewed as the ultimate sex act.

- *The orgasmic standard.* All sexual interaction should lead to orgasm.
- *The two-person standard.* Sex is an activity to be experienced by two.
- *The romantic standard.* Sex should be related to love.
- *The safer sex standard.* If we choose to be sexually active, we should act to prevent unintended pregnancy or disease transmission.[48]

These are not laws or rules, but rather social scripts that have been adopted over time. Sexual standards often shift over time, and many people choose not to follow them. We are a pluralistic nation, and that pluralism extends to our sexual practices. Rather than making blanket judgments about normal versus abnormal, Kelly suggests we ask the following questions:[49]

- Is a sexual behavior healthy and fulfilling for a particular person?
- Is it safe?
- Does it lead to the exploitation of others?
- Does it take place between responsible, consenting adults?

In this way, we can view behavior along a continuum that takes into account many individual factors. As you read about the options for sexual expression in the pages ahead, use these questions to explore your feelings about what is normal for you.

Options for Sexual Expression

The range of human sexual expression is virtually infinite. What you find enjoyable may not be an option for someone else. The ways you choose to meet your sexual needs today may have been very different two weeks ago or two years from now. Accepting yourself as a sexual person with individual desires and preferences is the first step in achieving sexual satisfaction.

Celibacy   Celibacy is avoidance of or abstention from sexual activities with others. Some individuals choose celibacy for religious or moral reasons. Others may be celibate for a period of time because of illness, the breakup of a long-term relationship, or lack of an acceptable partner. For some, celibacy is a lonely, agonizing state, but others find it an opportunity for introspection, values assessment, and personal growth.

Autoerotic Behaviors   Autoerotic behaviors involve sexual self-stimulation. The two most common are sexual fantasy and masturbation.

Homophobia   Irrational hatred or fear of homosexuals or homosexuality.

Celibacy   State of not being involved in a sexual relationship.

Autoerotic behaviors   Sexual self-stimulation.

Sexual fantasies are sexually arousing thoughts and dreams. Fantasies may reflect real-life experiences, forbidden desires, or the opportunity to practice new or anticipated sexual experiences. The fact that you may fantasize about a particular sexual experience does not mean that you want to, or have to, act that experience out. Sexual fantasies are just that—fantasy.

Masturbation is self-stimulation of the genitals. Although many people feel uncomfortable discussing masturbation, it is a common sexual practice across the life span. Masturbation is a natural, pleasure-seeking behavior in infants and children. It is a valuable and important means for adolescent males and females, as well as adults, to explore sexual feelings and responsiveness.

Kissing and Erotic Touching Kissing and erotic touching are two very common forms of nonverbal sexual communication. Both males and females have **erogenous zones,** areas of the body that when touched lead to sexual arousal. Erogenous zones may include genital as well as nongenital areas, such as the earlobes, mouth, breasts, and inner thighs. Almost any area of the body can be conditioned to respond erotically to touch. Spending time with your partner to explore and learn about his or her erogenous areas is another pleasurable, safe, and satisfying means of sexual expression.

Oral–Genital Stimulation Cunnilingus is the term used for oral stimulation of a female's genitals, and **fellatio** refers to oral stimulation of a male's genitals. Many partners find oral–genital stimulation intensely pleasurable. Seventy percent of college-aged men and women have had oral sex.[50] For some people, oral sex is not an option because of moral or religious beliefs. It is necessary to remember that HIV and other sexually transmitted infections (STIs) can be transmitted via unprotected oral–genital sex as well as via intercourse. Use of an appropriate barrier device is strongly recommended if either partner's health status is in question.

Vaginal Intercourse The term *intercourse* generally refers to **vaginal intercourse,** or insertion of the penis into the vagina. *Coitus* is another term for vaginal intercourse, which is the most often practiced form of sexual expression. A great variety of positions can be used during coitus. Examples include the missionary position (man on top facing the woman), woman on top, side by side, or man behind (rear entry). Many partners enjoy experimenting with different positions. Knowledge of yourself and your body, along with your ability to communicate effectively, will play a large part in determining the enjoyment or meaning of intercourse for you and your partner. Whatever your circumstance, you should practice safer sex to avoid disease and unwanted pregnancy.

Anal Intercourse The anal area is highly sensitive to touch, and some couples find pleasure in the stimulation of this area. **Anal intercourse** is insertion of the penis into the anus. Sixteen percent of college-aged men and women have had anal sex.[51] Stimulation of the anus by mouth or with the fingers is also practiced. As with all forms of sexual expression, anal stimulation or intercourse is not for everyone. If you do enjoy this form of sexual expression, remember to use condoms to prevent disease transmission. Also, anything inserted into the anus should not be directly inserted into the vagina, as bacteria commonly found in the anus can cause vaginal infections.

Variant Sexual Behavior

Although attitudes toward sexuality have changed radically since the Victorian era, some people still believe that any sexual behavior other than heterosexual intercourse is abnormal or perverted. People who study sexuality prefer to use the neutral term **variant sexual behavior** to describe sexual behaviors that are not engaged in by most people. For example:

- *Group sex.* Sexual activity involving more than two people. Participants in group sex run a higher risk of exposure to AIDS and other sexually transmitted infections.
- *Transvestism.* Wearing the clothing of the opposite sex. Most transvestites are male, heterosexual, and married.
- *Transsexualism.* Strong identification with the opposite sex in which men or women feel that they are "trapped in the wrong body." In some cases, transsexuals undergo sex-change operations. Since the 1960s, 4,000 of these operations have been performed in the United States.
- *Fetishism.* Sexual arousal achieved by looking at or touching inanimate objects, such as underclothing or shoes.

Some variant sexual behaviors can be harmful to the individual, to others, or to both. Many of the following activities are illegal in at least some states:

- *Exhibitionism.* Exposing one's genitals to strangers in public places. Most exhibitionists are seeking a reaction of shock or fear from their victims. Exhibitionism is a minor felony in most states.

Sexual fantasies   Sexually arousing thoughts and dreams.

Masturbation   Self-stimulation of genitals.

Erogenous zones   Areas of the body of both males and females that, when touched, lead to sexual arousal.

Cunnilingus   Oral stimulation of a female's genitals.

Fellatio   Oral stimulation of a male's genitals.

Vaginal intercourse   The insertion of the penis into the vagina.

Anal intercourse   The insertion of the penis into the anus.

Variant sexual behavior   A sexual behavior that is not engaged in by most people.

- *Voyeurism.* Observing other people for sexual gratification. Most voyeurs are men who attempt to watch women undressing or bathing. Voyeurism is an invasion of privacy and illegal in most states.
- *Sadomasochism.* Sexual activities in which gratification is received by inflicting pain (verbal or physical abuse) on a partner or by being the object of such infliction. A sadist is a person who receives gratification from inflicting pain, and a masochist is a person who receives gratification from experiencing it.
- *Pedophilia.* Sexual activity or attraction between an adult and a child. Any sexual activity involving a minor, including possession of child pornography, is illegal.
- *Autoerotic asphyxiation.* The practice of reducing or eliminating oxygen to the brain, usually by tying a cord around one's neck while masturbating to orgasm. Tragically, asphyxiation is usually discovered when people accidentally hang themselves.

What do you think?

How does our society define "normal" sexual behavior? ✳ *What behaviors do you consider normal or abnormal?* ✳ *Do you consider your own preferred forms of sexual expression to be normal?* ✳ *Why are some people more open than others to trying a variety of sexual behaviors?*

Difficulties That Can Hinder Sexual Functioning

Research indicates that **sexual dysfunction,** the problems that can hinder sexual functioning, are quite common. Don't feel embarrassed if you experience sexual dysfunction at some point in your life. The sexual part of you does not come with a lifetime warranty. You can have breakdowns involving your sexual function just as you can have breakdowns in any of your other body systems. Sexual dysfunction can be divided into four major classes: disorders of sexual desire, sexual arousal, orgasm, and sexual pain. All of them can be treated successfully.

Sexual Desire Disorders

The most frequent reason why people seek out a sex therapist is **ISD,** or **inhibited sexual desire.**[52] ISD is the lack of a sexual appetite or simply a lack of interest and pleasure in sexual activity. In some instances, it can result from stress or boredom with sex. **Sexual aversion disorder** is another type of desire dysfunction, characterized by sexual phobias (unreasonable fears) and anxiety about sexual contact. The psychological stress of a punitive upbringing, a rigid religious background, or a history of physical or sexual abuse may be sources of these desire disorders.

Sexual Arousal Disorders

The most common disorder in this category is erectile dysfunction. **Erectile dysfunction,** or **impotence,** is difficulty in achieving or maintaining a penile erection sufficient for intercourse. At some time in his life, every man experiences impotence. Causes are varied and include underlying diseases, such as diabetes or prostate problems; reactions to some medications (for example, medication for high blood pressure); depression; fatigue; stress; alcohol; performance anxiety; and guilt over real or imaginary problems (such as when a man compares himself to his partner's past lovers).

Some 30 million men in this country, half of them under age 65, suffer from impotence. Impotence generally becomes more of a problem as men age, affecting one in four men over the age of 65. Recently the FDA approved the drug Viagra (sildenafil citrate) to treat impotence. Response to the drug's release was record breaking. Taken by mouth one hour before sexual activity, Viagra was reported to manage erectile dysfunction successfully in 60 to 80 percent of cases during clinical trials.[53] The medication is not, however, without risk. The most commonly reported side effects include headache, flushing, stomachache, urinary tract infection, diarrhea, dizziness, rash, and mild and temporary visual changes. In addition, there have been several reported deaths in the United States among Viagra users, prompting more caution in prescribing it to patients with known cardiovascular disease and those taking commonly prescribed short- and long-acting nitrates, such as nitroglycerin.[54]

Orgasm Disorders

Premature ejaculation affects up to 50 percent of the male population at some time in their lives. **Premature ejaculation** is ejaculation that occurs prior to or very soon after the insertion of the penis into the vagina. Treatment for premature ejaculation involves a physical examination to rule out organic causes. If the cause of the problem is not physiological,

Sexual dysfunction   Problems associated with achieving sexual satisfaction.

Inhibited sexual desire (ISD)   Lack of sexual appetite or simply a lack of interest and pleasure in sexual activity.

Sexual aversion disorder   Type of desire dysfunction characterized by sexual phobias and anxiety about sexual contact.

Erectile dysfunction (impotence)   Difficulty in achieving or maintaining a penile erection sufficient for intercourse.

Premature ejaculation   Ejaculation that occurs prior to or almost immediately following penile penetration of the vagina.

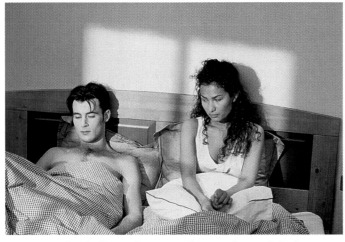

Recent studies indicate that some degree of sexual dysfunction is much more common than once thought. New treatments, such as Viagra, have helped many couples regain satisfying sexual relationships.

therapy is available to help a man learn how to control the timing of his ejaculation. Fatigue, stress, performance pressure, and alcohol use can all be contributing factors to orgasmic disorders in men.

In a woman, the inability to achieve orgasm is termed **female orgasmic disorder.** A woman with this disorder often blames herself and learns to fake orgasm to avoid embarrassment or preserve her partner's ego. Contributing to this response are the messages women have historically been given about sex as a duty rather than a pleasurable act for both parties. As with men who experience orgasmic disorders, the first step in treatment is a physical exam to rule out organic causes. However, the problem is often solved by simple self-exploration to learn more about what forms of stimulation are arousing enough to produce orgasm.

Masturbation is usually a primary focus in teaching a woman to become orgasmic. Through masturbation, a woman can learn how her body responds sexually to various types of touch. Once a woman has become orgasmic through masturbation, she learns to communicate her needs to her partner.

Female orgasmic disorder   A woman's inability to achieve orgasm.

Dyspareunia   Pain experienced by women during intercourse.

Vaginismus   A state in which the vaginal muscles contract so forcefully that penetration cannot be accomplished.

Rohypnol ("roofies," "rope," "forget pill")   A drug that is used in combination with alcohol to facilitate date rape by making a woman unaware of what is happening to her.

Sexual Pain Disorders

Two common disorders in this category are dyspareunia and vaginismus. **Dyspareunia** is pain experienced by a female during intercourse. This pain may be caused by diseases such as endometriosis, uterine tumors, chlamydia, gonorrhea, or urinary tract infections. Damage to tissues during childbirth and insufficient lubrication during intercourse may also cause discomfort. Dyspareunia can also be psychological in origin. As with other problems, dyspareunia can be treated with good results.

Vaginismus is the involuntary contraction of vaginal muscles, making penile insertion painful or impossible. Most cases of vaginismus are related to fear of intercourse or to unresolved sexual conflicts. Treatment involves teaching a woman to achieve orgasm through nonvaginal stimulation.

Seeking Help for Sexual Dysfunction

Many theories and treatment models can help people with sexual dysfunction. A first important step is choosing a qualified sex therapist or counselor. A national organization, the American Association of Sex Educators, Counselors, and Therapists (AASECT) has been in the forefront of establishing criteria for certifying sex therapists. These criteria include appropriate degree(s) in the helping professions, specialized coursework in human sexuality, and sufficient hours of practical therapy work under the direct supervision of a certified sex therapist. Lists of certified counselors and sex therapists, as well as clinics that treat sexual dysfunctions, can be obtained by contacting AASECT or SIECUS.

Drugs and Sex

Because psychoactive drugs affect the entire physiology, it is only logical that they affect sexual behavior. Promises of increased pleasure make drugs very tempting to those seeking greater sexual satisfaction. Too often, however, drugs become central to sexual activities and damage the relationship.

Alcohol is notorious for reducing inhibitions and promoting feelings of well-being and desirability. At the same time, alcohol inhibits sexual response; thus, the mind may be willing, but not the body.

Perhaps the greatest danger associated with use of drugs during sex is the tendency to blame the drug for negative behavior. "I can't help what I did last night because I was drunk" is a response that demonstrates sexual immaturity. A sexually mature person carefully examines risks and benefits and makes decisions accordingly. If drugs are necessary to increase erotic feelings, it is likely that the partners are being dishonest about their feelings for each other. Good sex should not depend on chemical substances.

Of growing concern in recent years is the increased use of "date rape drugs." These have become popular among college students and are often used in combination with alcohol.[55] Both **Rohypnol** ("roofies," "rope," "forget pill") and

GHB, or **gamma-hydroxybutrane** ("Liquid X," "Grievous Bodily Harm," "Easy Lay," "Mickey Finn") have been used to facilitate rape. The dangers of these drugs are discussed in more detail in Chapter 7.

> **What do you think?**
>
> *Why do we find it so difficult to discuss sexual dysfunction in our society?* ✳ *Do you think it is more difficult for men than for women to talk about dysfunction?* ✳ *Have you ever used alcohol or some other drug to enhance your sexual performance?* ✳ *Why are "date rape drugs" a major concern on college campuses?*

Being a sexually healthy adult is a process that requires a commitment to the ongoing assessment of your sexual attitudes and values, your relationships with others, your sexual actions, your communication skills, and all the new information to which you are exposed on a daily basis. Your challenge is to grow as you develop new skills and become more confident with your sexuality. Use the following questions to check your progress.

Gamma-hydroxybutrane (GHB) A "date rape drug" used in combination with alcohol to facilitate rape by making a woman unaware of what is happening to her.

Taking Charge

Managing Your Relationships and Sexual Behavior

Checklist for Change

Making Personal Choices

✓ What relationships are most important to you? How have these relationships affected your relationships with others?

✓ What positive things do you bring to a relationship?

✓ What do you expect in a long-term relationship? What behaviors would you consider acceptable and unacceptable in your committed partner?

✓ Do you feel comfortable with yourself sexually? Do you know the function and location of the structures that make up the male and female sexual anatomy?

✓ Make a list of the gender roles you have adopted to date. Do you feel limited or bound by any gender-role stereotypes? How might you change them?

✓ Do you know what your options are for expressing your sexuality? Have you reviewed the options and identified those you may be willing to try?

✓ Do you need to work on developing any new skills that will help you reach your goals regarding your sexual self?

Making Community Choices

✓ Do you reach out to friends who are having problems in their relationships?

✓ Do you try to work through your problems with others, or do you avoid problems?

✓ Have you taken the time to become informed about sexual issues and concerns in your community?

✓ What is your community's stand on sex education in the schools?

✓ Do you know what community resources are available to help people with questions about sexuality-related issues?

Summary

✳ Intimate relationships have several different characteristics, including behavioral interdependence, need fulfillment, emotional attachment, and emotional availability. These characteristics influence how we interact with others and the types of intimate relationships we form. Family, friends, and partners or lovers provide the most

common opportunities for intimacy. Each relationship may include healthy and unhealthy characteristics that may affect daily functioning.

✳ Gender differences in communication include conversation styles as well as differences in sharing feelings and disclosing personal facts and fears. These differences explain why men and women may relate differently in intimate relationships. Understanding these differences and learning how to deal with them are important aspects of healthy relationships.

✳ Barriers to intimacy often include the different emotional needs of both partners, jealousy, and emotional wounds that could result from being raised in a dysfunctional family.

✳ Commitment is an important ingredient in successful relationships for most people. The major types of committed relationships are marriage, cohabitation, and gay and lesbian partnerships.

✳ Success in committed relationships requires understanding the roles of partnering scripts, the importance of self-nurturance, and the elements of a good relationship.

✳ Deciding whether to marry or remain single or whether to have children requires serious consideration. Remaining single is more common than ever before. Most single people lead healthy, happy, and well-adjusted lives. Those who decide to have or not to have children can also lead rewarding, productive lives as long as they have given this decision the utmost thought, weighing the pros and cons of each alternative in the context of their lifestyle. Today's family structure may look different from that of previous generations, but love, trust, and commitment to a child's welfare continue to be the cornerstones of successful childrearing.

✳ Before relationships fail, often many warning signs appear. By recognizing these signs and taking action to change behaviors, partners may save and enhance their relationships.

✳ Sexual identity is determined by a complex interaction of genetic, physiological, and environmental factors. Biological sex, gender identity, gender roles, and sexual orientation are all blended into our sexual identity.

✳ The major components of the female sexual anatomy include the mons pubis, labia minora and majora, clitoris, urethral and vaginal openings, vagina, cervix, fallopian tubes, and ovaries. The major components of the male sexual anatomy are the penis, scrotum, testes, epididymides, vasa deferentia, ejaculatory ducts, and urethra.

✳ Physiologically, males and females experience four phases of sexual response: excitement/arousal, plateau, orgasm, and resolution.

✳ Humans can express their sexual selves in a variety of ways, including celibacy, autoerotic behaviors, kissing and erotic touch, oral–genital stimulation, vaginal intercourse, and anal intercourse. Sexual orientation refers to a person's enduring emotional, romantic, sexual, or affectionate attraction to other persons. Irrational hatred or fear of homosexuality or gay and lesbian persons is termed *homophobia*.

✳ Sexual dysfunctions can be classified into sexual desire disorders, sexual arousal disorders, orgasm disorders, and sexual pain disorders. Drug use can also lead to sexual dysfunction.

Discussion Questions

1. What are the characteristics of intimate relationships? What are behavioral interdependence, need fulfillment, emotional attachment, and emotional availability, and why is each important in relationship development?

2. Why are relationships with family important? Explain how your family unit was similar to or different from the traditional family unit in early America. Who made up your family of origin? Your nuclear family?

3. How can you tell the difference between a love relationship and one that is based primarily on attraction? What characteristics do love relationships share?

4. What problems can form barriers to intimacy? What actions can you take to reduce or remove these barriers?

5. What are common elements of good relationships? What are some common warning signs of trouble? What actions can you take to improve your own interpersonal relationships?

6. Name some common misconceptions about people who choose to remain single and about couples who choose not to have children. Do you want to have children? Why or why not? What characteristics show that a couple is ready to have children?

7. How have gender roles changed over the past 20 years? Do you view the changes as positive for both men and women?

8. Discuss the cycle of changes that occurs in our bodies in response to various hormones (e.g., sexual differentiation while in the womb, development of secondary sex characteristics at puberty, menopause).

9. What is "normal" sexual behavior? What criteria should we use to determine healthful sexual practice?

10. If scientists finally establish the combination of factors that interact to produce homosexual, heterosexual, or bisexual orientation, will that put an end to antigay prejudice? Why or why not?

11. How can we remove the stigma that surrounds sexual dysfunction so that individuals feel more open to seeking help? Are men and women impacted differently by sexual dysfunction?

Application Exercises

Reread the What Do You Think? scenario at the beginning of the chapter, and answer the following questions.

1. From what sources might Bob and Kathy be getting information that would lead them to question whether their sexual behaviors are normal?

2. Is there a "golden" standard for sexual behavior that fits all people and all situations? Explain your answer.

3. If Kathy and Bob are comfortable and satisfied with their current sexual behaviors, are they therefore normal?

4. What difficulties do people who wish to remain single experience in America today? Do you think its easier to remain single than it was in previous generations? Why or why not?

Accessing Your Health on the Internet `http`

Visit the following Internet sites to explore further topics and issues related to personal health. To visit an organization's website, go to the Companion Website for *Health: The Basics, Fifth Edition* at www.aw.com/donatelle, click on the book image, and select "Accessing Your Health on the Internet" from the navigation menu on the left.

1. ***Couples National Network.*** Link into a network for same-gender couples and singles, with resources about gay and lesbian issues.
2. ***University of Missouri Counseling Center Self-Help Area.*** Provides a bibliography on books and other resources on issues dealing with intimacy.
3. ***Mental Health Notes.*** User-friendly information about dysfunctional families from a licensed clinical psychologist. Includes links to related mental health articles.
4. ***ANWeb Resources—Peace and Conflict Resolution.*** Provides links to numerous sites dealing with conflict resolution.
5. ***Relationship Growth Online.*** Provides information, quizzes, games, advice, and links to more information on how to build better relationships.
6. ***Sexuality Information and Education Council of the United States (SIECUS).*** Information, guidelines, and materials for advancement of healthy and proper sex education.
7. ***American Association of Sex Educators, Counselors, and Therapists (AASECT).*** Professional organization providing standards of practice for treatment of sexual issues and disorders.
8. ***Go Ask Alice.*** An interactive question and answer line out of the Columbia University Health Services. "Alice" is available to answer questions each week about any health-related issues, including relationships, nutrition and diet, exercise, drugs, sex, alcohol, and stress.

Further Reading

Annual Editions. *Human Sexuality.* Guilford, CT: DPG/McGraw-Hill, 2001.
> *A volume of current articles covering a wide variety of topics in human sexuality; updated annually.*

Bullough, B., V. L. Bullough, and J. Elias. *Gender Blending.* Amherst, NY: Prometheus Books, 1997.
> *Every topic imaginable on gender and challenges to gender roles: transvestism, transsexualism, laws, etc.*

Chudacoff, H. P. *The Age of the Bachelor: Creating an American Culture.* Princeton, NJ: Princeton University Press, 1999.
> *Historical and sociological overview of what it means to be single and male in America.*

Galvin, K., and P. Cooper. *Making Connections.* Los Angeles: Roxbury Publishing, 2000.
> *Outstanding overview of the importance of interpersonal communication in everyday lives. Provides practical strategies to assist us at all stages of life.*

Gray, J. *Men Are from Mars, Women Are from Venus: A Practical Guide for Improving Communication and Getting What You Want in Your Relationships.* San Francisco: HarperCollins, 1998.
> *Overview of male and female communication styles and practical strategies for improving relationships. Available as both audiocassette and book.*

Koman, A. *How to Mend a Broken Heart: Letting Go and Moving On.* Chicago: Contemporary Books, 1997.
> *A step-by-step program for dealing with the end of a relationship, including working through the emotional stages, strategies for coping, and gaining strength to move on.*

SIECUS (Sexuality Information and Education Council of the United States) Report. A bimonthly journal. 130 West 42nd Street, New York, NY 10036.
> *Highly acclaimed and readable journal. Includes timely and thought-provoking articles on human sexuality, sexuality education, and AIDS.*

6

Birth Control, Pregnancy, and Childbirth

MANAGING YOUR FERTILITY

objectives

* List the different types of contraceptive methods, and discuss their effectiveness in preventing pregnancy and sexually transmitted infections.

* Summarize the legal decisions surrounding abortion and the various types of abortion procedures used today.

* Discuss some of the key issues to consider when planning a pregnancy.

* Explain the importance of prenatal care and the physical and emotional aspects of pregnancy.

* Describe the basic stages of childbirth, methods of managing childbirth, and the complications that can arise during labor and delivery.

* Review some of the primary causes of and possible solutions to infertility.

What do you think?

For the fourth time this year, Brittany is visiting her campus health service for emergency contraception. Her health care provider expressed concern that Brittany may be using emergency contraception for birth control instead of one of the many other contraceptive choices available to her. Brittany won't talk about the subject, nor will she agree to use a contraceptive such as the pill, Norplant, or an IUD.

Should limitations be placed on the dispensing of emergency contraception? ✱ *If so, what limitations would you propose?* ✱ *What would be the dangers of using this as one's sole method of contraception?* ✱ *Should a college health service offer access to emergency contraception?* ✱ *Should Brittany ask her partner to use a condom?*

Today, we not only understand the intimate details of reproduction but also possess technologies that can control or enhance our **fertility.** Along with information and technological advance comes choice, and choice goes hand in hand with responsibility. Choosing whether and when to have children is one of our greatest responsibilities. A woman and her partner have much to consider before planning or risking a pregnancy. Children, whether planned or unplanned, change people's lives. They require a lifelong personal commitment of love and nurturing.

Before you plan or risk a pregnancy, you have the responsibility to make certain you are physically, emotionally, and financially prepared to care for another human being. One measure of maturity is the ability to discuss reproduction and birth control with one's sexual partner before succumbing to sexual urges. Men often assume that their partners are taking care of birth control. Women often feel that bringing up the subject implies they are "easy" or "loose." Both may feel that this discussion interferes with romance and spontaneity. You will find embarrassment-free discussion a lot easier if you understand human reproduction and contraception and honestly consider your attitudes toward these matters before you find yourself in a compromising situation.

offer varying degrees of control over when and whether pregnancies occur. However, since people first associated sexual activity with pregnancy, society has searched for a simple, infallible, and risk-free way to prevent pregnancy. We have not yet found one.

To evaluate the effectiveness of a particular contraceptive method, you must be familiar with two concepts: perfect failure rate and typical use failure rate. *Perfect failure rate* refers to the number of pregnancies that are likely to occur in a year (per 100 uses of the method during sexual intercourse) if the method is used absolutely perfectly, that is, without any error. The *typical use failure rate* refers to the number of pregnancies that are likely to occur with typical use, that is, with the normal number of errors, memory lapses, and incorrect or incomplete use. This information is much more practical for people in helping them make informed decisions about contraceptive methods. See Table 6.1 to find ratings of various contraceptive methods. Many will be discussed in this chapter.

Many contraceptive methods can also protect, at least to some degree, against **sexually transmitted infections (STIs).** This is an important factor to consider in choosing a contraceptive. Table 6.2 compares the level of STI protection offered by various contraceptives.

Present methods of contraception fall into several categories. **Barrier methods** use a physical or chemical block to prevent the egg and sperm from joining. Hormonal methods

Methods of Fertility Management

Conception refers to the fertilization of an ovum by a sperm. The sperm enters the ovum. Its tail breaks off, and a protective chemical barrier secreted by the ovum surrounds the sperm and prevents other sperm from entering. The following conditions are necessary for conception:

1. A viable egg
2. A viable sperm
3. Possible access to the egg by the sperm

The term **contraception** (sometimes called *birth control*) refers to methods of preventing conception. These methods

---

Fertility   A person's ability to reproduce.

Conception   The fertilization of an ovum by a sperm.

Contraception   Methods of preventing conception.

Sexually transmitted infections (STIs)   A variety of infections that can be acquired through sexual contact.

Barrier methods   Contraceptive methods that block the meeting of egg and sperm by means of a physical barrier (e.g., condom, diaphragm, or cervical cap), a chemical barrier (e.g., spermicide), or both.

Table 6.1
Failure Rates of Various Contraceptions

METHOD	Percentage of Women Experiencing an Unintended Pregnancy Within the First Year of Use		% OF WOMEN CONTINUING USE AT ONE YEAR[3]
	TYPICAL USE[1]	PERFECT USE[2]	
Chance[4]	85	85	40
Spermicides[5]	26	6	63
Periodic abstinence	25		
Calendar		9	
Ovulation method		3	
Symptothermal[6]		2	
Post-ovulation		1	
Cap[7]			
Parous women (1 or more children)	40	26	42
Nulliparous women (no children)	20	9	56
Sponge			
Parous women	40	20	42
Nulliparous women	20	9	56
Diaphragm[7]	20	6	56
Withdrawal	19	4	
Condom[8]			
Female (Reality)	21	5	56
Male	14	3	61
Pill	5		71
Progestin only		0.5	
Combined		0.1	
IUD			
Progesterone T	2.0	1.5	81
Copper T 380A	0.8	0.6	78
LNg 20	0.1	0.1	81
Depo-Provera	0.3	0.3	70
Norplant and Norplant-2	0.05	0.05	88
Female sterilization	0.5	0.5	100
Male sterilization	0.15	0.10	100

Emergency Contraceptive Pills: Treatment initiated within 72 hours after unprotected intercourse reduces the risk of pregnancy by at least 75%.[9]

Lactational Amenorrhea Method: LAM is a highly effective, *temporary* method of contraception.[10]

[1]Among *typical* couples who initiate use of a method (not necessarily for the first time), the percentage who experience an accidental pregnancy during the first year if they do not stop use for any other reason.

[2]Among couples who initiate use of a method (not necessarily for the first time) and who use it perfectly (both consistently and correctly), the percentage who experience an accidental pregnancy during the first year if they do not stop use for any other reason.

[3]Among couples attempting to avoid pregnancy, the percentage who continue to use a method for 1 year.

[4]The percentages becoming pregnant in columns (2) and (3) are based on data from populations where contraception is not used and from women who cease using contraception in order to become pregnant. Among such populations, about 89% become pregnant within 1 year. This estimate was lowered slightly (to 85%) to represent the percentages who would become pregnant within 1 year among women now relying on reversible methods of contraception if they abandoned contraception altogether.

[5]Foams, creams, gels, vaginal suppositories, and vaginal film.

[6]Cervical mucus (ovulation) method supplemented by calendar in the pre-ovulatory and basal body temperature in the post-ovulatory phases.

[7]With spermicidal cream or jelly.

[8]Without spermicides.

[9]The treatment schedule is one dose within 72 hours after unprotected intercourse, and a second dose 12 hours after the first dose. The Food and Drug Administration has declared the following brands of oral contraceptives to be safe and effective for emergency contraception: Ovral (1 dose is 2 white pills), Alesse (1 dose is 5 pink pills), Nordette or Levlen (1 dose is 4 light-orange pills), Lo/Ovral (1 dose is 4 white pills), Triphasil or Tri-Levlen (1 dose is 4 yellow pills).

[10]However, to maintain effective protection against pregnancy, another method of contraception must be used as soon as menstruation resumes, the frequency or duration of breast-feeds is reduced, bottle feeds are introduced, or the baby reaches 6 months of age.

Source: R. Hatcher et al., *Contraceptive Technology,* 17th rev. ed. (New York: Ardent Media, Inc., 1998), 216, citing update of Trussell and Kost (1987) and Trussell et al. (1990c). See Chapter 31.

Table 6.2
Contraceptives and Protection Against Sexually Transmitted Infections

CONTRACEPTIVE METHOD	STI PROTECTION
Latex male condom	Excellent (if used correctly)
Female condom	Good
IUD	None
Pill/Norplant/Depo-Provera	None
Diaphragm/cervical cap	It may protect against STIs, but not HIV.
Abstinence	Excellent (if all activities involving fluid exchange are avoided)
Sterilization	None
Spermicides	Minimal
Fertility awareness methods	None

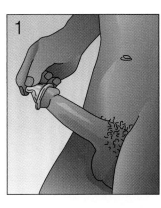 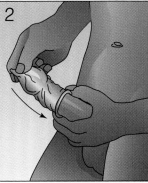

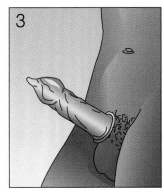 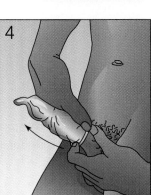

Figure 6.1
How to Use a Condom
The condom should be rolled over the erect penis before any penetration occurs. A small space (about $\frac{1}{2}$ inch) should be left at the end of the condom to collect the semen after ejaculation. Hold the tip of the condom, and unroll it all the way to the base of the penis. Hold the base of the condom before withdrawal to avoid spilling any semen.

ception may involve temporary or permanent abstinence, or planning intercourse in accordance with fertility patterns. (See the accompanying box, Assess Yourself.)

Barrier Methods

The Condom   The **condom** is a strong sheath of latex rubber or other material designed to fit over an erect penis. The condom catches the ejaculate, thereby preventing sperm from migrating toward the egg. It is the only temporary means of birth control available for men and the only barrier that effectively prevents the spread of STIs and HIV. Condoms come in a wide variety of styles: colored, ribbed for "extra sensation," lubricated, nonlubricated, and with or without reservoirs at the tip. All may be purchased with or without spermicide in pharmacies, in some supermarkets and public bathrooms, and in many health clinics. A new condom must be used for each act of intercourse or oral sex.

In addition to helping to prevent some sexually transmitted infections, including genital herpes and HIV, condoms may also slow or reduce the development of cervical abnormalities in women that can lead to cancer. A condom must be rolled onto the penis before the penis touches the vagina, and held in place when removing the penis from the vagina after ejaculation (Figure 6.1). For greatest efficacy, condoms should be used with a spermicide containing nonoxynol-9, the same agent found in many of the contraceptive foams and creams that women use. If necessary or desired, users can lubricate their own condoms with contraceptive foams, creams, and jellies or other water-based lubricants, such as

introduce synthetic hormones into the woman's system that prevent ovulation, thicken cervical mucus, or prevent a fertilized egg from implanting. Surgical methods can be used to permanently prevent pregnancy. Other methods of contra-

Condom   A single-use sheath of thin latex or other material designed to fit over an erect penis and to catch semen upon ejaculation.

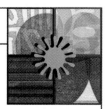

Contraceptive Comfort and Confidence Scale

The following series of questions is designed to help you assess whether the method of contraception you are using or may consider using in the future is or will be effective for you. Most individuals will have a few yes answers. Yes answers predict potential problems. If you have more than a few yes responses, you may want to talk to a health care provider, counselor, partner, or friend to decide whether to use this method or how to use it so that it will really be effective. In general, the more yes answers you have, the less likely you are to use this method consistently and correctly with every act of intercourse.

Method of contraception you are considering   _____

Answer yes or no to the following questions:

_____	1. Have I ever had problems using this method?
_____	2. Have I ever become pregnant while using this method?
_____	3. Am I afraid of using this method?
_____	4. Would I really rather not use this method?
_____	5. Will I have trouble remembering to use this method?
_____	6. Will I have trouble using this method correctly?
_____	7. Do I still have unanswered questions about this method?
_____	8. Does this method make menstrual periods longer or more painful?
_____	9. Does this method cost more than I can afford?
_____	10. Could this method cause serious complications?
_____	11. Am I opposed to this method because of any religious or moral beliefs?

Length of time you used this method in the past   _____

_____	12. Is my partner opposed to this method?
_____	13. Am I using this method without my partner's knowledge?
_____	14. Will using this method embarrass my partner?
_____	15. Will using this method embarrass me?
_____	16. Will I enjoy intercourse less because of this method?
_____	17. If this method interrupts lovemaking, will I avoid using it?
_____	18. Has a nurse or doctor ever told me not to use this method?
_____	19. Is there anything about my personality that could lead me to use this method incorrectly?
_____	20. Am I at risk of being exposed to HIV (the AIDS virus) or other sexually transmitted infections if I use this method?

_____ Total number of yes answers

Source: From R. A. Hatcher et al., *Contraceptive Technology,* 17th ed. (New York: Ardent Media, 1998), p. 238.

K-Y jelly, ForPlay Lubricants, Astroglide, or Wet or Aqua Lube, to name just a few. However, never use with a condom products such as baby oil, cold cream, petroleum jelly, vaginal yeast infection medications, or hand and body lotion. These products contain mineral oil and will make the latex begin to disintegrate within 60 seconds.

Condoms are less effective and more likely to break during intercourse if they are old or poorly stored. To maintain effectiveness, store them in a cool place (not in a wallet or hip pocket), and inspect them for small tears before use.

For some people, a condom ruins the spontaneity of sex. Stopping to put it on breaks the mood for them. Others report that the condom decreases sensation. These inconveniences contribute to improper use of the device. Couples who learn to put the condom on together as foreplay are generally more successful with this form of birth control.[1]

Foams, Suppositories, Jellies, and Creams Jellies, creams, suppositories, and foam, like condoms, do not require a prescription. Chemically, they are referred to as spermicides—substances designed to kill sperm. Foams, suppositories, jellies, and creams usually contain nonoxynol-9, a detergent believed also to be effective in killing viruses, bacteria, and other organisms. Although they are not recommended as the primary form of contraception, spermicides are often recommended for use with other forms of contraception. Though they help prevent the spread of certain STIs, they are most effective when used in conjunction with a condom.

Jellies and creams are packaged in tubes, and foams are available in aerosol cans. All have tubes designed for insertion into the vagina. They must be inserted far enough to cover the cervix, providing both a chemical barrier that kills sperm and a physical barrier that stops sperm from continuing toward an egg.

Suppositories are waxy capsules that are inserted deep in the vagina, where they melt. They must be inserted 10 to 20 minutes before intercourse to have time to melt but no longer than one hour prior to intercourse; otherwise, they lose their effectiveness. Additional contraceptive chemicals must be applied for each subsequent act of intercourse (Figure 6.2.).

The Female Condom The **female condom** is a single-use, soft, loose-fitting polyurethane sheath meant for internal use by women. It is designed as one unit with two diaphragm-like rings. One ring, which lies inside the sheath, serves as an insertion mechanism and internal anchor. The other ring, which 1remains outside the vagina once the device is inserted, protects the labia and the base of the penis from infection. Many women like the female condom because it gives them more control over reproduction than does the male condom. When used correctly, the female condom provides protection against HIV and STIs comparable to that of a latex male condom.

The Diaphragm, with Spermicidal Jelly or Cream Invented in the mid-nineteenth century, the **diaphragm** was the first widely used birth control method for women.

The diaphragm is a soft, shallow cup made of thin latex rubber. Its flexible, rubber-coated ring is designed to fit snugly behind the pubic bone in front of the cervix and over the back of the cervix on the other side. Diaphragms are manufactured in different sizes and must be fitted to the woman by a trained practitioner. The practitioner should also be certain that the user knows how to insert her diaphragm correctly before she leaves the practitioner's office.

Diaphragms must be used with spermicidal cream or jelly, which is applied to the inside of the diaphragm before insertion. The diaphragm holds the spermicide in place, creating a physical and chemical barrier against sperm. Additional spermicide must be applied before each subsequent act of intercourse, and the diaphragm must be left in place for six to eight hours after intercourse to allow the chemical to kill any sperm remaining in the vagina. When used with spermicidal jelly or cream, it offers significant protection against gonorrhea and possibly chlamydia and human papilloma virus (HPV) (Figure 6.3).

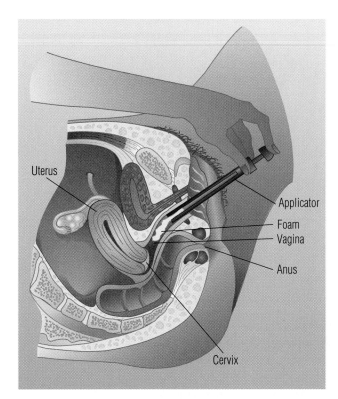

Figure 6.2
The Proper Method of Applying Spermicide Within the Vagina

Using the diaphragm during the menstrual period or leaving it in place beyond the recommended time slightly increases the user's risk of developing **toxic shock syndrome (TSS)**. This condition results from the multiplication of bacteria that spread to the bloodstream and cause sudden high fever, rash, nausea, vomiting, diarrhea, and a rapid drop in blood pressure. If not treated, TSS can be fatal. The diaphragm (as well as tampons left too long in place) creates conditions conducive to the growth of these bacteria. To reduce the risk of TSS, women should wash their hands carefully with soap and water before inserting or removing the diaphragm.

Spermicides Substances designed to kill sperm.

Female condom A single-use polyurethane sheath for internal use by women.

Diaphragm A latex, saucer-shaped device designed to cover the cervix and block access to the uterus; should always be used with spermicide.

Toxic shock syndrome (TSS) A potentially life-threatening disease that occurs when specific bacterial toxins are allowed to multiply unchecked in wounds or through improper use of tampons or diaphragms.

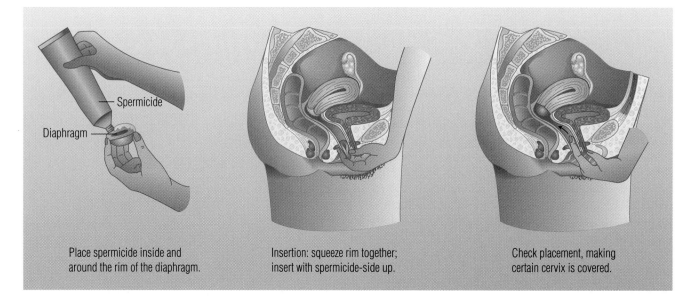

| Place spermicide inside and around the rim of the diaphragm. | Insertion: squeeze rim together; insert with spermicide-side up. | Check placement, making certain cervix is covered. |

Figure 6.3
The Proper Use and Placement of a Diaphragm

Another problem with the diaphragm is that it can put undue pressure on the urethra, blocking urinary flow and predisposing the user to bladder infections. A further disadvantage is that inserting the device can be awkward, especially if the woman is rushed. When inserted incorrectly, diaphragms are much less effective.

The Cervical Cap   One of the oldest methods used to prevent pregnancy, early cervical caps were made from beeswax, silver, or copper.

Today's **cervical cap** is a small cup made of latex that fits snugly over the entire cervix. It must be fitted by a practitioner and is designed for use with contraceptive jelly or cream. It is somewhat more difficult to insert than a diaphragm because of its smaller size.

The cap keeps sperm out of the uterus. It is held in place by suction created during application. Insertion may take place anywhere up to two days prior to intercourse, and the device must be left in place for six to eight hours after intercourse. The maximum length of time the cap can be left on the cervix is 48 hours. If removed and cleaned, it can be reinserted immediately. The cervical cap may offer protection against STIs but not HIV.

Cervical cap   A small cup made of latex that is designed to fit snugly over the entire cervix.

Oral contraceptives   Pills taken daily for three weeks of the menstrual cycle that prevent ovulation by regulating hormones.

Some women report unpleasant vaginal odors after use. Because the device can become dislodged during intercourse, placement must be checked frequently. It cannot be used during the menstrual period or for longer than 48 hours because of the risk of toxic shock syndrome.

Hormonal Methods

Oral Contraceptives   **Oral contraceptive** pills were first marketed in the United States in 1960. Their convenience quickly made them the most widely used reversible method of fertility control.

Most oral contraceptives work through the combined effects of synthetic estrogen and progesterone. Because the levels of estrogen in the pill are higher than those produced by the body, the pituitary gland is never signaled to produce follicle-stimulating hormone (FSH), without which ova will not develop in the ovaries. Progesterone in the pill prevents proper growth of the uterine lining and thickens the cervical mucus, forming a barrier against sperm.

Pills are meant to be taken in a cycle. At the end of each three-week cycle, the user discontinues the drug or takes a placebo pill for one week. The resultant drop in hormones causes the uterine lining to disintegrate, and the user will have a menstrual period, usually within one to three days. The same cycle is repeated every 28 days. Menstrual flow is generally lighter than it is for women who don't use the pill because the hormones in the pill prevent thick endometrial buildup.

Today's pill is different from the one introduced more than four decades ago. The original pill contained large amounts of estrogen, which caused certain risks for the user, whereas the current pill contains the minimal amount of estrogen necessary to prevent pregnancy.

Because the chemicals in oral contraceptives change the way the body metabolizes certain nutrients, all women using the pill should check with their prescribing practitioners regarding dietary supplements. The nutrients of concern include vitamin C and the B-complex vitamins—B_2, B_6, and B_{12}. A nutritious diet that includes whole grains, fresh fruits and vegetables, lean meats, fish and poultry, and nonfat dairy products is important.

Oral contraceptives can interact negatively with other drugs. For example, some antibiotics diminish the pill's effectiveness and may require an adjustment in dosage. Women in doubt should check with their prescribing practitioners or their pharmacists.

Return of fertility may be delayed after discontinuing the pill, but the pill is not known to cause infertility. Women who had irregular menstrual cycles before going on the pill are more likely to have problems conceiving, regardless of pill use.

The pill is convenient and does not interfere with lovemaking. It may lessen menstrual difficulties, such as cramps and premenstrual syndrome (PMS). Oral contraceptives also lower the risk of several health conditions, including endometrial and ovarian cancers, fibrocystic breast disease, ectopic pregnancies, ovarian cysts, pelvic inflammatory disease, and iron deficiency anemia.[2] But possible serious health problems associated with the pill include blood clots, which can lead to strokes or heart attacks, and an increased risk for high blood pressure. The risk is low for most healthy women under 35 who do not smoke; it increases with age and especially with cigarette smoking.

Outside these risk factors and certain associated side effects, the pill's greatest disadvantage is that it must be taken every day. If a woman misses one pill, she should use an alternative form of contraception for the remainder of that cycle. Another drawback is that the pill does not protect against sexually transmitted infections (STIs). Cost may also be a problem for some women. Finally, some teenagers report that the requirement to have a complete gynecological examination in order to get a prescription for the pill is a huge obstacle. Educating young women about what goes on in a gynecological exam would certainly help ease their anxiety.

Progestin-Only Pills   Progestin-only pills (or minipills) contain small doses of progesterone. Women who feel uncertain about using estrogen pills, who suffer from side effects related to estrogen, or who are nursing may choose these medications rather than combination pills. There is still some question about the specific ways in which progestin-only pills work. Current thought is that they change the composition of the cervical mucus, thus impeding sperm travel. They may also inhibit ovulation in some women. The effectiveness rate of progestin-only pills is 96 percent, which

is slightly lower than that of estrogen-containing pills. Also, their use usually leads to irregular menstrual bleeding. As with all oral contraceptives, the user has no protection against STIs.

Depo-Provera   **Depo-Provera** is a long-acting synthetic progesterone that is injected intramuscularly every three months. Researchers believe that the drug prevents ovulation. Depo-Provera encourages sexual spontaneity because the user does not have to remember to take a pill or insert a device. Those who want to start a family can usually do so without much of a waiting period. There are fewer health problems associated with Depo-Provera than with estrogen-containing pills. The main disadvantage is irregular bleeding, which can be troublesome at first, but within a year, most women are amenorrheic (have no menstrual periods). Weight gain (an average of five pounds in the first year) is common. Other possible side effects include dizziness, nervousness, and headache. Unlike other methods of contraception, this method cannot be stopped immediately if problems arise.

Norplant   With **Norplant,** six silicon capsules that contain progestin are surgically inserted under the skin of a woman's upper arm. For five years, they continuously release small amounts of progestin. The progestin in Norplant works the same way as oral contraceptives do; it suppresses ovulation, prevents growth of the uterine lining, and thickens the cervical mucus. Norplant is one of the most effective methods of birth control ever developed. A serious disadvantage, however, is its lack of protection against STIs.

A trained health care provider can insert Norplant in 10 to 15 minutes. This involves administering a local anesthetic to the upper arm, making a small incision, and with a special needle, placing the six capsules just under the skin in a fan shape. The capsules are similarly removed after five years or, if necessary, at any time after their insertion.

The capsules usually are invisible, and insertion does not leave a scar in most women. At this time, no serious side effects are known. Less serious side effects include irregular bleeding and irregular menstrual periods, acne, weight gain, breast tenderness, headaches, nervousness, depression, and nausea.

Depo-Provera   An injectable method of birth control that lasts for three months.

Norplant   A long-lasting contraceptive that consists of six silicon capsules surgically inserted under the skin in a woman's upper arm.

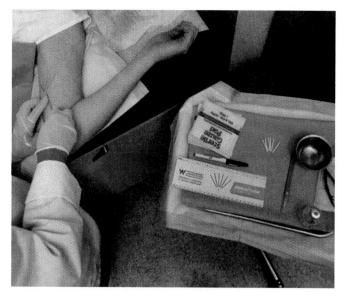

Norplant capsules are sugically implanted into the inside upper arm and provide a safe, long-term contraceptive option for women.

Surgical Methods

Sterilization has become the leading method of contraception for women (10.7 million women), closely followed by the oral contraceptive pill (10.4 million women).[3] Although newer surgical techniques make reversal of sterilization theoretically possible, anyone considering sterilization should assume that the operation is *not* reversible. Before becoming sterilized, people should think through possibilities, such as divorce and remarriage or a future improvement in their financial status, that might make a larger family realistic.

Female Sterilization **Tubal ligation** is one method of sterilization for females. In this surgical procedure, the fallopian tubes are either tied shut or cut and cauterized (burned) at the edges to seal the tubes, blocking sperm's access to released eggs. The operation is usually done in a hospital on an outpatient basis. First, the abdomen is inflated with carbon dioxide gas through a small incision in the navel. The surgeon then inserts a *laparoscope* into another incision just above the pubic bone. This specially designed instrument has a fiberoptic light source that enables the physician to see the

Sterilization Permanent fertility control achieved through surgical procedures.

Tubal ligation Sterilization of the female that involves the cutting and tying off or cauterizing of the fallopian tubes.

Hysterectomy The removal of the uterus.

Vasectomy Sterilization of the male that involves the cutting and tying off of both vasa deferentia.

fallopian tubes clearly. Once located, the tubes are cut and tied or cauterized.

Ovarian and uterine functions are not affected by a tubal ligation. The woman's menstrual cycle continues, and released eggs simply disintegrate and are absorbed by the lymphatic system. As soon as her incision heals, the woman may resume sexual intercourse with no fear of pregnancy.

As with any surgery, there are risks. Although rare, possible complications of a tubal ligation can include infection, pulmonary embolism, hemorrhage, and ectopic pregnancy.[4] Some patients are given general anesthesia, which itself presents a small risk; others receive local anesthesia. The procedure itself usually takes less than an hour, and the patient is generally allowed to return home within a short time after waking up. Women considering a tubal ligation should thoroughly discuss all the risks with their physician before the operation.

The **hysterectomy,** or removal of the uterus, is a method of sterilization requiring major surgery. It is usually done only when the patient's uterus is diseased or damaged.

Male Sterilization Sterilization in men is less complicated than in women. The procedure, called a **vasectomy,** is usually done on an outpatient basis, using a local anesthetic. The surgeon (generally a urologist) makes an incision on each side of the scrotum, locates the vas deferens on each side, and removes a piece from each. The ends are usually tied or sewn shut.

In a small percentage of cases, serious complications occur: formation of a blood clot in the scrotum (which usually disappears without medical treatment), infection, and inflammatory reactions. Because sperm are stored in other areas of the reproductive system besides the vasa deferentia, couples must use alternative methods of birth control for at least one month after the vasectomy. The man must check with his physician (who will do a semen analysis) to determine when unprotected intercourse can take place. The pregnancy rate in women whose partners have had vasectomies is about 15 in 10,000.

Many men are reluctant to consider sterilization because they fear the operation will affect their sexual performance. However, a vasectomy in no way affects sexual response. Because sperm constitute only a small percentage of the semen, the amount of ejaculate is not changed significantly. The testes continue to produce sperm, but the sperm can no longer enter the ejaculatory duct. After a time, sperm production may diminish. Any sperm that are manufactured disintegrate and are absorbed into the lymphatic system.

Although a vasectomy should be considered permanent, surgical reversal is sometimes successful in restoring fertility. Recent improvements in microsurgery techniques have resulted in annual pregnancy rates of between 40 and 60 percent for women whose partners have had reversals. The two major factors influencing the success rate of reversal are the doctor's expertise and the time elapsed since the vasectomy.

What do you think?

Who do you think is responsible for deciding which method of contraception should be used in a sexual relationship? ✴ *What are some examples of good opportunities for you and your partner to have a discussion about contraceptives?* ✴ *What do you think are the biggest barriers in our society to the use of condoms?*

Other Methods of Contraception

Intrauterine Devices   Women have been using **intrauterine devices (IUDs)** since 1909, but we still are not certain how they work. Although it was once thought that IUDs act by preventing implantation of a fertilized egg, most experts now believe that they interfere with the sperm's fertilization of the egg.

Two IUDs are currently available. One, called Progestasert, is a T-shaped plastic device that contains synthetic progesterone. It slowly releases the progesterone. The practitioner must remove this IUD and insert a new one every year. The other, ParaGuard, is also T-shaped, but it has copper wrapped around the shaft and does not contain any hormones. It can be left in place for four years before replacement.

A physician must fit and insert the IUD. For insertion, the device is folded and placed into a long, thin plastic applicator. The practitioner measures the depth of the uterus with a special instrument and then uses these measurements to place the IUD accurately so the arms of the T open out across the top of the uterus. One or two strings extend from the IUD into the vagina so the user can check to make sure that her IUD is in place. The device is removed by a practitioner when desired.

Disadvantages of IUDs include discomfort, cost of insertion, and potential complications. The device can cause heavy menstrual flow and severe cramps. Women using IUDs have a higher risk of uterine perforation, ectopic pregnancy, pelvic inflammatory disease, infertility, and tubal infections. If a pregnancy occurs while the IUD is in place, the chance of miscarriage is 25 to 50 percent. The device should be removed as soon as possible. Doctors often offer therapeutic abortion to women who become pregnant while using an IUD because of the serious risks (including premature delivery, infection, and congenital abnormalities) associated with continuing the pregnancy. For a comparison of contraceptive costs, see Table 6.3.

Withdrawal   The **withdrawal** method involves withdrawing the penis from the vagina just prior to ejaculation. This not very effective method of birth control is most commonly used by people who have not taken the time to consider alternatives. Because there can be up to half a million sperm in the drop of fluid at the tip of the penis before ejaculation, this method is unreliable. Timing withdrawal is also difficult; males concentrating on accurate timing may not be able to relax and enjoy intercourse.

Emergency Contraceptive Pills   There are more than 2.7 million unintended pregnancies per year in the United States, and nearly half are due to contraceptive failure. According to the Centers for Disease Control and Prevention, more than 11 million American women report using contraceptive methods associated with high failure rates, including condoms, withdrawal, periodic abstinence, and diaphragms.

Emergency contraception can be used when a condom breaks, after a sexual assault, or anytime unprotected sexual intercourse occurs. **Emergency contraceptive pills (ECPs)** are ordinary birth control pills containing the hormones estrogen and progestin. Although the therapy is commonly known as the "morning-after pill," the term is misleading; ECPs can be used up to 72 hours beyond and can reduce the risk of pregnancy by 75 percent.

Emergency contraceptives require a prescription. After a woman determines she is not already pregnant, by using the pregnancy test included in the kit, the first dose of two light blue emergency pills is taken as soon as possible, within 72 hours after intercourse. The second dose is taken 12 hours later.[5] The most common side effects related to ECPs are nausea, vomiting, menstrual irregularities, breast tenderness, headache, abdominal pain and cramps, and dizziness.

Emergency minipills contain progestin only. Like ECPs, minipills can be used immediately after unprotected intercourse and up to 72 hours beyond. Emergency minipills are equally as effective as ECPs, but nausea and vomiting are far less common. Emergency minipills are an excellent alternative for most women who cannot use ECPs that contain estrogen.

Abstinence and "Outercourse"   Strictly defined, abstinence means deliberately shunning intercourse. This strict definition would allow one to engage in such forms of sexual intimacy as massage, kissing, and solitary masturbation. But

---

Intrauterine device (IUD)   A T-shaped device that is implanted in the uterus to prevent pregnancy.

Withdrawal   A method of contraception that involves withdrawing the penis from the vagina before ejaculation. Also called "coitus interruptus."

Emergency contraceptive pills (ECPs)   Drugs taken within three days after intercourse to prevent fertilization or implantation.

Emergency minipills   Contraceptive pills containing only progestin that can be taken up to three days after unprotected intercourse.

Table 6.3
The Cost of Contraceptive Choices: An Example of Costs from a Student Health Service*

METHOD	PRODUCT	REGULAR PRICE
Oral contraceptives	Plan B	$ 10.00
	Ovral (MAT)	$ 10.00
	Alesse	$ 12.00
	Desogen	$ 12.00
	Estrostep	$ 12.00
	Loestrin FE	$ 12.00
	Loestrin FE	$ 12.00
	Lo-Orval	$ 12.00
	Mircette	$ 12.00
	Ortho Cyclen	$ 12.00
	Ortho Novum	$ 12.00
	Ortho TriCyclen	$ 12.00
	Triphasil	$ 12.00
	Zovia (Demulen)	$ 17.00
	Generic Modicon	$ 17.00
	NorQD	$ 29.00
	Ortho Cept	$ 17.00
	Ortho Novum	$ 17.00
	Generic Ortho Novum	$ 20.00
	Ovcon	$ 29.00
	Ovral	$ 42.00
	Yasmin	$ 25.00
Lunelle monthly injection		$ 21.50
Depo-Provera		$ 41.50
Diaphragms		$ 20.00
Spermicides	Encare Inserts	$ 7.75
	Delfen Foam	$ 7.50
	Gynol II Jelly	$ 7.95
	KY Plus Jelly	$ 7.05
	VCF Film	$ 9.58
Condoms	3/Pkg	$ 0.50
Female condoms	3/Pkg	$ 7.00
Non-latex condoms	6/Pkg	$ 5.85
Norplant		$425.00
Cervical cap		$ 56.70

*Most insurance companies do not cover the expenses of contraceptives, leaving the burden of payment on the user.

many people today have broadened the definition of abstinence to include all forms of sexual contact, even those that do not culminate in sexual intercourse.

Couples who go a step farther than massage and kissing and engage in activities such as oral–genital sex and mutual masturbation are sometimes said to be engaging in "outercourse." Like abstinence, outercourse can be 100 percent effective for birth control as long as the male does not ejaculate near the vaginal opening. Unlike abstinence, however, outercourse is not 100 percent effective against sexually transmitted infections (STIs). Oral–genital contact can result in transmission of an STI, although the practice can be made safer by using a condom on the penis or a dental dam on the vaginal opening.

Fertility awareness methods (FAM) Several types of birth control that require alteration of sexual behavior rather than chemical or physical intervention into the reproductive process.

Fertility Awareness Methods

Methods of fertility control that rely upon the alteration of sexual behavior are called **fertility awareness methods (FAM).** These techniques include observing female "fertile

The Contraceptive Horizon: Future Methods

The introduction of a new contraceptive may take years of research and clinical trials prior to winning approval from the Food and Drug Administration. However, it appears that within the next few years, our contraceptive options may be expanding. Here's a look at future contraceptives:

NEW BARRIER METHODS

- Lea's Shield is a one-size-fits-all silicon rubber device that covers the cervix. The FDA has asked for more clinical studies prior to approval.
- Disposable diaphragms and diaphragms made of silicone rather than latex are also upcoming.
- FemCap, already available in Europe, covers the cervix and forms a seal against the vaginal wall. It is used with spermicide and contains a groove that traps sperm. FemCap was expected to be submitted for FDA approval in 2001.

CONTRACEPTIVES FOR MEN

- The often-discussed "male pill" is probably still many years off. Researchers have tried a number of variations but found serious side effects, such as permanent sterility and blood pressure complications.
- An injectable contraceptive that stimulates the production of antibodies to male sex hormone production is in the works and will be tested more extensively within the next few years.
- A synthetic testosterone that would be delivered via a skin implant has been developed by the Population Council and is undergoing further testing to determine side effects.

IMPLANT REFINEMENTS

- The Population Council, which developed Norplant, is currently working on a single-rod implant delivery system that would inhibit ovulation for two years. The implant contains Nesterone, a synthetic progestin.

THE "PATCH"

- A transdermal patch delivering Nesterone is also in development by the Population Council. The patch would be affixed to a woman's abdomen and could be easily removed.

VAGINAL RINGS

- About the size of the outer ring of a diaphragm, a vaginal ring would be inserted into the vagina, where it would deliver synthetic hormones similar to those in a birth control pill. It contains lower hormone dose levels than oral contraceptives do and can be left in place for several weeks, then removed to initiate a menstrual period.

Sources: Population Council website, http://www.popcouncil.org/biomed/; Thrive Online website, http://www.thriveonline.oxygen.com/sex; Reproline website, http://www.reproline.jhu.edu/.

---

periods" by examining cervical mucus and/or keeping track of internal temperature, and then abstaining from sexual intercourse (penis–vagina contact) during these fertile times.

Two decades ago, the "rhythm method" was ridiculed because of its low effectiveness rates. However, it was the only method of birth control available to women belonging to religious denominations that forbid the use of oral contraceptives, barrier methods, and sterilization. Our present reproductive knowledge enables women and their partners to use natural methods of birth control with fewer risks of pregnancy, although these methods remain far less effective than others.

Fertility awareness methods rely upon basic physiology (Figure 6.4). A released ovum can survive for up to 48 hours after ovulation. Sperm can live for as long as five days in the vagina. Natural methods of birth control teach women to recognize their fertile times. Changes in cervical mucus prior to and during ovulation and a rise in basal body temperature are two frequently used indicators. Another method involves charting a woman's menstrual cycle and ovulation times on a calendar. Women may use any combination of these methods to determine their fertile times more accurately.

Cervical Mucus Method   The **cervical mucus method** requires women to examine the consistency and color of their normal vaginal secretions. Prior to ovulation, vaginal mucus becomes gelatinous and stretchy, and normal vaginal secretions may increase. Sexual activity involving penis–vagina contact must be avoided while this "fertile mucus" is present and for several days following the mucus changes.

Cervical mucus method   A birth control method that relies upon observation of changes in cervical mucus to determine when the woman is fertile so that the couple can abstain from intercourse during those times.

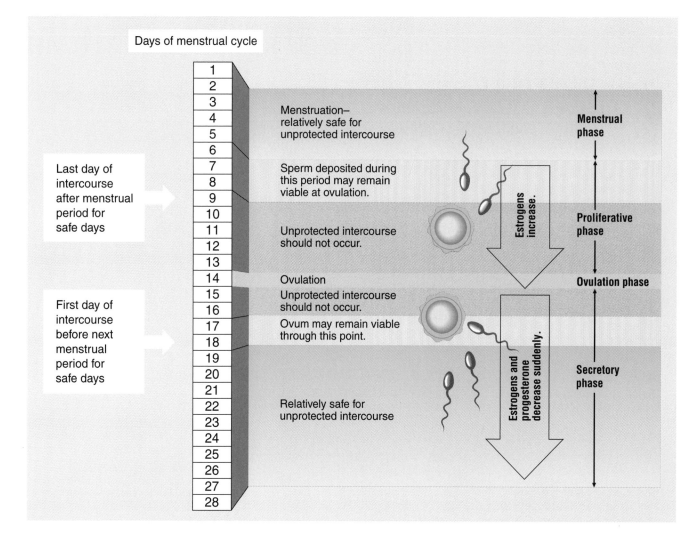

Figure 6.4

The Fertility Cycle

Fertility awareness methods can combine the use of a calendar, the cervical mucus method, and body temperature measurements to identify the fertile period. It is important to remember that most women do not have a consistent 28-day cycle.

Body Temperature Method The **body temperature method** relies on the fact that the female's basal body temperature rises between 0.4 and 0.8 degrees after ovulation has occurred. For this method to be effective, the woman must chart her temperature for several months to learn to recognize her body's temperature fluctuations. Abstinence from penis–vagina contact must be observed preceding the temperature rise until several days after the temperature rise was first noted.

The Calendar Method The **calendar method** requires the woman to record the exact number of days in her menstrual cycle. Because few women menstruate with complete regularity, this involves keeping a record of the menstrual cycle for 12 months, during which time some other method of birth control must be used. The first day of a woman's period counts as day 1. To determine the first fertile unsafe day of the cycle, she subtracts 18 from the number of days in the shortest cycle. To determine the last unsafe day of the cycle, she subtracts 11 from the number of days in the longest cycle. This method assumes that ovulation occurs during the midpoint of the cycle. The couple must abstain from penis–vagina contact during the fertile time.

Body temperature method A birth control method in which a woman monitors her body temperature for the rise that signals ovulation in order to abstain from intercourse around this time.

Calendar method A birth control method in which a woman's menstrual cycle is mapped on a calendar to determine presumed fertile times in order to abstain from penis–vagina contact during those times.

Abortion Access

The United States has had a long struggle over the issue of abortion. A review of laws and guidelines in other countries shows that different cultures have their own customs and beliefs. Here's a look at some international differences.

- Over 41 percent of the world's population live in countries that do not require women seeking abortion to meet specific "reason" requirements; that is, women don't have to provide an explanation for why they desire abortion.
- Fourteen countries (including India, Great Britain, and Zimbabwe) have laws that instruct health care providers to consider a woman's economic or social situation in providing abortion services. Women who can show that carrying a baby to term would cause hardship are permitted abortions.
- Thirteen percent of the world's population (53 nations) permit abortion only when the pregnancy poses a threat to the woman's health or safety. Some countries have specific guidelines for determining threat, whereas others allow room for interpretation. For example, in Jamaica, a woman's mental health can be considered, but in Peru there must be a physical threat of permanent injury if the woman carries to term.
- The most stringent laws—those prohibiting abortion completely or allowing abortion only in cases where the mother's life is endangered—are in place in 74 nations (representing 21 percent of the world's population), mainly in Africa and Latin America. In these nations, there can be criminal penalties for both the woman and the abortion provider.
- Fourteen countries require a husband to provide authorization before his wife can receive abortion services. These countries include Japan, Iraq, Syria, and Turkey.

Sources: From the Center for Reproductive Law and Policy, "Reproductive Rights 2000: Moving Forward," electronic edition, http://www.crlp.org/rr2k.html; A. Rahman, L. Katzive, and S. Fienshaw, "A Global Review of Laws on Induced Abortion, 1985–1997," *International Family Planning Perspectives* 24 (1998).

Women interested in fertility awareness methods of birth control are advised to take supervised classes in their use. Women who are untrained in these techniques run a high risk of unwanted pregnancy.

Abortion

In 1973, the landmark U.S. Supreme Court decision in *Roe v. Wade* stated that the "right to privacy . . . founded on the Fourteenth Amendment's concept of personal liberty . . . is broad enough to encompass a woman's decision whether or not to terminate her pregnancy."[6] The decision maintained that during the first trimester of pregnancy, a woman and her practitioner have the right to terminate the pregnancy through **abortion** without legal restrictions. It allowed individual states to set conditions for second-trimester abortions. Third-trimester abortions were ruled illegal unless the mother's life or health was in danger.

Prior to the legalization of first- and second-trimester abortions, women wishing to terminate a pregnancy had to travel to a country where the procedure was legal, consult an illegal abortionist, or perform their own abortions. Approximately 480,000 illegal abortions were performed in the United States each year, one-third of them on married women. These procedures led to death from hemorrhage or infection in some cases and to infertility from internal scarring in others.

People who oppose abortion believe that the embryo or fetus is a human being with rights that must be protected. The political debate continues as opponents of abortion pressure state and local governments to pass laws prohibiting the use of public funds for abortion and abortion counseling. In recent years, new legislation has given states the right to impose certain restrictions on abortions. In some states, abortions cannot be performed in publicly funded clinics, and other states have laws requiring parental notification before a teenager can obtain an abortion. Although *Roe v. Wade* has not been overturned, it faces many future challenges.

Although many opponents work through the courts and the political process, attacks on abortion clinics and on doctors who perform abortions are increasingly common. Nearly all clinics have faced some form of threats or acts of violence. Recent legal changes, such as the Freedom of Access to Clinic Entrance Act (FACE), offer some relief to the harassment and violence directed at abortion clinics. However, because of such acts, the biggest threat to a woman's access to an abortion now is finding a clinic rather than legal restrictions.[7]

The best birth control methods can fail. Women may be raped. Pregnancies can occur despite every possible precaution. When an unwanted pregnancy does occur, the woman must decide whether to terminate, carry to term and keep the baby, or carry to term and give the baby away. This

---

Abortion The medical means of terminating a pregnancy.

is a personal decision that each woman must make, based on her personal beliefs, values, and resources, after carefully considering all alternatives. For a discussion on how abortion is perceived in different countries, see the accompanying box, Health in a Diverse World.

Methods of Abortion

The type of abortion procedure is determined by how many weeks the woman has been pregnant. Length of pregnancy is calculated from the first day of a woman's last menstrual period.

If performed during the first trimester of pregnancy, abortion presents a relatively low risk to the mother. The most commonly used method of first-trimester abortion is **vacuum aspiration.** The procedure is usually performed under a local anesthetic. The cervix is dilated with instruments or by placing *laminaria,* a sterile seaweed product, in the cervical canal. The laminaria is left in place for a few hours or overnight and slowly dilates the cervix. After it is removed, a long tube is inserted into the uterus through the cervix, and gentle suction removes fetal tissue from the uterine walls.

Pregnancies that progress into the second trimester can be terminated through **dilation and evacuation (D&E),** a procedure that combines vacuum aspiration with a technique called **dilation and curettage (D&C).** For this procedure, the cervix is dilated with laminaria for one to two days, and a combination of instruments and vacuum aspiration is used to empty the uterus (Figure 6.5). Second-trimester abortions are frequently done under general anesthetic. Both procedures can be performed on an outpatient basis (usually in the physician's office), with or without pain medication. Gen-

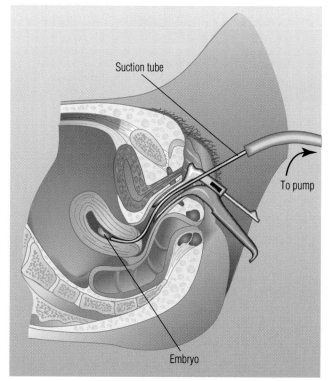

Figure 6.5
Vacuum Aspiration Abortion

erally, however, the woman is given a mild tranquilizer to help her relax. Both procedures may cause moderate to severe uterine cramping and blood loss.

Two other methods used in second-trimester abortions, though less common than the D&E, are prostaglandin or saline **induction abortions.** Prostaglandin hormones or a saline solution is injected into the uterus, which kills the fetus and initiates labor contractions. After 24 to 48 hours, the fetus and placenta are expelled from the uterus.

The **hysterotomy,** or surgical removal of the fetus from the uterus, may be used during emergencies, when the mother's life may be in danger, or when other types of abortions are deemed too dangerous.

The risks associated with abortions include infection, incomplete abortion (when parts of the placenta remain in the uterus), missed abortion (when the fetus is not actually removed), excessive bleeding, and cervical and uterine trauma. Follow-up and attention to dangerous signs decrease the chances of developing long-term problems.

The woman's mortality rate for first-trimester abortions averages one death for every 530,000 at 8 or fewer weeks. The rate for second-trimester abortions is higher than one per 17,000.[8] This higher rate later in the pregnancy is due to the increased risk of uterine perforation, bleeding, infection, and incomplete abortion due to the fact that the uterine wall becomes thinner as the pregnancy progresses.

One surgical method of performing abortion has been the subject of much controversy. **Intact dilation and**

Vacuum aspiration   The use of gentle suction to remove fetal tissue from the uterus.

Dilation and evacuation (D&E)   An abortion technique that combines vacuum aspiration with dilation and curettage; fetal tissue is both sucked and scraped out of the uterus.

Dilation and curettage (D&C)   An abortion technique in which the cervix is dilated with laminaria for one to two days, after which the uterine walls are scraped clean.

Induction abortion   A type of abortion in which chemicals are injected into the uterus through the uterine wall; labor begins, and the woman delivers a dead fetus.

Hysterotomy   The surgical removal of the fetus from the uterus.

Intact dilation and extraction (D&X)   A late-term abortion procedure in which the body of the fetus is extracted up to the head and then the contents of the cranium are aspirated.

extraction (D&X), sometimes referred to by the nonmedical term *partial-birth abortion,* is used only in certain cases, such as when other abortion methods could injure the mother. The procedure generally involves repositioning the fetus to a breech (feet first) position before extracting most of the body except for the head. The contents of the cranium are then aspirated, resulting in "vaginal delivery of a dead but otherwise intact fetus."[9] Thirty-one states have passed legislation attempting to ban intact dilation and extraction. However, the wording of the legislation in many states has been so general that it could be used to ban all types of abortion. For this reason, such legislation has often been challenged, and only ten states currently fully enforce the laws as written. Professional organizations such as the American College of Obstetrics and Gynecology and the American Medical Association state that physicians, acting in the best interests of their patients, should choose the safest and most appropriate method of abortion in each individual case.

Mifepristone (RU-486)

In September 2000, the U.S. Food and Drug Administration approved *mifepristone,* known as **RU-486,** after a 20-year odyssey. RU-486 is a steroid hormone that induces abortion by blocking the action of progesterone, a hormone produced by the ovaries and placenta that maintains the lining of the uterus. Similar in structure to progesterone, RU-486 binds to cell receptor sites normally occupied by progesterone, causing the uterine lining to break down. As a result, the uterine lining and the embryo are expelled from the uterus, terminating the pregnancy.

RU-486's nickname, "the abortion pill," may imply an easy process. However, this treatment actually involves more steps than a clinical abortion, which takes approximately 15 minutes followed by a physical recovery of about one day. With RU-486, a first visit to the clinic involves a physical exam and a dose of three mifepristone tablets, which may cause minor side effects such as nausea, headaches, weakness, and fatigue. The patient returns two days later for a dose of prostaglandins (trade name: Misoprostal), which cause uterine contractions that expel the fertilized egg. Women are required to stay under observation at the clinic for four hours.

Ninety-six percent of women who take RU-486 and prostaglandins during the first nine weeks of pregnancy will experience a complete abortion. A return visit is required 12 days later because the pills fail to expel the fetus completely in 4 percent of cases. In such an event, a clinical abortion becomes necessary.[10]

The side effects of this treatment are similar to those reported during heavy menstruation and include cramping, minor pain, and nausea. Approximately 1 in 1,000 women requires a blood transfusion because of severe bleeding. The procedure does not require hospitalization; women may be treated on an outpatient basis.

What do you think?

If you or your partner unexpectedly became pregnant, would you choose to terminate the pregnancy? ✻ *How might an abortion affect your relationship?* ✻ *What factors would you consider in making your decision?* ✻ *Why?*

Planning a Pregnancy

The many methods available to control fertility give you choices that did not exist when your parents—and even you—were born. If you are in the process of deciding whether to have children, take the time to evaluate your emotions, finances, and health.

Emotional Health

First and foremost, you need to evaluate why you want to have a child: to fulfill an inner need to carry on the family? To escape loneliness? Are there any other reasons? Can you care for this new human being in a loving and nurturing manner? Are you ready to make all the sacrifices necessary to bear and raise a child?

If you feel, based on your self-evaluation, that you are ready to be a parent, the next step is preparation. You can prepare for this change in your life in several ways: reading about parenthood, taking classes, talking to parents of children of all ages, and joining a support group. If you choose to adopt, you will find many support groups available to you as well.

Maternal Health

Before becoming pregnant, a woman should have a thorough medical examination. **Preconception care** should include assessment of potential complications. Medical problems such as diabetes and high blood pressure should be discussed, as should any genetic disorders that run in the family. Additional suggestions for a healthy pregnancy include the following:

- If you smoke and drink, stop.
- Reduce or eliminate caffeine intake.
- Avoid x-rays and environmental chemicals, such as lawn and garden chemicals.
- Maintain a normal weight; lose weight if necessary.
- Prior to becoming pregnant, get any dental x-ray examinations that will be needed for a checkup.[11]

RU-486 A steroid hormone that induces abortion by blocking the action of progesterone.

Preconception care Medical care received prior to becoming pregnant that helps a woman assess and address potential maternal health.

Paternal Health

It is common wisdom that mothers-to-be should steer clear of toxic chemicals that can cause birth defects. Even women who are trying to conceive are cautioned to avoid toxic environments, eat a nourishing diet, stop smoking and drinking alcohol, and avoid most medications. Now, similar precautions are recommended for fathers-to-be. New research suggests that a man's exposure to chemicals influences not only his ability to father a child but also the future health of his child.

Fathers-to-be have been overlooked in past preconception and prenatal studies for several reasons. Researchers assumed that the genetic damage leading to birth defects and other health problems occurred while a child was in the mother's womb. After all, they reasoned, that's where embryonic and fetal development takes place. Conventional medical wisdom also held that defective-looking sperm (those with misshapen heads, crooked tails, or retarded swimming ability) were incapable of fertilizing an egg.

Scientists have recently discovered that how sperm look has little to do with how they act. Misshapen sperm can penetrate an egg, and they do not necessarily carry defective genetic goods. Moreover, sperm that look healthy and swim well can be true genetic culprits. DNA fluorescent markers have identified normal-looking, yet genetically flawed, sperm that carry too many or too few chromosomes. Fathers contribute the extra chromosome 21 in about 6 percent of children with Down syndrome, which causes mental retardation; the extra X chromosome in 50 percent of boys with **Klinefelter's syndrome,** which causes abnormal sexual development; and the shortened chromosome 15 in about 85 percent of children with **Prader-Willi syndrome,** a disorder characterized by retardation and obesity.

Although some birth defects are caused by random errors of nature, it now appears that some disorders can be traced to sperm damaged by chemicals. Sperm are naturally vulnerable to toxic assault and genetic damage. Many drugs and ingested chemicals can readily invade the testes from the bloodstream; others ambush sperm after they leave the testes and pass through the epididymides, where they mature and are stored. By one route or another, half of 100 chemicals studied so far (including by-products of cigarette smoke) apparently harm sperm.

Some researchers believe that vitamin C is nature's way of protecting sex cells from damage. Bad diets, exposure to toxic chemicals, cigarette smoking, and diets low in vitamin C are implicated in sperm damage.[12]

Klinefelter's syndrome   A chromosome defect that causes abnormal sexual development.

Prader-Willi syndrome   A disorder characterized by mental retardation and obesity.

Financial Evaluation

Another important consideration in deciding whether to have a child is finances. First check your medical insurance: does it provide pregnancy benefits? If not, you can expect to pay between $1,500 and $5,000 for medical care during pregnancy and birth—and substantially more if complications arise. Both partners should find out about their employers' policies concerning parental leave, including length of leave available and conditions for returning to work.

The U.S. Department of Agriculture estimates that it will cost $160,140 to raise a child born in 1999 to the age of 17. When adjusted for inflation, the figure rises to $237,000! This equals a yearly cost of approximately $9,000. Housing costs and food are the two largest expenditures in raising children.[13] Can you afford to give your child the life you would like him or her to enjoy?

The cost of a college education is another consideration. If costs continue to rise by about 5 percent, the four-year cost of a college education at a public university will reach almost $120,000 by the year 2018.[14]

Also consider the cost and availability of quality child care. Prospective parents should realistically assess how much family assistance they can expect with a new baby as well as the availability of nonfamily child care. While you may be aware of the federal tax credit available for child care, you may not realize how little assistance it actually provides: between a maximum of $480 for one child in a family having income of over $28,000 to a maximum of $720 for one child in a family having income of under $10,000. A second child doubles the credit, but no further assistance is provided for a third child or more children. How much does full-time child care cost? It averages between $5,000 and $10,000 a year, depending on your location (urban areas tend to cost more).

Contingency Planning

A final consideration is how to provide for the child should something happen to you and your partner. If both of you were to die while the child is young, do you have relatives or close friends who would raise the child? If you have more than one child, would they have to be split up, or could they be kept together? Though unpleasant to think about, this sort of contingency planning is very important. Children who lose their parents are heartbroken and confused. A prearranged plan of action will smooth their transition into new families.

What do you think?

What factors will you consider in deciding whether or when to have children? ＊ *Is there a certain age at which you feel you will be ready to be a parent?* ＊ *What goals do you hope to achieve prior to undertaking parenthood?* ＊ *What are your biggest concerns about parenthood?*

Pregnancy

Pregnancy is an important event in a woman's life. The actions taken before a pregnancy begins, as well as behaviors during pregnancy, can have a significant effect on the health of both infant and mother.

Prenatal Care

A successful pregnancy requires the mother's ability to take good care of herself and her unborn child. It is essential to have regular medical checkups, beginning as soon as possible (certainly within the first three months). Early detection of fetal abnormalities and identification of high-risk mothers and infants are the major purposes of prenatal care. On the first visit, the practitioner should obtain a complete medical history of the mother and her family and note any hereditary conditions that could put a woman or her fetus at risk.

Regular checkups to measure weight gain and blood pressure and to monitor the size and position of the fetus should continue throughout the pregnancy. This early care reduces infant mortality and low birth weight. A study group for the American College of Obstetric and Gynecology recommends seven or eight prenatal visits for women with low-risk pregnancies. Unfortunately, prenatal care is not available to everyone. Approximately 30 percent of pregnant teenagers and unmarried women do not receive adequate prenatal attention. Babies of mothers who received no prenatal care are about 10 times more likely to die in the first month of life than babies of mothers who did get prenatal care.

Additional concerns include the mother's physical condition, her level of nutrition, her confidence in her ability to give birth, her use of drugs and medications, and the availability of a skilled practitioner who can oversee the pregnancy and delivery. A woman planning a pregnancy also needs a support system (spouse or partner, family, friends, community groups) willing to give her and her child love and emotional support during and after her pregnancy.

Choosing a Practitioner   A woman should carefully choose a practitioner to attend her pregnancy and delivery. If possible, this choice should be made before she becomes pregnant. Recommendations from friends are a good starting point. The woman's family physician may also be able to recommend a specialist.

When choosing a practitioner, parents should ask about credentials, professional qualifications, and experience. Besides this information, a pregnant woman must ask questions specific to her condition. Prospective parents should also inquire about the practitioner's experience in handling various complications, commitment to being at the mother's side during delivery, and beliefs and practices concerning the use of anesthesia, fetal monitoring, induced labor, and forceps delivery. What are the practitioner's attitudes toward birth control, abortion, and alternative birthing procedures?

The practitioner's approach to nutrition and medication during pregnancy should be similar to the woman's own. Finally, the parents must learn under what circumstances the practitioner would perform a cesarean section.

Two types of physicians can attend pregnancies and deliveries. The *obstetrician-gynecologist* (ob-gyn) is an M.D. who specializes in obstetrics (pregnancy and birth) and gynecology (care of women's reproductive organs). These practitioners are trained to handle all types of pregnancy- and delivery-related emergencies. A *family practitioner* is a licensed M.D. who provides comprehensive care for people of all ages. The majority of family practitioners have obstetrical experience but will refer a patient to a specialist if necessary. Unlike the ob-gyn, the family practitioner can serve as the baby's physician after attending the birth.

Midwives are also experienced practitioners who can attend both pregnancies and deliveries. *Certified nurse-midwives* are registered nurses having specialized training in pregnancy and delivery. Most midwives work in private practice or in conjunction with physicians. Those who work with physicians have access to traditional medical facilities to which they can turn in an emergency. *Lay midwives* may or may not have extensive training in handling an emergency. They may be self-taught rather than trained through formal certification procedures.

Alcohol and Drugs   A woman should avoid all types of drugs during pregnancy. Even common over-the-counter medications, such as aspirin, and beverages, such as coffee and tea, can damage a developing fetus.

During the first three months of pregnancy, the fetus is especially subject to the **teratogenic** (birth defect–causing) effects of some chemical substances. The fetus can also develop an addiction to or tolerance for drugs that the mother is using. Of particular concern to medical professionals is the use of tobacco and alcohol during pregnancy.

Women who are heavy drinkers may have normal first babies but subsequently deliver children having fetal alcohol syndrome. The symptoms of **fetal alcohol syndrome (FAS)** include mental retardation, slowed nerve reflexes, and small head size. The exact amount of alcohol necessary to cause FAS is not known, but researchers doubt that any alcohol is safe. Therefore, they recommend total abstinence from alcohol during pregnancy.

Midwife   Experienced practitioner who can attend both pregnancies and deliveries.

Teratogenic   Causing birth defects; may refer to drugs, environmental chemicals, x-rays, or diseases.

Fetal alcohol syndrome (FAS)   A collection of symptoms, including mental retardation, that can appear in infants of women who drink too much alcohol during pregnancy.

A doctor-approved exercise program during pregnacy can help control weight, make delivery easier, and have a healthy effet on the fetus.

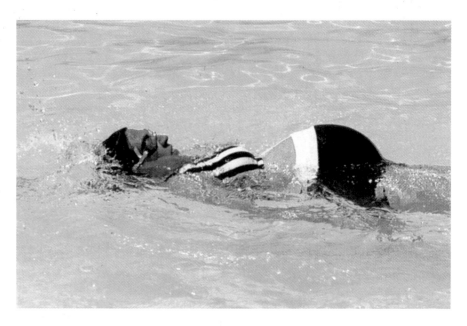

Studies have shown a 25 to 50 percent higher rate of fetal and infant deaths among women who smoke during pregnancy compared with those who do not.[15] Women who smoke more than 10 to 15 cigarettes a day during pregnancy have higher rates of miscarriage, stillbirth, premature births, and low-birth-weight babies than do nonsmokers. Smoking restricts the blood supply to the developing fetus and thus limits oxygen and nutrition delivery and waste removal. It appears to be a significant factor in the development of cleft lip and palate, and a significant relationship has been shown between both smoking and "secondhand" smoke and sudden infant death syndrome.[16] Fetal research on the effects of secondhand or sidestream smoke (inhaling smoke produced by others) is inconclusive, but babies whose parents smoke can be twice as susceptible as other babies to pneumonia, bronchitis, and related illnesses. Recent statistics for the United States show that tobacco use among pregnant women has steadily fallen since 1989, when about 20 percent of pregnant women smoked. In 1998, that rate had declined to 12.9 percent.[17]

X-rays X-rays present a clear danger to the fetus. Although most diagnostic tests produce minimal amounts of radiation, even low levels may cause birth defects or other problems, particularly if several low-dose x-rays are taken over a short time period. Pregnant women are advised to avoid x-rays unless absolutely necessary.

Nutrition and Exercise Pregnant women need additional protein, calories, vitamins and minerals, so their diets should be carefully monitored by a qualified practitioner. Special attention should be paid to getting enough folic acid (found in dark leafy greens), iron (dried fruits, meats, legumes, liver, egg yolks), calcium (nonfat or low-fat dairy products, some canned fish), and fluids.

Vitamin supplements can correct some deficiencies, but there is no substitute for a well-balanced diet. Babies born to poorly nourished mothers run high risks of substandard mental and physical development. Folic acid, when consumed before and during early pregnancy, reduces the risk of spina bifida, a common disabling birth condition resulting from failure of the spinal column to close. Manufacturers of breads, pastas, rice, and other grain products are now required to add folic acid to their products to reduce neural tube defects in newborns.

Weight gain during pregnancy helps nourish a growing baby. For a woman of normal weight before pregnancy, the recommended weight gain during pregnancy is 25–35 pounds. For obese or overweight women, weight gain of 15–25 pounds is recommended. Underweight women can gain 28–40 pounds, and women carrying twins should gain about 35–45 pounds. Gaining too much or too little weight can lead to complications. With higher weight gains, women may develop gestational diabetes, hypertension, or increased risk of delivery complications. Gaining too little weight increases the chance of a low-birth-weight baby.

Of the total number of pounds gained during pregnancy, about 6–8 are the baby's weight. The baby's birth weight is important, because low weight can mean health problems during labor and the baby's first few months. Pregnancy is not the time to think about losing weight—doing so may endanger the baby.[18]

As in all other stages of life, exercise is an important factor in weight control during pregnancy and overall maternal health. In one study, a balanced 45-minute exercise session three days per week was associated with heavier-birthweight babies, fewer surgical births, and shorter hospital stays after birth. Pregnant women should consult their physicians before starting any exercise program.

Other Factors   A pregnant woman should avoid exposure to toxic chemicals, heavy metals, pesticides, gases, and other hazardous compounds. She should not clean cat-litter boxes, because cat feces can contain organisms that cause a disease called **toxoplasmosis.** If a pregnant woman contracts this disease, her baby may be stillborn or suffer mental retardation or other birth defects.

Before becoming pregnant, a woman should be tested to determine whether she has had rubella (German measles). If she has not had the disease, she should be immunized for it and wait the recommended length of time before becoming pregnant. A rubella infection can kill the fetus or cause blindness or hearing disorders in the infant. If the woman has ever had genital herpes, she should inform her physician. The physician may want to deliver the baby by cesarean section, especially if the woman has active lesions. Contact with an active herpes infection during birth can be fatal to the infant.

A Woman's Reproductive Years

More than half of the average American woman's expected life span is spent between menarche (first menses) and menopause (last menses), a period of approximately 40 years. Deciding whether and when to have children, as well as how to prevent pregnancy when necessary, is a long-term concern.

Today, a woman over 35 who is pregnant has plenty of company. Whereas births to women in their 20s are declining, the rate of first births to women between the ages of 30 and 39 has doubled in the past decade, and births to women over 39 have increased by more than 50 percent. Many women who wait until their 30s to consider having a child find themselves wondering, "Am I too old to have a baby?" Statistically, the chances of having a baby with birth defects do rise after the age of 35. Researchers believe that there is a decline in both the quality and viability of eggs after this age.

Down syndrome, a condition characterized by mild to severe mental retardation and a variety of physical abnormalities, is the most common genetic condition. One in every 800 to 1,000 live births a year is a child with Down syndrome, representing approximately 5,000 births per year in the United States alone. A common myth is that most children with Down syndrome have older parents. The truth is that 80 percent of children born with Down syndrome are born to women younger than 35. However, the incidence does increase with age. The incidence of Down syndrome in babies born to a mother of age 20 is 1 in 10,000 births; it rises to 1 in 400 by age 35, to 1 in 110 by age 40, and to 1 in 35 when she is 45.[19]

Women who delay motherhood until their late 30s also worry about their physical ability to carry and deliver their babies. For these women, a comprehensive exercise program will assist in maintaining good posture and promoting a successful delivery. Despite these concerns, there are some advantages to having a baby later in life. In fact, many doctors note that older mothers tend to be more conscientious about following medical advice during pregnancy and more psychologically mature and ready to include an infant in their family than some younger women.

Pregnancy Testing

A woman may suspect she is pregnant before she has any pregnancy tests. A typical sign is a missed menstrual period, yet this is not always an accurate indicator. A woman can miss her period for a variety of reasons: stress, exercise, emotional upset. A pregnancy test scheduled in a medical office or birth control clinic will confirm the pregnancy. Women who wish to know immediately can purchase home pregnancy test kits, sold over the counter in drugstores. A positive test is based on the secretion of **human chorionic gonadotropin (HCG)** found in the woman's urine. Home test kits come equipped with a small sample of red blood cells coated with HCG antibodies to which the user adds a small amount of urine. If the concentration of HCG is great enough, it will clump together with the HCG antibodies, indicating that the user is pregnant.

Home pregnancy test kits are about 85 to 95 percent reliable. If done too early in the pregnancy, they may show a false negative. Other causes of false negatives are unclean test tubes, ingestion of certain drugs, and vaginal or urinary tract infections. Accuracy also depends on the quality of the test itself and the user's ability to perform it and interpret the results. Blood tests administered and analyzed by a medical laboratory give more accurate results.

The Process of Pregnancy

Pregnancy begins the moment a sperm fertilizes an ovum in the fallopian tubes (Figure 6.6.). From there, the single cell multiplies, becoming a sphere-shaped cluster of cells as it travels toward the uterus, a journey that may last three to four days. Upon arrival, the embryo burrows into the thick, spongy endometrium and is nourished from this carefully prepared lining.

Early Signs of Pregnancy   The first sign of pregnancy is usually a missed menstrual period (although some women "spot" in early pregnancy, and such spotting may be mistaken for a period). Other signs of pregnancy include the following:

Toxoplasmosis   A disease caused by an organism found in cat feces that, when contracted by a pregnant woman, may result in stillbirth or an infant with mental retardation or birth defects.

Down syndrome   A condition characterized by mental retardation and a variety of physical abnormalities.

Human chorionic gonadotropin (HCG)   Hormone detectable in blood or urine samples of a mother within the first few weeks of pregnancy.

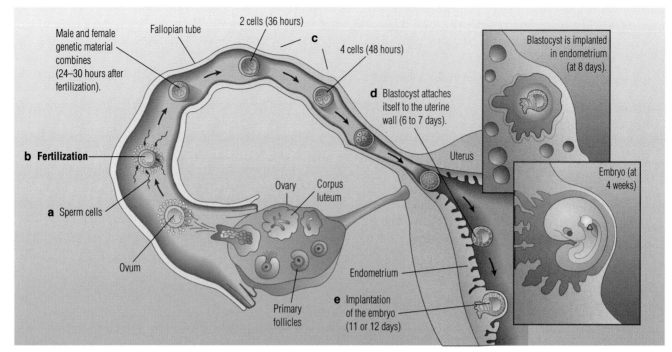

Figure 6.6
Fertilization
(a) The efforts of hundreds of sperm may allow one sperm to penetrate the ovum's corona radiata, an outer layer of cells, and then the zona pellucida, a thick inner membrane. (b) The sperm nucleus fuses with the egg nucleus at fertilization, producing a zygote. (c) The zygote divides first into two cells, then four cells, and so on. (d) The blastocyst attaches itself to the uterine wall. (e) The blastocyst implants itself in the endometrium.

- Breast tenderness
- Emotional upset
- Extreme fatigue
- Nausea
- Sleeplessness
- Vomiting (especially in the morning)

Pregnancy typically lasts 40 weeks. The due date is calculated from the expectant mother's last menstrual period. Pregnancy is typically divided into three phases, or **trimesters,** of approximately three months each.

Trimester A three-month segment of pregnancy; used to describe specific developmental changes that occur in the embryo or fetus.

Embryo The fertilized egg from conception until the end of two months' development.

Fetus The name given the developing baby from the third month of pregnancy until birth.

Placenta The network of blood vessels, connected to the umbilical cord, that carries nutrients to the developing infant and carries wastes away.

The First Trimester During the first trimester, few noticeable changes occur in the mother's body. The expectant mother may urinate more frequently and experience morning sickness, swollen breasts, or undue fatigue. But these symptoms may not be frequent or severe, so she may not even realize she is pregnant unless she has a pregnancy test.

During the first two months after conception, the **embryo** differentiates and develops its various organ systems, beginning with the nervous and circulatory systems. At the start of the third month, the embryo is called a **fetus,** indicating that all organ systems are in place. For the rest of the pregnancy, growth and refinement occur in each major body system so that they can function independently, yet in coordination, at birth. The accompanying photos illustrate physical changes during fetal development.

The Second Trimester At the beginning of the second trimester, physical changes in the mother become more visible. Her breasts swell, and her waistline thickens. During this time, the fetus makes greater demands upon the mother's body. In particular, the **placenta,** the network of blood vessels that carry nutrients and oxygen to the fetus and fetal waste products to the mother, becomes well established.

The Third Trimester The time from the end of the sixth month through the ninth is considered the third trimester. This is the period of greatest fetal growth, when the fetus

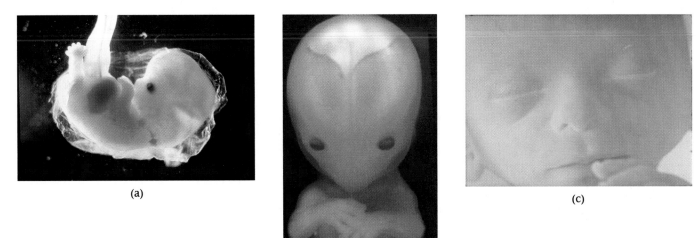

(a)

(b)

(c)

This series of fetoscopic photographs shows the development of a fetus from the first (a), second (b), and third (c), trimesters of pregnancy.

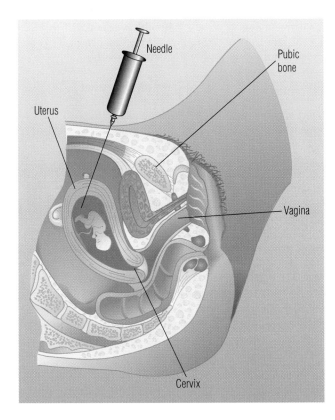

Figure 6.7
Amniocentesis
The process of amniocentesis can detect certain congenital problems as well as the sex of the fetus.

gains most of its weight. During the third trimester, the fetus must get large amounts of calcium, iron, and nitrogen from the food the mother eats. Approximately 85 percent of the calcium and iron the mother digests goes into the fetal bloodstream.

Although the fetus may live if it is born during the seventh month, it needs the layer of fat it acquires during the eighth month and time for the organs (especially the respiratory and digestive organs) to develop to their full potential. Babies born prematurely usually require intensive medical care.

Of course, the process of pregnancy involves much more than the changes in a woman's body. Many important emotional changes occur from the time a woman learns she is pregnant through the **"fourth trimester"** (the first six weeks of an infant's life outside the womb). Table 6.4 outlines common emotions and emotional challenges that may arise over the course of pregnancy.

Prenatal Testing and Screening

Modern technology enables medical practitioners to detect health defects in a fetus as early as the fourteenth to eighteenth weeks of pregnancy. One common testing procedure, **amniocentesis,** which is strongly recommended for women over age 35, involves inserting a long needle through the mother's abdominal and uterine walls into the **amniotic sac,** the protective pouch surrounding the baby (Figure 6.7). The

"Fourth trimester"   The first six weeks of an infant's life outside the womb.

Amniocentesis   A medical test in which a small amount of fluid is drawn from the amniotic sac to test for Down syndrome and genetic diseases.

Amniotic sac   The protective pouch surrounding the baby.

Table 6.4
Common Emotions Experienced Throughout the Pregnancy Process

FIRST TRIMESTER	SECOND TRIMESTER	THIRD TRIMESTER	FOURTH TRIMESTER
Disbelief that one is actually pregnant	Sense that the pregnancy feels "real"	Development of emotional relationship with baby —beginning to view baby as a person as more fetal movement occurs	Sense of being overwhelmed at new responsibility—"What do we do now?"
Fear of miscarriage	Less fear of miscarriage	Fear of labor, labor complications, possible defects	Difficulty in settling limits on friend and family visits; learning to negotiate everyone's roles in baby's life
Feeling of being overwhelmed by changes	Wonder at hearing the heartbeat, feeling movement, bulging tummy	Possible tiredness of pregnancy (Pregnancy seems to take over identity—"Is that all people want to talk about?")	Exhaustion and emotional vacillation due to sleep deprivation, breast-feeding
Tendency to be more emotional, crying more easily, for example	Frustration when symptoms make fulfilling other responsibilities difficult	Impatience for due date to arrive, possible frustration with limited mobility	Surprise at how slow the physical healing process may be, impatient to get back to pre-pregnancy shape
Apprehension about upcoming decisions (screening tests, etc.)	Differing emotions about weight gain (Some enjoy it; others struggle with it.)	Interest in others' birth experiences (especially one's mother's) and parenting styles	Amazement at the birth process
Excitement about telling others about pregnancy if waiting until the end of first trimester	Excitement and anxiety in making plans for future	Excitement in making final preparations for baby, baby showers, which makes the event seem more real	Excitement about future; apprehension about post–maternity leave transition, if applicable —"How will I balance everything?"
Anxiety about being a parent	Anxiety about being a parent	Anxiety about being a parent	Anxiety about being a parent

Source: Information for second through fourth trimesters adapted from C. M. Peterson and N. L. Stotland, "Physical and Emotional Changes," *Lamaze Parents Magazine,* 2000 spring/summer issue.

needle draws out three to four teaspoons of fluid, which is analyzed for genetic information about the baby. This test can reveal the presence of 40 genetic abnormalities, including Down syndrome, Tay-Sachs disease (a fatal disorder of the nervous system common among Jewish people of Eastern European descent), and sickle-cell anemia (a debilitating blood disorder found primarily among people of African descent). Amniocentesis can also reveal the sex of the child, a fact many parents choose not to know until the birth. Although widely used, amniocentesis is not without risk. Chances of fetal damage and miscarriage as a result of testing are 1 in 400.

Another procedure, *ultrasound,* or *sonography,* uses high-frequency sound waves to determine the size and position of the fetus. Ultrasound can also detect defects in the central nervous system and digestive system of the fetus. Knowing the position of the fetus assists practitioners in performing amniocentesis and delivering the child. New three-dimensional ultrasound techniques clarify images and improve doctors' efforts to detect and treat defects prenatally.

A third procedure, *fetoscopy,* involves making a small incision in the abdominal and uterine walls and inserting an optical viewer into the uterus to view the fetus directly. This device is used with ultrasound to determine fetal age and location of the placenta. This method is still experimental and involves some risk. It causes miscarriage in approximately 5 percent of cases.

A fourth procedure, *chorionic villus sampling (CVS)*, involves snipping tissue from the developing fetal sac. CVS can be used at 10 to 12 weeks of pregnancy, and the test results are available in 12 to 48 hours. This test is an attractive option for couples who are at high risk for having a baby with Down syndrome or a debilitating hereditary disease.

If any of these tests reveals a serious birth defect, parents are advised to undergo genetic counseling. In the case of a chromosomal abnormality such as Down syndrome, the parents are usually offered the option of a therapeutic abortion. Some parents choose this option; others research their unborn child's disability and decide to go ahead with the birth and offer the baby the love and support all children deserve.

> ### What do you think?
> *In looking at your current lifestyle, what behaviors (e.g., nutritional choices, fitness) would you cease or begin in order to promote a healthy pregnancy?* ✱ *What characteristics or skills would you look for in selecting a health care provider for care during your own or your partner's pregnancy?* ✱ *What are your thoughts on prenatal testing?* ✱ *Would you want to know whether you are carrying a child with a genetic defect or other abnormality? Why or why not?*

Childbirth

Making decisions that will affect a newborn baby begins long before the baby is born. Prospective parents need to make a number of key decisions. These include where to have the baby, whether to use drugs during labor and delivery, which childbirth method to use, and whether to breast-feed or bottle-feed. Having answers to these questions will ensure a smoother passage into parenthood.

Choosing Where to Have Your Baby

Today's prospective mothers have many delivery options, ranging from traditional hospital birth to home birth. Parental values are important. Many couples, for instance, feel that the modern medical establishment has dehumanized the birth process; thus, they choose to deliver at home or at a *birthing center,* a homelike setting outside a hospital where women can give birth and receive postdelivery care by a team of professional practitioners, including physicians and registered nurses.

However, hospitals have responded to the desire for a more relaxed, less medically oriented birthing process. Many hospitals now offer labor–delivery–postpartum birthing rooms, which allow patients with noncomplicated deliveries to spend the entire process in one room. In addition, "rooming-in," or keeping the baby in the same room with the mother at all times, is encouraged to facilitate bonding and breast-feeding. Partners are generally encouraged to "room-in" with mother and baby as well.

Labor and Delivery

The birth process has three stages (Figure 6.8). The exact mechanisms that signal the mother's body that the baby is ready to be born are unknown. During the few weeks preceding delivery, the baby normally shifts and turns to a head-down position, and the cervix begins to dilate (widen). The junction of the pubic bones also loosens to permit expansion of the pelvic girdle during birth.

In the first stage of labor, the amniotic sac breaks, causing a rush of fluid from the vagina (commonly referred to as "breaking of the waters"). Contractions in the abdomen and lower back also signal the beginning of labor. Early contractions push the baby downward, putting pressure on the cervix and dilating it further. The first stage of labor may last from a couple of hours to more than a day for a first birth, but it is usually much shorter during subsequent births.

The end of the first stage of labor, called **transition,** is the process during which the cervix becomes fully dilated and the baby's head begins to move into the vagina, or the birth canal. Contractions usually come quickly during transition, which generally lasts 30 minutes or less.

The second stage of labor (the *expulsion stage*) follows transition when the cervix has become fully dilated. Contractions become rhythmic, stronger, and more painful as the uterus works to push the baby through the birth canal. The expulsion stage lasts one to four hours and concludes when the infant is finally pushed out of the mother's body. In some cases, the attending practitioner will do an **episiotomy,** a straight incision in the mother's **perineum,** to prevent the baby's head from tearing vaginal tissues and speed the baby's exit from the vagina. Sometimes women can avoid the need for an episiotomy by exercising and getting good nutrition throughout pregnancy, by trying different birth positions, or by having an attendant massage the perineal tissue. However, the skin's natural elasticity and the baby's size are limiting factors.

After delivery, the attending practitioner cleans the baby's mucus-filled breathing passages, and the baby takes

---

Transition   The process during which the cervix becomes nearly fully dilated and the head of the fetus begins to move into the birth canal.

Episiotomy   A straight incision in the mother's perineum.

Perineum   The area between the vulva and the anus.

its first breath, generally accompanied by a loud wail. (The traditional "slap" on the baby's buttocks, often romanticized in old movies, is no longer a common practice because of the trauma associated with it.) The umbilical cord is then tied and severed. The stump of cord attached to the baby's navel dries up and drops off within a few days.

In the meantime, the mother continues into the third stage of labor, during which the placenta, or **afterbirth,** is expelled from the womb. This stage is usually completed within 30 minutes after delivery.

Most mothers prefer to have their new infants next to them following the birth. Together with their spouse or partner, they feel a need to share this time of bonding with their infant.

Managing Labor: Medical and Nonmedical Approaches

Because pain-killing drugs given to the mother during labor can cause sluggish responses in the newborn and other complications, many women choose drug-free labor and delivery. But it is important to keep a flexible attitude about pain relief because each labor is different. Working in partnership with a health care provider to make the best decision for mother and baby is the best plan. Use of pain-killing medication during a delivery is not a sign of weakness. One person is not a "success" for delivering without medication while another is a "failure" for using medical measures. Remember, pain is to be expected. In fact, many experts say that the pain of labor is the most difficult in the human experience. However, there is no one right answer in managing that pain.

Birth Alternatives

Expectant parents have several options for the setting of their infant's birth and their participation in it. Although several of these methods have decreased in popularity, all continue to be used.

The Lamaze Method The Lamaze method is the most popular birth alternative in the United States. Prelabor education classes teach the mother to control her pain through special breathing patterns, focusing exercises, and relaxation. Lamaze births usually take place in a hospital or birthing center with a physician or midwife in attendance. The partner (or labor coach) assists by giving emotional support, physical comfort (massage and ice chips), and coaching for proper breath control during contractions. Lamaze proponents discourage the use of drugs.

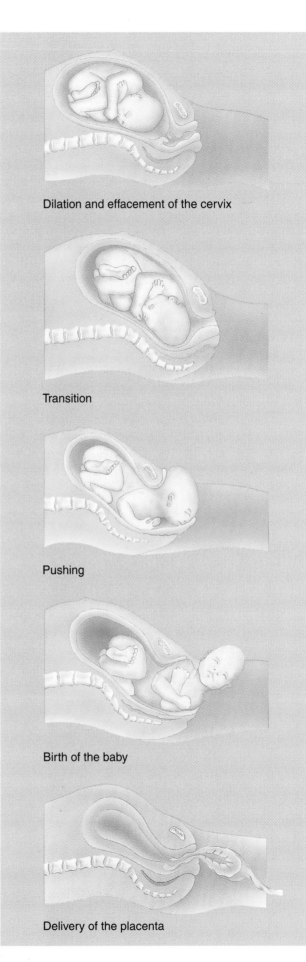

Dilation and effacement of the cervix

Transition

Pushing

Birth of the baby

Delivery of the placenta

Figure 6.8
The Birth Process

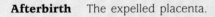

Afterbirth   The expelled placenta.

The Harris Method   Parents using the Harris method are taught by registered nurses. Gentle touching and controlled breathing are stressed. Partners provide emotional support while a physician–nurse team essentially controls the labor and delivery. Drugs are not prohibited.

Childbirth Without Fear   Sometimes called the Read method, Childbirth Without Fear advocates relaxation and education for understanding the birth process. Mothers are taught to recognize that anticipating pain creates more pain. The partner provides emotional support, and drugs are not prohibited.

The Leboyer Method   Leboyer proponents believe that birth in the standard delivery room is a traumatic experience for the baby. The Leboyer method allows the mother to deliver in a dark and quiet setting. Immediately after delivery, the infant is placed in a warm bath to ease its transition to life outside the womb. Drug use is discouraged.

The Bradley Method   The Bradley method emphasizes little to no pain medication and as little medical intervention in the birthing process as possible. Good nutrition and physical activity patterns throughout pregnancy are stressed, and deep relaxation methods are taught. This method also focuses on the partner's role in a satisfying labor experience.

Water Birth   Proponents of this method recommend giving birth in a dimly lighted, relaxed environment. The mother is placed in a warm tub. The partner may join the woman in the tub to help massage and guide her through contractions. The baby is delivered into the water and then placed at the mother's breast. Many water births take place in the home, generally with no painkillers.

Breast-Feeding and the Postpartum Period

Although the new mother's milk will not begin to flow for two or more days, her breasts secrete a thick yellow substance called *colostrum*. Because this fluid contains vital antibodies to help fight infection, the newborn baby should be allowed to suckle.

As a result of recent scientific findings, the American Academy of Pediatrics strongly recommends that full-term newborns be breast-fed. This recommendation does not mean, however, that breast milk is the only way to nourish a baby. Prepared formulas can provide nourishment that allows a baby to grow and thrive.

Still, there are many advantages to breast-feeding. Breast milk is perfectly suited to a baby's nutritional needs. Breast-fed babies have fewer illnesses and a much lower hospitalization rate because breast milk contains maternal antibodies and immunological cells that stimulate the infant's immune system. When breast-fed babies do get sick, they recover more quickly. They are also less likely to be obese than babies fed on formulas, and they have fewer allergies.

When deciding whether to breast- or bottle-feed, mothers need to consider their own desires and preferences. Both feeding methods can supply the physical and emotional closeness so essential to the parent–child relationship.

A recent study by Avery and colleagues found that women who were able to breast-feed successfully for longer periods of time generally viewed breast-feeding as more positive, had more knowledge about the process, and had higher self-efficacy in their ability to breast-feed.[20]

The *postpartum period* lasts from four to six weeks after delivery. During this time, the mother's reproductive organs revert to a nonpregnant state. Many women experience energy depletion, anxiety, mood swings, and depression during this period. This experience, known as **postpartum depression,** appears to be a normal end-product of the birth process. For most women, the symptoms gradually disappear as their bodies return to normal. For others, the symptoms, coupled with the stresses of managing a new family, can cause more severe depression that lasts for several months.

> **What do you think?**
> *What are your thoughts on medical versus natural management of labor and delivery?* ✳ *Do you have strong preferences for how you'd like to manage your own birthing process? If so, what are they?* ✳ *What might be the advantages and disadvantages of breast-feeding?*

Complications

Problems and complications can occur during labor and delivery, even following a successful pregnancy. Such possibilities should be discussed with the practitioner prior to labor so the mother understands what medical procedures may be necessary for her safety and that of her child. Although pregnancy still involves a certain amount of risk, the risk is lower than for many other common activities.

Cesarean Section (C-Section)   If labor lasts too long or if a baby is presenting wrong (about to exit the uterus in any way but head first), a **cesarean section (C-section)** may be necessary. This surgical procedure involves making an incision across the mother's abdomen and through the uterus to remove the baby. This operation is also performed in cases in

---

Postpartum depression   The experience of energy depletion, anxiety, mood swings, and depression that women may feel during the postpartum period.

Cesarean section (C-section)   A surgical procedure in which a baby is removed through an incision made in the mother's abdominal and uterine walls.

which labor is extremely difficult, maternal blood pressure falls rapidly, the placenta separates from the uterus too soon, the mother has diabetes, or other problems occur.

A cesarean section can be traumatic for the mother if she is not prepared for it. The rate of delivery by cesarean section in the United States increased from 5 percent in the mid-1960s to more than 25 percent by 1988 but leveled off to approximately 17 percent in 1999.[21] Risks to the mother are the same as for any major abdominal surgery, and recovery from birth takes considerably longer after a C-section. Although a cesarean section may be necessary in certain cases, some physicians and critics feel that the option has been used too frequently in this country. The federal government's Centers for Disease Control and Prevention (CDC) believes that about one in three of the cesarean deliveries performed in 1991 were unnecessary. The CDC had hoped to lower the rate of cesareans in the United States to 15 per 100 births by the year 2000, a level the agency considers to be medically appropriate. Unfortunately, the goal has not been met.

Now, however, surgical techniques allow some women who have had a cesarean section to deliver later children vaginally. Guidelines published by the American College of Obstetricians and Gynecologists give an estimated 50 to 80 percent of women the option of a vaginal birth after cesarean (VBAC). Cesarean sections will still be necessary, however, if the original incision runs from the top to the bottom of the uterus (as opposed to across); if the baby is over 9 pounds; if the birth is multiple; or if the mother has a medical condition that would make vaginal delivery difficult or dangerous, such as a very small pelvis, chronic high blood pressure, or diabetes.

Miscarriage   One in 10 pregnancies does not end in delivery. Loss of the fetus before it is viable is called a **miscarriage** (also referred to as spontaneous abortion). An estimated 70 to 90 percent of women who miscarry eventually become pregnant again.

Reasons for miscarriage vary. In some cases, the fertilized egg has failed to divide correctly. In others, genetic abnormalities, maternal illness, or infections are responsible. Maternal hormonal imbalance may also cause a miscarriage, as may a weak cervix or toxic chemicals in the environment. In most cases, the cause is not known.

A blood incompatibility between mother and father can cause **Rh factor** problems, sometimes resulting in miscarriage. Rh is a blood protein. Rh problems occur when the mother is Rh-negative and the fetus is Rh-positive. During a first birth, some of the baby's blood passes into the mother's bloodstream. An Rh-negative mother may manufacture antibodies to destroy the Rh-positive blood introduced into her bloodstream at the time of birth. Her first baby will be unaffected, but subsequent babies with positive Rh factor will be at risk for a severe anemia called *hemolytic disease* because the mother's Rh antibodies will attack the fetus's red blood cells.

Medical advances now offer both prevention and treatment for this condition. If testing reveals Rh incompatibility, intrauterine transfusions can be given or an early delivery by cesarean section can be done, depending upon the individual case. Prevention is preferable to treatment. All women with Rh-negative blood should be injected with a medication called RhoGAM within 72 hours of any birth, miscarriage, or abortion. This injection will prevent them from developing the Rh antibodies.

Another cause of miscarriage is **ectopic pregnancy,** or implantation of a fertilized egg outside the uterus. A fertilized egg may implant itself in the fallopian tube or, occasionally, in the pelvic cavity. Because these structures are not capable of expanding and nourishing a developing fetus, the pregnancy cannot continue. Such pregnancies are surgically terminated. Most often, the affected fallopian tube is also removed.

Ectopic pregnancy is generally accompanied by pain in the lower abdomen or aching in the shoulders as the blood flows up toward the diaphragm. If bleeding is significant, blood pressure drops, and the woman can go into shock. If an ectopic pregnancy goes undiagnosed and untreated, the fallopian tube will rupture, putting the woman at great risk of hemorrhage, peritonitis (infection in the abdomen), and even death.

Over the past 12 years, the incidence of ectopic pregnancy has tripled, and no one really understands why. We do know that ectopic pregnancy is a potential side effect of pelvic inflammatory disease (PID), which has become increasingly common in recent years. The scarring or blockage of the fallopian tubes characteristic of this disease prevents the fertilized egg from passing to the uterus. About 50 percent of women who have had an ectopic pregnancy conceive again. But women who have had one ectopic pregnancy run a higher risk of having another.

Stillbirth is one of the most traumatic events a couple can face. A stillborn baby is one that is born dead, often for no apparent reason. The grief experienced following a stillbirth is usually devastating. Nine months of happy anticipation have been thwarted. Family, friends, and other children may be in a state of shock, needing comfort and not knowing where to turn. The mother's breasts produce milk, and there is no infant to be fed. A room with a crib and toys is left empty.

Miscarriage   Loss of the fetus before it is viable; also called spontaneous abortion.

Rh factor   A blood protein related to the production of antibodies. If an Rh-negative mother is pregnant with an Rh-positive fetus, the mother will manufacture antibodies that can kill the fetus, causing miscarriage.

Ectopic pregnancy   Implantation of a fertilized egg outside the uterus, usually in a fallopian tube; a medical emergency that can end in death from hemorrhage for the mother.

Stillbirth   The birth of a dead baby.

The grief can last for years, and both partners may blame themselves or each other. In many cases, no amount of reassurance from the attending physician, relatives, or friends can assuage the grief or guilt. Well-intended comments such as, "Oh, you'll have another baby someday," may only create uncomfortable feelings.

Some communities have groups called the Compassionate Friends to help parents and other family members through this grieving process. This nonprofit organization is for parents who have lost a child of any age for any reason.

Sudden Infant Death Syndrome (SIDS) The sudden death of an infant under one year of age, for no apparent reason, is called **sudden infant death syndrome (SIDS).** Though SIDS is the leading cause of death for children aged one month to one year, affecting about 1 in 1,000 infants in the United States each year, it is not a disease. Rather, it is ruled the cause of death after all other possibilities are ruled out. A SIDS death is sudden and silent; death occurs quickly, often associated with sleep and no signs of suffering.

Because SIDS is a diagnosis of exclusion, doctors do not know what causes it. However, research done in countries including England, New Zealand, Australia, and Norway has shown that placing children on their backs or sides to sleep cuts the rate of SIDS by as much as half. The American Academy of Pediatrics advises parents to lay infants on their backs. Additional precautions against SIDS include having a firm surface for the infant's bed, not allowing the infant to become too warm, maintaining a smoke-free environment, having regular pediatric visits, breast-feeding, and seeking prenatal care.

Infertility

An estimated one in six American couples experiences **infertility,** or difficulties in conceiving. Reasons include the trend toward delaying childbirth (as a woman gets older, she is less likely to conceive), endometriosis, and the rising incidence of pelvic inflammatory disease.

Causes in Women

Endometriosis is the leading cause of infertility in women in the United States. With this disorder, parts of the endometrial lining of the uterus implant themselves outside the uterus—in the fallopian tubes, lungs, intestines, outer uterine walls or ovarian walls, and/or on the ligaments that support the uterus. The disorder can be treated surgically or with hormonal preparations. Success rates vary.

Another cause of infertility is **pelvic inflammatory disease (PID),** a serious infection that scars the fallopian tubes and blocks sperm migration. PID is a collective name for any extensive bacterial infection of the female pelvic organs, particularly the uterus, cervix, fallopian tubes, and ovaries. PID is often the result of chlamydia or gonorrheal

infections that spread to the fallopian tubes or ovaries. Symptoms of PID include severe pain, fever, and sometimes vaginal discharge.

The past 30 years have brought a tremendous increase in the annual number of PID cases, from 17,800 to about 1 million per year. During the reproductive years, one in seven women reports having been treated for PID,[22] and tens of thousands have been rendered sterile. One episode of PID causes sterility in 10 to 15 percent of women, and 50 to 75 percent become sterile after three or four infections.[23]

Causes in Men

Among men, the single largest fertility problem is **low sperm count.** Although only one viable sperm is needed for fertilization, research has shown that all the other sperm in the ejaculate aid in the fertilization process. There are normally 60 to 80 million sperm per milliliter of semen. When the count drops below 60 million, fertility declines.

Low sperm count may be attributable to environmental factors, such as exposure of the scrotum to intense heat or cold, radiation, or altitude, or even to wearing excessively tight underwear or outerwear. However, other factors, such as the mumps virus, can damage the cells that make sperm. Varicose veins above one or both testicles can also render men infertile. Male infertility problems account for around 40 percent of infertility cases.

Treatment

For the couple desperately wishing to conceive, the road to parenthood may be frustrating. Fortunately, medical treatment can identify the cause of infertility in about 90 percent of affected couples. The chances of becoming pregnant range from 30 to 70 percent, depending on the reason for

---

Sudden infant death syndrome (SIDS) The sudden death of an infant under one year of age for no apparent reason.

Infertility Difficulties in conceiving.

Endometriosis A disorder in which uterine lining tissue establishes itself outside the uterus; the leading cause of infertility in the United States.

Pelvic inflammatory disease (PID) An infection that scars the fallopian tubes and consequently blocks sperm migration, causing infertility.

Low sperm count A sperm count below 60 million sperm per milliliter of semen; the leading cause of infertility in men.

infertility. The countless tests and the invasion of privacy that characterize some couples' efforts to conceive can put stress on an otherwise strong, healthy relationship. Before starting fertility tests, couples should reassess their priorities. Some will choose to undergo counseling to help them clarify their feelings about the fertility process. A good physician or fertility team will take the time to ascertain the couple's level of motivation.

Fertility workups can be very expensive, and the costs are not usually covered by insurance companies. Fertility workups for men include a sperm count, a test for sperm motility, and analysis of any disease processes present. Such procedures should be undertaken only by a qualified urologist. Women are thoroughly examined by an obstetrician–gynecologist for the composition of cervical mucus, extent of tubal scarring, and evidence of endometriosis.

Complete fertility workups may take four to five months and can be unsettling. The couple may be instructed to have sex "by the calendar" to increase their chances of conceiving. In some cases, surgery can correct structural problems, such as tubal scarring. In others, administering hormones can improve the health of ova and sperm. Sometimes pregnancy can be achieved by collecting the man's sperm from several ejaculations and inseminating the woman at a later time.

When all surgical and hormonal methods fail, the couple still has some options. These, too, can be very expensive. **Fertility drugs,** such as Clomid and Pergonal, stimulate ovulation in women who are not ovulating. Ninety percent of women who use these drugs will begin to ovulate, and half will conceive.

Fertility drugs can have many side effects, including headaches, irritability, restlessness, depression, fatigue, edema (fluid retention), abnormal uterine bleeding, breast tenderness, vasomotor flushes (hot flashes), and visual difficulties. Women using fertility drugs are also at increased risk of developing multiple ovarian cysts (fluid-filled growths) and liver damage. The drugs sometimes trigger the release of more than one egg. Thus a woman treated with one of these drugs has a one in ten chance of having multiple births. Most such births are twins, but triplets and even quadruplets are not uncommon.

Alternative insemination of a woman with her partner's sperm is another treatment option. This technique has led to an estimated 250,000 births in the United States, primarily for couples in which the man is infertile. If this procedure fails, the couple may choose insemination by an anonymous donor through a "sperm bank." Many men sell their sperm to such banks. The sperm are classified according to the physical characteristics of the donor (for example, blonde hair, blue eyes) and then frozen for future use. Frozen sperm can survive for up to five years. The woman being inseminated usually chooses sperm from a man whose physical characteristics resemble those of her partner or match her own personal preferences.

In the last few years, concern has been expressed about the possibility of transmitting the AIDS virus through alternative insemination. As a result, donors are routinely screened for the disease.

In vitro fertilization, often referred to as "test tube" fertilization, involves collecting a viable ovum from the prospective mother and transferring it to a nutrient medium in a laboratory, where it is fertilized with sperm from the woman's partner or a donor. After a few days, the embryo is transplanted into the mother's uterus, where, it is hoped, it will develop normally. Until 1984, in vitro fertilization was classified as experimental. Since then, it has moved into the mainstream of standard infertility treatments. Since 1984, the in vitro process has been responsible for 26,000 births in the United States alone.

In **gamete intrafallopian transfer (GIFT),** the egg is "harvested" from the woman's ovary and placed in the fallopian tube with the man's sperm. Less expensive and time consuming than in vitro fertilization, GIFT mimics nature by allowing the egg to be fertilized in the fallopian tube and migrate to the uterus according to the normal timetable.

Intracytoplasmic sperm injection (ICSI) was first performed successfully in 1992. Basically, a sperm cell is injected into an egg. This complex procedure required researchers to learn how to manipulate both egg and sperm without damaging them. This technique can help men with low sperm counts or motility, and even those who cannot ejaculate or have no live sperm in their semen as a result of vasectomy, chemotherapy, or a medical disorder. Scientists have examined a thousand babies born using this technique and have found no higher rate of birth defects than in the general population. Nonetheless, ICSI is still considered experimental.

Fertility drugs   Hormones that stimulate ovulation in women who are not ovulating; often responsible for multiple births.

Alternative insemination   Fertilization accomplished by depositing a partner's or a donor's semen into a women's vagina via a thin tube; almost always done in a doctor's office.

In vitro fertilization   Fertilization of an egg in a nutrient medium and subsequent transfer back to the mother's body.

Gamete intrafallopian transfer (GIFT)   Procedure in which an egg harvested from the female partner's ovary is placed with the male partner's sperm in her fallopian tube, where it is fertilized and then migrates to the uterus for implantation.

Intracytoplasmic sperm injection (ICSI)   Fertilization accomplished by injecting a sperm cell directly into an egg.

In **nonsurgical embryo transfer,** a donor egg is fertilized by the man's sperm and implanted in the woman's uterus. This procedure may also be used in cases involving the transfer of an already fertilized ovum into the uterus of another woman.

In **embryo transfer,** an ovum from a donor's body is artificially inseminated by the male partner's sperm, allowed to stay in the donor's body for a time, and then transplanted into the female partner's body.

Some laboratories are experimenting with **embryo freezing,** in which a fertilized embryo is suspended in a solution of liquid nitrogen. When desired, it is gradually thawed and implanted into the prospective mother. The first U.S. birth of a frozen embryo was reported in 1986. In the future, this technique may make it possible for young couples to produce an embryo and save it for later implantation when they are ready to have a child, thus reducing the risks of fertilizing older eggs.

Infertile couples, whose only prior hope for children was adoption, have a new alternative—**embryo adoption programs.** The embryos are originally collected from couples who want children via in vitro fertilization. These couples often donate and freeze extra embryos in case the procedure fails or they want to have more children at a later time. These couples can now donate their unneeded embryos to others. The adopting couple can enjoy the experience of pregnancy and control prenatal care. The cost is approximately $4,000 for the embryos to be thawed and transferred to an infertile woman's uterus or fallopian tubes.

The ethical and moral questions surrounding experimental infertility treatments are staggering. Before moving forward with any of these treatments, individuals need to ask themselves a few important questions. Has infertility been absolutely confirmed? Are reputable infertility counseling services accessible? Have they explored all possible alternatives and considered potential risks? Have all affected parties examined their attitudes, values, and beliefs about conceiving a child in this manner? Finally, individuals need to consider what and how they will tell the child about their method of conception.

Surrogate Motherhood

Between 60 and 70 percent of infertile couples are able to conceive after treatment. The rest decide to live without children, to adopt, or to attempt surrogate motherhood. In this option, the couple hires a woman to be alternatively inseminated by the husband. The surrogate then carries the baby to term and surrenders it upon birth to the couple. Surrogate mothers are reportedly paid about $10,000 for their services and are reimbursed for medical expenses. Legal and medical expenses can run as high as $30,000 for the infertile couple.

Couples considering surrogate motherhood are advised to consult a lawyer regarding contracts. Most of these legal documents stipulate that the surrogate mother must undergo amniocentesis and that if the fetus is defective, she must consent to an abortion. In that case, or if the surrogate miscarries, she is reimbursed for her time and expenses. The prospective parents must also agree to take the baby if it is carried to term, even if it is unhealthy or has physical abnormalities.

Adoption

For couples who have decided that biological childbirth is not an option for them, adoption provides an alternative to bearing a child. Currently, about 50,000 children are available for adoption in the United States every year. This is far fewer than the number of couples seeking adoptions. By some estimates, only 1 in 30 couples receives the children they want. On average, couples spend two years on the adoption process. Some couples choose to adopt orphans or refugees from other countries.

Because the number of American children available for adoption is limited, women who consider placing their child for adoption have gained new leverage. Increasingly, couples wishing to adopt have turned to independent adoptions arranged by a lawyer, or they may directly negotiate with the birth mother. Independent adoptions now surpass those arranged by social service agencies.

> ### What do you think?
> *How much time and money would you be willing to invest in infertility treatments if you were to find that you and your partner had infertility problems? ❋ Do you think that single women and lesbians should have equal access to alternative methods of insemination? Why or why not? ❋ Do you think single women or men and gay males or lesbians should have equal opportunities at adoption? ❋ How do you think society views these types of adoptions? Why?*

Nonsurgical embryo transfer   In vitro fertilization of a donor egg by the male partner's (or donor's) sperm and subsequent transfer to the female partner's or another woman's uterus.

Embryo transfer   Artificial insemination of a donor with male partner's sperm; after a time, the embryo is transferred from the donor to the female partner's body.

Embryo freezing   The freezing of an embryo for later implantation.

Embryo adoption programs   A procedure whereby an infertile couple is able to purchase frozen embryos donated by another couple.

Reproduction Choices: Making Responsible Decisions

After reading this chapter, you should realize that pregnancy, childbirth, and reproductive issues are not to be taken lightly. The choices between different types of birth control and the ethical issues surrounding fertility are complex. It's important to take control of your own fertility and to share this responsibility in your relationships. Is birth control an option for you? If so, have you considered which birth control options would be most appropriate for you? Be sure to examine all potential side effects and drug interactions. The following questions can help you determine your level of readiness regarding reproduction and sexual health.

Checklist for Change

Making Personal Choices

✓ If you are in a stable relationship and are considering having a child, is it something both you and your partner want?

✓ Do you know and feel comfortable with your philosophical beliefs about children?

✓ Do you feel comfortable discussing birth control with your partner?

✓ Do you feel comfortable choosing a method of birth control that meets the needs of both yourself and your partner?

✓ Are you familiar with the resources available if you have trouble conceiving?

✓ Have you discussed alternatives should you or your partner becomes pregnant?

Making Community Choices

✓ Have you taken the time to become educated about the issues and concerns related to parenting?

✓ Do you listen with an open mind to issues involving reproduction and sexual health and then make informed decisions?

✓ When you think about having children, do you think in terms of long-range planning?

✓ Do you advocate for allowing people to make choices that are in their best interest, regardless of your own personal philosophy or opinions?

✓ Do you believe in providing support for community agencies and social services that assist in meeting the sexual and reproductive health needs of your community?

✓ Do you try to volunteer your time to other people or agencies that may need your assistance?

Summary

* Latex condoms and the female condom, when used correctly for oral sex or intercourse, provide the most effective protection in preventing sexually transmitted infections. Other contraceptive methods include abstinence, outercourse, oral contraceptives, foams, jellies, suppositories, creams, the diaphragm, the cervical cap, intrauterine devices, withdrawal, Norplant, and Depo-Provera. Fertility awareness methods rely on altering sexual practices to avoid pregnancy. Whereas all these methods of contraception are reversible, sterilization is permanent.

* Abortion is currently legal in the United States through the second trimester. Abortion methods include vacuum aspiration, dilation and evacuation (D&E), dilation and curettage (D&C), intact dilation and extraction (D&X), hysterotomy, induction abortion, and RU-486 "abortion pills."

* Parenting is a demanding job that requires careful planning. Emotional health, maternal health, paternal health, financial evaluation, and contingency planning all need to be taken into account.

* Prenatal care includes a complete physical exam within the first trimester and avoidance of alcohol and drugs, cigarettes, x-rays, and chemicals having teratogenic effects. Full-term pregnancy covers three trimesters.

* Childbirth occurs in three stages. Birth alternatives include the Lamaze method, the Harris method, Childbirth Without Fear, the Leboyer method, the Bradley method, and water birth. Partners should jointly choose a labor method early in the pregnancy to be better prepared for labor when it occurs. Complications of pregnancy and childbirth include miscarriage, ectopic pregnancy, stillbirth, and cesarean section.

* Infertility in women may be caused by pelvic inflammatory disease or endometriosis. In men, it may be caused by low sperm count. Treatment may include alternative insemination, in vitro fertilization, gamete intrafallopian transfer, nonsurgical embryo transfer, and embryo transfer. Surrogate motherhood involves hiring a fertile woman to be alternatively inseminated by the male partner.

Discussion Questions

1. List the most effective contraceptive methods. What are their drawbacks? What medical conditions would keep a person from using them? What are the characteristics of the methods that you think would be most effective for you, and why?
2. What are the various methods of abortion? What are the two opposing viewpoints concerning abortion? What is *Roe v. Wade,* and what impact did it have on the abortion debate?
3. What are the most important considerations in deciding whether the time is right to become a parent? What factors will you consider regarding the number of children you will have?
4. Discuss the growth of the fetus through the three trimesters. What medical checkups or tests should be done during each trimester?
5. Discuss the emotional aspects of pregnancy. What types of emotional reactions are common in each trimester and the postpartum period (the "fourth trimester")?
6. Discuss the medical and nonmedical (natural) management of childbirth. What options are available to manage labor? Discuss the various types of alternative birthing practice.

Application Exercise

Reread the What Do You Think? scenario at the beginning of the chapter, and answer the following questions.

1. What contraceptive options might Brittany consider other than emergency contraception?
2. What are the positive and negative aspects of emergency contraception methods? What potential risks is Brittany taking by using only these methods?

Accessing Your Health on the Internet

Visit the following Internet sites to explore further topics and issues related to personal health. To visit an organization's website, go to the Companion Website for *Health: The Basics, Fifth Edition* at www.aw.com/donatelle, click on the book image, and select "Accessing Your Health on the Internet" from the navigation menu on the left.

1. ***The National Parenting Center.*** This site invites parents to expand their parenting skills and strengths by sharing information in chat rooms and in an online newsletter.
2. ***Safer Sex.*** Provides information on safer sex issues. Discusses such issues as what is safer sex, whether oral sex is safe, and women and safer sex. Provides links to other websites.
3. ***Childbirth.Org.*** Information to encourage parents to be good consumers, knowing their options and how to provide themselves with the best possible care essential to a healthy pregnancy.

Further Reading

Boston Women's Health Collective. *Our Bodies, Ourselves for the New Century: A Book by and for Women.* New York: Simon and Schuster, 1998.
Like its earlier editions, this volume contains information about women's health from a decidedly feminist angle. Every aspect of health is covered, including nutrition, emotional health, fitness, relationships, reproduction, contraception, and pregnancy.

Firestone, Robert and Joyce Cattlet. *Fear of Intimacy,* 2001 American Psychological Association.
Provides insightful information about how we think about relationships and family and why relationships fail or thrive.

Hatcher, R. A., et al., *Contraceptive Technology.* 17th rev. ed. New York: Ardent Media, 1998.
Perhaps the best primary reference concerning birth control for physicians, family planning centers, student health services, and educators. Contributions include many staff members of the Centers for Disease Control and Prevention.

Stoppard, Miriam. *Conceptions, Pregnancy and Birth.* DK Publishing. ISBN 0789451158. (2000).
Overview of facts, issues, and concerns that pregnant women have during pregnancy and throughout the birthing process.

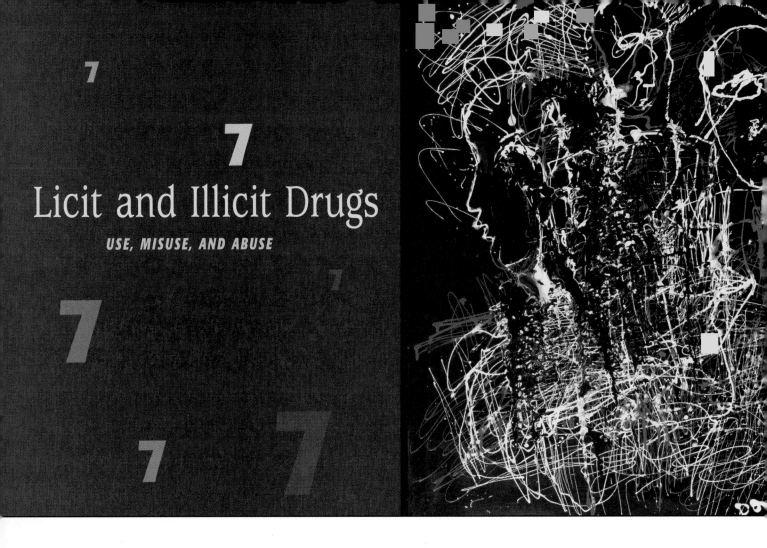

7

Licit and Illicit Drugs

USE, MISUSE, AND ABUSE

objectives

* List the six categories of drugs, and explain their routes of administration.

* Compare and contrast choices in prescription and over-the-counter drugs, and identify actions that will maximize the benefit received from such drugs.

* Discuss proper drug use, and explain how hazardous drug interactions occur.

* Discuss patterns of illicit drug use, including who uses illicit drugs and why.

* Describe the use and abuse of controlled substances, including cocaine, amphetamines, marijuana, opiates, psychedelics, deliriants, designer drugs, and inhalants.

* Profile overall illegal drug use in the United States, including frequency, financial impact, arrests for drug offenses, and impact on the workplace.

* Identify the signs of addiction.

Greg and some of his friends were smoking marijuana in Greg's residence hall room. They used fans to blow the smoke out the window, air freshener candles to mask the smell, and a towel at the bottom of the door to prevent the smoke from escaping. However, the residence hall assistant smelled the scent and immediately called security. Greg and his friends were arrested and eventually kicked out of the residence hall, left to find new housing during midsemester. Greg felt this measure was extremely unfair because underage students caught drinking alcohol in their rooms were rarely written up.

Do you think Greg has a valid point? ✳ How common is marijuana use on your campus? ✳ Do you know the penalty for smoking marijuana in your residence halls on campus? ✳ What are the substance abuse policies on your campus? ✳ Do you think your school's substance abuse policies are enough to deter students from using controlled substances?

D rug misuse and abuse are problems of staggering proportions in our society. Each year drug and alcohol abuse contributes to the deaths of over 120,000 Americans. They also cost taxpayers more than $294 billion in preventable health care costs, extra law enforcement, auto crashes, crime, and lost productivity.[1] It's impossible to put a dollar amount on the pain, suffering, and dysfunction that drugs cause in our everyday lives.

While overall use of drugs in the United States has fallen by 50 percent in the last 20 years, the past 10 years have shown an increase of use of certain drugs by adolescents.[2] Why so many people use drugs, and the mechanisms by which drugs cause harm are topics of ongoing research. Human beings appear to have a need to alter their consciousness, or mental state. We like to feel good, to escape, and to feel different. Consciousness can be altered in many ways: Children spinning until they become dizzy and adults enjoying the rush of thrilling high-intensity activities are examples. To change our awareness, many of us listen to music, skydive, ski, skate, read, daydream, meditate, pray, or have sexual relations. Others turn to illicit drugs to alter consciousness.

Drug Dynamics

Drugs work because they physically resemble the chemicals produced naturally within the body (Figure 7.1). Most bodily processes result from chemical reactions or from changes in electrical charge. Because drugs possess an electrical charge and a chemical structure similar to those of chemicals that occur naturally in the body, they can affect physical functions in many different ways. For example, many painkillers resemble the endorphins ("morphine within") that are manufactured in the body.

A current explanation of how drugs work is the *receptor site theory*. According to this theory, drugs bind to specific **receptor sites** in the body: specialized cells to which, because of their size, shape, electrical charge, and chemical properties, drugs can attach themselves. Most drugs can attach to multiple receptor sites located throughout the body in places such as the heart and blood system and the lungs, liver, kidneys, brain, and gonads (testicles or ovaries).

Types of Drugs

Scientists divide drugs into six categories: prescription, over-the-counter (OTC), recreational, herbal, illicit, and commercial drugs. These classifications are based primarily on drug action, although some are based on the source of the chemical in question. Each category includes some drugs that stimulate the body, some that depress body functions, and others that produce **hallucinations,** images (auditory or visual) that are perceived but are not real. Each category also includes **psychoactive drugs,** which have the potential to alter a person's mood or behavior.

- **Prescription drugs** are those substances that can be obtained only with the written prescription of a licensed physician. More than 10,000 types of prescription drugs are sold in the United States.

Receptor sites   Specialized cells to which drugs can attach themselves.

Hallucination   An image, auditory or visual, that is perceived but is not real.

Psychoactive drugs   Drugs that have the potential to alter mood or behavior.

Prescription drugs   Medications that can be obtained only with the written prescription of a licensed physician.

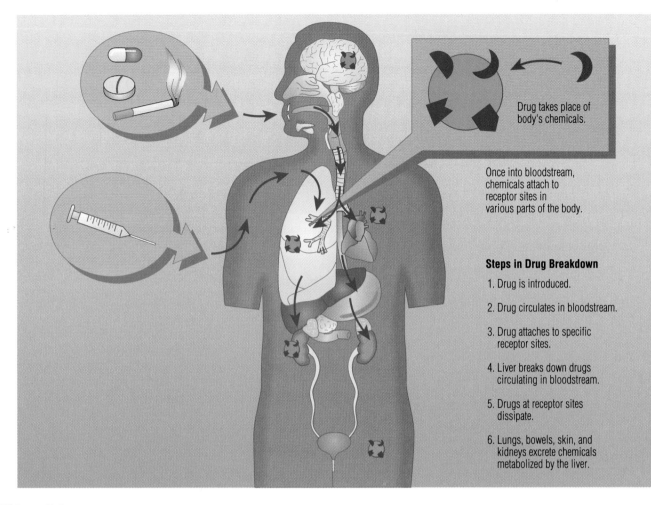

Figure 7.1
How the Body Metabolizes Drugs

Drug takes place of body's chemicals.

Once into bloodstream, chemicals attach to receptor sites in various parts of the body.

Steps in Drug Breakdown

1. Drug is introduced.

2. Drug circulates in bloodstream.

3. Drug attaches to specific receptor sites.

4. Liver breaks down drugs circulating in bloodstream.

5. Drugs at receptor sites dissipate.

6. Lungs, bowels, skin, and kidneys excrete chemicals metabolized by the liver.

- **Over-the-counter (OTC) drugs** can be purchased in pharmacies, supermarkets, and discount stores. Each year, Americans spend over $14 billion on OTC products, and the market is increasing at the rate of 20 percent annually. More than 300,000 OTC products are available, and an estimated three out of four people routinely self-medicate with them.

- **Recreational drugs** belong to a somewhat vague category whose boundaries depend on how people define *recreation*. Generally, these drugs contain chemicals used to help people relax or socialize. Most of them are legally sanctioned even though they are psychoactive. Alcohol, tobacco, coffee, tea, and chocolate products are usually included in this category.

- **Herbal preparations** form another vague category. Included among these approximately 750 substances are herbal teas and other products of plant origin that are believed to have medicinal properties.

- **Illicit (illegal) drugs** are the most notorious type of drug. Although laws governing their use, possession, cultivation, manufacture, and sale differ from state to state, illicit drugs are generally recognized as harmful. All of them are psychoactive.

- **Commercial preparations** are the most universally used yet least commonly recognized chemical substances having drug action. More than 1,000 of these substances exist, including seemingly benign items such as perfumes,

Over-the-counter (OTC) drugs   Medications that can be purchased in pharmacies or supermarkets without a physician's prescription.

Recreational drugs   Legal drugs that contain chemicals that help people relax or socialize.

Herbal preparations   Substances of plant origin that are believed to have medicinal properties.

Illicit (illegal) drugs   Drugs whose use, possession, cultivation, manufacture, and/or sale is against the law because they are generally recognized as harmful.

Commercial preparations   Commonly used chemical substances, including cosmetics, household cleaning products, and industrial by-products.

cosmetics, household cleansers, paints, glues, inks, dyes, gardening chemicals, pesticides, and industrial by-products.

Routes of Administration of Drugs

Route of administration refers to the way in which a given drug is taken into the body. Common routes are oral ingestion, injection, inhalation, inunction, and suppository.

Oral ingestion is the most common route of administration. Drugs that are swallowed include tablets, capsules, and liquids. Oral ingestion generally results in relatively slow absorption compared to other methods of administration because the drug must pass through the stomach, where digestive juices act upon it, and then move on to the small intestine before it enters the bloodstream. Several things affect drug absorption.

Many oral preparations are coated to keep them from being dissolved too quickly by corrosive stomach acids before they reach the intestine, as well as to protect the stomach lining from irritating chemicals in the drugs. Food in the stomach also slows the absorption of drugs. Some drugs must not be taken with certain foods because the food will inhibit their action, whereas others must be taken with food to prevent stomach irritation.

Depending on the drug and the amount of food in the stomach, drugs taken orally produce their effects within 20 minutes to one hour after ingestion. The only exception is alcohol, which takes effect sooner because some of it is absorbed directly into the bloodstream from the stomach. Age, metabolism and drug characteristics also effect speed of absorption.

Injection, another common form of drug administration, involves using a hypodermic syringe to introduce a drug into the body. **Intravenous injection,** or injection directly into a vein, puts the chemical in its most concentrated form directly into the bloodstream. Effects will be felt within three minutes, making this route extremely effective, particularly in medical emergencies. But injection of many substances into the bloodstream may cause serious or even fatal reactions. In addition, some serious diseases, such as hepatitis and AIDS, can be transferred in this way. For this reason, intravenous injection can be one of the most dangerous routes of administration.

Intramuscular injection places the hypodermic needle into muscular tissue, usually in the buttocks or the back of the upper arm. Normally used to administer antibiotics and vaccinations, this route of administration results in much slower absorption than intravenous injection, but ensures slow and consistent dispersion of the drug into body tissues.

Subcutaneous injection puts the drug into the layer of fat directly beneath the skin. Its common medical uses include administration of local anesthetics and insulin replacement therapy. A drug injected subcutaneously will circulate even more slowly than an intramuscularly injected drug because it takes longer to be absorbed into the bloodstream.

Inhalation refers to administration of drugs through the nostrils. This method transfers the drug rapidly into the bloodstream through the alveoli (air sacs) in the lungs. Examples of illicit inhalation include cocaine sniffing and inhaling aerosol sprays, gases, or fumes from solvents. Effects are frequently immediate but do not last as long as effects associated with slower routes of administration because only small amounts of a drug can be absorbed and metabolized in the lungs.

Inunction introduces chemicals into the body through the skin. A common example is the small adhesive patch that is used to alleviate motion sickness. This patch, which contains a prescription medicine, is applied to the skin behind one ear, where it slowly releases its chemicals to provide relief for nauseated travelers. Another example is the nicotine patch.

Suppositories are drugs that are mixed with a waxy medium designed to melt at body temperature. The most common type is inserted into the anus past the rectal sphincter muscles, which hold the suppository in place. As the wax melts, the drug is released and absorbed through the rectal walls into the bloodstream. Because this area of the anatomy contains many blood vessels, the effects of the drug are usually felt within 15 minutes. Other types of suppositories are for use in the vagina. Vaginal suppositories usually release drugs, such as antifungal agents, that treat problems in the vagina itself rather than drugs meant to travel in the bloodstream.

Using, Misusing, and Abusing Drugs

Although drug abuse is usually referred to in connection with illicit psychoactive drugs, many people abuse and misuse prescription and OTC medications. **Drug misuse** involves the

---

Route of administration   The manner in which a drug is taken into the body.

Oral ingestion   Intake of drugs through the mouth.

Injection   The introduction of drugs into the body via a hypodermic needle.

Intravenous injection   The introduction of drugs directly into a vein.

Intramuscular injection   The introduction of drugs into muscles.

Subcutaneous injection   The introduction of drugs into the layer of fat directly beneath the skin.

Inhalation   The introduction of drugs through the nostrils.

Inunction   The introduction of drugs through the skin.

Suppositories   Mixtures of drugs and a waxy medium designed to melt at body temperature that are inserted into the anus or vagina.

Drug misuse   The use of a drug for a purpose for which it was not intended.

use of a drug for a purpose for which it was not intended. For example, taking a friend's high-powered prescription painkiller for your headache is a misuse of that drug. This is not too far removed from **drug abuse,** or the excessive use of any drug, and may result in serious harm.

The misuse and abuse of any drug may lead to *addiction*. Both risks and benefits are involved in the use of any chemical substance. Intelligent decision making requires a clear-headed evaluation of these risks and benefits.

> ### What do you think?
> *What are some situations in which students misuse drugs?* ✳ *Other than alcohol, what drugs (prescription or OTC) do students tend to abuse while they are at college?*

Defining Addiction

Addiction is continued involvement with a substance or activity despite ongoing negative consequences. Addictive behaviors initially provide a sense of pleasure or stability that is beyond the addict's power to achieve in other ways. Eventually, the addicted person needs to be involved in the behavior in order to feel normal.

Physiological dependence is only one indicator of addiction. Psychological dynamics play an important role, which explains why behaviors not related to the use of chemicals—gambling, for example—may also be addictive. In fact, psychological and physiological dependence are so in-

tertwined that it is not really possible to separate the two. For every psychological state, there is a corresponding physiological state. In other words, everything you feel is tied to a chemical process occurring in your body.[3] Thus, addictions once thought to be entirely psychological in nature are now understood to have physiological components.

To be addictive, a behavior must have the potential to produce a positive mood change. Chemicals are responsible for the most profound addictions, not only because they produce dramatic mood changes, but also because they cause cellular changes to which the body adapts so well that it eventually requires the chemical in order to function normally. Yet other behaviors, such as gambling, spending money, working, and engaging in sex, also create changes at the cellular level along with positive mood changes. Although the mechanism is not well understood, all forms of addiction probably reflect dysfunction of certain biochemical systems in the brain.[4]

Traditionally, diagnosis of an addiction was limited to drug addiction and was based on three criteria: (1) the presence of an abstinence syndrome, or **withdrawal**—a series of temporary physical and psychological symptoms that occurs when the addicted person abruptly stops using the drug; (2) an associated pattern of pathological behavior (deterioration in work performance, relationships, and social interaction); and (3) **relapse,** the tendency to return to the addictive behavior after a period of abstinence. Furthermore, until recently, health professionals were unwilling to diagnose an addiction until medical symptoms appeared in the patient. Now we know that although withdrawal, pathological behavior, relapse, and medical symptoms are valid indicators of addiction, they do not characterize all addictive behavior.

Signs of Addiction

If you asked ten people to define addiction, you would quite possibly get ten different responses. Studies show that all animals share the same basic pleasure and reward circuits in the brain that turn on when they come into contact with addictive substances or engage in something pleasurable, such as eating or orgasm. We all engage in potentially addictive behaviors to some extent because some are essential to our survival and are highly reinforcing, such as eating, drinking, and sex. At some point along the continuum, however, some individuals are not able to engage in these behaviors moderately, and they become addicted.

All addictions are characterized by four common symptoms: (1) **compulsion,** which is characterized by **obsession,** or excessive preoccupation with the behavior and an overwhelming need to perform it; (2) **loss of control,** or the inability to predict reliably whether any isolated occurrence of the behavior will be healthy or damaging; (3) **negative consequences,** such as physical damage, legal trouble, financial problems, academic failure, or family dissolution, which do not occur with healthy involvement in any behavior; and

---

Drug abuse   The excessive use of a drug.

Addiction   Continued involvement with a substance or activity despite ongoing negative consequences.

Withdrawal   A series of temporary physical and biopsychosocial symptoms that occur when the addict abruptly abstains from an addictive chemical or behavior.

Relapse   The tendency to return to the addictive behavior after a period of abstinence.

Compulsion   Obsessive preoccupation with a behavior and an overwhelming need to perform it.

Obsession   Excessive preoccupation with an addictive object or behavior.

Loss of control   Inability to predict reliably whether a particular instance of involvement with the addictive object or behavior will be healthy or damaging.

Negative consequences   Physical damage, legal trouble, financial ruin, academic failure, family dissolution, and other severe problems associated with addiction.

(4) **denial,** or the inability to perceive that the behavior is self-destructive. These four components are present in all addictions, whether chemical or behavioral.

What do you think?

Have you ever seen signs of addiction in a friend or family member? ✳ What types of negative consequences have you witnessed? ✳ Can you think of any habits you have that could potentially become addictive?

Prescription Drugs

Even though prescription drugs are administered under medical supervision, the wise consumer still takes precautions. Hazards and complications arising from the use of prescription drugs are common.

Types of Prescription Drugs

Antibiotics are drugs used to fight bacterial infection. Bacterial infections continue to be among the most common serious diseases in the United States and throughout the world. The vast majority of these can be cured with antibiotic treatment. There are currently close to 100 different antibiotics, which may be dispensed by intramuscular injection or in tablet or capsule form. Some, called broad-spectrum antibiotics, are designed to control disease caused by a number of bacterial species. These medications may also kill off helpful bacteria in the body, thus triggering secondary infections. For example, some vaginal infections are related to long-term use of antibiotics.

Sedatives are central nervous system depressants that induce sleep and relieve anxiety. Because of the high incidence of anxiety and sleep disorders in the United States, drugs that encourage relaxation and drowsiness are frequently prescribed. The potential for addiction is high. Detoxification can be life-threatening and must be medically supervised. Because doctors do not prescribe sedatives as frequently as they did in past decades, users often purchase them illegally.

Tranquilizers, another form of central nervous system depressant, are classified as major and minor tranquilizers. The most powerful tranquilizers are used to treat major psychiatric illnesses. When used appropriately, these strong sedatives can reduce violent aggressiveness and self-destructive impulses.

The so-called minor tranquilizers gained much notoriety in the late 1960s and early 1970s when consumer groups discovered that these drugs—known by their trade names Valium, Librium, and Miltown—were the most commonly prescribed medications in the United States. They were often prescribed for women who suffered from anxiety. These drugs have a high potential for addiction, and many people became physically and psychologically dependent on them. When the media reported on the widespread and casual prescribing of these drugs, physicians were forced to reevaluate the practice. Today a doctor is more likely to suggest psychotherapy or counseling for patients suffering from anxiety.

Antidepressants are medications typically used to treat major depression, although occasionally they are used to treat other forms of depression that may be resistant to conventional therapy. There are several groups of antidepressant medications approved for use in the United States. Prozac, Zoloft, and Paxil are among the most frequently prescribed antidepressants.

Generic Drugs

Generic drugs, medications sold under a chemical name rather than under a brand name, have gained popularity in recent years. They contain the same active ingredients as brand-name drugs but are less expensive.

Generic drugs can help reduce health care costs because their price is often less than half that of brand-name medications. If your doctor prescribes a drug, always ask whether a generic equivalent exists and whether it would be safe and effective for you to try.

There is some controversy about the effectiveness of some generic drugs because substitutions are often made in minor ingredients that can affect the way the drug is absorbed, causing discomfort or even allergic reactions in some users. Always note any reactions you have to medications, and tell your doctor. Also, not all drugs are available as generics.

Over-the-Counter Drugs

Over-the-counter drugs are nonprescription substances we use in the course of self-diagnosis and self-medication. More than one-third of the time people treat their routine health problems with OTC medications. Most OTC drugs are

---

Denial   Inability to perceive or accurately interpret the effects of the addictive behavior.

Antibiotics   Prescription drugs designed to fight bacterial infection.

Sedatives   Central nervous system depressants that induce sleep and relieve anxiety.

Tranquilizers   Central nervous system depressants that relax the body and calm anxiety.

Antidepressants   Prescription drugs used to treat clinically diagnosed depression.

Generic drugs   Drugs marketed by chemical name rather than brand name.

Preserving the Usefulness of Antibiotics

In the 1300s, the scourge known as the bubonic plague killed up to one-third of Europe's population. In modern times, we've been told that such a plague isn't possible. It would be controlled handily with the help of antibiotic drugs such as streptomycin, gentamicin, and chloramphenicol, drugs once thought to be invincible—that is, until 1995, when a 16-year-old boy from Madagascar, infected with bubonic plague, failed to respond to the usual antibiotic treatments. This was the first documented case of antibiotic-resistant plague, which did eventually succumb to another antibiotic.

Throughout the world, many other infectious germs, including those that cause pneumonia, ear infections, acne, gonorrhea, urinary tract infections, meningitis, and tuberculosis, can now outwit some of the most commonly used antibiotics and their synthetic counterparts, antimicrobials. According to specialists at the Mayo Clinic in Rochester, Minnesota, drug resistance may have contributed to the 58 percent rise in infectious disease deaths among Americans between 1980 and 1992.

Every time a patient takes penicillin or another antibiotic for a bacterial infection, the drug kills most of the bacteria. But a few tenacious germs may survive by mutating or acquiring resistance genes from other bacteria. These surviving genes can multiply quickly, creating drug-resistant strains. The presence of these strains may mean the patient's next infection will not respond to the first-choice antibiotic therapy. Also, the resistant bacteria may be transmitted to other people in the community.

What's behind these drug-resistant strains? Two factors. One relates to individual patients; the other reflects practices of the medical community. On an individual level, patients who are prescribed antibiotics don't always follow instructions properly. To be completely effective, antibiotics are to be taken for a specific number of days. Many people, however, stop taking the drug after symptoms have cleared or they start feeling better. Unfortunately, some of the bacteria may still be present in the system, free to attack again and able to mutate. In addition, doctors are sometimes too quick to prescribe antibiotics for all sorts of symptoms, even though antibiotics work only against bacterial infections, not viral infections such as the common cold. It is estimated that more than 50 to 150 million antibiotic prescriptions written for patients each year outside of hospitals are unnecessary. Organisms that have already developed defenses against antibiotic attack include the following:

✓ *Staphylococcus aureus.* One of the primary causes of infections in patients in U.S. hospitals; can infect burns, skin, and surgical wounds.
✓ *Enterococcus.* Can cause everything from urinary tract infections to heart valve infections.

✓ *Streptococcus pneumoniae.* Up to 30 percent of the strains of this bacterium, which can cause pneumonia, meningitis, and ear infections, are at least partially resistant to antibiotics in the penicillin family.

Other bacteria that have grown resistant to antibiotics once considered reliable are *Neisseria gonorrhoeae,* which causes the sexually transmitted infection gonorrhea; *Salmonella,* and *Escherichia coli (E. coli),* the culprits behind food poisoning; and *Mycobacterium tuberculosis,* which causes tuberculosis.

What can you do to help curb the problem of antibiotic-resistant bacteria?

✓ Don't demand an antibiotic when the health care provider determines that one is not appropriate.
✓ Finish each prescription. Even when your symptoms have disappeared, some bacteria may still survive and reproduce if you don't complete the course of treatment.
✓ Don't take leftover antibiotics or antibiotics prescribed for someone else.

Source: FDA Consumer Magazine (November–December 1998); downloaded October 22, 1998.

---

manufactured from a basic group of 1,000 chemicals. The many different products available to us are produced by combining as few as two and as many as ten substances.

How Prescription Drugs Become OTC Drugs

The Food and Drug Administration (FDA) regularly reviews prescription drugs to evaluate how suitable they would be as OTC products. For a drug to be switched from prescription to OTC status, it must meet the following criteria:

1. The drug has been marketed as a prescription drug for at least three years.
2. The use of the drug has been relatively high during the time it was available as a prescription drug.
3. Adverse drug reactions are not alarming, and the frequency of side effects has not increased during the time the drug was available to the public.

Since this policy has been in effect, the FDA has switched hundreds of drugs from prescription to OTC status. Some examples are the analgesic/anti-inflammatory medicines ibuprofen (Advil, Motrin, Nuprin) and naproxen sodium (Aleve, Anaprox), the antihistamine Benadryl, the vaginal antifungal Gyne-Lotrimin, the bronchodilator Bronkaid Mist, and the hydrocortisone Cortaid. Many more prescription drugs are currently being considered for OTC status.

Types of OTC Drugs

The FDA has categorized 26 types of OTC preparations. Those most commonly used are analgesics, cold/cough/allergy and asthma relievers, stimulants, sleeping aids and relaxants, and dieting aids.

Analgesics   We spend more than $2 billion annually on **analgesics** (pain relievers), the largest sales category of OTC drugs in the United States. Although these pain relievers come in several forms, aspirin, acetaminophen (Tylenol, Pamprin, Panadol), ibuprofen (Advil, Motrin, Nuprin), and ibuprofen-like drugs such as naproxen sodium (Aleve, Anaprox) and ketoprofen (Orudis) are the most common.

Most pain relievers work at receptor sites by interrupting pain signals. Some are categorized as NSAIDs (nonsteroidal anti-inflammatory drugs). NSAIDs are sometimes called **prostaglandin inhibitors.** Prostaglandins are chemicals that resemble hormones and are released by the body in response to pain. (Scientists believe that the additional pain caused by the release of prostaglandins signals the body to begin the healing process.) Prostaglandin inhibitors restrain the release of prostaglandins, thereby reducing the pain. Common NSAIDs include ibuprofen (Advil, Motrin, Nuprin), naproxen sodium (Aleve, Anaprox), and aspirin.

In addition to relieving pain, aspirin lowers fever by increasing the flow of blood to the skin surface, which causes sweating, thereby cooling the body. Aspirin has also long been used to reduce the inflammation and swelling associated with arthritis. Recently it has been discovered that aspirin's anticoagulant effects (interference with blood clotting) make it useful for reducing the risk of heart attack and stroke.

Although aspirin has been popular for nearly a century, it is not as harmless as many people think. Possible side effects—for it and many other NSAIDS—include allergic reactions, ringing in the ears, stomach bleeding, and ulcers. Combining aspirin with alcohol can compound aspirin's gastric irritant properties. As with all drugs, read the labels. Some analgesic labels caution against driving or operating heavy machinery when using the drug, and most warn that analgesics should not be taken with alcohol.

In addition, research has linked aspirin to a potentially fatal condition called *Reye's syndrome*. Children, teenagers, and young adults (up to age 25) who are treated with aspirin while recovering from the flu or chickenpox are at risk for developing the syndrome. Aspirin substitutes are recommended for people in these age groups.

Acetaminophen is an aspirin substitute found in Tylenol and related medications. Like aspirin, acetaminophen is an effective analgesic and antipyretic (fever-reducing drug). It does not, however, relieve inflamed or swollen joints. The side effects associated with acetaminophen are generally minimal, though overdose can cause liver damage.

Several analgesics are available as prescription or OTC drugs. Generally, the OTC drugs (for example, Nuprin, Advil, and Aleve) are milder versions of the prescription varieties. Aleve's main distinction is its lasting effect: whereas other analgesics must be taken every 4 to 6 hours, once every 8 to 12 hours is sufficient for Aleve.

Cold, Cough, Allergy, and Asthma Relievers   The operative word in the category of cough, cold, and asthma relievers is *reliever*. Most of these medications are designed to alleviate the discomforting symptoms associated with maladies of the upper respiratory tract. Unfortunately, no drugs exist to cure the actual diseases. The drugs available provide only temporary relief until the sufferer's immune system prevails over the disease. Both aspirin and acetaminophen are on the government's lists of medications in this category that are **Generally Recognized as Safe (GRAS)** and **Generally Recognized as Effective (GRAE).** Basic types of OTC cold, cough, and allergy relievers include the following:

- *Expectorants*. These drugs loosen phlegm, allowing the user to cough it up and clear congested respiratory passages. GRAS and GRAE reviewers found no expectorants to be both safe and effective.
- *Antitussives*. These OTC drugs calm or curtail the cough reflex. They are most effective when the cough is "dry," or does not produce phlegm. Oral codeine, dextromethorphan, and diphenhydramine are the most common antitussives that are on both the GRAE and GRAS lists.
- *Antihistamines*. These central nervous system depressants dry runny noses, clear postnasal drip, clear sinus congestion, and reduce tears.
- *Decongestants*. These remedies reduce nasal stuffiness due to colds.
- *Anticholinergics*. These substances are often added to cold preparations to reduce nasal secretions and tears. None of

Analgesics   Pain relievers.

Prostaglandin inhibitors   Drugs that inhibit the production and release of prostaglandins, hormone-like substances associated with arthritis or menstrual pain.

Generally Recognized as Safe (GRAS)   A list of drugs generally recognized as safe, which seldom cause side effects when used properly.

Generally Recognized as Effective (GRAE)   A list of drugs generally recognized as effective, which work for their intended purpose when used properly.

the preparations tested was found to be GRAE/GRAS. Some cold compounds contain alcohol in concentrations that may exceed 40 percent.

Stimulants   Nonprescription stimulants are sometimes used by college students who have neglected assignments and other obligations until the last minute. The active ingredient in OTC stimulants is caffeine, which heightens wakefulness, increases alertness, and relieves fatigue. None of the OTC stimulants has been judged GRAS or GRAE.

Sleeping Aids   In 2000, nearly 50 percent of the U.S. population experienced insomnia at least five nights each month. About 1 percent of the adult population routinely treat their insomnia with OTC sleep aids (such as Nytol, Sleep-Eze, and Sominex) that are advertised as providing a "safe and restful" sleep.[5] These drugs are often used to induce the drowsy feelings that precede sleep. The principal ingredient in OTC sleeping aids is an antihistamine called pyrilamine maleate. Chronic reliance on sleeping aids may lead to addiction; people accustomed to using these products may eventually find it impossible to sleep without them.

Dieting Aids   In the United States, there is a $200 million market for dieting aids that are designed to help people lose weight. Some of these drugs (e.g., Acutrim, Dexatrim) are advertised as "appetite suppressants." The FDA has pulled several appetite suppressants off the market because their active ingredient was phenylpropanolamine (PPA), which has been linked to increased risk of stroke.[6]

Estimates show that when taken as recommended, even the best OTC dieting aids significantly reduce appetite in fewer than 30 percent of users and tolerance occurs in only one to three days of use. Manufacturers of appetite suppressants often include a written diet to complement their drug. Many of these diets contain 1,200 calories. However, most people who limit themselves to 1,200 calories per day will lose weight—without any help from appetite suppressants. Clearly, these products have no value in treating obesity.

Some people rely on **laxatives** and **diuretics** ("water pills") to lose weight. Frequent use of laxatives disrupts the body's natural elimination patterns and may cause constipa-

tion or even obstipation (inability to have a bowel movement). The use of laxatives to produce weight loss has generally unspectacular results and can rob the body of needed fluids, salts, and minerals.

Taking diuretics to lose weight is also dangerous. Not only will the user gain the weight back upon drinking fluids, but diuretic use may also contribute to dangerous chemical imbalances. The potassium and sodium eliminated by diuretics play important roles in maintaining electrolyte balance. Depletion of these vital minerals may cause weakness, dizziness, fatigue, and sometimes death.

Rules for Proper OTC Drug Use

Despite a common belief that OTC products are safe and effective, indiscriminate use and abuse can occur with these drugs as with all others. For example, people who frequently drop medication into their eyes to "get the red out" or pop antacids after every meal are likely to be addicted. Many people also experience adverse side effects because they ignore the warning on the labels or simply do not read them.

OTC medications are far more powerful than ever before, and the science behind them is stronger as well. Therefore, when you use any type of medication, do your homework. Observe the following rules when taking nonprescription drugs:

1. Always know what you are taking. Identify the active ingredients in the product.
2. Know the effects. Be sure you know both the desired and potentially undesired effects of each active ingredient.
3. Read the warnings and cautions.
4. Don't use anything for more than one or two weeks.
5. Be particularly cautious if you are also taking prescription drugs.
6. If you have questions, ask your pharmacist.
7. *If you don't need it, don't take it!*

Drug Interactions

Sharing medications, using outdated prescriptions, taking higher doses than recommended, or using medications as a substitute for dealing with personal problems may result in serious health consequences. So may **polydrug use**: taking several medications or illegal drugs simultaneously. This may result in very dangerous problems associated with drug interactions. The most hazardous interactions are synergism, antagonism, inhibition, and intolerance.

Synergism, also known as potentiation, is an interaction of two or more drugs in which the effects of the individual drugs are multiplied beyond what would normally be expected if they were taken alone. Synergism can be expressed mathematically as 2 + 2 = 10.

A synergistic interaction is most likely to occur when *central nervous system depressants* are combined. Included in this category are alcohol, opiates (morphine, heroin), antihistamines (cold remedies), sedative hypnotics (Quaaludes), minor

---

Laxative   Medication used to soften stool and relieve constipation.

Diuretic   Drug that increases the excretion of urine from the body.

Polydrug use   The simultaneous use of multiple medications or illicit drugs.

Synergism   An interaction of two or more drugs that produces more profound effects than would be expected if the drugs were taken separately.

---

tranquilizers (Valium, Librium, and Xanax), and barbiturates. The worst possible combination is alcohol and barbiturates (sleeping preparations such as Seconal and phenobarbital) because combining these depressants slows down brain centers that normally control vital functions. Respiration, heart rate, and blood pressure can drop to the point of inducing coma and even death.

Prescription and OTC drugs carry labels warning the user not to combine the drug with certain other drugs or with alcohol. Because the dangers associated with synergism are so great, you should always verify any possible drug interactions before using a prescribed or OTC drug. Pharmacists, physicians, drug information centers, or community drug education centers can answer your questions. Even if one of the drugs in question is an illegal substance, you should still attempt to determine the dangers involved in combining it with other drugs. Health care professionals are legally bound to maintain confidentiality even when they know that a client is using illegal substances.

Antagonism, although not usually as serious as synergism, can produce unwanted and unpleasant effects. In an antagonistic reaction, drugs work at the same receptor site so that one drug blocks the action of the other. The "blocking" drug occupies the receptor site and prevents the other drug from attaching, thus altering its absorption and action.

With **inhibition,** the effects of one drug are eliminated or reduced by the presence of another drug at the receptor site. One common inhibitory reaction occurs between antacid tablets and aspirin. The antacid inhibits the absorption of aspirin, making it less effective as a pain reliever. Other inhibitory reactions occur between alcohol and contraceptive pills and between antibiotics and contraceptive pills. Alcohol and antibiotics may make birth control pills less effective.

Intolerance occurs when drugs combine in the body to produce extremely uncomfortable reactions. The drug Antabuse, used to help alcoholics give up alcohol, works by producing this type of interaction. It binds liver enzymes (the chemicals the liver produces to break down alcohol), making it impossible for the body to metabolize alcohol. As a result, an Antabuse user who drinks alcohol experiences nausea, vomiting, and, occasionally, fever.

Cross-tolerance occurs when a person develops a physiological tolerance to one drug and shows a similar tolerance to selected other drugs as a result. Taking one drug may actually increase the body's tolerance to another drug. For example, cross-tolerance can develop between alcohol and barbiturates, two depressant drugs.

Illicit Drugs

Whereas some people become addicted to prescription drugs and painkillers, others use illicit drugs—those drugs that are illegal to possess, produce, or sell. The problem of illicit drug use touches us all. We may use illicit substances ourselves, watch someone we love struggle with drug abuse, or become the victim of a drug-related crime. At the very least, we are forced to pay increasing taxes for law enforcement and drug rehabilitation. An estimated 9.4 percent of full-time employees of the U.S. workforce is under the influence of illicit drugs or alcohol on any given day.[7] When our co-workers use drugs, the effectiveness of our own work is diminished. If the car we drive was assembled by drug-using workers at the plant, we are in danger. A drug-using bus driver, train engineer, or pilot jeopardizes our safety.

The good news is overall the use of illicit drugs has declined significantly in recent years. Use of most drugs increased from the early 1970s to the late 1970s, peaked between 1979 and 1986, and declined until 1996, from which point it has not changed. In 1999, an estimated 14.8 million Americans were illicit drug users, about half the 1979 peak level of 25 million users. However, several age groups have increased their use of illicit drugs. Among youth, for example, illicit drug use, notably of marijuana, has been increasing in recent years.[8]

Who Uses Illicit Drugs?

Illicit drug users come from all walks of life. A 2000 survey conducted by the National Institute on Drug Abuse (NIDA) noted that 9.7 percent of the population aged 12–17 had reported using illicit drugs during the past year.[9] Rates of illicit drug abuse typically increase with age and peak in the early college years (ages 18–20) at 19.6 percent. After age 20, rates generally decline with age. The only exception to this is the 40–44 year old group, with rates higher than the 35–39 age group; probably due to the fact that these young 40-year-olds were in their teens during the 1970s, when drug use was on a dramatic increase in America.[10]

The reasons for using drugs vary from one situation to another and from one person to another. Factors such as geographic location, age, gender, race, socioeconomic status, religious affiliation, genetic background, physiology, personality, experiences, and expectations are just a few of the many factors that influence whether a person chooses to use or not use illicit drugs.

Patterns of drug use among college-aged students vary considerably from one college campus to another and

---

Antagonism   A type of interaction in which two or more drugs work at the same receptor site.

Inhibition   A type of interaction in which the effects of one drug are eliminated or reduced by the presence of another drug at the receptor site.

Intolerance   A type of interaction in which two or more drugs produce extremely uncomfortable symptoms.

Cross-tolerance   The development of a tolerance to one drug that reduces the effects of another similar drug.

Table 7.1
Annual Prevalence of Use for Various Types of Drugs, 2000: Full-Time College Students Versus Respondents 1–4 Years Beyond High School

	Total	
	FULL-TIME COLLEGE (%)	OTHERS (%)
Any illicit drug	36.1	40.9
Any illicit drug other than marijuana	15.6	22.0
Marijuana	34.0	36.7
Inhalants	2.9	3.4
Hallucinogens	6.7	9.2
LSD	4.3	7.4
Cocaine	4.8	7.9
Crack	0.9	2.6
MDMA (Ecstasy)	9.1	10.0
Heroin	0.5	0.7
Other narcotics	4.5	7.0
Amphetamines, adjusted	6.6	9.3
Ice	0.5	2.3
Barbiturates	3.7	5.4
Tranquilizers	4.2	6.8
Alcohol	83.2	82.5
Cigarettes	41.3	50.4
Approximate Weighted N =	1350	990

Source: National Institute on Drug Abuse, National Survey Results on Drug Use 1975–2000: College Students & Adults, Ages 19–40. *The Monitoring the Future Study* (Washington, D.C.: National Institutes of Health, 2001).

between young adults who choose to attend college and those who do not. For example, a nationwide sample of over 40,000 students from all over the United States suggests that rates may be higher than previously reported, particularly for drugs like marijuana. In this study, approximately 34 percent of full-time students had tried marijuana during the previous year. In comparison, nearly, 37 percent of similar-age young adults who did not attend college had used marijuana. Approximately 4.8 percent of college students surveyed reported using cocaine in the past year (see Table 7.1), whereas 7.9 percent of the non-students said they had used cocaine during the previous year. Nationally, the number of college students who had tried any form of illicit drug was over 36 percent. These numbers, particularly when combined with legal use of alcohol, have many college administrators concerned, even though numbers have gone down from previous years.

> **Cocaine** A powerful stimulant drug made from the leaves of the South American coca shrub.

In spite of years of efforts aimed at prevention and intervention, most anti-drug programs have not been effective because they have focused on only one aspect of drug abuse. *Just Say NO* campaigns are prime examples of programs that focus only on the willpower of a population pressured by peers and the media to have fun and to fit in socially. The pressures to use drugs are often tremendous and the reasons for using them are complex. Only programs that take a comprehensive, multidimensional approach to drug prevention are likely to be successful. That means that we must consider policies, programs, and support services in interventions, rather than just relying on the willpower of the individual. See the Assess Yourself box.

> **What do you think?**
> *What factors do you believe influence trends of illicit drug use in the United States?* ✳ *What is the attitude toward drug use on your college campus?* ✳ *Are some drugs considered more acceptable than others?* ✳ *Is drug use considered more acceptable at certain times or on certain occasions? Explain your answer.*

Controlled Substances

Drugs are classified into five "schedules," or categories, based on their potential for abuse, their medical uses, and accepted standards of safe use (Table 7.2). Schedule I drugs, those with the highest potential for abuse, are considered to have no valid medical uses. Although Schedule II, III, IV, and V drugs have known and accepted medical applications, many of them present serious threats to health when abused or misused. Penalties for illegal use are tied to the drugs' schedule level.

Hundreds of illegal drugs exist. For general purposes, they can be divided into five representative categories: stimulants, such as cocaine; marijuana and its derivatives; depressants, such as the opiates; hallucinogens and dissociative drugs; and so-called designer drugs. All are Schedule I or Schedule II drugs. These categories include the drugs that are illegal to grow, manufacture, sell, or distribute in any form in the United States.

Cocaine

Cocaine ("coke") is a white crystalline powder derived from the leaves of the South American coca shrub (not related to cocoa plants). Cocaine has been described as one of the most powerful naturally occurring stimulants.

Methods of Cocaine Use Cocaine can be taken in several ways. The powdered form of the drug is "snorted" through the nose. When cocaine is snorted, it can damage mucous

Recognizing a Drug Problem

ARE YOU CONTROLLED BY DRUGS?

How do you know whether you are chemically dependent? A dependent person can't stop using drugs. This abuse hurts the user and everyone around him or her. Take the following assessment. The more "yes" checks you make, the more likely you have a problem.

Yes No

☐ ☐ Do you use drugs to handle stress or escape from life's problems?
☐ ☐ Have you unsuccessfully tried to cut down or quit using your drug?
☐ ☐ Have you ever been in trouble with the law or been arrested because of your drug use?
☐ ☐ Do you think a party or social gathering isn't fun unless drugs are available?
☐ ☐ Do you avoid people or places that do not support your usage?
☐ ☐ Do you neglect your responsibilities because you'd rather use your drug?
☐ ☐ Have your friends, family, or employer expressed concern about your drug use?
☐ ☐ Do you do things under the influence of drugs that you would not normally do?
☐ ☐ Have you seriously thought that you might have a chemical dependence problem?

ARE YOU CONTROLLED BY A DRUG USER?

Is your life controlled by a chemical abuser? Your love and care (codependence) may actually be enabling the chemical abuser to continue the abuse, hurting you and others. Try this assessment; the more "yes" checks you make, the more likely there's a problem.

Yes No

☐ ☐ Do you often have to lie or cover up for the chemical abuser?
☐ ☐ Do you spend time counseling the person about the problem?
☐ ☐ Have you taken on additional financial or family responsibilities?
☐ ☐ Do you feel that you have to control the chemical abuser's behavior?
☐ ☐ At the office, have you done work or attended meetings for the abuser?
☐ ☐ Do you often put your own needs and desires after the user's?
☐ ☐ Do you spend time each day worrying about your situation?
☐ ☐ Do you analyze your behavior to find clues to how it might affect the chemical abuser?
☐ ☐ Do you feel powerless and at your wit's end about the abuser's problem?

Source: Reprinted by permission of Krames Communications, 1100 Grundy Lane, San Bruno, CA 94066-3030.

---

membranes in the nose and cause sinusitis. It can destroy the user's sense of smell, and occasionally it even eats a hole in the septum.

Smoking (known as *freebasing*) and intravenous injections are even more dangerous means of taking cocaine. Freebasing has become more popular than injecting in recent years because people fear contracting diseases such as AIDS and hepatitis by sharing contaminated needles. But freebasing involves other dangers in addition to those posed by the cocaine itself. Because the volatile mixes it requires are very explosive, some people have been killed or seriously burned. Smoking cocaine can also cause lung and liver damage.

Many cocaine users still occasionally "shoot up," which introduces large amounts into the body rapidly. Within seconds, an incredible sense of euphoria sets in. This intense high lasts for 15 to 20 minutes, and then the user heads into a "crash." To prevent the unpleasant effects of the crash, users must shoot up frequently, which can severely damage veins. Users who inject place themselves at risk not only for AIDS and hepatitis but also for skin infections, inflamed arteries, and infection of the lining of the heart.

Physical Effects of Cocaine   The effects of cocaine are felt rapidly. Snorted cocaine enters the bloodstream through the

Table 7.2
How Drugs Are Scheduled

SCHEDULE	CHARACTERISTICS	EXAMPLES
Schedule I	High potential for abuse and addiction; no accepted medical use	Amphetamine (DMA, STP) Heroin Phencyclidine (PCP) LSD Marijuana Methaqualone
Schedule II	High potential for abuse and addiction; restricted medical use	Cocaine Codeine* Methadone Morphine Opium Secobarbital (Seconal) Pentobarbital (Nembutal)
Schedule III	Some potential for abuse and addiction; currently accepted medical use	Butalbital combinations (Fiorinal) Nalorphine Noludar
Schedule IV	Low potential for abuse and addiction; currently accepted medical use	Chlorpromazine (Thorazine) Phenobarbital Minor tranquilizers
Schedule V	Lowest potential for abuse; accepted medical use	Robitussin A-C OTC preparations

*Can also be Schedule III or Schedule IV, depending on use.

Source: Information from Drug Enforcement, July 1979; National Institute on Drug Abuse, Statistical Series, Annual Data Report, 1989 (Rockville, MD: U.S. OHHS, 1989), pp. 228–236.

lungs in less than one minute and reaches the brain in less than three minutes. When cocaine binds at its receptor sites in the central nervous system, it produces intense pleasure. The euphoria quickly abates, however, and the desire to regain the pleasurable feelings makes the user want more cocaine (Figure 7.2).

Cocaine is both an anesthetic and a central nervous system stimulant. In tiny doses, it can slow heart rate. In larger doses, the physical effects are dramatic: increased heart rate and blood pressure, loss of appetite that can lead to dramatic weight loss, convulsions, muscle twitching, irregular heartbeat, and even eventual death due to overdose. Other effects of cocaine include temporary relief of depression, decreased fatigue, talkativeness, increased alertness, and heightened self-confidence. Again, however, as the dose increases, users become irritable and apprehensive, and their behavior may turn paranoid or violent.

Cocaine-Affected Babies   Because cocaine rapidly crosses the placenta (as virtually all drugs do), the fetus is vulnerable when a pregnant woman snorts, freebases, or shoots up. It is estimated that between 2.4 and 3.5 percent of pregnant women between the ages of 12 and 34 abuse cocaine. It is

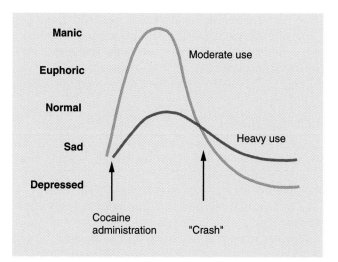

Figure 7.2
Ups and Downs of a Typical Dose of Cocaine
Source: C. Levingthal, Drugs, Behavior, and Modern Society (Boston: Allyn and Bacon, 1999), p. 76.

difficult to gauge how many newborns have been exposed to cocaine, because pregnant users are reluctant to discuss their drug habit with health care providers for fear of prosecution. The most threatening problem during pregnancy is the increased risk of a miscarriage.

Fetuses exposed to cocaine or crack in the womb are more likely to suffer a small head, premature delivery, reduced birth weight, increased irritability, and subtle learning and cognitive deficits. Recent research suggests that a significant number of these children develop problems with learning and language skills that require remedial attention.[11] It is critical that these children be identified early and receive immediate intervention. For both financial and humane reasons, developing prenatal care and education programs for mothers at risk should be a priority for state and local government.[12]

Freebase Cocaine Freebase is a form of cocaine that is more powerful and costly than the powder or chip (crack) form. Street cocaine (cocaine hydrochloride) is converted to pure base by removing the hydrochloride salt and many of the "cutting agents." The end product, freebase, is smoked through a water pipe.

Because freebase cocaine reaches the brain within seconds, it is more dangerous than snorted cocaine. It produces a quick, intense high that disappears quickly, leaving an intense craving for more. Freebasers typically increase the amount and frequency of the dose. They often become severely addicted and experience serious health problems.

Side effects of freebasing cocaine include weight loss, increased heart rate and blood pressure, depression, paranoia, and hallucinations. Freebase cocaine is an extremely dangerous drug and is responsible for a large number of cocaine-related hospital emergency-room visits and deaths.

Crack Crack is the street name given to freebase cocaine processed from cocaine hydrochloride by using ammonia or sodium bicarbonate (baking soda), water, and heat to remove the hydrochloride. (Crack can also be processed with ether, but this is much riskier because ether is flammable.) The mixture (90 percent pure cocaine) is then dried. The soapy-looking substance that results can be broken into "rocks" and smoked. These rocks are approximately five times as strong as cocaine. Crack gets its name from the popping noises it makes when burned. Crack is also sometimes called "rock," an alias that should not be confused with rock cocaine. Rock cocaine is a cocaine hydrochloride substance that is primarily sold in California. White in color, it is about the shape of a pencil eraser and is typically snorted.

Because crack is such a pure drug, it takes much less time to achieve the desired high. One puff of a pebble-sized rock produces an intense high that lasts for approximately 20 minutes. The user can usually get three or four hits off a rock before it is used up. Crack is typically sold in small vials, folding papers, or heavy aluminum foil containing two or three rocks, and costing between $10 and $20.

A crack user may quickly become addicted. Addiction is accelerated by the speed at which crack is absorbed through

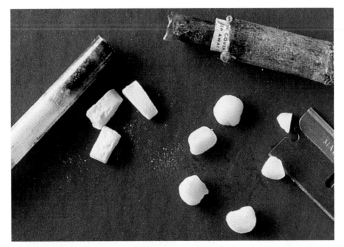

Although new "drugs of choice" make the news frequently, the availability of crack cocaine continues to be a major problem.

the lungs (it hits the brain within seconds after use) and by the intensity of the high. It is not uncommon for crack addicts to spend over $1,000 a day on the habit. Although there is no definitive way of estimating the extent of crack use in the United States, most authorities agree that it is highly popular.

Cocaine Addiction and Society Cocaine addicts often suffer both physiological damage and serious disruption in lifestyle, including loss of employment and self-esteem. It is estimated that the annual cost of cocaine addiction in the United States exceeds $3.8 billion. However, there is no way to measure the cost in wasted lives. An estimated 5 million Americans from all socioeconomic groups are addicted to cocaine. Every day, 5,000 new users try cocaine or crack. Federal agencies estimate that 3 to 4 million people had used the drug at least once in the past year. Experts suggest that 10 percent of recreational users will go on to heavy use.[13]

The Drug Enforcement Agency (DEA) has to date found no successful method to fight cocaine and crack in the United States. Cocaine has been called unpredictable by drug experts, deadly by coroners, dangerous by former users, and disastrous by the media. Apparently, the risks associated with the use of the drug do not override users' desire to experience the euphoria it produces.

Because cocaine is illegal, a complex underground network has developed to manufacture and sell the drug. Buyers may not always get the product they think they are purchasing. Cocaine marketed for snorting may be only 60 percent pure. Usually, it is mixed, or "cut," with other white powdery

---

Freebase The most powerful distillate of cocaine.

Crack A distillate of powdered cocaine that comes in small, hard "chips" or "rocks."

Table 7.3
Effects of Amphetamines on the Body and Mind

	BODY	MIND
Low Dose	Increased heartbeat	Decreased fatigue
	Increased blood pressure	Increased confidence
	Decreased appetite	Increased feeling of alertness
	Increased breathing rate	Restlessness, talkativeness
	Inability to sleep	Increased Irritability
	Sweating	Fearfulness, apprehension
	Dry mouth	Distrust of people
	Muscle twitching	Behavioral stereotypy
	Convulsions	Hallucinations
	Fever	Psychosis
	Chest pain	
	Irregular heartbeat	
High Dose	Death due to overdose	

Source: G. Hanson and P. Venturelli, Drugs and Society (Sudbury, MA: Jones and Bartlett, 1998), p. 259.

substances such as mannitol or sugar, though occasionally it is cut with arsenic or other cocaine-like powders that may themselves be highly dangerous.

What do you think?

Have all segments of society been affected by crack use? ✳ *If not, which segments of the U.S. population experience the greatest impact from crack use?* ✳ *Why might this be the case?* ✳ *Is there a difference in the profile of a person who uses crack rather than cocaine? Explain your answer.*

Amphetamines

The **amphetamines** include a large and varied group of synthetic agents that stimulate the central nervous system. Small doses of amphetamines improve alertness, lessen fatigue, and generally elevate mood. With repeated use, however, physical and psychological dependency develop. Sleep

Amphetamines A large and varied group of synthetic agents that stimulate the central nervous system.

Rebound effects Severe withdrawal effects, including depression, nausea, and violent behavior, which are experienced by users of stimulants.

Methamphetamine A powerfully addictive drug that strongly activates certain areas of the brain and affects the central nervous system.

patterns are affected (insomnia); heart rate, breathing rate, and blood pressure increase; and restlessness, anxiety, appetite suppression, and vision problems are common. High doses over long time periods can produce hallucinations, delusions, and disorganized behavior. Abusers become paranoid, fearing everything and everyone. Some become very aggressive or antisocial (Table 7.3.)

Tolerance to these powerful stimulants develops rapidly, and the user trying to cut down or quit may experience unpleasant **rebound effects.** These severe withdrawal symptoms, which are peculiar to stimulants, include depression, irritability, violent behavior, headaches, nausea, and deep fatigue.

Amphetamines for recreational use are sold under a variety of names. "Bennies" (amphetamine/Benzedrine), "dex" (dextroamphetamine/Dexedrine), and "meth" or "speed" (methamphetamine/Methedrine) are some of the most common. Other street terms for amphetamines are "cross tops," "uppers," "wake-ups," "lid poppers," "cartwheels," and "blackies." Amphetamines do have therapeutic uses in the treatment of attention deficit/hyperactivity disorder in children (Ritalin, Cylert) and of obesity (Pondimin).

Newer-Generation Stimulants

Methamphetamine is a powerfully addictive drug that strongly activates certain areas of the brain and affects the central nervous system in general. Methamphetamine is closely related chemically to amphetamine, but its central nervous system effects are greater.

Methamphetamine is relatively easy to make. People nicknamed "cookers" produce methamphetamine batches using cookbook-style recipes that often include common over-the-counter ingredients, such as ephedrine, pseudoephedrine, and phenylpropanolamine. Since 1996, laws have increased the penalties associated with manufacturing methamphetamine.

The effects of methamphetamine last six to eight hours, considerably longer than those produced by crack and cocaine. The immediate effects can include irritability and anxiety; increased body temperature, heart rate, and blood pressure; and possible death. The high state of irritability and agitation has been associated with violent behavior among some users.

Ice is a potent methamphetamine that is imported primarily from Asia, particularly from South Korea and Taiwan. It is purer and more crystalline than the version manufactured in many large U.S. cities. Because it is odorless, public use of ice often goes unnoticed.

Typically, ice quickly becomes addictive. Some users have reported severe cravings after using it only once. The effects of ice are long lasting. They include wakefulness, mood elevation, and excitability, all of which appeal to work-addicted young adults, particularly those who must put in long hours in high-stress jobs. Because the drug is very inexpensive and produces such an intense high (lasting from 4 to 14 hours), it has become popular among young people looking for a quick high. A penny-sized plastic bag, called a "paper," may cost $50, but when smoked, it can keep a person high for a few days or for as long as a week. In contrast, an ounce of cocaine causes a high that lasts only about 20 minutes.

The sensation caused by smoking ice is called *amping,* for the amplified euphoria it produces. However, as is true of other methamphetamines, the "down" side of this drug is devastating. Prolonged use can cause fatal lung and kidney damage as well as long-lasting psychological damage. In some instances, major psychological dysfunction has lasted as long as $2^{1}/_{2}$ years after last use. Aggressive behavior is also associated with the drug, as evidenced by the dramatic increase in the number of ice-related violent crimes.[14] The number of babies born severely addicted to the drug is also increasing at an alarming rate.

Marijuana

Although archaeological evidence documents the use of **marijuana** ("grass," "weed," "pot") as far back as 6,000 years, the drug did not become popular in the United States until the 1960s. Marijuana receives less media attention today than it did then, but it still is the illicit drug used most frequently by far. Nearly one of every three Americans over the age of 12 has tried marijuana at least once. Some 12 million Americans have used it; more than 1 million cannot control their use.

Physical Effects of Marijuana Marijuana is derived from either the *Cannabis sativa* or *Cannabis indica* (hemp) plants. Current American-grown marijuana is a turbocharged version of the hippie weed of the late 1960s. Developed using cross-breeding, genetic engineering, and American farming ingenuity, top-grade cannabis packs a punch very similar to that of hashish. **Tetrahydrocannabinol (THC)** is the psychoactive sub-

stance in marijuana, and the key to determining how powerful a high it will produce. Whereas marijuana from three decades ago ranged in potency from 1 to 2 percent THC, a current crop averages between 4 and 6 percent. The more refined varieties, usually grown without seeds (such as sinsemilla and Northern Lights), vary between 6 and 8 percent.[15]

Hashish, a potent cannabis preparation derived mainly from the thick, sticky resin of the plant, contains high concentrations of THC. Hash oil, a substance produced by percolating a solvent such as ether through dried marijuana to extract the THC, is a tarlike liquid that may contain up to 70 percent THC.

Marijuana can be brewed and drunk in tea or baked into quickbreads or brownies. THC concentrations in such products are impossible to estimate. Most of the time, however, marijuana is rolled into cigarettes (joints), or smoked in a pipe or water pipe (bong). Effects are generally felt within 10 to 30 minutes and usually wear off within three hours.

The most noticeable effect of THC is the dilation of the eyes' blood vessels, which produces the characteristic bloodshot eyes. Smokers of the drug also exhibit coughing, dry mouth and throat ("cotton mouth"), increased thirst and appetite, lowered blood pressure, and mild muscular weakness, primarily exhibited in drooping eyelids. Those users who take a high dose in an unfamiliar or uncomfortable setting may experience anxiety.

Users can experience intensified reactions to various stimuli. Colors and sounds, as well as the speed at which things move, may seem magnified, and high doses of hashish may produce vivid visual hallucinations.

> **What do you think?**
>
> *Why do you think that marijuana is the most popular illicit drug on college campuses?* ✳ *How widespread is marijuana use on your campus?*

Effects of Chronic Marijuana Use Because marijuana is illegal in most parts of the United States and has been widely used only since the 1960s, long-term studies of its effects have been difficult to conduct. Also, studies conducted in the

---

Ice A potent, inexpensive methamphetamine that has long-lasting effects.

Marijuana Chopped leaves and flowers of the *Cannabis indica* or *Cannabis sativa* plant (hemp); a psychoactive stimulant that intensifies reactions to environmental stimuli.

Tetrahydrocannabinol (THC) The chemical name for the active ingredient in marijuana.

Hashish The sticky resin of the cannabis plant, which is high in THC.

1960s involved marijuana with THC levels constituting only a fraction of today's plant levels, so their results may not apply to the more toxic forms available today. Most current information about chronic marijuana use comes from countries such as Jamaica and Costa Rica, where the drug is not illegal. These studies of long-term use (ten or more years) indicate that it causes lung damage comparable to that caused by tobacco smoking. Indeed, smoking a single joint may be as damaging to the lungs as smoking five tobacco cigarettes. The chemicals themselves do not injure the heart, but the effects of inhaling burning material do. Inhalation of marijuana transfers carbon monoxide to the bloodstream. Because the blood has a greater affinity for carbon monoxide than it does for oxygen, this diminishes the oxygen-carrying capacity of the blood. The heart must work harder to pump the vital element to oxygen-starved tissues.

Other risks associated with marijuana include suppression of the immune system, blood pressure changes, and impaired memory function. Recent studies suggest that pregnant women who smoke marijuana are at a higher risk for stillbirth or miscarriage and for delivering low-birth-weight babies and babies with abnormalities of the nervous system. Babies born to marijuana smokers are five times more likely to have features similar to those exhibited by children with fetal alcohol syndrome.

Debates concerning the effects of marijuana on the reproductive system have yet to be resolved. Studies conducted in the mid-1970s suggested that marijuana inhibited testosterone (and thus sperm) production in males and caused chromosomal breakage in both ova and sperm. Subsequent research in these areas is inconclusive. The question of whether the high-level THC plants currently available

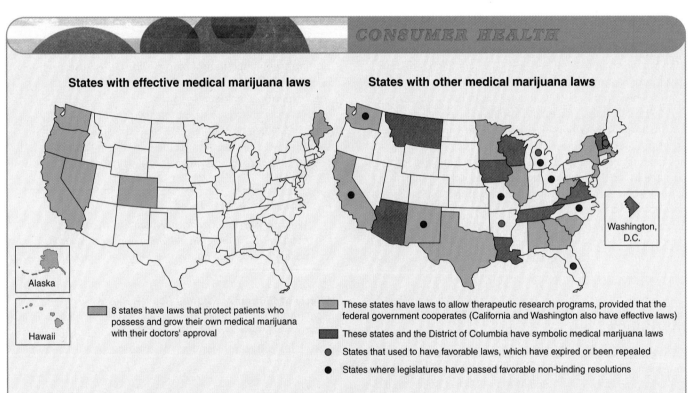

CONSUMER HEALTH

States with effective medical marijuana laws

States with other medical marijuana laws

Alaska

Hawaii

Washington, D.C.

8 states have laws that protect patients who possess and grow their own medical marijuana with their doctors' approval

These states have laws to allow therapeutic research programs, provided that the federal government cooperates (California and Washington also have effective laws)

These states and the District of Columbia have symbolic medical marijuana laws

States that used to have favorable laws, which have expired or been repealed

States where legislatures have passed favorable non-binding resolutions

Medicinal Use of Marijuana: Legal Challenges Continue

For a number of years, marijuana's legal status for use for medicinal purposes has been hotly debated. So far, 30 states and the District of Columbia have laws on the books that recognize marijuana's medical value. Twelve states with "Therapeutic Research Program" laws are nevertheless unable to give patients legal access to medical marijuana because of the federal laws. Ten states and the District of Columbia have symbolic laws that recognize marijuana's medical value but fail to provide patients with protection from arrest for possession of an illegal drug. Voters in Alaska, California, Colorado, Hawaii, Maine, Oregon, Nevada, and Washington state have chosen to legalize marijuana for medicinal uses (see the accompanying figures). These new state laws, however, conflict with federal laws against the possession of marijuana and have led to new battles in courts. In February 1999, attorneys general from a number of western states met with federal officials to discuss reclassifying marijuana as a Schedule II drug. Reclassification would allow marijuana to be prescribed by physicians and would clear up some of the conflict.

Source: R. Schmitz and C. Thomas, "State By State Medical Marijuana Laws: How To Remove the Threat of Arrest," June 2001, http://mmp.org/statelaw/index.html.

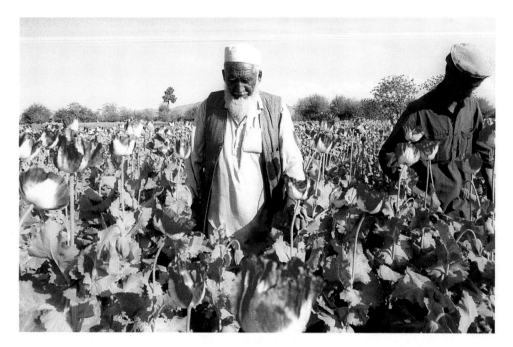

Despite its beautiful flower and innocent appearance, the poppy is the source of opium, a powerful narcotic.

will increase the risks associated with this drug is, as yet, unanswered.

Marijuana and Medicine   Although recognized as a dangerous drug by the U.S. government, marijuana has several medical purposes. It has been used to help control the side effects, such as severe nausea and vomiting, produced by chemotherapy (chemical treatment for cancer). It improves appetite and forestalls the loss of lean muscle mass associated with AIDS-related wasting syndrome. Marijuana reduces the muscle pain and spasticity caused by diseases such as multiple sclerosis.[16] It also temporarily relieves the eye pressure of glaucoma, although it is unclear whether it is any more effective than legal glaucoma drugs.[17]

Marijuana and Driving   Marijuana use presents clear hazards for drivers of motor vehicles as well as others on the road. The drug substantially reduces a driver's ability to react and make quick decisions. Studies reveal that 60 to 80 percent of marijuana users sometimes drive while high.[18] Studies of automobile accident victims show that 6 to 12 percent of nonfatally injured drivers and 4 to 16 percent of fatally injured drivers had THC in their bloodstreams. Perceptual and other performance deficits resulting from marijuana use may persist for some time after the high subsides, though users who attempt to drive, fly, or operate heavy machinery often fail to recognize their impairment.

Opiates

Opiates cause drowsiness, relieve pain, and induce euphoria. Also called **narcotics,** they are derived from the parent drug **opium,** a dark, resinous substance made from the milky juice of the opium poppy. Other opiates include *morphine, codeine, heroin,* and *black tar heroin.*

During the late nineteenth and early twentieth centuries, many patent medicines contained opiates. Suppliers advertised these concoctions as cures for everything from menstrual cramps to teething pains. More powerful than opium, **morphine** (named after Morpheus, the Greek god of sleep) was widely used as a painkiller during the Civil War. **Codeine,** a less powerful analgesic derived from morphine, also became popular.

As the use of opiates became more common, physicians noted that patients tended to become dependent on these substances. Contrary to earlier belief, all of the opiates are highly addictive. Growing concern about addiction led to government controls of narcotic use. Today, physicians are still subject to audits of their prescriptions of these agents.

Some opiates are still used for medical purposes. Doctors sometimes prescribe morphine for severe pain. Codeine is found in prescription cough syrups and other painkillers. Several prescription drugs, including Percodan, Demerol, and Dilaudid, contain synthetic opiates. All opiate use is strictly regulated.

Physical Effects of Opiates   Opiates are powerful depressants of the central nervous system. In addition to relieving

---

Narcotics   Drugs that induce sleep and relieve pain; primarily the opiates.

Opium   The parent drug of the opiates; made from the seedpod resin of the opium poppy.

Morphine   A derivative of opium; sometimes used by medical practitioners to relieve pain.

Codeine   A drug derived from morphine; used in cough syrups and certain painkillers.

pain, these drugs lower heart rate, respiration, and blood pressure. Side effects include weakness, dizziness, nausea, vomiting, euphoria, decreased sex drive, visual disturbances, and lack of coordination. The following section discusses the progression of heroin addiction; addiction to any other opiate follows a similar path.

Heroin Addiction   Heroin is a white powder derived from morphine. **Black tar heroin** is a sticky, dark brown, foul-smelling substance. It is estimated that 600,000 Americans are addicted to heroin, with men outnumbering women addicts by three to one.[19] Authorities believe that the United States is at the beginning of a new heroin epidemic. There is concern that this epidemic will be worse than previous ones because the drug is now two to three times more available than ever before. The contemporary version of heroin is so potent that users can get high by snorting or smoking the drug rather than by injecting it and putting themselves at risk for AIDS; however, most heroin addicts continue to inject themselves. Once an inner-city drug, heroin is becoming more widespread among middle-class people who tend to try whatever drug is new and trendy. Many have switched from cocaine to heroin because the heroin high is not so stimulating and the drug is less expensive than cocaine.

Once considered a cure for morphine dependency, heroin was later discovered to be even more addictive and potent than morphine. Today, heroin has no medical use.

Heroin is a depressant that produces drowsiness and a dreamy, mentally slow feeling. It can cause drastic mood swings, with euphoric highs followed by depressive lows. Heroin also slows respiration and urinary output and constricts the pupils of the eyes. In fact, pupil constriction is a classic sign of narcotic intoxication—hence the stereotype of the drug user hiding behind a pair of dark sunglasses. Symptoms of tolerance and withdrawal can appear within three weeks of first use.

The most common route of administration for heroin addicts is "mainlining"—intravenous injection of powdered heroin mixed in a solution. Many users describe the "rush" they feel when injecting themselves as intensely pleasurable, whereas others report unpredictable and unpleasant side effects. The temporary nature of the rush contributes to the drug's high potential for addiction—many addicts shoot up four or five times a day. Mainlining can cause veins to scar and eventually collapse. Once a vein has collapsed, it can no longer be used to introduce heroin into the bloodstream. Addicts become expert at locating new veins to use: in the feet, the legs, even the temples. When they do not want their needle tracks (scars) to show, they inject themselves under the tongue or in the groin.

The physiology of the human body could be said to encourage opiate addiction. Opiate-like substances called **endorphins** are manufactured in the body and have multiple receptor sites, particularly in the central nervous system. When endorphins attach themselves at these points, they create feelings of painless well-being. Medical researchers have referred to endorphins as "the body's own opiates." When endorphin levels are high, people feel euphoric. The same euphoria occurs when opiates or related chemicals are active at the endorphin receptor sites.

Treatment for Heroin Addiction   Programs to help heroin addicts kick the habit have not been very successful. The rate of *recidivism* (tendency to return to previous behaviors) is high. Some addicts resume drug use even after years of drug-free living because the craving for the injection rush is very strong. It takes a great deal of discipline to seek alternative, nondrug highs.

Heroin addicts experience a distinct pattern of withdrawal. They begin to crave another dose four to six hours after their last dose. Symptoms of withdrawal include intense desire for the drug, yawning, a runny nose, sweating, and crying. About 12 hours after the last dose, addicts experience sleep disturbance, dilated pupils, loss of appetite, irritability, goose bumps, and muscle tremors. The most difficult time in the withdrawal process occurs 24 to 72 hours following last use. All of the preceding symptoms continue, along with nausea, abdominal cramps, restlessness, insomnia, vomiting, diarrhea, extreme anxiety, hot and cold flashes, elevated blood pressure, and rapid heartbeat and respiration. Once the peak of withdrawal has been passed, all these symptoms begin to subside. Still, the recovering addict has many hurdles to jump.

Methadone maintenance is one treatment available for people addicted to heroin or other opiates. Methadone is a synthetic narcotic that blocks the effects of opiate withdrawal. It is chemically similar enough to the opiates to control the tremors, chills, vomiting, diarrhea, and severe abdominal pains of withdrawal. Methadone dosage is decreased over a period of time until the addict is weaned off the drug.

Methadone maintenance is controversial because of the drug's own potential for addiction. Critics contend that the program merely substitutes one addiction for another. Proponents argue that people on methadone maintenance are less likely to engage in criminal activities to support their habits than heroin addicts are. For this reason, many methadone maintenance programs are financed by state or federal government and are available to clients free of charge or at reduced costs.

Heroin   An illegally manufactured derivative of morphine, usually injected into the bloodstream.

Black tar heroin   A dark brown, sticky substance made from morphine.

Endorphins   Opiate-like hormones that are manufactured in the human body and contribute to natural feelings of well-being.

Methadone maintenance   A treatment for people addicted to opiates that substitutes methadone, a synthetic narcotic, for the opiate of addiction.

A number of new drug therapies for opiate dependence are emerging. Naltrexone (Trexan), an opiate antagonist, has been approved as a treatment. While on Naltrexone, recovering addicts do not have the compulsion to use heroin, and if they do use, they don't get high, so there is no point in using the drug. More recently, researchers have reported promising results with Temgesic (buprenorphine) a mild, nonaddicting synthetic opiate, which, like heroin and methadone, bonds to certain receptors in the brain, blocks pain messages, and persuades the brain that its cravings for heroin have been satisfied. Addicts report that while they are taking buprenorphine, they do not crave heroin anymore.

Hallucinogens (Psychedelics)

Hallucinogens are also commonly referred to as psychedelics. The term **psychedelic** was adapted from a Greek phrase meaning "mind manifesting." Psychedelics are a group of drugs whose primary pharmacological effect is to alter feelings, perceptions, and thoughts in the user. The major receptor sites for most of these drugs are in the part of the brain that is responsible for interpreting outside stimuli before allowing these signals to travel to other parts of the brain. This area, the **reticular formation,** is located in the brain stem at the upper end of the spinal cord (Figure 7.3). When a hallucinogenic drug is present at a reticular formation receptor site, messages become scrambled, and the user may see wavy walls instead of straight ones or may smell colors and hear tastes. This mixing of sensory messages is known as **synesthesia.**

In addition to synesthetic effects, users may recall events long buried in the subconscious mind or become less inhibited than they are in a nondrug state. The most widely recognized hallucinogenic drugs are LSD, mescaline, psilocybin, and psilocin. All are illegal and carry severe penalties for manufacture, possession, transportation, or sale.

LSD Of all the hallucinogens, **lysergic acid diethylamide (LSD)** has achieved the most notoriety. First synthesized in the late 1930s by Swiss chemist Albert Hoffman, LSD resulted from experiments to derive medically useful drugs from the ergot fungus found on rye and other cereal grains. Because LSD seemed capable of unlocking the secrets of the mind, psychiatrists initially felt it could be beneficial to patients unable to remember suppressed traumas. From 1950 through 1968, the drug was used for such purposes.

Media attention was drawn to LSD in the late 1960s. Young people were using the drug to "turn on" and "tune out" the world that gave them the war in Vietnam, race riots, and political assassinations. In 1970, federal authorities, under intense pressure from the public, placed LSD on the list of controlled substances (Schedule I). LSD's popularity peaked in 1972, then tapered off, primarily because of users' inability to control dosages accurately.

Because of the recent wave of nostalgia for the 1960s, this dangerous psychedelic drug has been making a come-

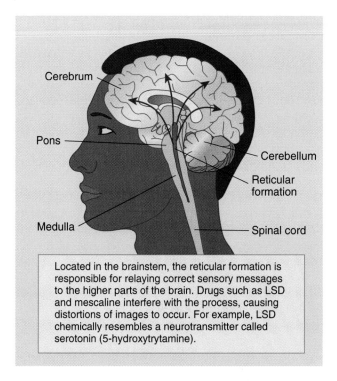

Located in the brainstem, the reticular formation is responsible for relaying correct sensory messages to the higher parts of the brain. Drugs such as LSD and mescaline interfere with the process, causing distortions of images to occur. For example, LSD chemically resembles a neurotransmitter called serotonin (5-hydroxytrytamine).

Figure 7.3
Reticular Formation

back. Known on the street as "acid," LSD is now available in virtually every state. Over 10 million Americans, most of them under age 35, have tried LSD at least once. LSD especially attracts younger users. In 1999, approximately 10 percent of high school seniors reported having tried LSD at least once. A national survey of college students showed that 5.4 percent had used it.[20]

An odorless, tasteless, white crystalline powder, LSD is most frequently dissolved in water to make a solution that can then be used to manufacture the street forms of the drug: tablets, blotter acid, and windowpane. What the LSD consumer usually buys is blotter acid—small squares of blotter-like paper that have been impregnated with the liquid. The blotter is swallowed or chewed briefly. LSD also comes

Psychedelics Drugs that distort the processing of sensory information in the brain.

Reticular formation An area in the brain stem that is responsible for relaying messages to other areas in the brain.

Synesthesia A (usually) drug-created effect in which sensory messages are incorrectly assigned—for example, hearing a taste or smelling a sound.

Lysergic acid diethylamide (LSD) Psychedelic drug causing sensory disruptions; also called acid.

in tiny thin squares of gelatin called windowpane and in tablets called microdots, which are less than an eighth of an inch across (it would take ten or more to add up to the size of an aspirin tablet). Microdots and windowpane are just a sideshow; blotter is the medium of choice. It comes decorated with a mind-boggling array of designs, some of them copied from characters created by Disney and other cartoon studios. As with any illegally purchased drug, users run the risk of buying an impure product.

LSD is one of the most powerful drugs known to science and can produce strong effects in doses as low as 20 micrograms. (To give you an idea of how small a dose this is, the average postage stamp weighs approximately 60,000 micrograms.) The potency of the typical dose of LSD currently ranges from 20 to 80 micrograms, compared to 150 to 300 micrograms commonly used in the 1960s.

Despite its reputation for being primarily a psychedelic, LSD produces a large number of physical effects, including slightly increased heart rate, elevated blood pressure and temperature, gooseflesh (roughened skin), increased reflex speeds, muscle tremors and twitches, perspiration, increased salivation, chills, headaches, and mild nausea. Because the drug also stimulates uterine muscle contractions, it can lead to premature labor and miscarriage in pregnant women.

The psychological effects of LSD vary. Euphoria is the common psychological state produced by the drug, but the user may also experience *dysphoria* (a sense of evil and foreboding). The drug also shortens attention span, causing the mind to wander. Thoughts may be interposed and juxtaposed, so the user experiences several different thoughts simultaneously. Synesthesia occurs occasionally. Users become introspective, and suppressed memories may surface, often taking on bizarre symbolism. Many more effects are possible, including decreased aggressiveness and enhanced sensory experiences.

Although some LSD users report hallucinations, it is more likely that they are experiencing illusions. These distortions of ordinary perceptions may include movement of stationary objects. "Bad trips," the most publicized risk of LSD, are commonly related to the user's mood. The user, for example, may interpret increased heart rate as a heart attack (a "bad body trip"). Often bad trips result when a user confronts a suppressed emotional experience or memory (a "bad head trip").

Although there is no evidence that LSD creates physical dependence, it may well create psychological dependence. Many LSD users become depressed for one or two days following a trip and turn to the drug to relieve this depression. The result is a cycle of using LSD to relieve post-LSD depression, which often leads to psychological addiction.

> **What do you think?**
> *Are people today using LSD for the same reasons it was used in the 1960s? ✳ What are the perceived attractions and the real dangers of LSD use?*

Mescaline Mescaline is one of hundreds of chemicals derived from the **peyote** cactus, a small, buttonlike cactus that grows in the southwestern United States and parts of Latin America. Natives of these regions have long used the dried peyote buttons for religious purposes. In fact, members of the Native American Church (a religion practiced by thousands of North American Indians) have been granted special permission to use the drug during religious ceremonies in some states.

Users normally swallow 10 to 12 dried peyote buttons. These buttons taste bitter and generally induce immediate nausea or vomiting. Long-time users claim that the nausea becomes less noticeable with frequent use.

Those who are able to keep the drug down begin to feel the effects within 30 to 90 minutes, when mescaline reaches maximum concentration in the brain. (It may persist for up to nine or ten hours.) Unlike LSD, mescaline is a powerful hallucinogen. It is also a central nervous system stimulant.

Products sold on the street as mescaline are likely to be synthetic chemical relatives of the true drug. Street names of these products include DOM, STP, TMA, and MMDA. Any of these can be toxic in small quantities.

Psilocybin Psilocybin and *psilocin* are the active chemicals in a group of mushrooms sometimes called "magic mushrooms." Psilocybe mushrooms, which grow throughout the world, can be cultivated from spores or harvested wild. Because many mushrooms resemble the psilocybe variety, people who use wild mushrooms for any purpose should be certain of what they are doing. Mushroom varieties can easily be misidentified, and mistakes can be fatal. Psilocybin is similar to LSD in its physical effects, which generally wear off within four to six hours.

Dissociative Drugs

Dissociative drugs distort perceptions of sight and sound, and produce feelings of detachment—dissociation from the environment and oneself. These mind-altering effects are not the hallucinations or illusions that may be found with LSD or psilocybin. The dissociative drugs act by altering the distribution of neurotransmitter glutamate throughout the brain.

Mescaline A hallucinogenic drug derived from the peyote cactus.

Peyote A cactus with small "buttons" that, when ingested, produce hallucinogenic effects.

Psilocybin The active chemical found in psilocybe mushrooms; it produces hallucinations.

Dissociative Producing an anesthetic effect characterized by a feeling of being detached from the physical self.

Addiction Across Cultures

Like the United States, many countries are struggling with epidemic rates of drug addiction. In fact, demand for addiction treatment services is increasing in many nations. Here's a look at current drug addiction treatment data from around the world:

- In India, more people are seeking treatment for heroin addiction, based on estimates that up to 1 million people became addicted to the substance during the 1980s.
- Political upheaval and the resulting disintegration of the family appear to be strongly related to rising drug abuse. A study in Ireland found that as many as 10 percent of young people (aged 15–20) in Dublin were addicted to heroin.
- In the Americas as a whole, cocaine and cocaine derivatives account for almost 60 percent of the demand for drug treatment.
- In contrast, in European nations, opiates, primarily heroin, are the drug of choice for nearly three-quarters of individuals seeking treatment.
- Opiates are also the leading drug of choice for about two-thirds of addicted individuals in Asian nations.
- Amphetamine use is higher in Nordic nations, such as Sweden and Finland, where it accounts for 20 percent and 40 percent of treatment needs, respectively.
- Treatment for cannabis (marijuana, hashish) is much higher in the Caribbean, including Jamaica, where it accounts for over 50 percent of treatment demand.

Sources: From United Nations Office for Drug Control and Crime Prevention, "The Social Impact of Drug Abuse" (New York: Author, 1995); and "Global Illicit Drug Trends" (New York: Author, 1999).

Glutamate is involved in perception of pain, responses to the environment, and memory.

PCP Phencyclidine, or **PCP,** is one of the best known dissociative drugs. It is a synthetic substance that became a black-market drug in the early 1970s. PCP was originally developed as a "disassociative anesthetic," which means that patients administered this drug could keep their eyes open, apparently remain conscious, and feel no pain during a medical procedure. Patients would afterward experience amnesia for the time the drug was in their system. Such a drug had obvious advantages as an anesthetic, but its unpredictability and drastic effects (postoperative delirium, confusion, and agitation) made doctors abandon it, and it was withdrawn from the legal market.

On the illegal market, PCP is a white, crystalline powder that users often sprinkle onto marijuana cigarettes. It is dangerous and unpredictable regardless of the method of administration. Common street names for PCP are "angel dust" for the crystalline powdered form, and "peace pill" and "horse tranquilizer" for the tablet form.

The effects of PCP depend on the dosage. A dose as small as 5 mg will produce effects similar to those of strong central nervous system depressants—slurred speech, impaired coordination, reduced sensitivity to pain, and reduced heart and respiratory rate. Doses between 5 and 10 mg cause fever, salivation, nausea, vomiting, and total loss of sensitivity to pain. Doses greater than 10 mg result in a drastic drop in blood pressure, coma, muscular rigidity, violent outbursts, and possible convulsions and death.

Psychologically, PCP may produce either euphoria or dysphoria. It is also known to produce hallucinations as well as delusions and overall delirium. Some users experience a prolonged state of "nothingness." The long-term effects of PCP use are unknown.

Designer Drugs (Club Drugs)

Designer drugs are produced in chemical laboratories, often manufactured in homes, and sold illegally. These drugs are easy to produce from available raw materials. The drugs themselves were once technically legal because the law had to specify the exact chemical structure of an illicit drug. However, there is now a law in place that bans all chemical cousins of illegal drugs.

Collectively known as *club drugs,* these dangerous substances include *Ecstasy, GHB, Special K,* and *Rohypnol.* Although users may think them harmless, research has shown that club drugs can produce a range of unwanted effects, including hallucinations, paranoia, amnesia, and in

---

Phencyclidine (PCP) A deliriant commonly called "angel dust."

Designer drug A synthetic analog (a drug that produces similar effects) of an existing illicit drug.

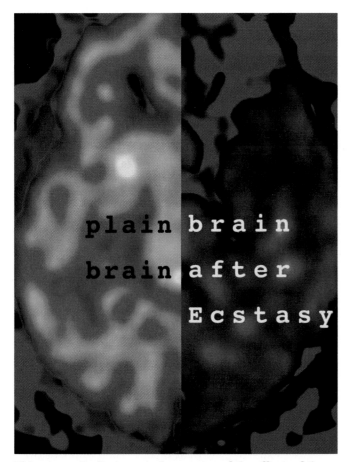

plain brain
brain after
Ecstasy

This composite brain scan shows some of the effects of the drug Ecstasy. The left side shows healthy serotonin sites. The dark sections on the right are serotonin sites no longer present even after three weeks without Ecstasy. Serotonin helps regulate mood, learning, and sleep.

some cases, death. Some club drugs work on the same brain mechanisms as alcohol and therefore can dangerously boost the effects of both substances. Because the drugs are odorless and tasteless, people can easily slip them into drinks. Some of them have been associated with sexual assaults and for that reason are referred to as "date rape drugs."

Ecstasy (3,4 methylenedioxymethamphetamine, also known as XTC or *MDMA*), once dubbed the "LSD of the 80s," has had a resurgence of popularity on many college campuses. At some universities, almost one of every four students report having used it largely due to the Rave party or club drug settings found in many campus communities. Ecstasy creates feelings of openness and warmth, combined with the mind-expanding characteristics of hallucinogens. Effects begin within 30 minutes and can last for four to six

Inhalants Products that are sniffed or inhaled in order to produce highs.

hours. Young people may use Ecstasy initially to improve mood or get energized so they can keep dancing; it also raises heart rate and blood pressure and may lead to an elevated body temperature that can cause kidney and/or cardiovascular failure. Chronic use appears to damage the brain's ability to think and regulate emotion, memory, sleep, and pain. While it is not as addictive as heroin or cocaine, adverse effects may include nausea, hallucinations, chills, sweating, tremors, teeth clenching, severe muscle cramps, and blurred vision. In addition to those already mentioned anxiety attacks, panic attacks, paranoia, and depression may occur. Particularly when combined with alcohol, loss of consciousness, seizures, stroke, and coma may also occur. Combined with alcohol, Ecstasy can be extremely dangerous and sometimes fatal. Recent studies indicate that Ecstasy may produce long-lasting neurotoxic effects in the brain. It appears that Ecstasy damages brain cells that produce serotonin, and it is unknown whether these brain cells will regenerate.[21] While MDMA abuse currently is not as widespread as other drugs, its use has gone up over 500 percent in the last five years.[22]

Inhalants

Inhalants are chemicals that produce vapors that, when inhaled, can cause hallucinations and create intoxicating and euphoric effects. They are not commonly recognized as drugs. They are legal to purchase and universally available but are potentially dangerous when used incorrectly. These drugs generally appeal to young people who can't afford illicit substances.

Some of these agents are organic solvents representing the chemical by-products of the distillation of petroleum products. Rubber cement, model glue, paint thinner, lighter fluid, varnish, wax, spot removers, and gasoline belong to this group. Most of these substances are sniffed by users in search of a quick, cheap high.

Because they are inhaled, the volatile chemicals in these products reach the bloodstream within seconds. An inhaled substance is not diluted or buffered by stomach acids or other body fluids and thus is more potent than it would be if swallowed. This characteristic, along with the fact that dosages are extremely difficult to control because everyone has unique lung and breathing capacities, makes inhalants particularly dangerous.

The effects of inhalants usually last for fewer than 15 minutes. Users may experience dizziness, disorientation, impaired coordination, reduced judgment, and slowed reaction times. Signs of inhalant use include the following: unjustifiable collection of glues, paints, lacquer thinner, cleaning fluid, and ether; sniffles similar to those produced by a cold; and a smell on the breath similar to the inhalable substance. The effects of inhalants resemble those of central nervous system depressants, and combining inhalants with alcohol produces a synergistic effect. In addition, these substances in combination can cause severe liver damage that can be fatal.

An overdose of fumes from inhalants can cause unconsciousness. If the user's oxygen intake is reduced during the inhaling process, death can result within five minutes. Whether a user is a first-time or chronic user, sudden sniffing death (SSD) syndrome can be a fatal consequence. This syndrome can occur if a user inhales deeply and then participates in physical activity or is startled.

Amyl Nitrite   Sometimes called "poppers" or "rush," **amyl nitrite** is packaged in small, cloth-covered glass capsules that can be crushed to release the active chemical. The drug is often prescribed to alleviate chest pain in heart patients, because it dilates small blood vessels and reduces blood pressure. Dilation of blood vessels in the genital area is thought to enhance sensations or perceptions of orgasm. It also produces fainting, dizziness, warmth, and skin flushing.

Nitrous Oxide   **Nitrous oxide** is sometimes used as an adjunct to dental anesthesia or minor surgical anesthesia. It is also a propellant chemical in aerosol products such as whipped toppings. Users experience a state of euphoria, floating sensations, and illusions. Effects also include pain relief and a "silly" feeling, demonstrated by laughing and giggling (hence its nickname, "laughing gas"). Regulating dosages of this drug can be difficult. Sustained inhalation can lead to unconsciousness, coma, and death.

Steroids

Public awareness of **anabolic steroids** has been heightened by media stories about their use by amateur and professional athletes, including Arnold Schwarzenegger during his competitive bodybuilding days. Anabolic steroids are artificial forms of the male hormone testosterone that promote muscle growth and strength. These **ergogenic drugs** are used primarily by young men to increase their strength, power, bulk (weight), speed, and athletic performance.

Most steroids are obtained through the black market. It was once estimated that approximately 17 to 20 percent of college athletes used steroids. Now that the National Collegiate Athletic Association (NCAA) has instituted much stricter drug-testing policies, reported use of anabolic steroids among intercollegiate athletics has dropped to 1.1 percent. However, a recent survey among high school students found a significant increase in the use of anabolic steroids since 1991. Few data exist, however, on the extent of steroid abuse by adults. It has been estimated that hundreds of thousands of people aged 18 and older abuse anabolic steroids at least once a year. Among both adolescents and adults, steroid abuse is higher among males than females. However, steroid abuse is growing most rapidly among young women.[23]

Steroids are available in two forms: injectable solution and pills. Anabolic steroids produce a state of euphoria, diminished fatigue, and increased bulk and power in both sexes. These qualities give steroids an addictive quality. When users stop, they appear to undergo psychological withdrawal, mainly caused by the disappearance of the physique they have become accustomed to.

Adverse effects occur in both men and women who use steroids. These drugs cause mood swings (aggression and violence), sometimes known as "roid rage"; acne; liver tumors; elevated cholesterol levels; hypertension; kidney disease; and immune system disturbances. There is also a danger of AIDS transmission through shared needles. In women, large doses of anabolic steroids may trigger the development of masculine attributes, such as lowered voice, increased facial and body hair, and male pattern baldness; they may also result in an enlarged clitoris, decreased breast size, and changes in or absence of menstruation. When taken by healthy males, anabolic steroids shut down the body's production of testosterone, causing men's breasts to grow and testicles to atrophy.

To combat the growing problem of steroid use, Congress passed the Anabolic Steroids Control Act (ASCA) of 1990. This law makes it a crime to possess, prescribe, or distribute anabolic steroids for any use other than the treatment of specific diseases. Anabolic steroids are now classified as a Schedule III drug. Penalties for their illegal use include up to five years' imprisonment and a $250,000 fine for the first offense, and up to ten years' imprisonment and a $500,000 fine for subsequent offenses.

A new and alarming trend is the use of other drugs to achieve the "performance-enhancing" effects of steroids. The two most common steroid alternatives are gamma-hydroxybutyrate (GHB) and clenbuterol. GHB is a deadly, illegal drug that is a primary ingredient in many "performance-enhancing" formulas. GHB does not produce a high. It does, however, cause headaches, nausea, vomiting, diarrhea, seizures and other central nervous system disorders, and possibly death. Clenbuterol is used in some countries for certain veterinary treatments, but it is not approved for any use—in animals or humans—in the United States.

In 1998 new attention was drawn to the issue of steroids and related substances when St. Louis Cardinals slugger Mark McGwire admitted to using a supplement containing androstenedione (andro), an adrenal hormone that is produced naturally in both men and women. Andro raises levels of testosterone, which helps build lean muscle mass and promotes quicker recovery after injury. McGwire had

---

Amyl nitrite   A drug that dilates blood vessels and is properly used to relieve chest pain.

Nitrous oxide   The chemical name for "laughing gas," a substance properly used for surgical or dental anesthesia.

Anabolic steroids   Artificial forms of the hormone testosterone that promote muscle growth and strength.

Ergogenic drug   Substance that enhances athletic performance.

done nothing illegal, as the supplement can be purchased over the counter (with sales estimated at up to $800 million a year). Moreover, its use is legal in baseball, although banned by the NFL, NCAA, and International Olympic Committee. A recent study found that when men take 100 milligrams of andro three times daily, it increases estrogen levels by up to 80 percent, enlarges the prostate gland, and increases heart disease by 10 to 15 percent. This finding may or may not affect its use in major league baseball—no decision has yet been made.

Other muscle-building supplements are also common. Though andro has been banned by many sports organizations, visits to the locker rooms of many teams belonging to these organizations would disclose large containers of other supplements, such as creatine, intended to help athletes build muscle mass. Although they are legal, questions remain whether enough research has been done concerning the safety of these supplements. Some people worry that they may bring consequences similar to those of steroids, such as liver damage and heart problems.

> **What do you think?**
>
> *Do you think androstenedione should be declared illegal?* ✳ *Would you consider using supplements for the sole purpose of increasing your body build and potentially your athletic performance?* ✳ *Are steroid users stigmatized in our society in the same way as users of other illicit drugs?* ✳ *Do you think they should be? Why or why not?*

Illegal Drug Use in the United States

Stories of people who have tried illegal drugs, enjoyed them, and suffered no consequences may tempt you to try them yourself. You may tell yourself it's "just this once," convincing yourself that one-time use is harmless. Given the dangers surrounding these substances, however, you should think twice. The risks associated with drug use extend beyond the personal. The decision to try any illicit substance encourages illicit drug manufacture and transport, thus contributing to the national drug problem. The financial burden of illegal drug use on the U.S. economy is staggering, with an estimated economic cost of around $97.7 billion.[24] This estimate includes substance abuse treatment and prevention costs, other health care costs, costs associated with reduced job productivity or lost earnings, and social costs, such as crime and social welfare.

In addition, roughly one-half of all expenditures to combat crime are related to illegal drugs. The burden of these costs is absorbed primarily by the government, followed by those who abuse drugs and members of their households, and taxpayers who must subsidize extra

police/law enforcement, prisons, and property damage. Additionally, there is also a significant incalculable "cost" to citizens who live in fear of being victimized and may avoid areas of a city or refuse to go out after dark in areas where drug traffic is a serious problem.

Drugs in the Workplace

Results of the National Household Survey on Drug Abuse estimates that 9.4 percent of all U.S. workers use illicit drugs on the job on any given day. With approximately 77 percent of illicit drug users in the United States employed to some degree, the cost to American businesses soars into the billions of dollars annually.[25] These costs reflect reduced work performance and efficiency, lost productivity, increased absenteeism and turnover, increased use of health benefits, accidents, and indirect losses from impaired judgment.

The highest rates of illicit drug use exist among workers in the construction, food preparation, restaurant, transportation, and material-moving industries. Workers who require a considerable amount of public trust, such as police officers, teachers, and child-care workers, report the lowest use. In addition, younger employees (18 to 24 years old) are more likely to report drug use than employees 25 and older. Drug users are 1.6 times more likely than nonusers to quit their jobs or be fired, and 1.5 times more likely to be disciplined by their supervisors.[26]

Many companies have instituted drug testing for their employees. Mandatory drug urinalysis is controversial. Critics argue that such testing violates Fourth Amendment rights of protection from unreasonable search and seizure. Proponents believe the personal inconvenience entailed in testing pales in comparison to the problems caused by drug use in the workplace. Several court decisions have affirmed the right of employers to test their employees for drug use. They contend that Fourth Amendment rights pertain only to employees of government agencies, not to those of private businesses. Most Americans apparently support some type of drug testing for certain types of job categories.

Drug testing is expensive, with costs running as high as $100 per individual test. Moreover, some critics question the accuracy and reliability of the results. Both false positives and false negatives can occur. As drug testing becomes more common in the work environment, it is gaining greater acceptance by employees, who see testing as a step to improving safety and productivity.

> **What do you think?**
>
> *What do you believe are the moral and ethical issues surrounding drug testing?* ✳ *Are you in a high-risk job?* ✳ *Is it the employer's legal right to conduct drug testing at the worksite?* ✳ *If so, do you think it is morally or ethically justified? Explain your answer.*

Solutions to the Problem

The most popular antidrug strategies for many years were total prohibition and "scare tactics." Both approaches proved ineffective. Prohibition of alcohol during the 1920s created more problems than it solved, as did prohibition of opiates in 1914. Outlawing other illicit drugs has neither eliminated them nor curtailed their traffic across U.S. borders.

In general, researchers in the field of drug education agree that a multimodal approach is best. Students should be taught the difference between drug use and abuse. Factual information that is free of scare tactics must be presented; lecturing and moralizing about drug use and abuse do not work. Emphasis should be placed on things that are important to young people. Telling adolescent males that girls will find them disgusting if their breath stinks of cigarettes or pot will get their attention. Likewise, lecturing on the negative effects of drug use is a much less effective deterrent than teaching young people how to negotiate the social scene. DARE, one program intended to educate students, has been largely ineffective. Education efforts need to focus on achieving better outcomes for preventing drug use.

We must target at-risk groups for study so we can better understand the circumstances that make them suscepti-ble to drug use. Time, money, and effort by educators, parents, and policy makers are needed to ensure that today's youth are given the love and security essential for building productive and meaningful lives.

Among the strategies suggested for combating drug abuse are stricter border surveillance to reduce drug trafficking, longer prison sentences for drug pushers, increased government spending on preventing and enforcing antidrug laws, and greater cooperation between government agencies and private groups and individuals. All of these approaches will probably help up to a point, but neither alone nor in combination do they offer a total solution to the problem. Drug abuse has been a part of human behavior for thousands of years, and it is not likely to disappear in the near future. For this reason, it is necessary to educate ourselves and to develop the self-discipline necessary to avoid dangerous drug dependence.

> ### What do you think?
>
> *Do you feel the public has a social responsibility to fight drug abuse?* ✳ *Other than financial costs, what other "costs" to society as a whole does drug abuse cause?* ✳ *Is it accurate to say that drug abuse is someone else's problem? Why or why not?*

Taking Charge

Managing Drug Use Behavior

A college environment offers many opportunities for a young person, most of which are good. Unfortunately, other opportunities can be dangerous, including the availability of drugs. Are you aware of the drug culture on your campus? Have drugs had an effect on your life? Before you try a new drug, take a moment to think about what you're doing. Think about what you want to experience or why you want to change your mental state. Then ask yourself whether the drug will really achieve that. Are there alternatives for reaching the desired change? What are the potential side effects? Are the risks worth the momentary high? Are you willing to risk potential addiction?

Checklist for Change

✓ What drugs are most popular among your peers? What is it about these drugs that makes them popular?

✓ How do you and your peers feel about illicit drug use? Is it condoned or condemned? Has this viewpoint changed in the past few years? What has led to these feelings?

✓ Are you prepared for the challenge of refusing to use illicit drugs that you may be offered and for dealing with the consequences associated with that decision?

✓ Do you practice assertiveness? Do you practice speaking up and voicing your opinion regardless of the subject?

✓ Do you have strategies for coping with stress? Do you use exercise, meditation, or some other healthy activity to reduce stress?

✓ Do you take the time to find out about the current drug problems on your campus and in your community?

✓ Would you be willing to assist a friend in combating his or her substance abuse problem? Would you take your friend or accompany him or her to support groups or recommend that they get help? Have you given any thought to how you might approach this issue with them?

✓ Would you be willing to be a role model in community programs such as Big Brothers or Big Sisters?

Summary

* The six categories of drugs are prescription drugs, OTC drugs, recreational drugs, herbal preparations, illicit drugs, and commercial preparations. Routes of administration include oral ingestion, injection (intravenous, intramuscular, and subcutaneous), inhalation, inunction, and suppositories.
* Prescription drugs are administered under medical supervision. There are dozens of categories, including antibiotics, sedatives, tranquilizers, and antidepressants. Generic drugs can often be substituted for more expensive brand-name drugs. Over-the-counter drug categories include analgesics, cold/cough/allergy and asthma relievers, stimulants, sleeping aids and relaxants, and dieting aids. Exercise personal responsibility by reading directions for OTC drugs and asking your pharmacist or doctor whether any special precautions are advised when taking these substances.
* Addiction is the continued involvement with a substance or activity despite ongoing negative consequences.
* People from all walks of life use illicit drugs, although college students report higher usage rates than does the general population. Drug use has declined since the mid-1980s.
* Controlled substances include cocaine and its derivatives, amphetamines, newer-generation stimulants, marijuana, the opiates, the psychedelics, the deliriants, designer drugs, inhalants, and steroids. Users tend to become addicted quickly to such drugs.
* The drug problem reaches everyone through crime and elevated health care costs. Drugs are a major problem in the workplace; workplace drug testing is one proposed solution to this problem.

Discussion Questions

1. What is the name of the current theory that explains how drugs work in the body? Explain how this theory works.
2. Explain the terms *synergism, antagonism,* and *inhibition.*
3. What are the advantages and disadvantages associated with use of generic drugs?
4. Do you think there is such a thing as responsible use of illicit drugs? Would you change any of the current laws governing drugs? How would you determine what is legitimate use and illegitimate use?
5. Why do you think that many people today feel that marijuana use is not dangerous? What are the arguments in favor of legalizing marijuana? What are the arguments against legalization? How common is the use of marijuana on your campus?
6. How do you and your peers feel about illicit drug use? How and why has your opinion changed in recent years, if it has?
7. Debate the issue of workplace drug testing. Would you apply for a job that had drug testing as an interview requirement? As a continuing requirement?
8. What could you do to help a friend who is fighting a substance abuse problem? What resources on your campus could help you?
9. What types of programs do you think would be effective in preventing drug abuse among high school and college students? How would programs for high school students differ from those for college students?
10. Discuss how addiction affects family and friends. What role do family and friends play in helping the addict get help and maintain recovery?

Application Exercise

Reread the What Do You Think? scenario at the beginning of the chapter and answer the following questions.

1. What are some of the health risks associated with smoking marijuana? How frequently do you think marijuana use contributes to students' academic problems?
2. Do you think that Greg and his friends were treated fairly? Why or why not? Do you think more students come to your campus having used marijuana in the past, or do you think they more typically begin using marijuana when they get to campus? Do you think marijuana should continue to be a Schedule I drug? Why or why not?

Accessing Your Health on the Internet

Visit the following Internet sites to explore further topics and issues related to personal health. To visit an organization's website, go to the Companion Website for *Health: The Basics, Fifth Edition* at www.aw.com/donatelle, click on the book image, and select "Accessing Your Health on the Internet" from the navigation menu on the left.

1. ***Join Together.*** An excellent site for the most current information related to substance abuse. This site also includes information on gun violence and provides advice on organizing and taking political action.

2. ***National Institute on Drug Abuse (NIDA).*** The home page of this U.S. government agency has information on the latest statistics and findings in drug research.

3. ***Club Drugs.*** A website designed to disseminate science-based information about club drugs.

4. ***Substance Abuse and Mental Health Services Administration (SAMHSA).*** Outstanding resource for information about national surveys, ongoing research and national drug interventions.

Further Reading

Elster, J. (ed.). *Addiction: Entries and Exits.* New York: Russell Sage Foundation, 2000.

Addresses current addiction controversies from an international perspective, with authors from the United States and Norway. Topics include whether addicts have a choice in their behavior and current addiction theories.

Goldstein, Avram. *Addiction: From Biology to Drug Policy.* New York: Oxford University Press, 2001.

This book is divided into three parts—how drugs impact the brain, how each drug causes addiction, and how addictive drugs impact society. The author offers an explanation about what we know about drug addiction in each of these three areas, how we know what we know, and what we can and cannot do about the drug problem.

Greenburg, S. *2001 Physician's Desk Reference for Nonprescription Drugs,* 20th ed. Oradell, NJ: Medical Economics Data, 2001.

Outlines proper uses, possible dangers, and effective ingredients of nonprescription medications.

Griffith, W. H. *Complete Guide to Prescription and Nonprescription Drugs,* 16th ed. Berkeley, CA: Berkeley Publishing Group, 2000.

This essential guide answers every conceivable question about prescription and nonprescription drugs—information about dosages, side effects, precautions, interactions, and more. More than 5,000 brand-name and 700 generic drugs are profiled in an easy-to-use format.

West, J. W. *The Betty Ford Center Book of Answers: Help for Those Struggling with Substance Abuse and the People Who Love Them.* New York: Pocket Books, 1997.

Written by the former director of the Betty Ford Center, one of the leading alcohol and drug treatment centers in the United States. Provides answers to the most frequently asked questions about treatment and recovery; includes comprehensive coverage of drug abuse issues for addicts and their families.

U.S. Department of Health and Human Services. *Research Report Series.* Washington, D.C.: National Institute on Drug Abuse.

The Research Report Series is available through the National Institute on Drug Abuse. These booklets provide a current overview of research and practical information regarding illicit and licit drug use in the United States.

8

Alcohol, Tobacco, and Caffeine

DAILY PLEASURES, DAILY CHALLENGES

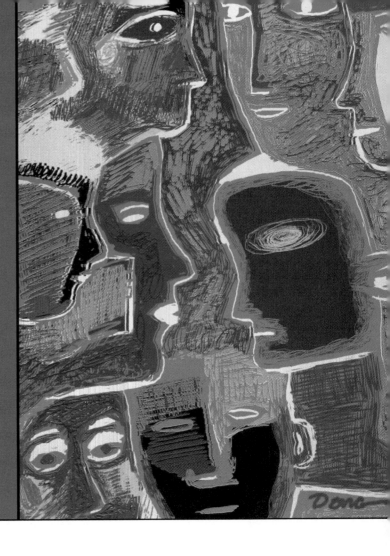

objectives

* Summarize the alcohol use patterns of college students, and discuss overall trends in consumption.

* Explain the physiological and behavioral effects of alcohol, including blood alcohol concentration, absorption, metabolism, and immediate and long-term effects of alcohol consumption.

* Explain the symptoms and causes of alcoholism, its cost to society, and its effects on the family.

* Explain the treatment of alcoholism, including the family's role, varied treatment methods, and whether or not alcoholics can be cured.

* Discuss the social and political issues involved in tobacco use.

* Discuss how the chemicals in tobacco products affect a smoker's body.

* Review the health effects of smoking and smokeless tobacco, and identify the adverse effects of tobacco on a fetus's health.

* Evaluate the risks that environmental tobacco smoke may pose to nonsmokers.

* Compare the benefits and risks associated with caffeine, and summarize the health consequences of long-term caffeine use.

Usually the word *drug* conjures up images of people abusing illegal substances. We use the term to describe dangerous chemicals such as heroin or cocaine, without recognizing that socially accepted substances can be drugs, too—for example, alcohol, tobacco, and caffeine.

Alcohol: An Overview

Moderate use of alcohol can enhance celebrations or special times. Research shows that very low levels of use may actually decrease some health risks. However, always remember that alcohol is a chemical substance that affects your physical and mental behavior.

An estimated 70 percent of Americans consume alcoholic beverages regularly, though consumption patterns are unevenly distributed throughout the drinking population. Ten percent are heavy drinkers, and they account for half of all the alcohol consumed. The remaining 90 percent of the drinking population are infrequent, light, or moderate drinkers.

Alcohol and College Students

Alcohol is the most widely used (and abused) recreational drug in our society. It is also the most popular drug on college campuses, where approximately 84 percent of students consume alcoholic beverages.[1] About one-third of college students are classified as heavy drinkers, meaning that they consume large amounts of alcohol per drinking occasion. Therefore, students who might go out and drink only once a week are considered heavy drinkers if they

consume a great deal of alcohol. In a new trend on college campuses, women's consumption of alcohol is close to equaling men's. Exactly how much does a typical college student consume? Colleges and universities have been described as among the "alcohol-drenched institutions." See the accompanying Reality Check box. Every year, America's 12 million undergraduates drink 4 billion cans of beer, averaging 55 six-packs per person, and spend $446 on alcoholic beverages—more than they spend on soft drinks and textbooks combined.[2]

Despite these figures, fewer students are drinking alcohol than in the past. In 1980, 9.5 percent of students nationwide said they abstained from alcohol; in 1999, 19 percent were abstainers.[3] According to the University of Michigan's Institute for Social Research, the percentage of students who report drinking daily also has declined, from 6.5 percent in 1980 to 4.8 percent.[4]

College is a critical time to become aware of and responsible for drinking. There is little doubt that drinking is a part of campus culture and tradition. Students are away from home, often for the first time, and many are excited by their newfound independence. For some students, this independence and the rite of passage into the college culture are symbolized by the use of alcohol. It provides the answer to one of the most commonly heard statements on any college campus: "There is nothing to do." Additionally, many students suggest they drink "to have fun." Having fun, which often means drinking to simply get drunk, may really be a way of coping with stress, boredom, anxiety, or pressures created by academic and social demands.

Statistics about college students' drinking may not always reflect the actual incidence of alcohol consumption. Students consistently report that their friends drink much more than they do and that average drinking within their

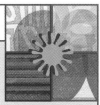

The Facts About College Students and Drinking

Perhaps you've heard conflicting reports in the media about the prevalence and effects of drinking on campus. What are the real facts? The following statistics reveal the scope of the problem.

✓ Alcohol kills more people below age 21 than cocaine, marijuana, and heroin combined.

✓ One night of heavy drinking can impair the ability to think abstractly for up to 30 days, limiting a student's ability to relate textbook reading to a professor's lecture, or to think through a football play.

✓ College administrators estimate that alcohol is involved in 29 percent of dropouts, 38 percent of academic failures, 64 percent of violent behaviors, and 6 percent of unsafe sexual practices.

✓ Heavier drinking, tougher law enforcement, and better reporting caused alcohol-related arrest rates to shoot up by 24.3 percent in 1999.

✓ The National Bureau of Economic Research found that areas of a college campus offering cheap beer prices had more violent and nonviolent crime, including trouble between students and police or other campus authorities, arguments, physical fight-ing, property damage, false fire alarms, and sexual misconduct.

✓ Alcohol is involved in more than two-thirds of suicides among college students, one-third of all emotional and academic problems, 90 percent of campus rapes and sexual assaults, and 95 percent of violent crime on campus.

✓ Close to 40 percent of students surveyed reported binge drinking in high school.

✓ Women who drink heavily are 40 percent more likely to experience unwanted sexual advances than are those who drink less.

✓ Seventy-five percent of male students and 55 percent of female students involved in acquaintance rape had been drinking or using drugs at the time.

✓ College binge drinking occurs more frequently among male students, students who reside on campus, intercollegiate athletes, and members of fraternities and sororities.

✓ Approximately 40 percent of fraternity and sorority members report being frequent binge drinkers.

✓ As many as 360,000 of the nation's 12 million undergraduates will die from alcohol-related causes while in school. This is more than the number who will receive M.A. and Ph.D. degrees.

✓ College students under the age of 21 are more prone to binge drinking and pay less for their alcohol than their older classmates do, according to researchers at the Harvard University School of Public Health.

✓ Though underage students are likely to drink less often, they consume more per occasion than students aged 21 and older who are allowed to drink legally.

✓ College students who have serious alcohol problems and engage in dangerous behaviors are more likely than other students to have guns with them at school.

Source: Data were compiled from the numerous studies cited throughout this chapter and from: L. D. Johnson, P. M. O'Malley, and J. G. Bachman, *The Monitoring the Future Study, 1975–1999*, Vol. II (Rockville, MD: NIDA, 2000); H. Wechsler, et al., "College Binge Drinking in the 1990s: A Continuing Problem," *Journal of American College Health* 48 (2000); A. Cohen, "Battle of the Binge," *Time* (September 8, 1997).

---

own social living group is higher than actual self-reports. Such misinformation may promote or be used to excuse excessive drinking practices among college students. In a survey of students at a large Midwestern university, 42 percent reported not having a hangover in the past six months. Yet that same group of surveyed students believed that only 3 percent of their peers had not had a hangover in the past month. Many colleges have begun to make efforts to reduce the misperception of what is normal drinking behavior among college students. It is hoped that providing students with accurate information about their peers and their peers' drinking behavior will reduce the pressure on students who feel as though they need to drink or to drink in excess.

High-Risk "Binge" Drinking and College Students

Binge drinking is defined as five drinks in a row by men and four in a row by women on a single occasion. The stakes of binge drinking are high because of the increased risk for alcohol-related injuries or death. An estimated 50 students die annually from alcohol poisonings. In a single month,

Binge drinking   Drinking for the express purpose of becoming intoxicated; five drinks in a single sitting for men and four drinks in a sitting for women.

November 1997, five college students died in alcohol-related accidents in the state of Virginia alone.

According to a 1999 study by the Harvard School of Public Health, 44 percent of students were found to be binge drinkers, and of those, 22.7 percent were reported as frequent bingers, that is, people who binge drink three times or more in a two-week period[5] (Table 8.1). Compared with non-binge drinkers, frequent binge drinkers were more likely to have an array of problems on campus. For example, frequent binge drinkers are 16 times more likely to miss class, 8 times more likely to get behind in their school work, and more apt to get into trouble with campus or local police.[6]

Although everyone is at some risk for alcohol-related problems, college students seem to be particularly vulnerable for the following reasons:

- Alcohol exacerbates their already high risk for suicide, automobile crashes, and falls.
- Many college and university customs, norms, traditions, and mores encourage certain dangerous practices and patterns of alcohol use.
- University campuses are heavily targeted by advertising and promotions from the alcoholic beverage industry.
- It is more common for college students than their noncollegiate peers to drink recklessly and to engage in drinking games and other dangerous drinking practices.
- College students are particularly vulnerable to peer influences and have a strong need to be accepted by their peers.
- There is institutional denial by college administrators that alcohol problems exist on their campuses.

Table 8.1
College Students' Patterns of Alcohol Use, 1999

CATEGORY	TOTAL (%)	MEN (%)	WOMEN (%)
Abstainer (past year)	19.2	20.1	18.7
Non-binge drinker	36.6	29.3	41.3
Occasional binge drinker	21.4	24.7	19.4
Frequent binge drinker	22.7	26.0	20.6

Source: H. Wechsler, College Alcohol Survey, unpublished data, 1999.

To prevent alcohol abuse, many colleges and universities are instituting strong policies against drinking. University presidents have formed a leadership group to help curb the problem of alcohol abuse. Many fraternities have elected to have dry houses. At the same time, colleges and universities are making more help available to students with drinking problems. Today, both individual counseling and group counseling are offered on most campuses, and more attention is being directed toward preventing alcohol abuse. Student organizations such as BACCHUS (Boost Alcohol Consciousness Concerning the Health of University Students) promote responsible drinking and party hosting.

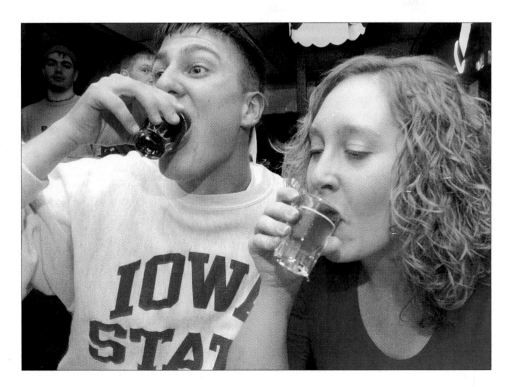

Deciding when to drink, and how much, is no small matter. Irresponsible consumption of alcohol can easily result in disaster.

Trends in Consumption

In general, alcohol consumption levels among Americans have been steadily declining since the late 1970s. In 1998, the estimated per capita consumption was the equivalent of 2.19 gallons of pure alcohol per person.[7] This represents a substantial decline from 2.64 gallons in 1977. (This measure indicates the amount of alcohol that a person would obtain by drinking approximately 50 gallons of beer, 20 gallons of wine, or more than 4 gallons of distilled spirits.)

This downward trend has been tied to a growing attention to weight, personal health, and physical activity. The alcohol industry has responded by introducing beer and wines with fewer calories and reduced alcohol content.

> ### What do you think?
> *For what reasons do college students drink excessive amounts of alcohol? ✱ Are there particular traditions related to when and why students drink on your campus? ✱ Have you ever had your sleep or studies interrupted or have you had to baby-sit a friend because of drinking? ✱ Did you say anything about it to your friend? ✱ How did the person respond?*

Physiological and Behavioral Effects of Alcohol

The Chemical Makeup of Alcohol

The intoxicating substance found in beer, wine, liquor, and liqueurs is **ethyl alcohol,** or **ethanol.** It is produced during a process called **fermentation,** whereby yeast organisms break down plant sugars, yielding ethanol and carbon dioxide. Fermentation continues until the solution of plant sugars (called mash) reaches a concentration of 14 percent alcohol. At this point, the alcohol kills the yeast and halts the chemical reactions that produce it.

For beers and ales, which are fermented from malt barley, the process stops when the alcohol concentration is 14 percent. Manufacturers then add other ingredients that dilute the alcohol content of the beverage. Other alcoholic beverages are produced through further processing called **distillation,** during which alcohol vapors are released from the mash at high temperatures. The vapors are then condensed and mixed with water to make the final product.

The **proof** of an alcoholic drink is a measure of the percentage of alcohol in the beverage. "Proof" comes from "gunpowder proof," a reference to the gunpowder test, whereby potential buyers would test the distiller's product by pouring it on gunpowder and attempting to light it. If the alcohol content was at least 50 percent, the gunpowder would burn; otherwise the water in the product would put out the flame. Thus, alcohol percentage is 50 percent of the given proof. For example, 80 proof whiskey or scotch is 40 percent alcohol by volume, and 100 proof vodka is 50 percent alcohol by volume. The proof of a beverage indicates its strength. Lower-proof drinks will produce fewer alcohol effects than the same amount of higher-proof drinks.

Most wines are between 12 and 15 percent alcohol, and ales are between 6 and 8 percent. The alcoholic content of beers is between 2 and 6 percent, varying according to state laws and type of beer.

Behavioral Effects

Blood alcohol concentration (BAC) is the ratio of alcohol to total blood volume. It is the factor used to measure the physiological and behavioral effects of alcohol. Despite individual differences, alcohol produces some general behavioral effects depending on BAC (Table 8.2). At a BAC of 0.02, a person feels slightly relaxed and in a good mood. At 0.05, relaxation increases, there is some motor impairment, and a willingness to talk becomes apparent. At 0.08, the person feels euphoric and experiences further motor impairment. At 0.10, the depressant effects of alcohol become apparent, drowsiness sets in, and motor skills are further impaired, followed by a loss of judgment. Thus, a driver may not be able to estimate distances or speed, and some drinkers lose their ability to make value-related decisions and may do things they would not do when sober. As BAC increases, the drinker suffers increased physiological and psychological effects. All these changes are negative. Alcohol ingestion does not enhance any physical skills or mental functions.

People can acquire physical and psychological tolerance to the effects of alcohol through regular use. The nervous system adapts over time, so greater amounts of alcohol are required to produce the same physiological and

---

Ethyl alcohol (ethanol)   An addictive drug produced by fermentation and found in many beverages.

Fermentation   The process whereby yeast organisms break down plant sugars to yield ethanol.

Distillation   The process whereby mash is subjected to high temperatures to release alcohol vapors, which are then condensed and mixed with water to make the final product.

Proof   A measure of the percentage of alcohol in a beverage.

Blood alcohol concentration (BAC)   The ratio of alcohol to total blood volume; the factor used to measure the physiological and behavioral effects of alcohol.

Table 8.2

Psychological and Physical Effects of Various Blood-Alcohol Concentration Levels*

NUMBER OF DRINKS[†]	BLOOD-ALCOHOL CONCENTRATION (%)	PSYCHOLOGICAL AND PHYSICAL EFFECTS
1	0.02–0.03	No overt effects, slight mood elevation
2	0.05–0.06	Feeling of relaxation, warmth; slight decrease in reaction time and in fine-muscle coordination
3	0.08–0.09	Balance, speech, vision, and hearing slightly impaired; feelings of euphoria, increased confidence; loss of motor coordination
	0.10	Legal intoxication in most states; some have lower limits
4	0.11–0.12	Coordination and balance becoming difficult; distinct impairment of mental faculties, judgment
5	0.14–0.15	Major impairment of mental and physical control; slurred speech, blurred vision, lack of motor skills
7	0.20	Loss of motor control—must have assistance in moving about; mental confusion
10	0.30	Severe intoxication; minimal conscious control of mind and body
14	0.40	Unconsciousness, threshold of coma
17	0.50	Deep coma
20	0.60	Death from respiratory failure

*For each hour elapsed since the last drink, subtract 0.015 percent blood-alcohol concentration, or approximately one drink.
[†]One drink = one beer (4 percent alcohol, 12 ounces), one highball (1 ounce whiskey), or one glass table wine (5 ounces).

Source: Modified from data given in Ohio State Police Driver Information Seminars and the National Clearinghouse for Alcohol and Alcoholism Information, Rockville, MD.

psychological effects. Some people can learn to modify their behavior so that they appear to be sober even when their BAC is quite high. This ability is called **learned behavioral tolerance.**

Absorption and Metabolism

Unlike the molecules found in most other ingestible foods and drugs, alcohol molecules are sufficiently small and fat soluble to be absorbed throughout the entire gastrointestinal system. A negligible amount of alcohol is absorbed through the lining of the mouth. Approximately 20 percent of ingested alcohol diffuses through the stomach lining into the bloodstream, and nearly 80 percent passes through the linings of the upper third of the small intestine. Absorption into the bloodstream is rapid and complete.

Several factors influence how quickly your body will absorb alcohol: the alcohol concentration in your drink, the amount of alcohol you consume, the amount of food in your stomach, pylorospasm (spasm of the pyloric valve in the digestive system), and your mood. The higher the concentration of alcohol in your drink, the more rapidly it will be absorbed in your digestive tract. As a rule, wine and beer are absorbed more slowly than distilled beverages. Carbonated alcoholic beverages—such as champagne and sparkling wines—are absorbed more rapidly than those containing no sparkling additives, or fizz. Carbonated beverages and drinks served with mixers cause the pyloric valve—the opening from the stomach into the small intestine—to relax, thereby emptying the contents of the stomach more rapidly into the small intestine. Because the small intestine is the site of the greatest absorption of alcohol, carbonated beverages increase the rate of absorption. In contrast, if your stomach is full, absorption is slowed because the surface area exposed to alcohol is smaller. A full stomach also retards the emptying of alcoholic beverages into the small intestine.

In addition, the more alcohol you consume, the longer absorption takes. Alcohol can irritate the digestive system, causing a spasm in the pyloric valve (pylorospasm). When the pyloric valve is closed, nothing can move from the stomach to the upper third of the small intestine, which slows absorption. If the irritation continues, it can cause vomiting.

Learned behavioral tolerance   The ability of heavy drinkers to modify behavior so that they appear to be sober even when they have high BAC levels.

Mood is another factor, because emotions affect how long it takes for the contents of the stomach to empty into the intestine. Powerful moods, such as stress and tension, are likely to cause the stomach to "dump" its contents into the small intestine. That is why alcohol is absorbed much more rapidly when people are tense than when they are relaxed.

Alcohol is metabolized in the liver, where it is converted by the enzyme alcohol dehydrogenase to acetaldehyde. It is then rapidly oxidized to acetate, converted to carbon dioxide and water, and eventually excreted from the body. Acetaldehyde is a toxic chemical that can cause immediate symptoms, such as nausea and vomiting, as well as long-term effects, such as liver damage. A very small portion of alcohol is excreted unchanged by the kidneys, lungs, and skin.

Like food, alcohol contains calories. Proteins and carbohydrates (starches and sugars) each contain 4 kilocalories (kcal) per gram. Fat contains 9 kcal per gram. Alcohol, although similar in structure to carbohydrates, contains 7 kcal per gram. The body uses the calories in alcohol in the same manner it uses those found in carbohydrates: for immediate energy or for storage as fat if not immediately needed.

When compared to the variable breakdown rates of foods and other beverages, the breakdown of alcohol occurs at a fairly constant rate of 0.5 ounce per hour. This amount of alcohol is equivalent to 12 ounces of 5 percent beer, 5 ounces of 12 percent wine, or 1.5 ounces of 40 percent (80 proof) liquor. Legal limits of BAC for operating motor vehicles vary from state to state. Most states set the legal limit at 0.08 to 0.10 percent. A driver whose BAC exceeds the state's legal limit is considered legally intoxicated.

A drinker's BAC depends on weight and body fat, the water content in body tissues, the concentration of alcohol in the beverage consumed, the rate of consumption, and the volume of alcohol consumed. Heavier people have larger body surfaces through which to diffuse alcohol; therefore, they have lower concentrations of alcohol in their blood than do thin people after drinking the same amount. Because alcohol does not diffuse as rapidly into body fat as into water, alcohol concentration is higher in a person with more body fat. Because a woman is likely to have more body fat and less water in her body tissues than a man of the same weight, she will be more intoxicated than a man after drinking the same amount of alcohol.

Alcohol Poisoning

Alcohol Poisoning Alcohol poisoning occurs much more frequently than people realize, and all too often it can be fatal. Drinking large amounts of alcohol in a short period of time can cause the blood alcohol level to reach the lethal range relatively quickly. Alcohol, either used alone or in combination with other drugs, is probably responsible for more toxic overdose deaths than any other substance.

Death from alcohol poisoning can be caused by either central nervous system (CNS) and respiratory depression or the inhalation of vomit or fluid into the lungs. The amount of alcohol it takes for a person to become unconscious is dangerously close to the lethal dose. Signs of alcohol poisoning include the following: inability to be roused; a weak, rapid pulse; an unusual or irregular breathing pattern; and cool (possibly damp), pale, or bluish skin. If you are with someone who has been drinking heavily and who exhibits these conditions, or if you are unsure about the person's condition, call 911 for emergency help right away.

Women and Alcohol Body fat is not the only contributor to the differences in alcohol's effects on men and women. Compared to men, women appear to have half as much alcohol hydrogenase, the enzyme that breaks down alcohol in the stomach before it has a chance to get to the bloodstream and the brain. Therefore, if a man and a woman drink the same amount of alcohol, the woman's BAC will be approximately 30 percent higher than the man's, leaving her more vulnerable to slurred speech, careless driving, and other drinking-related impairments.

Breathalyzer and Other Tests The Breathalyzer tests used by law enforcement officers determine BAC based on the amount of alcohol exhaled in the breath. Urinalysis can also yield a BAC based on the concentration of unmetabolized alcohol in the urine. Both breath analysis and urinalysis are used to determine whether a driver is legally intoxicated, but blood tests are more accurate measures. An increasing number of states are requiring blood tests for people suspected of driving under the influence of alcohol. In some states, refusal to take the breath or urine test results in immediate revocation of the person's driver's license.

What do you think?

Have you noticed that some types of alcoholic beverages affect people more quickly than others? ✷ *What factors affect BAC levels?* ✷ *Are these factors different for men and women?* ✷ *If so, how?*

Immediate Effects

The most dramatic effects produced by ethanol occur within the central nervous system (CNS). The primary action of the drug is to reduce the frequency of nerve transmissions and impulses at synaptic junctions. This depresses CNS functions, with resulting decreases in respiratory rate, pulse rate, and blood pressure. As CNS depression deepens, vital functions become noticeably depressed. In extreme cases, coma and death can result.

Table 8.3
Drugs and Alcohol: Actions and Interactions

DRUG CLASS / TRADE NAME(S)	EFFECTS WITH ALCOHOL
Antialcohol: Antabuse	Severe reactions to even small amounts; headache, nausea, blurred vision, convulsions, coma, possible death.
Antibiotics: Penicillin, Cyantin	Reduced therapeutic effectiveness.
Antidepressants: Elavil, Sinequan, Tofranil, Nardil	Increased central nervous system (CNS) depression, blood pressure changes. Combined use of alcohol and MAO inhibitors, a specific type of antidepressant, can trigger massive increases in blood pressure, even brain hemorrhage and death.
Antihistamines: Allerest, Dristan	Drowsiness and CNS depression. Driving ability impaired.
Aspirin: Anacin, Excedrin, Bayer	Irritates stomach lining. May cause gastrointestinal pain, bleeding.
Depressants: Valium, Ativan, Placidyl	Dangerous CNS depression, loss of coordination, coma. High risk of overdose and death.
Narcotics: heroin, codeine, Darvon	Serious CNS depression. Possible respiratory arrest and death.
Stimulants: caffeine, cocaine	Masks depressant action of alcohol. May increase blood pressure, physical tension.

Source: Reprinted by permission from *Drugs and Alcohol: Simple Facts about Alcohol and Drug Combinations* (Phoenix: DIN Publications, 1988), no. 121.

Alcohol is a diuretic, causing increased urinary output. Although this effect might be expected to lead to automatic **dehydration** (loss of water), the body actually retains water, most of it in the muscles or in the cerebral tissues. The reason is that water is usually pulled out of the **cerebrospinal fluid** (fluid within the brain and spinal cord), leading to what is known as mitochondrial dehydration at the cellular level within the nervous system. Mitochondria are miniature organs within cells that are responsible for specific functions. They rely heavily upon fluid balance. When mitochondrial dehydration occurs from drinking, the mitochondria cannot carry out their normal functions, resulting in symptoms that include the "morning-after" headaches suffered by some drinkers.

Alcohol irritates the gastrointestinal system and may cause indigestion and heartburn if taken on an empty stomach. Long-term use of alcohol causes repeated irritation that has been linked to cancers of the esophagus and stomach. In addition, people who engage in brief drinking sprees during which they consume unusually high amounts of alcohol put themselves at risk for irregular heartbeat or even total loss of heart rhythm, which can disrupt blood flow and damage the heart muscle.

A **hangover** is often experienced the morning after a drinking spree. The symptoms of a hangover are familiar to most people who drink: headache, muscle aches, upset stomach, anxiety, depression, and thirst. **Congeners** are thought to play a role in the development of a hangover. Congeners are forms of alcohol that are metabolized more slowly than ethanol and are more toxic. The body metabolizes the congeners after the ethanol is gone from the system, and their toxic by-products may contribute to the hangover. In addition, alcohol upsets the water balance in the body, resulting in excess urination and thirst the next day. Increased production of hydrochloric acid can irritate the stomach lining and cause nausea. It usually takes 12 hours to recover from a hangover. Bed rest, solid food, and aspirin may help relieve its discomforts, but unfortunately, nothing cures it but time.

When you use any drug (and alcohol is a drug), you need to be aware of the possible interactions with any other drugs, whether prescription or over-the-counter. Table 8.3 summarizes possible interactions. Note that alcohol may cause a negative interaction even with aspirin.

Long-Term Effects

Alcohol is distributed throughout most of the body and may affect many different organs and tissues. Problems associated

Dehydration   Loss of fluids from body tissues.

Cerebrospinal fluid   Fluid within and surrounding the brain and spinal cord tissues.

Hangover   The physiological reaction to excessive drinking, including symptoms such as headache, upset stomach, anxiety, depression, diarrhea, and thirst.

Congeners   Forms of alcohol that are metabolized more slowly than ethanol and produce toxic by-products.

with long-term, habitual use of alcohol include diseases of the nervous system, cardiovascular system, and liver, and some cancers.

Effects on the Nervous System

The nervous system is especially sensitive to alcohol. Even people who drink moderately experience shrinkage in brain size and weight and a loss of some degree of intellectual ability. The damage that results from alcohol use is localized primarily in the left side of the brain, which is responsible for written and spoken language, logic, and mathematical skills. The degree of shrinkage appears to be directly related to the amount of alcohol consumed. In terms of memory loss, the evidence suggests that having one drink every day is better than saving up for a binge and consuming seven or eight drinks in a night. The amount of alcohol consumed at one time is critical. Alcohol-related brain damage can be partially reversed with good nutrition and staying sober.

Cardiovascular Effects

Alcohol affects the cardiovascular system in a number of ways. Numerous studies have associated light to moderate alcohol consumption (no more than two drinks a day) with a reduced risk of coronary artery disease. Several mechanisms have been proposed to explain how this might happen. The strongest evidence favors an increase in high-density lipoprotein (HDL) cholesterol, which is known as the "good" cholesterol. Studies have shown that drinkers have higher levels of HDL. Another factor that might help is an *antithrombotic* effect. Alcohol consumption is associated with a decrease in clotting factors that contribute to the development of atherosclerosis.

However, alcohol consumption is not recommended as a preventive measure against heart disease because it causes many more cardiovascular health hazards than benefits. Alcohol contributes to high blood pressure and slightly increased heart rate and cardiac output. Those who report drinking three to five drinks a day, regardless of race or sex, have higher blood pressure than those who drink less.

Liver Disease

One of the most common diseases related to alcohol abuse is **cirrhosis** of the liver. It is among the top ten causes of death in the United States. One result of heavy drinking is that the liver begins to store fat—a condition known as fatty liver. If there is insufficient time between drinking episodes, this fat cannot be transported to storage sites, and the fat-filled liver cells stop functioning. Continued drinking can cause a further stage of liver deterioration called fibrosis, in which the damaged area of the liver develops fibrous scar tissue. Cell function can be partially restored at this stage with proper nutrition and abstinence from alcohol. If the person continues to drink, however, cirrhosis results. At this point, the liver cells die and the damage becomes permanent.

Alcoholic hepatitis is a serious condition resulting from prolonged use of alcohol. A chronic inflammation of the liver develops, which may be fatal in itself or progress to cirrhosis.

Cancer

The repeated irritation caused by long-term use of alcohol has been linked to cancers of the esophagus, stomach, mouth, tongue, and liver. Research has also shown a link between breast cancer and moderate levels of alcohol consumption in women. One compelling report has demonstrated that "drinkers of three or more glasses of alcoholic beverages per day appear to be at greater risk for breast cancer."[8] A 1994 Harvard Medical School study of male drinkers showed a 12 percent higher risk of cancer for those who had only one drink a day and a 123 percent higher risk for those who had two drinks a day. It is unclear how alcohol exerts its carcinogenic effects, though it is thought that it inhibits the absorption of carcinogenic substances, permitting them to be taken to sensitive organs.

Other Effects

As stated earlier, alcohol is an irritant to the gastrointestinal system and thus may cause indigestion and heartburn if ingested on an empty stomach. Alcohol also damages the mucous membranes and can cause inflammation of the esophagus, chronic stomach irritation, problems with intestinal absorption, and chronic diarrhea.

Alcohol abuse is a major cause of chronic inflammation of the pancreas, the organ that produces digestive enzymes and insulin. Chronic abuse of alcohol inhibits enzyme production, which further inhibits the absorption of nutrients. Drinking alcohol can block the absorption of calcium, a nutrient that strengthens bones. This should be of particular concern to women because as women age, their risk for osteoporosis (bone thinning and calcium loss) increases. Heavy consumption of alcohol worsens this condition.

Evidence also suggests that alcohol impairs the body's ability to recognize and fight foreign bodies, such as bacteria and viruses. The relationship between alcohol and AIDS is unclear, especially because some of the populations at risk for AIDS are also at risk for alcohol abuse. But any stressor with a known effect on the immune system—not just alcohol—would probably contribute to the development of the disease.

Cirrhosis The last stage of liver disease associated with chronic heavy use of alcohol during which liver cells die and damage becomes permanent.

Alcoholic hepatitis Condition resulting from prolonged use of alcohol, in which the liver is inflamed. It can result in death.

Alcohol and Pregnancy

Of the 30 known **teratogens** in the environment, alcohol is one of the most dangerous and common. Alcohol can harm fetal development.

More than 10 percent of all children have been exposed to high levels of alcohol in utero. All will suffer varying degrees of effects, ranging from mild learning disabilities to major physical, mental, and intellectual impairment. It takes very little alcohol to cause serious damage. Research has shown that even a single exposure to high levels of alcohol can cause significant brain damage in the infant.[9] A disorder called **fetal alcohol syndrome (FAS)** is associated with alcohol consumption during pregnancy. Alcohol consumed during the first trimester poses the greatest threat to organ development; exposure during the last trimester, when the brain is developing rapidly, is most likely to affect CNS development. FAS is the third most common birth defect and the second leading cause of mental retardation in the United States. The incidence of FAS is estimated to be 1 to 2 of every 1,000 live births. It is the most common preventable cause of mental impairment in the Western world.

FAS occurs when alcohol ingested by the mother passes through the placenta into the infant's bloodstream. Because the fetus is so small, its BAC will be much higher than that of the mother. Among the symptoms of FAS are mental retardation, small head, tremors, and abnormalities of the face, limbs, heart, and brain.

Children with a history of prenatal alcohol exposure but with fewer than the full physical or behavioral symptoms of FAS may be categorized as having **fetal alcohol effects (FAE).** FAE is estimated to occur three to four times as often as FAS, although it is much less recognized. The signs of FAE in newborns are low birth weight and irritability, and there may be permanent mental impairment. Infants whose mothers habitually consumed more than three ounces of alcohol (approximately six drinks) in a short time period when pregnant are at high risk for FAE. Risk levels for babies whose mothers consume smaller amounts are uncertain.

Alcohol can also be passed to a nursing baby through breast milk. For this reason, most doctors advise nursing mothers not to drink for at least four hours before nursing their babies and preferably to abstain altogether.

What do you think?

Why do we hear so little about FAS in this country when it is the third most common birth defect and second leading cause of mental retardation? ✴ *Is this a reflection of our society's denial of alcohol as a dangerous drug?*

Drinking and Driving

The leading cause of death for all age groups from 5 to 45 years old (including college students) is traffic accidents. Ap-proximately 40 percent of all traffic fatalities are alcohol related.[10] Unfortunately, college students are overrepresented in alcohol-related crashes. The College Alcohol Study findings indicated that 20 percent of non-binge drinkers, 43 percent of occasional bingers, and 59 percent of frequent bingers reported driving while intoxicated.[11] Furthermore, it is estimated that three out of every ten Americans will be involved in an alcohol-related accident at some time in their lives.[12] Studies show that those involved in car crashes who had been drinking have a 40 to 50 percent higher chance of dying than nondrinkers involved in car crashes.

In 2000, there were 16,653 alcohol-related traffic fatalities (ARTFs), a 30 percent reduction from the ARTF data reported in 1990. This number represents an average of one alcohol-related fatality every 32 minutes.[13] From 1990 to 2000, intoxication rates (BAC of 0.10 percent or greater) decreased for drivers of all age groups involved in fatal crashes. The highest intoxication rates in fatal crashes in 2000 were recorded for drivers 21 to 24 years old (27.0 percent), followed by ages 25 to 34 (24.0 percent) and 35 to 44 (22.0 percent). Approximately 1.5 million drivers were arrested in 1999 for driving under the influence of alcohol. This is an arrest rate of 1 for every 121 licensed drivers in the United States.[14]

Several factors probably contributed to these reductions in ARTFs: laws that raised the drinking age to 21; stricter law enforcement; increased emphasis on zero tolerance (laws prohibiting those under 21 from driving with *any* detectable BAC); and the educational and other prevention programs designed to discourage drinking and driving. Most states have set 0.10 percent as the BAC at which drivers are considered to be legally drunk (refer to Table 8.2). However, several states have lowered the standard to 0.08 percent, and others are likely to follow.

Laboratory and test track research shows that the vast majority of drivers, even experienced drinkers, are impaired at a BAC of 0.08 percent with regard to critical driving tasks. Braking, steering, lane changing, judgment, and divided attention, among other measures, are all affected significantly at 0.08 BAC. National groups such as MADD (Mothers

---

Teratogens   Certain chemicals, some therapeutic and illicit drugs, radiation, and intrauterine viral infections that cause fetal malformations.

Fetal alcohol syndrome (FAS)   A disorder that may affect the fetus when the mother consumes alcohol during pregnancy. Among its effects are mental retardation, small head, tremors, and abnormalities of the face, limbs, heart, and brain.

Fetal alcohol effects (FAE)   A syndrome describing children with a history of prenatal alcohol exposure but without all the physical or behavioral symptoms of FAS. Among its symptoms are low birth weight, irritability, and possible permanent mental impairment.

Against Drunk Driving), started by a mother whose child was killed by a drunk driver, go as far as tracking drunk driving cases through the court systems to ensure that drunk drivers are punished. Members of the high school group SADD (Students Against Drunk Driving) educate their peers about the dangers of drinking and driving.

Despite all these measures, the risk of being involved in an alcohol-related automobile crash remains substantial. Researchers have shown a direct relationship between the amount of alcohol in a driver's bloodstream and the likelihood of a crash. A driver with a BAC level of 0.10 percent is approximately ten times more likely to be involved in a car accident than a driver who has not been drinking. At a BAC of 0.15 on weekend nights, the likelihood of dying in a single-vehicle crash is more than 380 times higher than for non-drinkers. Alcohol involvement is highest during nighttime (9:00 P.M. to 6:00 A.M.) single-vehicle crashes, in which 53 percent of fatally injured passenger vehicle drivers in 2000 had BACs at or over 0.10 percent. Only 27 percent of fatally injured drivers involved in nighttime single-vehicle crashes had no alcohol in their blood. Not only does the time of day increase risk of being involved in an alcohol-related crash, but whether it is a weekday or weekend also makes a difference. In 2000, 30 percent of all fatal crashes during the week were alcohol-related, compared with 53 percent on weekends.[15]

Alcohol Abuse and Alcoholism

Alcohol use becomes **alcohol abuse** or **alcoholism** when it interferes with work, school, or social and family relationships or when it entails any violation of the law, including driving under the influence (DUI).

Identifying a Problem Drinker

As in other drug addictions, tolerance, psychological dependence, and withdrawal symptoms must be present to qualify a drinker as an addict. Addiction results from chronic use over a period of time that may vary from person to person. Problem drinkers or irresponsible users are not necessarily alcoholics. The stereotype of the alcoholic on skid row applies to only 5 percent of the alcoholic population. The remaining 95 percent of alcoholics live in some type of extended family unit. They can be found at all socioeconomic levels and in all professions, ethnic groups, geographical locations, religions, and races.

Studies suggest that the lifetime risk of alcoholism in the United States is about 10 percent for men and 3 percent for women. Moreover, 25 percent of the American population (50 million people) is affected by the alcoholism of a friend or family member. The 2000 National Household Survey on Drug Abuse found that 5.6 percent of Americans were heavy drinkers and 20.6 percent were binge drinkers.

Recognizing and admitting the existence of an alcohol problem are often extremely difficult. Alcoholics themselves deny their problem, often making statements such as, "I can stop any time I want to. I just don't want to right now." Their families also tend to deny the existence of a problem, saying things such as, "He really has been under a lot of stress lately. Besides, he only drinks beer." The fear of being labeled a "problem drinker" often prevents people from seeking help.

Women are the fastest-growing population of alcohol abusers. They tend to become alcoholic at a later age and after fewer years of heavy drinking than do male alcoholics. Women at highest risk for alcohol-related problems are those who are unmarried but living with a partner, are in their 20s or early 30s, or have a husband or partner who drinks heavily.

> **What do you think?**
> *What do you think the legal BAC for drivers should be? Explain your answer.* ✳ *Why do you think that many states have not lowered the legal limit to 0.08?* ✳ *What should the penalty be for people arrested for driving under the influence of alcohol (DUI) for the first offense? The second offense? The third offense?*

The Causes of Alcohol Abuse and Alcoholism

We know that alcoholism is a disease with biological and social/environmental components, but we do not know what role each component plays in the disease.

Biological and Family Factors Research into the hereditary and environmental causes of alcoholism has found higher rates of alcoholism among family members of alcoholics. In fact, according to researchers, alcoholism is four to five times more common among children of alcoholics than in the general population.

Male alcoholics, especially, are more likely than nonalcoholics to have alcoholic parents and siblings. Two distinct subtypes of alcoholism have provided important information about the inheritance of alcoholism. *Type 1 alcoholics* are drinkers who had at least one parent of either sex who was a problem drinker and who grew up in an environment that encouraged heavy drinking. Their drinking is reinforced by environmental events during which there is heavy drinking. Type 1 alcohol abusers share certain personality characteristics. They avoid novelty and harmful situations and are concerned about the thoughts and feelings of others. *Type 2 alcoholism* is seen in males only. These alcoholics are

---

Alcohol abuse (alcoholism) Use of alcohol that interferes with work, school, or personal relationships or that entails violations of the law.

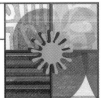

Alcohol Abuse and Alcoholism: Common Questions

Although many people think that they have a clear understanding of the disease alcoholism, there is much that remains in question. Answering the following questions may indicate your own level of knowledge about the disease. For further information, particularly as it relates to alcohol use on college campuses, check out the National Institute of Alcohol Abuse and Alcoholism.

1. Alcoholism is a disease characterized by which four symptoms?
2. Is alcoholism an inherited trait?   Yes   Probably   No
3. Do you have to be an alcoholic to experience problems?   Yes   No
4. Which groups of individuals tend to have the most problems with alcoholism?

ANSWERS:

1. The four symptoms of alcoholism include:

   Craving (a strong need or urge to drink alcohol)

   Loss of control (not being able to stop drinking once drinking begins)

   Physical dependence (withdrawal symptoms, such as nausea, sweating, shakiness, and anxiety after stopping drinking)

   Tolerance: (the need to drink greater amounts of alcohol to get high)

   (See also, the Diagnostic Statistical Manual IV published by the American Psychological Association for more information.)

2. Probably yes. The risk for developing alcoholism does indeed run in families. While part of this may be explained by genetics, lifestyle is a major factor. Currently, researchers are trying to locate the actual genes that put you at risk. Your friends, the amount of stress in your life, and how readily available alcohol is are also factors that increase risk. Remember that risk is not destiny. A child of an alcoholic won't automatically become an alcoholic. Others develop alcoholism even though no one in their family is an alcoholic. If you know you are at risk, you can take steps to protect yourself.

3. No. Alcoholism is only one type of alcohol problem. Alcohol abuse can be just as harmful. A person can abuse alcohol without being an alcoholic—that is, he or she may drink too much, too often and still not be dependent on alcohol. Some of the problems of alcohol abuse include: not being able to meet work, school, or family responsibilities; drunk driving arrests and car crashes; and drinking-related medical conditions. Under some circumstances, even social or moderate drinking is dangerous—for example, when driving, during pregnancy, or when taking certain medications.

4. Alcohol abuse and alcoholism cut across gender, race, and nationality. Nearly 1 in 3 adults abuse alcohol in the United States today. In general, more men than women are alcohol dependent or have alcohol problems. Alcohol problems are highest among young adults, aged 18–29, and lowest among adults ages 65 and older. We also know that the younger you start the more likely that you will have a problem.

Source: NIAAA web site: http://www.collegedrinkingprevention.gov/facts/qa.aspx. College Drinking: FAQ's on Alcohol abuse and Alcoholism.

typically the biological sons of alcoholic fathers who have a history of both violence and drug use. Type 2 alcoholics display the opposite characteristics of Type 1 alcoholics. They do not seek social approval, they lack inhibition, and they are prone to novelty-seeking behavior.[16]

One study found a strong relationship between alcoholism and alcoholic patterns within the family.[17] Children with one alcoholic parent had a 52 percent chance of becoming alcoholics themselves. With two alcoholic parents, the chances of becoming alcoholic jumped to 71 percent. The researchers felt that both heredity and environment were significant factors in the development of alcoholism but were reluctant to specify precisely how these factors worked.

Social and Cultural Factors Although a family history of alcoholism may predispose a person to problems with alcohol, numerous other factors may mitigate or exacerbate that tendency. Social and cultural factors may trigger the affliction for many people who are not genetically predisposed to alcoholism. Some people begin drinking as a way to dull the pain of an acute loss or an emotional or social problem. For example, college students may drink to escape the stress of college life, disappointment over unfulfilled expectations, difficulties in forming relationships, or loss of the security of home, loved ones, and close friends. Involvement in a painful relationship, death of a family member, and other problems may trigger a search for an anesthetic. Unfortunately, the emotional discomfort that causes many people to turn to alcohol also ultimately causes them to become even more uncomfortable as the depressant effect of the drug begins to take its toll. Thus, the person who is already depressed may become even more depressed, antagonizing friends and other social supports until they begin to turn away. Eventually, the drinker becomes physically dependent on the drug.

Family attitudes toward alcohol also seem to influence whether a person will develop a drinking problem. It has been clearly demonstrated that people who are raised in cultures in which drinking is a part of religious or ceremonial activities or in which alcohol is a traditional part of the family meal are less prone to alcohol dependence. In contrast, in societies in which alcohol purchase is carefully controlled and drinking is regarded as a rite of passage to adulthood, the tendency for abuse appears to be greater.

Certain social factors have been linked with alcoholism as well. These include urbanization, the weakening of links to the extended family and a general loosening of kinship ties, increased mobility, and changing religious and philosophical values. Apparently, then, some combination of heredity and environment plays a decisive role in the development of alcoholism. Some ethnic and racial groups also have special alcohol abuse problems.

Effects of Alcoholism on the Family

Only recently have people begun to recognize that it is not only the alcoholic but also the alcoholic's entire family that suffers. Although most research focuses on family effects during the late stages of alcoholism, the family unit actually begins to react early on as the person starts to show symptoms of the disease.

An estimated 76 million Americans (about 43 percent of the U.S. adult population) have been exposed to alcoholism in the family.[18] Twenty-two million members of alcoholic families are aged 18 or older, and many have carried childhood emotional scars into adulthood. Approximately one in four children under age 18 lives in an atmosphere of anxiety, tension, confusion, and denial.[19]

In dysfunctional families, children learn certain rules from a very early age: don't talk, don't trust, and don't feel. These unspoken rules allow the family to avoid dealing with real problems and real issues. Family members unconsciously adapt to the alcoholic's behavior by adjusting their own behavior. Unfortunately, these behaviors actually help keep the alcoholic drinking. Children in such dysfunctional families generally assume at least one of the following roles:

- *Family hero.* Tries to divert attention from the problem by being too good to be true.
- *Scapegoat.* Draws attention away from the family's primary problem through delinquency or misbehavior.
- *Lost child.* Becomes passive and quietly withdraws from upsetting situations.
- *Mascot.* Disrupts tense situations by providing comic relief.

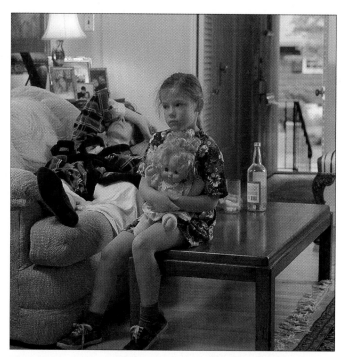

Though no clear proof exists, health officials suspect that a person's attitudes about alcohol use may be influenced by the behavior patterns witnessed while growing up.

For children in alcoholic homes, life is a struggle. They have to deal with constant stress, anxiety, and embarrassment. Because the alcoholic is the center of attention, the children's wants and needs are often ignored. It is not uncommon for these children to be victims of violence, abuse, neglect, or incest. As we have seen, when such children grow up, they are much more prone to alcoholic behaviors themselves than are children from nonalcoholic families.

In the past decade, we have come to recognize the unique problems of adult children of alcoholics whose difficulties in life stem from a lack of parental nurturing during childhood. Among these problems are an inability to develop social attachments, a need to be in control of all emotions and situations, low self-esteem, and depression. Fortunately, not all individuals who have grown up in alcoholic families are doomed to have lifelong problems. As many of these people mature, they develop a resilience in response to their families' problems. They thus enter adulthood armed with positive strengths and valuable career-oriented skills, such as the ability to assume responsibility, strong organizational skills, and realistic expectations of their jobs and others.

> **What do you think?**
>
> *How was alcohol used in your family when you were growing up? ✳ Was alcohol used only on special occasions or not at all? ✳ How much do you think your family's attitudes and behaviors toward alcohol have shaped your behavior?*

Costs to Society

The entire society suffers the consequences of individuals' alcohol abuse. Close to half of all traffic fatalities are attributable to alcohol. According to the National Institute on Alcohol Abuse and Alcoholism, in 1998, alcohol-related costs to society were at least $184.6 billion, after factoring in health insurance, criminal justice, treatment costs, and lost productivity. Reportedly, alcoholism is directly and indirectly responsible for over 25 percent of the nation's medical expenses and lost earnings. Well over 50 percent of all child abuse cases are the result of alcohol-related problems. Finally, the costs in emotional health are impossible to measure.[20]

Women and Alcoholism

In the past, women have consumed less alcohol and have had fewer alcohol-related problems than have men. But now, greater percentages of women, especially college-aged women, are choosing to drink and are drinking more heavily. Studies indicate that there are now almost as many female as male alcoholics. Risk factors for drinking problems among *all women* include the following:

- A family history of drinking problems
- Pressure to drink from a peer or spouse
- Depression
- Stress

Risk factors among *young women* include the following:

- College attendance: women in college drink more, and more frequently, than they do after they graduate
- Nontraditional, low-status, and part-time jobs; unemployment
- Being single, divorced, or separated

Risk factors among *middle-aged women* include the following:

- Loss of social roles (e.g., through divorce, children growing up and leaving the home)
- Abuse of prescription drugs
- Heavy drinking by spouse
- Presence of other disorders, such as depression

Risk factors among *older women* include the following:

- Heavy- or problem-drinking spouse
- Retirement, with a loss of social networks centered on the workplace

Drinking patterns among *different age groups* also differ in these ways:

- Younger women drink more overall, drink more often, and experience more alcohol-related problems, such as drinking and driving, assaults, suicide attempts, and difficulties at work.
- Middle-aged women are more likely to develop drinking problems in response to a traumatic or life-changing event, such as divorce, surgery, or death of a significant other.
- Older women are more likely than are older men to have developed drinking problems within the past 10 years.[21]

It is estimated that only 14 percent of women who need treatment get it. In one study, women cite the following reasons for not seeking treatment: potential loss of income, not wanting others to know they may have a problem, inability to pay for treatment, and the fear that treatment would not be confidential.[22] Another major obstacle is child care; most residential treatment centers do not allow women to bring their children with them.

> **What do you think?**
>
> *Why do you think women appear to be drinking more heavily today than they did in the past? ✳ Does society look at men's and women's drinking habits in the same way? ✳ Can you think of ways to increase support for women in their recovery process?*

Recovery

The Family's Role

Despite growing recognition of our national alcohol problem, fewer than 10 percent of alcoholics in the United States receive any care. Factors contributing to this low figure include an inability or unwillingness to admit to an alcohol problem; the social stigma attached to alcoholism; breakdowns in referral and delivery systems (failure of physicians or psychotherapists to follow up on referrals, client failure to follow through with recommended treatments, or failure of rehabilitation facilities to give quality care); and failure of the professional medical establishment to recognize and diagnose alcoholic symptoms among their patients.

Most alcoholics and problem drinkers who seek help have experienced a turning point or dramatic occurrence: a spouse walks out, taking children and possessions; the boss issues an ultimatum to dry out or ship out. The alcoholic ready for treatment has, in most cases, reached a low point. Devoid of hope, physically depleted, and spiritually despairing, the alcoholic has finally recognized that alcohol controls his or her life. The first step on the road to recovery is to regain that control and assume responsibility for personal actions.

Members of an alcoholic's family sometimes take action before the alcoholic does. They may go to an organization or a treatment facility to seek help for themselves and their relative. An effective method of helping an alcoholic to confront the disease is a process called **intervention.** Essentially, an intervention is a planned confrontation with the alcoholic that involves several family members plus professional counselors. The family members express their love and concern, telling the alcoholic that they will no longer refrain from acknowledging the problem and affirming their support for appropriate treatment. A family intervention is the turning point for a growing number of alcoholics.

Treatment Programs

The alcoholic who is ready for help has several avenues of treatment: psychologists and psychiatrists specializing in the treatment of alcoholism, private treatment centers, hospitals specifically designed to treat alcoholics, community mental health facilities, and support groups such as Alcoholics Anonymous.

Intervention   A planned confrontation with an alcoholic in which family members or friends express their concern about the alcoholic's drinking.

Delirium tremens (DTs)   A state of confusion brought on by withdrawal from alcohol. Symptoms include hallucinations, anxiety, and trembling.

Private Treatment Facilities   Private treatment facilities have been making concerted efforts to attract patients through radio and television advertising. On admission to the treatment facility, the patient is given a complete physical exam to determine whether underlying medical problems will interfere with treatment. Alcoholics who decide to quit drinking will experience withdrawal symptoms, including the following:

- Hyperexcitability
- Confusion
- Sleep disorders
- Convulsions
- Agitation
- Tremors of the hands
- Brief hallucinations
- Depression
- Headache
- Seizures

For a small percentage of people, alcohol withdrawal results in a severe syndrome known as **delirium tremens (DTs).** Delirium tremens is characterized by confusion, delusions, agitated behavior, and hallucinations.

For any long-term addict, medical supervision is usually necessary. *Detoxification,* the process by which addicts end their dependence on a drug, is commonly carried out in a medical facility, where patients can be monitored to prevent fatal withdrawal reactions. Withdrawal takes from 7 to 21 days. Shortly after detoxification, alcoholics begin their treatment for psychological addiction. Most treatment facilities keep their patients from three to six weeks. Treatment at private treatment centers costs several thousand dollars, but some insurance programs or employers will assume most of this expense.

Family Therapy, Individual Therapy, and Group Therapy
In family therapy, the person and family members gradually examine the psychological reasons underlying the addiction. In individual and group therapy with fellow addicts, alcoholics learn positive coping skills for situations that have regularly caused them to turn to alcohol. On some college campuses, the problems associated with alcohol abuse are so great that student health centers are opening their own treatment programs.

Other Types of Treatment   Two other treatments are drug and aversion therapy. Disulfiram (trade name: Antabuse) is the drug of choice for treating alcoholics. If alcohol is consumed, the drug causes unpleasant effects such as headache, nausea, vomiting, drowsiness, and hangover. These symptoms discourage the alcoholic from drinking. Aversion therapy is based on conditioning therapy. It works on the premise that the sight, smell, and taste of alcohol will acquire aversive properties if repeatedly paired with a noxious stimulus. For a period of ten days, the alcoholic takes drugs that induce vomiting when combined with several drinks. These treatments work best in conjunction with some type of counseling.

Alcoholics Anonymous (AA) is a private, nonprofit, self-help organization founded in 1935. The organization, which relies upon group support to help people stop drinking, currently has over 1 million members and has branches all over the world. At meetings, last names are never used and no one is forced to speak. Members are taught to believe that their alcoholism is a lifetime problem and they may never use alcohol again. They share their struggles with each other and talk about the devastating effects alcoholism has had on their personal and professional lives. All members are asked to place their faith and control of the habit into the hands of a "higher power." The road to recovery is taken one step at a time. AA offers specialized meetings for gay, atheist, HIV-positive, and professional individuals with alcohol problems.

Alcoholics Anonymous also has auxiliary groups to help spouses or partners, friends, and children of alcoholics. *Al-Anon* is the group dedicated to helping adult relatives and friends of alcoholics understand the disease and how they can contribute to the recovery process. Spouses and other adult loved ones often play an unwitting role in perpetuating the alcoholic's problems. For example, the adult relative may call the alcoholic's boss and lie about why the alcoholic missed work. At Al-Anon, these people's roles in their loved one's alcoholism are examined and explored, and alternative behaviors are suggested.

Alateen, another AA-related organization, helps adolescents live with alcoholic parents. They are taught that they are not at fault for their parents' problems. They develop their self-esteem to overcome guilt and function better socially.

Other self-help groups include Women for Sobriety and Secular Organizations for Sobriety (SOS). Women for Sobriety addresses the differing needs of female alcoholics, who often have more severe problems than males. Unlike AA meetings, where attendance can be quite large, each group has no more than ten members. Secular Organizations for Sobriety was founded to help people who are uncomfortable with AA's spiritual emphasis.

Relapse

Success in recovery from alcoholism varies with the individual. A return to alcoholic habits often follows what appears to be a successful recovery. Some alcoholics never recover. Some partially recover and improve other parts of their lives but remain dependent on alcohol. Many alcoholics refer to themselves as "recovering" throughout their lifetime; they never use the word *cured.*

Roughly 60 percent of alcoholics relapse (resume drinking) within the first three months of treatment. Why is the relapse rate so high? Treating an addiction requires more than getting the addict to stop using a substance; it also requires getting the person to break a pattern of behavior that has dominated his or her life.

People who are seeking to regain a healthy lifestyle must not only confront their addiction, but also must guard against the tendency to relapse. Drinkers with compulsive

personalities need to learn to understand themselves and take control. Others need to view treatment as a long-term process that takes a lot of effort beyond attending a weekly self-help group meeting. In order to work, a recovery program must offer the alcoholic ways to increase self-esteem and resume personal growth. Alcoholics most likely to recover completely are those who developed their dependence after the age of 20, those with intact and supportive family units, and those who have reached a high level of personal disgust coupled with strong motivation to recover.

Our Smoking Society

Tobacco use is the single most preventable cause of death in the United States.[23] While tobacco companies publish full-page advertisements refuting the dangers of smoking, nearly 430,000 Americans die each year of tobacco-related diseases.[24] This is 50 times as many as will die from all illegal drugs combined. In addition, 10 million will suffer from diseases caused by tobacco. To date, tobacco is known to be the probable cause of about 25 diseases. One in every five deaths in the United States is smoking related. New studies estimate that about half of all regular smokers die of smoking-related diseases. Therefore, any contention by the tobacco industry that tobacco use is not dangerous is irresponsible and ignores the growing weight of scientific evidence.

How many teenagers smoke? In 1991, the Youth Risk Assessment Survey (YRAS), which includes only middle and high school students, indicated that 27.5 percent of teenagers smoke; by 1999, 34.8 percent were current smokers. The most recent survey of adolescent smokers has shown a downward trend from the 1997 survey, with the exception of 12th grade. Currently, the percentage of teenage males and females smoking is equal, at approximately 34.8 percent.[25] The number of teenagers who become daily smokers before the age of 18 is estimated to be more than 3,000 per day. Every day another 6,000 teens under the age of 18 smoke their first cigarette. The increase in cigarette use is attributed in part to the ready availability of tobacco products through vending machines and the aggressive drive by tobacco companies to entice young people to smoke.

Tobacco and Social Issues

The production and distribution of tobacco products in the United States and abroad involve many political and economic issues. During the 1980s, tobacco products were one of the top five U.S. exports. Tobacco-growing states derive

---

Alcoholics Anonymous (AA)   An organization whose goal is to help alcoholics stop drinking; includes auxiliary branches such as Al-Anon and Alateen.

Cigarettes and Society

Marketing and consumption of tobacco products vary from neighborhood to neighborhood and from country to country. The following statistics show how the tobacco industry targets different populations and how smoking affects people worldwide.

- Billboards advertising tobacco products are placed in African-American communities four to five times more often than in white communities. In 1985, tobacco companies spent $5.8 million for advertisements on eight-foot billboards in African-American communities, accounting for 37 percent of total advertising in this medium.

- Cigarette companies advertise heavily in popular African-American magazines. They also successfully target the African-American community by sponsoring entertainment, sporting, and cultural events and political and literacy campaigns.

- Developing nations often lack the legislative controls necessary to regulate tobacco use. In many of these countries, cigarettes are sold without the warning label required in the countries where they are manufactured. American cigarettes sold in the Philippines contain more tar and nicotine and produce more carbon monoxide than the same brands sold in the United States. Cigarettes sold in Asia have a higher tar content than cigarettes sold in Western countries.

- To increase sales in developing countries, promotional ads are often aimed at women. The reason for this is simple: Half the men in developing countries already smoke, whereas only 5 percent of the women do. In contrast, in most industrialized countries the percentages of men and women who smoke are roughly the same, about 30 percent.

- As the smoking of tobacco has become a popular habit around the world, it has taken a tremendous toll. Worldwide, tobacco use is responsible for 90 percent of all lung cancer deaths, 75 percent of bronchitis deaths, and 25 percent of cardiovascular deaths. The World Health Organization (WHO) estimates that every year over 2.5 million people die prematurely as a result of smoking cigarettes.

- In China, a research team has declared a "public health emergency" due to smoking-related diseases. Cases of lung cancer are increasing by 4.5 percent a year. It is estimated that some 300 million Chinese smoke—about 60 percent of men but fewer than 10 percent of women. Smoking is so popular in China that the Chinese are willing to spend up to 60 percent of their personal income on cigarettes. "There are more smokers in China than there are people in the U.S.," notes Tom Houston, director of the American Medical Association's Department of Preventive Medicine.

- In developing countries, many smokers are unaware of the risks. For example, a study in China showed that most smokers thought smoking did little or no harm.

- Smoking is declining among men in most high-income countries. In contrast, it is increasing among men in most low- and middle-income countries and among women worldwide.

- It is estimated that the number of children and young people taking up smoking ranges from 68,000 to 84,000 in low- and middle-income countries every day.

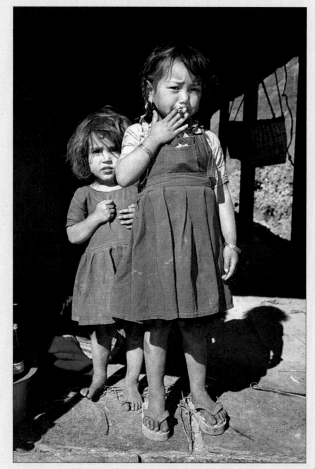

substantial income from tobacco production, and federal, state, and local governments benefit enormously from cigarette taxes. More recently, nationwide health awareness has led to a decrease in the use of tobacco products among U.S. adults.

Advertising According to estimates, the tobacco industry spends $18 million per day on advertising and promotional materials. With the number of smokers declining by about 1 million each year, the industry must actively recruit new smokers. Campaigns are directed at all age, social, and ethnic groups, but because children and teenagers constitute 90 percent of all new smokers, much of the advertising has been directed toward them. Evidence of product recognition with underage smokers is clear: 86 percent of underage smokers prefer one of the three most heavily advertised brands—Marlboro, Newport, or Camel. One of the most blatant campaigns aimed at young adults was the popular Joe Camel ad campaign. After R. J. Reynolds introduced the cartoon figure, Camel's market share among underage smokers jumped from 3 to 13.3 percent in three years.

Advertisements in women's magazines imply that smoking is the key to financial success, independence, and social acceptance. Many brands also have thin spokeswomen pushing "slim" and "light" cigarettes to cash in on women's fear of gaining weight. These ads have apparently been working. From the mid-1970s through the late 1990s, cigarette sales to women increased dramatically. By 1987, statistics indicated that cigarette-induced lung cancer had surpassed breast cancer as the leading form of cancer death among women.

Women are not the only targets of gender-based cigarette advertisements. Males are depicted changing clothes in a locker room, charging over rugged terrain in off-road vehicles, or riding bay stallions into the sunset in blatant appeals to a need to feel and appear masculine. In addition, minorities are often targeted.

Apparently, 18- to 24-year-olds have become the new target for tobacco advertisers. The tobacco industry has set up very aggressive marketing promotions specifically targeted to this age group in bars, at music festivals, and the like. Additionally, modeling and peer influence have an impact on smoking initiation. This potential impact is heightened by the fact that although over half of campuses are considered smoke-free, they do permit smoking in residence hall rooms, student centers, and cafeterias, and many sell tobacco products in campus stores and student lounges.

Financial Costs to Society   The use of tobacco products is costly to all of us in terms of lost productivity and lost lives. In 1996, smoking-related illnesses cost the nation more than $100 billion. The economic burden of tobacco use was more than $50 billion in medical expenditures (including hospital, physician, and nursing home expenditures, prescription drugs, and home health care expenditures) and $50 billion in indirect costs (absenteeism, added cost of fire insurance, training costs to replace employees who die prematurely, disability payments, and so on).[26] Based on these figures, smoking costs each American approximately $398 per year.

College Students and Smoking

College and university students are especially vulnerable when they are placed in a new, often stressful social and academic environment. For many, the college years are their initial taste of freedom from parental supervision. Smoking

may begin earlier, but most college students are a part of the significant age group in which people initiate smoking and become hooked.

A recent study found that cigarette smoking among U.S. college students increased by 32 percent between 1991 and 1999. In 1999, researchers surveyed more than 14,000 students from 119 U.S. colleges. This poll took into account all types of tobacco use, including cigars, smokeless tobacco, and pipe smoking, rather than just cigarettes. Researchers found that cigarette smoking rates had not changed between 1997 and 1999; however, more than 60 percent of college students had tried some tobacco product. One-third of students had used tobacco in the month before the study, and just under half had used tobacco in the past year. Among current smokers, the survey found that 32 percent smoked less than a cigarette a day, and 13 percent smoked a pack or more per day. Furthermore, the study found students who used tobacco products were more likely to smoke marijuana, binge drink, have multiple sex partners, earn lower grades, rate parties as more important than academic activities, and spend more time socializing with friends.[27]

A common perception is that students are not interested in smoking cessation efforts. However, a recent study reported that 70 percent of cigarette smokers had tried to quit smoking. Unfortunately, three out of four were still smokers.[28] It is important that colleges and universities engage in antismoking efforts, strictly control tobacco advertising, provide smoke-free residence halls, and offer greater access to smoking cessation programs.

> **What do you think?**
> *Have you noticed an increase in the number of your friends who have become smokers or occasional smokers?* ✸ *How many of them smoked prior to coming to college, and how many picked up the habit at college?* ✸ *What are their reasons for smoking?* ✸ *What barriers keep your friends from quitting?*

Tobacco and Its Effects

The chemical stimulant **nicotine** is the major psychoactive substance in all tobacco products. In its natural form, nicotine is a colorless liquid that turns brown upon oxidation (exposure to oxygen). When tobacco leaves are burned in a cigarette, pipe, or cigar, nicotine is released and inhaled into the lungs. Sucking or chewing a quid (a pinch of snuff typically tucked between the gum and lower lip) of tobacco

Nicotine   The stimulant chemical in tobacco products.

More than 4,000 chemicals, including these:

CANCER-CAUSING AGENTS	METALS	OTHER CHEMICALS	
Nitrosamines	Aluminum	Acetone (nail polish remover)	Hexamine (barbecue lighter)
Crysenes	Zinc	Acetic acid (vinegar)	Hydrogen cyanide (gas chamber poison)
Cadmium	Magnesium	Ammonia (floor/toilet cleaner)	
Benzo(a)pyrene	Mercury	Arsenic (poison)	Methane (swamp gas)
Polonium 210	Gold	Butane (cigarette lighter fluid)	Methanol (rocket fuel)
Nickel	Silicon	Cadmium (rechargeable batteries)	Naphthalene (mothballs)
PAHs	Silver		Nicotine (insecticide/addictive drug)
Diberiz acidine	Titanium	Carbon monoxide (car exhaust fumes)	
B-Naphthylamine	Lead		Nitrobenzene (gasoline additive)
Urethane	Copper	DDT/dieldrin (insecticides)	Nitrous oxide phenols (disinfectant)
N. nitrosonornicotine		Ethanol (alcohol)	Stearic acid (candle wax)
Toluidine		Formaldehyde (preserver of body tissue and fabric)	Toluene (industrial solvent)
			Vinyl chloride (makes PVC)

releases nicotine into the saliva, and the nicotine is then absorbed through the mucous membranes in the mouth.

Smoking is the most common form of tobacco use. Smoking delivers a strong dose of nicotine to the user, along with an additional 4,000 chemical substances (Table 8.4). Among these chemicals are various gases and vapors that carry particulate matter in concentrations that are 500,000 times greater than those of the most air-polluted cities in the world.[29]

Particulate matter condenses in the lungs to form a thick, brownish sludge called **tar.** Tar contains various carcinogenic (cancer-causing) agents such as benzo(a)pyrene and chemical irritants such as phenol. Phenol has the potential to combine with other chemicals to contribute to the development of lung cancer.

In healthy lungs, millions of tiny hairlike tissues called cilia sweep away foreign matter, to be expelled from the lungs by coughing. Nicotine impairs the cleansing function of the cilia by paralyzing them for up to one hour following the smoking of a single cigarette. This allows tars and other solids in tobacco smoke to accumulate and irritate sensitive lung tissue.

Tar and nicotine are not the only harmful chemicals in cigarettes. In fact, tars account for only 8 percent of tobacco smoke. The remaining 92 percent consists of various gases, the most dangerous of which is **carbon monoxide.** In to-

bacco smoke, the concentration of carbon monoxide is 800 times higher than the level considered safe by the U.S. Environmental Protection Agency (EPA). In the human body, carbon monoxide reduces the oxygen-carrying capacity of the red blood cells by binding with the receptor sites for oxygen. This causes oxygen deprivation in many body tissues.

The heat from tobacco smoke, which can reach 1,616 degrees Fahrenheit, is also harmful. Inhaling hot gases exposes sensitive mucous membranes to irritating chemicals that weaken the tissues and contribute to cancers of the mouth, larynx, and throat.

Tobacco Products

Tobacco comes in several forms. Cigarettes, cigars, pipes, and bidis are used for burning and inhaling tobacco. Smokeless tobacco is inhaled or placed in the mouth.

Filtered cigarettes designed to reduce levels of gases such as hydrogen cyanide and hydrocarbons may actually deliver more hazardous carbon monoxide to the user than do nonfiltered brands. Some smokers use low-tar and low-nicotine products as an excuse to smoke more cigarettes. This practice is self-defeating because smokers wind up exposing themselves to more harmful substances than they would with regular-strength cigarettes.

Clove cigarettes contain about 40 percent ground cloves (a spice) and about 60 percent tobacco. Many users mistakenly believe that these products are made entirely of ground cloves and that smoking them eliminates the risks associated with tobacco. In fact, clove cigarettes contain higher levels of tar, nicotine, and carbon monoxide than do regular cigarettes. In addition, the numbing effect of eugenol, the active ingredient in cloves, allows smokers to inhale the smoke more deeply.

Tar   A thick, brownish substance condensed from particulate matter in smoked tobacco.

Carbon monoxide   A gas found in cigarette smoke that binds at oxygen receptor sites in the blood.

Cigars Those big stogies that we see celebrities and government figures puffing on these days are nothing more than tobacco fillers wrapped in more tobacco. Since 1991, cigar sales in the United States have increased by 250 percent. This growing fad is especially popular among young men and women, fueled in part by the willingness of celebrities to be photographed puffing on one. Among some women, cigar smoking symbolizes an impulse to be slightly outrageous and liberated. Many people believe that cigars are safer than cigarettes, when in fact nothing could be further from the truth.[30] Cigar smoke contains 23 poisons and 43 carcinogens.

Smoking as little as one cigar per day can increase the risk of several cancers, including cancer of the oral cavity (lip, tongue, mouth, and throat), esophagus, larynx, and lungs. Daily cigar smoking, especially for people who inhale, also increases the risk of heart disease (cigar smokers double their risk of heart attack and stroke) and a type of lung disease known as chronic obstructive pulmonary disease (COPD). Smoking one or two cigars doubles the risk for oral cancers and esophageal cancer, compared with risk for someone who has never smoked. The risks increase with the number of cigars smoked per day.

A common question asked is whether cigars are addictive. Most cigars have as much nicotine as several cigarettes, and nicotine is highly addictive. When cigar smokers inhale, nicotine is absorbed as rapidly as it is with cigarettes. For those who don't inhale, nicotine is still absorbed through the mucous membranes in the mouth.

Bidis Bidis are small hand-rolled, flavored cigarettes, generally made in India or Southeast Asia. They come in a variety of flavors, such as vanilla, chocolate, and cherry, and cost $2 to $4 for a pack of 20. Bidis look similar to a marijuana joint or a clove cigarette and have become increasingly popular with college students, who view them as safer, cheaper, and easier to obtain than cigarettes. However, they are far more toxic than cigarettes. A study by the Massachusetts Department of Health found that bidis produced three times more carbon monoxide and nicotine and five times more tar than cigarettes during an identical testing process. The tendu leaf wrappers are nonporous, meaning that smokers have to pull harder to inhale and inhale more to keep the bidi lit. During testing, it took an average of 28 puffs to smoke a bidi, compared to only 9 puffs for a regular cigarette. This results in much more exposure to the higher amounts of tar, nicotine, and carbon monoxide, and bidis lack any sort of filter to lessen the levels. Research clearly indicates that bidi smokers are at the same, if not higher, risk for coronary heart disease and cancer due to smoking.[31]

Smokeless Tobacco Approximately 5 million U.S. adults use smokeless tobacco. Most of them are teenage (20 percent of male high school students) and young adult males, who are often emulating a professional sports figure or family member. There are two types of smokeless tobacco—chewing tobacco and snuff.

Chewing tobacco is placed between the gums and teeth for sucking or chewing. It comes in three forms: loose leaf, plug, or twist. Chewing tobacco contains tobacco leaves treated with molasses and other flavorings. The user places a "quid" of tobacco in the mouth between the teeth and gums and then sucks or chews the quid to release the nicotine. Once the quid becomes ineffective, the user spits it out and inserts another. **Dipping** is another method of using chewing tobacco. The dipper takes a small amount of tobacco and places it between the lower lip and teeth to stimulate the flow of saliva and release the nicotine. Dipping rapidly releases nicotine into the bloodstream.

Snuff is a finely ground form of tobacco that can be inhaled, chewed, or placed against the gums. It comes in dry or moist powdered form or sachets (tea bag–like pouches). Usually snuff is placed inside the cheek. Inhaling dry snuff is more common in Europe than in the United States.[32]

Smokeless tobacco is just as addictive as cigarettes because of its nicotine content. There is nicotine in all tobacco products, but smokeless tobacco contains even more than cigarettes. Holding an average-sized dip or chew in the mouth for 30 minutes delivers as much nicotine as smoking four cigarettes. A two-can-a-week snuff dipper gets as much nicotine as a one-and-a-half-pack-a-day smoker.

Smokeless tobacco also contains 10 times the amount of cancer-producing substances found in cigarettes and 100 times more than the Food and Drug Administration allows in foods and other substances used by the public. A major risk of chewing tobacco is **leukoplakia,** a condition characterized by leathery white patches inside the mouth produced by contact with irritants in tobacco juice. Between 3 and 17 percent of diagnosed leukoplakia cases develop into oral cancer. It is estimated that 75 percent of the 30,000 oral cancer cases in 1999 resulted from either smokeless tobacco or cigarettes. Users of smokeless tobacco are 50 times more likely to develop oral cancers than are nonusers. Warning signs of oral cancers include lumps in the jaw or neck; color changes or lumps inside the lips; white, smooth, or scaly patches in the mouth or on the neck, lips, or tongue; a red spot or sore on

Bidis Hand-rolled flavored cigarettes.

Chewing tobacco A stringy type of tobacco that is placed in the mouth and then sucked or chewed.

Dipping Placing a small amount of chewing tobacco between the front lip and teeth for rapid nicotine absorption.

Snuff A powdered form of tobacco that is sniffed and absorbed through the mucous membranes in the nose or placed inside the cheek and sucked.

Leukoplakia A condition characterized by leathery white patches inside the mouth produced by contact with irritants in tobacco juice.

the lips or gums or inside the mouth that does not heal in two weeks; repeated bleeding in the mouth; and difficulty or abnormality in speaking or swallowing.

The lag time between first use and contracting cancer is shorter for smokeless tobacco users than for smokers because absorption through the gums is the most efficient route of nicotine administration. A growing body of evidence suggests that long-term use of smokeless tobacco also increases the risk of cancer of the larynx, esophagus, nasal cavity, pancreas, kidney, and bladder. Moreover, many smokeless tobacco users eventually "graduate" to cigarettes.

The stimulant effects of nicotine may create the same circulatory and respiratory problems for chewers as for smokers. Chronic smokeless tobacco use also results in delayed wound healing, peptic ulcer disease, and reproductive disturbances.

Like smoked tobacco, smokeless tobacco also impairs the senses of taste and smell, causing the user to add salt and sugar to food, which may contribute to high blood pressure and obesity. Some smokeless tobacco products contain high levels of sodium (salt), which also contributes to high blood pressure. In addition, dental problems are common among users of smokeless tobacco. Contact with tobacco juice causes receding gums, tooth decay, bad breath, and discolored teeth. Damage to both the teeth and jawbone can contribute to early loss of teeth. Users of any tobacco products may not be able to use the vitamins and other nutrients in food effectively.

Smokeless tobacco users have the same problems that smokers do when trying to quit. Withdrawal symptoms are almost universal; relapse is common. Symptoms that often accompany nicotine withdrawal include headache, gastrointestinal discomfort, sleeping problems, irritability, anxiety, aggressiveness, craving for tobacco, and a reduction in heart rate, blood pressure, and hormone secretions.

Physiological Effects of Nicotine

Nicotine is a powerful central nervous system stimulant that produces a variety of physiological effects. Its stimulant action in the cerebral cortex produces an aroused, alert mental state. Nicotine also stimulates the adrenal glands, increasing the production of adrenaline. The physical effects of nicotine stimulation include increased heart and respiratory rate, constricted blood vessels, and subsequent increased blood pressure because the heart must work harder to pump blood through the narrowed vessels.

Nicotine poisoning Symptoms often experienced by beginning smokers, including dizziness, diarrhea, lightheadedness, rapid and erratic pulse, clammy skin, nausea, and vomiting.

Nicotine decreases blood sugar levels and the stomach contractions that signal hunger. These factors, along with decreased sensation in the taste buds, reduce appetite. For this reason, many smokers eat less than nonsmokers do and weigh, on average, seven pounds less than nonsmokers. Beginning smokers usually feel the effects of nicotine with their first puff. These symptoms, called **nicotine poisoning,** include dizziness, lightheadedness, rapid and erratic pulse, clammy skin, nausea, vomiting, and diarrhea. The effects of nicotine poisoning cease as soon as tolerance to the chemical develops. Medical research indicates that tolerance develops almost immediately in new users, perhaps after the second or third cigarette. In contrast, tolerance to most other drugs, such as alcohol, develops over a period of months or years. Regular smokers often do not experience the "buzz" of smoking. They continue to smoke simply because stopping is too difficult.

What do you think?
Because nicotine is highly addictive, should it be regulated as a controlled substance? ✴ How could tobacco be regulated effectively? ✴ Should more resources be used for research into nicotine addiction? Why or why not?

Health Hazards of Smoking

Cigarette smoking adversely affects the health of every person who smokes. Each day cigarettes contribute to over 1,000 deaths from cancer, cardiovascular disease, and respiratory disorders.

Cancer

The American Cancer Society estimates that tobacco smoking causes more than 85 to 90 percent of all cases of lung cancer. Lung cancer is the leading cause of cancer deaths in the United States. It is estimated that there were 164,100 *new* cases of lung cancer in the United States in 2000 alone, and an estimated 156,900 Americans *died* of lung cancer in 2000. Fewer than 10 percent of lung cancers occur among nonsmokers.[33] Figure 8.1 illustrates how tobacco smoke damages the lungs.

Lung cancer can take 10 to 30 years to develop. The outlook for victims of this disease is poor. Most lung cancer is not diagnosed until it is fairly widespread in the body; at that point, the five-year survival rate is only 13 percent. When a malignancy is diagnosed and recognized while still localized, the five-year survival rate rises to 47 percent.

If you are a smoker, your risk of developing lung cancer depends on several factors. First, the number of cigarettes you smoke per day is important. Someone who smokes two packs a day is 15 to 25 times more likely to develop lung cancer than a nonsmoker. If you started smoking in your

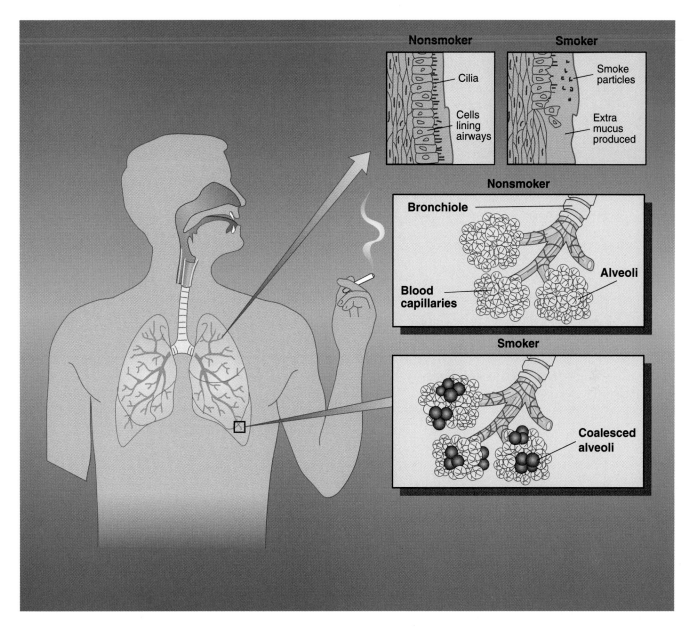

Figure 8.1

How Cigarette Smoking Damages the Lungs

Smoke particles irritate the lung airways, causing excess mucus production (top right). They also indirectly destroy the walls of the lungs' alveoli, which coalesce (above). Both factors reduce lung efficiency. In addition, tar in tobacco smoke has a direct cancer-causing action.

teens, you have a greater chance of developing lung cancer than people who started later. If you inhale deeply when you smoke, you also increase your chances. Occupational or domestic exposure to other irritants, such as asbestos and radon, will also increase your likelihood of developing lung cancer.[34]

Tobacco is linked to other cancers as well. Cigarette smoking increases the risk of pancreatic cancer by 70 percent. Smokers can reduce those odds by 30 percent if they quit for 11 years or more.[35] Cancers of the lip, tongue, salivary glands, and esophagus are five times more likely to

occur among smokers than among nonsmokers. Smokers are also more likely to develop kidney, bladder, and larynx cancers.

Cardiovascular Disease

Half of all tobacco-related deaths occur as a result of some form of heart disease.[36] Smokers have a 70 percent higher death rate from heart disease than nonsmokers do, and heavy smokers have a 200 percent higher death rate than moderate smokers. In fact, smoking cigarettes poses as great a risk for developing heart disease as high blood pressure and high cholesterol levels do.

Smoking contributes to heart disease by adding the equivalent of 10 years of aging to the arteries.[37] One explanation is that smoking encourages atherosclerosis, the buildup of fatty deposits in the heart and major blood vessels. For unknown reasons, smoking decreases blood levels of HDLs (high-density lipoproteins), which help protect against heart attacks. Smoking also contributes to **platelet adhesiveness,** the sticking together of red blood cells that is associated with blood clots. The oxygen deprivation associated with smoking decreases the oxygen supply to the heart and can weaken tissues. Smoking also contributes to irregular heart rhythms, which can trigger a heart attack. Both carbon monoxide and nicotine in cigarette smoke can precipitate angina attacks (pain spasms in the chest when the heart muscle does not get the blood supply it needs).

The number of years a person has smoked does not seem to bear much relation to cardiovascular risk. If a person quits smoking, the risk of dying from a heart attack is reduced by half after only one year without smoking and declines gradually thereafter. After about 15 years without smoking, the ex-smoker's risk of cardiovascular disease is similar to that of people who have never smoked.

Stroke Smokers are twice as likely to suffer strokes as nonsmokers are. A stroke occurs when a small blood vessel in the brain bursts or is blocked by a blood clot, denying oxygen and nourishment to vital portions of the brain. Depending on the area of the brain supplied by the vessel, stroke can result in paralysis, loss of mental functioning, or death. Smoking contributes to strokes by raising blood pressure, thereby increasing the stress on vessel walls. Platelet adhesiveness contributes to clotting. Five to 15 years after they stop smoking, the risk of stroke for ex-smokers is the same as that of people who have never smoked.

Respiratory Disorders

Smoking quickly impairs the respiratory system. Smokers can feel its impact in a relatively short period of time—they are more prone to breathlessness, chronic cough, and excess phlegm production than nonsmokers their age. Smokers tend to miss work one-third more often than nonsmokers do,

primarily because of respiratory diseases, and they are up to 18 times more likely to die of lung disease.

Chronic bronchitis is the presence of a productive cough that persists or recurs frequently. It may develop in smokers because their inflamed lungs produce more mucus and constantly try to rid themselves of this mucus and foreign particles. The effort to do so results in "smoker's hack," the persistent cough experienced by most smokers. Smokers are more prone than nonsmokers to respiratory ailments such as influenza, pneumonia, and colds.

Emphysema is a chronic disease in which the alveoli (the tiny air sacs in the lungs) are destroyed, impairing the lungs' ability to obtain oxygen and remove carbon dioxide. As a result, breathing becomes difficult. Whereas healthy people expend only about 5 percent of their energy in breathing, people with advanced emphysema spend nearly 80 percent of their energy. A simple movement such as rising from a seated position becomes painful and difficult for the emphysema patient. Because the heart has to work harder to do even the simplest tasks, it may become enlarged, and the person may die from heart damage. There is no known cure for emphysema. Approximately 80 percent of all cases are related to cigarette smoking.

Smoking and Your Sex Life

Despite attempts by tobacco advertisers to make smoking appear sexy, research shows just the opposite: It can cause impotence in men. A number of recent studies have found that male smokers are about two times more likely than nonsmokers to suffer from some form of impotence. Toxins in cigarette smoke damage blood vessels, reducing blood flow to the penis and leading to an inadequate erection. It is thought that impotence could indicate oncoming cardiovascular disease.

Other Health Effects of Smoking

Gum disease is three times more common among smokers than among nonsmokers, and smokers lose significantly more teeth.[38] Smokers are also likely to use more medications. Nicotine and the other ingredients in cigarettes interfere with the metabolism of drugs: nicotine speeds up the process by which the body uses and eliminates drugs, so that medications become less effective. The smoker may therefore have to take a higher dosage of a drug or take it more frequently.

Platelet adhesiveness   Stickiness of red blood cells associated with blood clots.

Emphysema   A chronic lung disease in which the tiny air sacs in the lungs are destroyed, making breathing difficult.

> ### What do you think?
> *Most people are very aware of the long-term hazards associated with tobacco use, yet despite prevention efforts, people continue to smoke. Why do you think this is so?* ✳ *What strategies might be effective at reducing the number of people who begin smoking?*

Environmental Tobacco Smoke (ETS)

Although fewer than 30 percent of Americans are smokers, air pollution from smoking in public places continues to be a problem. **Environmental tobacco smoke (ETS)** is divided into two categories: mainstream and sidestream smoke (also called secondhand smoke). **Mainstream smoke** refers to smoke drawn through tobacco while inhaling; **sidestream smoke** refers to smoke from the burning end of a cigarette or smoke exhaled by a smoker. People who breathe smoke from someone else's smoking product are said to be *involuntary* or *passive* smokers. Nearly nine out of ten nonsmoking Americans are exposed to environmental tobacco smoke. In fact, measurable levels of nicotine were found in the blood of 88 percent of all nontobacco users.

Risks from ETS

Although involuntary smokers breathe less tobacco than active smokers do, they still face risks from exposure to tobacco smoke. Sidestream smoke actually contains more carcinogenic substances than the smoke that a smoker inhales. According to the American Lung Association, sidestream smoke has about two times more tar and nicotine, five times more carbon monoxide, and 50 times more ammonia than mainstream smoke. ETS is estimated to be responsible for approximately 3,000 lung cancer deaths, 37,000 cardiovascular disease deaths, and 13,000 deaths from other cancers.[39] The Environmental Protection Agency (EPA) has designated secondhand tobacco smoke a *group A cancer-causing agent* that is even worse than other group A threats, such as benzene, arsenic, and radon. There is also evidence that sidestream smoke poses an even greater risk for death due to heart disease than for death due to lung cancer.[40]

Sidestream smoke is estimated to cause more deaths per year than any other environmental pollutant. The risk of dying because of exposure to passive smoking is 100 times greater than the risk that requires the EPA to label a pollutant as carcinogenic and 10,000 times greater than the risk that requires the labeling of a food as carcinogenic.[41]

Lung cancer and heart disease are not the only risks involuntary smokers face. Exposure to ETS among children increases their risk of infections of the lower respiratory tract. An estimated 300,000 children are at greater risk of pneumonia and bronchitis as a result.[42] Children exposed to sidestream smoke have a greater chance of developing other respiratory problems, such as cough, wheezing, asthma, and chest colds, along with a decrease in lung function. The greatest effects of sidestream smoke are seen in children under the age of five. Children exposed to sidestream smoke daily in the home miss 33 percent more school days and have 10 percent more colds and acute respiratory infections than those not exposed. A recent study found that 31.2 percent of children are exposed to cigarette smoke daily in the home. This study found wide regional, income, and education differences: children of high-income, high-education-level parents in California are exposed far less than are children of low-income, low-education-level parents in the Midwest.[43]

Cigarette, cigar, and pipe smoke in enclosed areas presents other hazards. Ten to 15 percent of nonsmokers are extremely sensitive (hypersensitive) to cigarette smoke. These people experience itchy eyes, difficulty in breathing, painful headaches, nausea, and dizziness in response to minute amounts of smoke. The level of carbon monoxide in cigarette smoke contained in enclosed places is 4,000 times higher than the clean air standard recommended by the EPA.

Efforts to reduce the hazards associated with passive smoking have been gaining momentum in recent years. Groups such as GASP (Group Against Smokers' Pollution) and ASH (Action on Smoking and Health) have been working since the early 1970s to reduce smoking in public places. In response to their efforts, some 44 states have enacted laws restricting smoking in public places such as restaurants, theaters, and airports. The federal government has restricted smoking in all government buildings. Hotels and motels now set aside rooms for nonsmokers, and car rental agencies designate certain vehicles for nonsmokers. Since 1990, smoking has been banned on all domestic airline flights.

> **What do you think?**
>
> *What rights, if any, should smokers have with regard to smoking in public places?* ✳ *Does your campus allow smoking in residence halls?* ✳ *Does your community have nonsmoking restaurants, or only restaurants that have nonsmoking sections?* ✳ *Do you think your community would support nonsmoking restaurants and bars? Why or why not?*

Tobacco and Politics

It has been nearly 40 years since the government began warning that tobacco use is hazardous to the health of the nation. Today the tobacco industry is under fire—46 states have sued to recover health care costs related to treating smokers.

In 1998, the tobacco industry reached a Master's Settlement Agreement with these states. Key provisions include the following:[44]

Environmental tobacco smoke (ETS)   Smoke from tobacco products, including sidestream and mainstream smoke.

Mainstream smoke   Smoke that is drawn through tobacco while inhaling.

Sidestream smoke   The cigarette, pipe, or cigar smoke breathed by nonsmokers; also called secondhand smoke.

Tobacco Reinvents Itself

Philip Morris is the world's largest producer and marketer of consumer packaged goods and the largest food company in the nation. It is also the world's largest and most profitable tobacco corporation. To many Americans, Philip Morris, which owns Kraft Foods, is firmly linked to the more than 400,000 people in the United States and 3.4 million worldwide who die each year from smoking-related illnesses. This company has also led the way, in the United States and internationally, in spreading the tobacco epidemic, in particular to girls and women, especially in regions where they traditionally have not smoked. In addition, Philip Morris and other tobacco companies have been charged with deliberately deceiving the public regarding the safety of tobacco and creating and marketing a chemical addiction for profit.

However, a visit to the Philip Morris headquarters in New York paints a different picture. Philip Morris is aggressively promoting its charitable work, in particular its youth smoking-prevention program. The company houses the Whitney Museum exhibit of an Indian artist and sponsors the Thurgood Marshall Scholars. Furthermore, Philip Morris employees are involved in efforts to fight hunger and combat domestic violence. The company donates $60 million a year to charity and spends another $100 million in advertising to inform the public about its good deeds. The advertising campaign is a concerted strategy to improve Philip Morris's corporate image and build credibility. In addition to the advertising campaign, the company has established a speakers' bureau where top company executives go on the road to talk to PTA meetings and other group gatherings about the company's charitable work.

What is the ethical dilemma associated with this corporation? What is the tobacco company's ethical obligation to society? Do you think Philip Morris is doing the right thing by changing its focus, or is this change merely a public relations effort?

- The tobacco payments will total approximately $206 billion to be paid over 25 years nationwide.
- The industry will pay $1.5 billion over 10 years to support antismoking measures, including education and advertising. An additional $250 million will fund research to determine the most effective ways to stop kids from smoking.
- The industry is barred from billboard advertising, including advertisements on transit systems. In-store ads are still permitted but will be limited in size.
- All outdoor advertising is banned, including billboards, signs, and placards larger than a poster in arenas, stadiums, shopping malls, and video arcades.
- The agreement bans young people's access to free samples, proof-of-purchase gifts, and sale and distribution of "branded" merchandise, such as T-shirts, hats, and other items bearing tobacco brand names or logos.
- There is a ban on the use of cartoon characters, such as Joe Camel, in advertising. (Such advertising is considered particularly appealing to young children.)
- Tobacco company sponsorship of concerts, athletic events, or any event in which a significant portion of the audience consists of young people is forbidden.
- The industry agreed not to market cigarettes to children and not misrepresent the health effects of cigarettes.

Other states and communities are advocating for stricter tobacco control. A number of states have imposed extra taxes on cigarette sales in an effort to discourage use. The monies are then used for various purposes, including prevention and cessation programs and school health programs. Two community-based programs, ASSIST (American Stop Smoking Intervention Study) and IMPACT (Initiatives to Mobilize for the Prevention and Control of Tobacco Use), are tobacco control initiatives focused on creating legislation to help prohibit the sale of tobacco to minors and assist with enforcement.

Quitting

Quitting smoking isn't easy. Smokers must break both the physical addiction to nicotine, and the habit of lighting up at certain times of the day.

From what we know about successful quitters, quitting is often a lengthy process involving several unsuccessful attempts before success is finally achieved. Even successful quitters suffer occasional slips, emphasizing the fact that quitting smoking is a dynamic process that occurs over time.

Approximately one-third of smokers attempt to quit each year. Unfortunately, 90 percent or more of those attempts fail. The person who wishes to quit smoking has several options. Most try to quit "cold turkey"—that is, they decide simply not to smoke again. Others resort to short-term quitting programs, such as those offered by the American Cancer Society, which are based on behavior modification and a system of self-rewards. Still others turn to treatment centers that are part of large franchises or of a local medical clinic's community outreach plan. Finally, some people work privately with their physicians to reach their goal.

Prospective quitters must decide which method or combination of methods will work best for them. Programs that combine several approaches have shown the most promise. Financial considerations, personality characteristics, and level of addiction are all factors to consider.

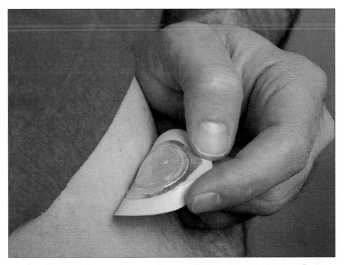

A nicotine patch can lessen the unpleasant symptoms of nicotine withdrawal. The patch delivers nicotine through the skin. Success rates for quitting are highest when the patch is combined with counseling or a behavior modification program.

Breaking the Nicotine Addiction

Nicotine addiction may be one of the toughest addictions to overcome. Smokers' attempts to quit lead to withdrawal symptoms. Symptoms of **nicotine withdrawal** include irritability, restlessness, nausea, vomiting, and intense cravings for tobacco.

Nicotine Replacement Products   Nontobacco products that replace depleted levels of nicotine in the bloodstream have helped some people stop using tobacco. The two most common are nicotine chewing gum and the nicotine patch, both of which are available over-the-counter. The FDA has also approved a nicotine nasal spray, a nicotine inhaler, and a nicotine pill.

Some patients use Nicorette, a chewing gum containing nicotine, to reduce nicotine consumption over time. Under the guidance of a physician, the user chews between 12 and 24 pieces of gum per day for up to six months. Nicorette delivers about as much nicotine as a cigarette does, but because it is absorbed through the mucous membrane of the mouth, it doesn't produce the same rush. Users experience no withdrawal symptoms and fewer cravings for nicotine as the dosage is reduced until they are completely weaned.

The nicotine patch, first marketed in 1991, is generally used in conjunction with a comprehensive smoking-behavior cessation program. A small, thin, 24-hour patch placed on the smoker's upper body delivers a continuous flow of nicotine through the skin, helping to relieve cravings. The patch is worn for 8 to 12 weeks under the guidance of a physician. During this time, the dose of nicotine is gradually reduced until the smoker is fully weaned from nicotine. Occasional side effects include mild skin irritation, insomnia, dry mouth, and nervousness. The patch costs the equivalent of two packs of cigarettes a day—about $4—and some insurance plans will pay for it.

How effective is the nicotine patch? According to an analysis of 17 studies involving 5,098 people, the nicotine patch was at least twice as effective as placebo (fake) patches. At the end of treatment periods lasting at least four weeks, 27 percent of nicotine patch wearers were free of cigarettes versus 13 percent of placebo patch users. Six months later, 22 percent of the nicotine patch users were abstinent compared with only 9 percent of the placebo users. The study also showed that the patch was effective with or without intensive counseling.[45]

The nasal spray, which requires a prescription, is much more powerful and delivers nicotine to the bloodstream faster than gum or the patch. Patients are warned to be careful not to overdose; as little as 40 milligrams of nicotine taken at once could be lethal. The spray is somewhat unpleasant to use. The FDA has advised that it should be used for no more than three months and never for more than six months, so that smokers don't find themselves as dependent on nicotine in spray form as they were on cigarettes. The FDA also advises that no one who experiences nasal or sinus problems, allergies, or asthma should use it.

The nicotine inhaler, which also requires a prescription, consists of a mouthpiece and cartridge. By puffing on the mouthpiece, the smoker inhales air saturated with nicotine, which is absorbed through the lining of the mouth, not the lungs. This nicotine enters the body much more slowly than the nicotine in cigarettes does. Using the inhaler mimics the hand-to-mouth actions used in smoking and causes the back of the throat to feel as it would when inhaling tobacco smoke. Each cartridge last for 80 long puffs, and each cartridge is designed for 20 minutes of use.

Approved in 1997 by the FDA, Zyban, the smoking cessation pill, offers new hope to many who thought they could never quit. Zyban is thought to work on dopamine and norepinephrine receptors in the brain to decrease craving and withdrawal symptoms. Because of the way this prescription medication works, it is important to start the pills 10 to 14 days before the targeted quit date; it requires planning ahead.

Breaking the Habit

For many smokers, the road to quitting includes antismoking therapy. Among the more common techniques are aversion therapy, operant conditioning, and self-control therapy.

Aversion Therapy   Aversion techniques attempt to reduce smoking by pairing the act of smoking with a noxious stimulus so that smoking itself is perceived as unpleasant. For

Nicotine withdrawal   Symptoms, including nausea, headaches, and irritability, suffered by smokers who cease using tobacco.

example, the technique of rapid smoking instructs patients to smoke rapidly and continuously until they exceed their tolerance for cigarette smoke, producing unpleasant sensations. Short-term rates of success are high, but many patients relapse over time.

Operant Strategies Pairing the act of smoking with an external stimulus is a typical example of this method. For example, one technique requires smokers to carry a timer that sounds a buzzer at different intervals. When the buzzer sounds, the patient is required to smoke a cigarette. Once

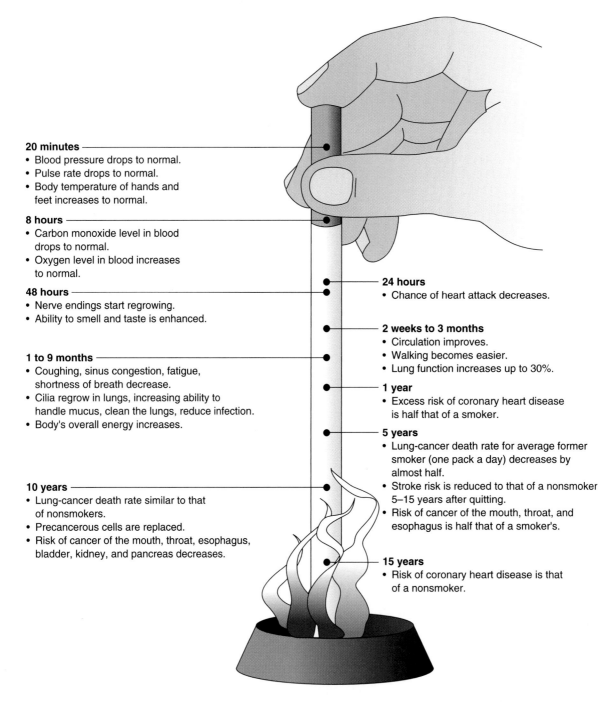

20 minutes
• Blood pressure drops to normal.
• Pulse rate drops to normal.
• Body temperature of hands and feet increases to normal.

8 hours
• Carbon monoxide level in blood drops to normal.
• Oxygen level in blood increases to normal.

48 hours
• Nerve endings start regrowing.
• Ability to smell and taste is enhanced.

1 to 9 months
• Coughing, sinus congestion, fatigue, shortness of breath decrease.
• Cilia regrow in lungs, increasing ability to handle mucus, clean the lungs, reduce infection.
• Body's overall energy increases.

10 years
• Lung-cancer death rate similar to that of nonsmokers.
• Precancerous cells are replaced.
• Risk of cancer of the mouth, throat, esophagus, bladder, kidney, and pancreas decreases.

24 hours
• Chance of heart attack decreases.

2 weeks to 3 months
• Circulation improves.
• Walking becomes easier.
• Lung function increases up to 30%.

1 year
• Excess risk of coronary heart disease is half that of a smoker.

5 years
• Lung-cancer death rate for average former smoker (one pack a day) decreases by almost half.
• Stroke risk is reduced to that of a nonsmoker 5–15 years after quitting.
• Risk of cancer of the mouth, throat, and esophagus is half that of a smoker's.

15 years
• Risk of coronary heart disease is that of a nonsmoker.

Figure 8.2
When Smokers Quit
Within 20 minutes of smoking that last cigarette, the body begins a series of changes that continues for years. However, by smoking just one cigarette a day, the smoker loses all these benefits, according to the American Cancer Society.
Source: G. Hanson and P. Venturelli, *Drugs and Society,* 5th ed. (Sudbury, MA: Jones and Bartlett, 1998), p. 320.

the smoker is conditioned to associate the buzzer with smoking, the buzzer is eliminated, and, one hopes, so is the smoking.

Self-Control Self-control strategies view smoking as a learned habit associated with specific situations. Therapy is aimed at identifying these situations and teaching smokers the skills necessary to resist smoking.

> **What do you think?**
> *Do you know people who have tried to quit smoking recently?* ✳ *What was this experience like for them?* ✳ *Were they successful? If not, what factors contributed to relapse?*

Benefits of Quitting

According to the American Cancer Society, many tissues damaged by smoking can repair themselves. As soon as smokers stop, the body begins the repair process (Figure 8.2). Within eight hours, carbon monoxide and oxygen levels return to normal, and "smoker's breath" disappears. Often, within a month of quitting, the mucus that clogs airways is broken up and eliminated. Circulation and the senses of taste and smell improve within weeks. Many ex-smokers say they have more energy, sleep better, and feel more alert. By the end of one year, the risk for lung cancer and stroke decreases. In addition, smokers reduce considerably their risks of developing cancers of the mouth, throat, esophagus, larynx, pancreas, bladder, and cervix. They also cut their risk of peripheral artery disease, chronic obstructive lung disease, coronary heart disease, and ulcers. Women are less likely to bear babies with low birth weight. Within two years, the risk for heart attack drops to near normal. At the end of 10 smoke-free years, the ex-smoker can expect to live out his or her normal life span.

Caffeine

Caffeine is the most popular and widely consumed drug in the United States. Almost half of all Americans drink coffee every day, and many others use caffeine in some other form, mainly for its well-known "wake-up" effect. Drinking coffee is legal, even socially encouraged. Many people believe caffeine is not a drug and not really addictive. Coffee and other caffeine-containing products seem harmless; with no cream or sugar added, they are calorie-free and therefore a good way to fill up if you are dieting. If you share these attitudes, you should think again because research in the past decade has linked caffeine to certain health problems.

Caffeine is a drug derived from the chemical family called **xanthines.** Two related chemicals, *theophylline* and *theobromine,* are found in tea and chocolate, respectively. The xanthines are mild central nervous system stimulants that enhance mental alertness and reduce feelings of fatigue.

Other stimulant effects include increases in heart muscle contractions, oxygen consumption, metabolism, and urinary output. These effects are felt within 15 to 45 minutes of ingesting a product that contains caffeine.

Side effects of the xanthines include wakefulness, insomnia, irregular heartbeat, dizziness, nausea, indigestion, and sometimes mild delirium. Some people also experience heartburn. As with some other drugs, the user's psychological outlook and expectations will influence the effects.

Different products contain different concentrations of caffeine. A 5-ounce cup of coffee contains between 65 and 115 milligrams of caffeine. Caffeine concentrations vary with the brand of the beverage and the strength of the brew. Small chocolate bars contain up to 15 milligrams of caffeine and theobromine. Table 8.5 compares various caffeine containing products.

Caffeine Addiction

As the effects of caffeine wear off, users may feel let down—mentally or physically depressed, exhausted, and weak. To counteract this, people commonly choose to drink another cup of coffee. Habitually engaging in this practice leads to tolerance and psychological dependence. Until the mid-1970s, caffeine was not medically recognized as addictive. Chronic caffeine use and its attendant behaviors were called "coffee nerves." This syndrome is now recognized as *caffeine intoxication,* or **caffeinism.** Symptoms of caffeinism include chronic insomnia, jitters, irritability, nervousness, anxiety, and involuntary muscle twitches. Withdrawing the caffeine may compound the effects and produce severe headaches. (Some physicians ask their patients to take a simple test for caffeine addiction: don't consume anything containing caffeine, and if you get a severe headache within four hours, you are addicted.) Because caffeine meets the requirements for addiction—tolerance, psychological dependence, and withdrawal symptoms—it can be classified as addictive.

Although you would have to drink between 67 and 100 cups of coffee in a day to produce a fatal overdose of caffeine, you may experience sensory disturbances after consuming only 10 cups of coffee within a 24-hour period. These symptoms include tinnitus (ringing in the ears), spots before the eyes, numbness in arms and legs, poor circulation, and visual hallucinations. Because 10 cups of coffee is not an extraordinary amount to drink in one day, caffeine use clearly poses health threats.

> **Caffeine**   A stimulant found in coffee, tea, chocolate, and some soft drinks.
>
> **Xanthines**   The chemical family of stimulants to which caffeine belongs.
>
> **Caffeinism**   Caffeine intoxication brought on by excessive caffeine use; symptoms include chronic insomnia, irritability, anxiety, muscle twitches, and headaches.

Table 8.5
Caffeine Content of Various Products

PRODUCT	CAFFEINE CONTENT (AVERAGE MG PER SERVING)
Coffee (5-oz. cup)	
Regular brewed	65–115
Decaffeinated brewed	3
Decaffeinated instant	2
Tea (6-oz. cup)	
Hot steeped	36
Iced	31
Soft Drinks (12-oz. servings)	
Jolt Cola	100
Dr. Pepper	61
Mountain Dew	54
Coca-Cola	46
Pepsi-Cola	36–38
Chocolate	
1 oz. baking chocolate	25
1 oz. chocolate candy bar	15
½ cup chocolate pudding	4–12
Over-the-Counter Drugs	
No Doz (2 tablets)	200
Excedrin (2 tablets)	130
Midol (2 tablets)	65
Anacin (2 tablets)	64

What do you think?

How much caffeine do you consume? ✳ *What is your pattern of caffeine consumption for the day?* ✳ *Why do you consume caffeine?* ✳ *Have you ever experienced any ill effects after avoiding caffeine for a period of time?*

The Health Consequences of Long-Term Caffeine Use

Long-term caffeine use has been suspected of being linked to a number of serious health problems, ranging from heart disease and cancer to mental dysfunction and birth defects. However, no strong evidence exists to suggest that moderate caffeine use (less than 500 milligrams daily, approximately 5 cups of coffee) produces harmful effects in healthy, nonpregnant people.

It appears that caffeine does not cause long-term high blood pressure and has not been linked to strokes. Nor is there any evidence of a relationship between coffee and heart disease.[46] However, people who suffer from irregular heartbeat are cautioned against caffeine because the resultant increase in heart rate might be life-threatening. Both decaffeinated and caffeinated coffee products contain ingredients that can irritate the stomach lining and be harmful to people with stomach ulcers.

For years, caffeine consumption was linked with fibrocystic breast disease, a condition characterized by painful, noncancerous lumps in the breast. Reports claim that caffeine promotes cyst formation in female breasts. Although these conclusions have been challenged, many clinicians advise patients with mammillary cysts to avoid caffeine. In addition, some reports indicate that very high doses of caffeine given to pregnant laboratory animals can cause stillbirths or offspring with low birth weight or limb deformations. Studies have found that moderate consumption of caffeine (less than 300 milligrams per day) did not significantly affect human fetal development.[47] Mothers are usually advised to avoid or at least reduce caffeine use during pregnancy.

Taking Charge

Managing the Use of Alcohol, Tobacco, and Caffeine

Making healthy behavior changes is never easy but always beneficial. After reading this chapter, you have a better understanding of the potential dangers—and the responsibilities—of using what many people consider recreational drugs. Being aware of the risks will make you more thoughtful when you are confronted with these substances. Do you have an appropriate relationship with alcohol, tobacco, and caffeine?

Checklist for Change

Making Personal Choices

A social drinker typically

✓ Drinks slowly and knows when to stop (does not drink to get drunk).

✓ Eats before or while drinking.

✓ Never drives after drinking.

✓ Respects nondrinkers and laws related to drinking.

A problem drinker

✓ Drinks to get drunk.

✓ Tries to solve problems by drinking alcohol.

✓ Experiences changes in personality and may become loud, angry, or violent, or silent, remote, and reclusive.

✓ Drinks when he or she should not—before driving or going to class or work.

✓ Causes other problems—harms himself or herself, family, friends, and strangers.

✓ Needs "liquid courage" before parties or dates.

Do you smoke? Here's how to quit:

✓ Identify your smoking habits. Keep a daily journal for one to two weeks; record when and where you smoked and whom you were with at the time.

✓ Get support. Phone your local chapter of the American Cancer Society or community hospital to find out about programs and support groups.

✓ Begin by tapering off. For a period of one to two weeks, cut down or change to a lower-nicotine brand (in the latter case, be careful not to increase the number of cigarettes you smoke). Stop carrying matches.

Don't buy a new pack until you finish the one you're smoking, and never buy a carton.

✓ Set a quit date. Announce to family and friends when you are going to stop.

✓ Stop. A week before you quit, cut your cigarette consumption down to a few cigarettes per day. Smoke these in the late day or evening. By this time, you may be able to notice some of the negative effects of smoking. On the day you quit, treat yourself to something nice.

✓ Continue to seek support from your support group. Increase your physical activity. Avoid situations you associate most closely with smoking.

✓ If you fail to stop despite your best efforts, don't beat yourself up. Try again soon.

To reduce caffeine consumption:

✓ Cut back gradually. Mix caffeinated with decaffeinated products.

✓ Be aware that caffeinated products often play a central role in social customs ("Let's meet for coffee").

Summary

❋ Alcohol is a central nervous system depressant used by 70 percent of all Americans and more than 84 percent of all college students. Although consumption trends are slowly creeping downward, college students are still under extreme pressure to consume alcohol.

❋ Alcohol's effect on the body is measured by the blood alcohol concentration (BAC), the ratio of alcohol to total blood volume. The higher the BAC, the greater the impairment of judgment and coordination and the greater the drowsiness. Some negative consequences associated with alcohol use and college students are lower grade-point averages, academic problems, traffic accidents, dropping out of school, unplanned sex, hangovers, and injury. Long-term alcohol overuse includes damage to the nervous system, cardiovascular damage, liver disease, and increased risk for cancer. Use during pregnancy can cause fetal alcohol effects (FAE) or fetal alcohol syndrome (FAS).

❋ Alcohol use becomes alcoholism when it interferes with school, work, or social and family relationships or entails violations of the law. Causes of alcoholism include biological and family factors and social and cultural factors. Alcoholism has far-reaching effects on families, especially on children.

❋ Treatment options for alcoholism include detoxification at private medical facilities, therapy (family, individual, or group), and programs such as Alcoholics Anonymous.

* The use of tobacco involves many social and political issues, including advertising targeted at youth and women, the largest growing populations of smokers. Health care and lost productivity resulting from smoking cost the nation as much as $100 billion per year.
* Tobacco is available in smoking and smokeless forms, both containing addictive nicotine (a psychoactive substance). Smoking also delivers 4,000 other chemicals to the lungs of smokers.
* Health hazards of smoking include markedly higher rates of cancer, heart and circulatory disorders, respiratory diseases, and gum diseases. Smoking while pregnant presents risks for the fetus, including miscarriage and low birth weight.

* Smokeless tobacco contains more nicotine than do cigarettes and dramatically increases risks for oral cancer and other oral problems.
* Environmental tobacco smoke (sidestream smoke) puts nonsmokers at risk for cancer and heart disease.
* Nicotine replacement products (gum and the patch) can help wean smokers off nicotine. Several therapy methods can help smokers break the habit.
* Caffeine is a widely used central nervous system stimulant. No long-term ill-health effects have been proven, although chronic users who try to quit may experience withdrawal.

Discussion Questions

1. When it comes to drinking alcohol, how much is too much? How can you avoid drinking amounts that will affect your judgment? When you see a friend having "too many" drinks at a party, what actions do you normally take? What actions could you take?
2. What are some of the most common negative consequences college students experience as a result of drinking? What are secondhand effects of binge drinking? Why do students tolerate negative behaviors of students who have been drinking?
3. Determine what your BAC would be if you drank four beers in two hours (assume they are spaced at equal intervals). What physiological effects will you feel after each drink? Would a person of similar weight show greater effects after having four gin and tonics instead of beer? Why or why not? At what point in your life should you start worrying about the long-term effects of alcohol abuse?
4. Describe the difference between a problem drinker and an alcoholic. What factors can cause someone to slide from responsibly consuming alcohol to becoming an alcoholic? What effect does alcoholism have on an alcoholic's family?

5. Does anyone ever recover from alcoholism? Why or why not? Do you think society's views on drinking have changed over the years? Explain your answer.
6. New research suggests that genetic factors might be more influential than environmental factors in smoking initiation and nicotine dependence. How might this information change current prevention efforts? How would you design smoking prevention strategies targeted at adolescents?
7. Discuss short-term and long-term health hazards associated with tobacco. How will increased tobacco use among adolescents and college students impact the medical system in the future? Who should be responsible for the medical expenses of smokers? Insurance companies? Smokers themselves?
8. Restrictions on smoking are increasing in our society. Do you think these restrictions are fair? Do they infringe on people's rights? Are the restrictions too strict or not strict enough?
9. Describe the pros and cons of each method of tobacco cessation. Which would be most effective for you? Explain why.
10. Discuss problems related to the ingestion of caffeine. How much caffeine do you consume? Why?

Application Exercise

Reread the What Do You Think? scenarios at the beginning of the chapter and answer the following questions.

1. What is it about a college environment that encourages drinking games?
2. What dangers are associated with these games? What signs show that someone might be developing alcohol poisoning?

3. What do you think the legal drinking age should be? What responsibility does Mark have for his brother's safety? In what ways do people "learn how to drink"?

Accessing Your Health on the Internet

Visit the following Internet sites to explore further topics and issues related to personal health. To visit an organization's website, go to the Companion Website for *Health: The Basics, Fifth Edition* at www.aw.com/donatelle, click on the book image, and select "Accessing Your Health on the Internet" from the navigation menu on the left.

1. ***Drinking: A Student's Guide.*** This website is designed exclusively for student use and oriented to answering questions and concerns that students have about drinking. An online knowledge test provides immediate feedback about alcohol intake. This website also provides facts and statistics, guidelines to low-risk drinking, and risk reduction techniques.

2. ***Higher Education Center for Alcohol and Other Drug Prevention.*** This website is funded through the U.S. Department of Education and provides information relevant to colleges and universities. A specific site exists for students who are seeking information regarding alcohol.

3. ***Had Enough.*** This entertaining website is designed for college students who have suffered the secondhandeffects (baby-sitting a roommate who has been drinking, having sleep interrupted, and so on.) of other students' drinking. It offers suggestions for taking action and being proactive about policy issues on your campus.

Further Reading

Kuhn, C., S. Swartzwelder, W. Wilson, J. Foster, and L. Wilson. *Buzzed: The Straight Facts About the Most Used and Abused Drugs from Alcohol to Ecstasy.* New York: Norton, 1998.
A straightforward, informative book. The first part consists of chapters on each of 12 kinds of drugs: alcohol, caffeine, enactogens, hallucinogens, herbal drugs, inhalants, marijuana, nicotine, opiates, sedatives, steroids, and stimulants. The second part of the book describes the complex neurochemistry with great clarity.

Nuwer, H. *Wrongs of Passage: Fraternities, Sororities, Hazing, and Binge Drinking.* Bloomington: Indiana University Press, 1999.
A comprehensive exposé on the continuing crisis of death and injury among fraternity and sorority pledges. The book provides an overview of Greek customs and demands that encouraged hazing as well as the recent deaths of students at some of the nation's most prestigious universities. The author argues that we need to control the Greek system as well as other organizations that employ similar, sometimes deadly, hazing practices.

Glantz, S. A., and E. D. Balbach. *The Tobacco War: Inside the California Battles.* Berkeley: University of California Press, 2000.
Charts the dramatic and complex history of tobacco politics in California over the past quarter century. Shows how the accomplishments of tobacco-control advocates have changed how people view the tobacco industry and its behavior.

Kluger, R. *Ashes to Ashes: America's Hundred-Year Cigarette War, the Public Health, and the Unabashed Triumph of Philip Morris.* New York: Vintage Books, 1997.
A definitive history of America's controversial tobacco industry, focusing on Philip Morris. Traces the development of the cigarette, revelations of its toxicity, and the impact of political and corporate shenanigans on the battle over smoking.

Whelan, E. *Cigarettes: What the Warning Label Doesn't Tell You—The First Comprehensive Guide to the Health Consequences of Smoking.* New York: Prometheus Books, 1997.
From impotence to diabetes, cataracts to psoriasis, the proven dangers of smoking go well beyond heart and lung disease. This book details all the known health threats of smoking. Twenty-one experts explain how smoking can affect the body.

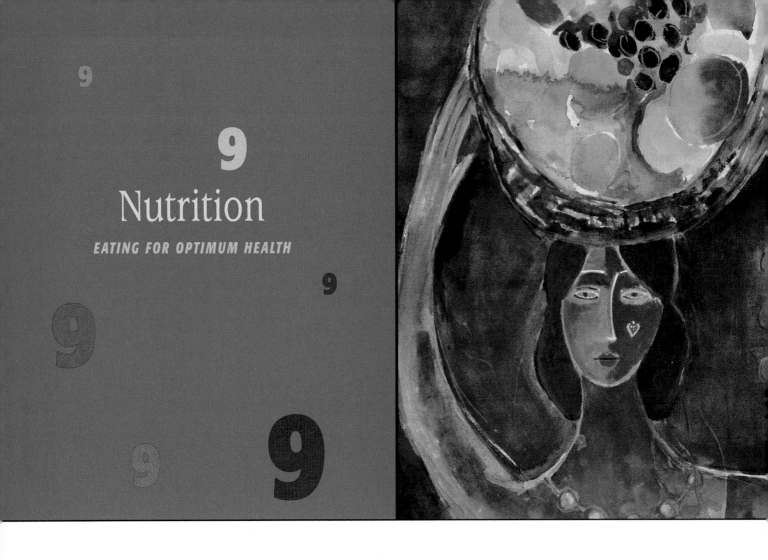

9
Nutrition

EATING FOR OPTIMUM HEALTH

objectives

* Examine the factors that influence dietary choices.

* Discuss how to change old eating habits, including using the Food Guide Pyramids appropriately, eating nutrient-dense foods, and other behaviors that enhance health.

* Describe the major essential nutrients, indicating what purpose they serve in maintaining overall health. Explain any controversies related to these substances.

* Discuss the role of food as a form of medicine. Discuss the facts related to new trends in nutrition and food supplements and their roles in health and well-being.

* Distinguish among the various forms of vegetarianism, discussing possible health benefits and risks from these dietary alternatives.

* Discuss issues surrounding gender and nutrition, food

safety, and the unique dietary issues facing college students.

* Discuss the unique problems that college students may have when trying to eat healthy foods and the actions they can take to comply with the Food Guide Pyramid.

* Explain some of the food safety concerns facing Americans and people from other regions of the world.

Roberto is a fitness enthusiast who runs five to ten miles daily, lifts weights three to four times per week, and constantly talks about his quest for the perfect body. He criticizes anyone who puts butter on bread or eats any kind of fast food. He worries constantly about his food intake and the "fuel" that supplies his body with energy.

How would you assess Roberto's dietary behavior? ✳ *What factors might contribute to his concerns?* ✳ *What, if anything, do you think he should do differently? Why?*

Do you ever get frustrated by conflicting information about diet and nutritional supplements? If so, you are like millions of other Americans. In fact, three out of four Americans say that there is far too much contradictory information about nutrition and complain that they are overwhelmed by the daunting task of trying to distinguish fact from fiction.[1] Just when we think we know the answers, a new research study tells us that what we thought was true probably isn't.

Today, we face dietary choices and nutritional challenges that our grandparents never dreamed of—exotic foreign foods; dietary supplements; artificial sweeteners; no-fat, low-fat, and artificial-fat alternatives; cholesterol-free, high-protein, high-carbohydrate, and low-calorie products. Thousands of alternatives bombard us daily. Caught in the crossfire of advertised claims by the food industry and advice provided by health and nutrition experts, most of us find it difficult to make wise dietary decisions.

When you are living away from home for the first time, suddenly having to make your own choices about food may seem a formidable task. A study of more than 2,000 college students indicated that students often face considerable difficulty planning healthy menus and having the resources to prepare balanced meals.[2] On the other hand, a subsequent study showed that college students and graduates tend to practice more healthful habits and make healthier food choices than nonstudents.[3] Many of the eating behaviors from both of these studies appear to mirror eating patterns that students learned in their homes.

seeing, and tasting foods, can stimulate appetite even if we're not hungry. Finding the right balance between eating to maintain body function (eating to live) and eating to satisfy appetite (living to eat) is a constant struggle for many of us. The following are among the most powerful influences that make us who we are, nutritionally:[4]

- *Personal preferences.* We all choose certain foods because we like the taste.
- *Habit.* Many of us select foods because they are familiar and provide comfort.
- *Ethnic heritage or tradition.* People eat the foods they grew up eating.
- *Social interactions.* For many of us, eating and socializing go hand in hand.
- *Availability, convenience, and economy.* Those with lower incomes find some foods too expensive, whereas others with higher incomes have more choice. Most of us eat foods that are readily available, quick and easy to prepare, and friendly to our budgets.
- *Emotional comfort.* We learn from birth that eating is a pleasant experience associated with warmth, pleasure, and sensory delights.
- *Values.* Food choices often reflect one's religious or spiritual beliefs, political views, or environmental concerns.
- *Body image.* Many people select certain foods because they believe they will enhance appearance, improve health, or act as a preventive agent.
- *Nutrition.* Many people make nutrition choices based purely on health concerns.

Nutrition is the science that investigates the relationship between physiological function and the essential elements of

Assessing Eating Behaviors

Although we have all undoubtedly experienced **hunger** before mealtime, few Americans have experienced the type of hunger that continues for days and threatens survival. Most of us do not eat to sustain physical survival. Instead, we eat because we experience **appetite**—the desire to eat—or because some inner signal tells us that it's time to eat. Appetite may cause a person to eat even when the person is quite full.

Many factors influence when we eat, what we eat, and how much we eat. Sensory stimulation, such as smelling,

Hunger   The feeling associated with the physiological need to eat.

Appetite   The desire to eat; normally accompanies hunger but is more psychological than physiological.

Nutrition   The science that investigates the relationship between physiological function and the essential elements of foods eaten.

What's Your EQ (Eating Quotient)?

Keeping up with the latest on what to eat—or not to eat—isn't easy. If you think a few facts might have slipped past you, this quiz should help. There's only one correct answer for each question.

1. Which of these foods is most likely to help prevent the most common form of blindness in older Americans?

a.	b.	c.	d.	e.
carrots	oranges	spinach	tomato juice	zucchini

2. Which is worst for you?

a.	b.	c.	d.	e.
butter	tub margarine	stick margarine	whipped butter	light tub margarine

3. Which claim is backed by the best research?

a.	b.	c.	d.	e.
Hot dogs increase the risk of childhood leukemia.	Carnitine helps you lose weight.	Cranberry juice can help treat urinary tract infections.	Garlic strengthens your immune system.	Coenzyme Q10 helps prevent heart disease.

4. Breast cancer kills more women than any other disease.

a.	b.
true	false

5. Which disease has not been linked to diets that are rich in red meat?

a.	b.	c.	d.
colon cancer	heart disease	prostate cancer	stomach cancer

6. A diet rich in fruits and vegetables has not been clearly linked to a lower risk of:

a.	b.	c.	d.
breast cancer	colon cancer	lung cancer	stroke

7. A healthy Mediterranean diet has very little:

a.	b.	c.	d.	e.
bread	olive oil	beans	vegetables	cheese

8. If you're in your 50s or 60s and your blood pressure is normal, it will stay that way.

a.	b.
true	false

9. Four of these strategies have been clearly shown to keep blood pressure from rising. Which hasn't?

a.	b.	c.	d.	e.
cutting salt	losing excess weight	eating potassium-rich foods	getting enough vitamin C	exercising regularly

10. Which is not a good source of potassium?

a.	b.	c.	d.	e.
cantaloupe	yogurt	brown rice	squash	kidney beans

11. Which has not been linked to a high-salt diet?

a.	b.	c.	d.
stroke	stomach cancer	osteoporosis	diabetes

12. There's evidence that the B vitamin folic acid cuts the risk of all but:

a.	b.	c.	d.	e.
birth defects, such as spina bifida	stroke	colon cancer	heart disease	prostate cancer

13. Which of the following foods is not a good source of folic acid?

a.	b.	c.	d.	e.
tuna fish	corn flakes	asparagus	lentils	orange juice

14. The evidence is strongest that vitamin C can:

a.	b.	c.	d.	e.
prevent cancer	lower blood pressure	reduce the duration of colds	prevent colds	prevent cataracts

15. Which of the following does not appear to be dangerous in high doses?

a.	b.	c.	d.
vitamin B_6	vitamin B_{12}	niacin	vitamin D

16. Most multivitamin supplements contain far less than a day's worth of:

a.	b.	c.	d.	e.
zinc	vitamin A	iron	calcium	vitamin D

17. Which food poisoning symptoms warrant calling the doctor?

a.	b.	c.	d.
bloody diarrhea	a stiff neck, severe headache, and fever	excessive vomiting	any of the above

18. Which is least likely to cause food poisoning?

a.	b.	c.	d.	e.
undercooked chicken	Caesar salad dressing	raw oysters	rare hamburger	mayonnaise

19. Which is least likely to have contaminants?

a.	b.	c.	d.	e.
flounder	swordfish	raw clams	bluefish	lake trout

20. What poisons the most children under the age of six?

a.	b.	c.	d.
eating moldy food	drinking household cleaners	taking an overdose of iron pills	chewing poisonous houseplant leaves

ANSWERS

1. c. Two carotenoids found in spinach—lutein and zeaxanthin—appear to protect eyes more than beta-carotene and other carotenoids. Other good sources: red bell pepper, okra, and leafy greens, such as kale, collard greens, and romaine lettuce.

2. a. Butter's saturated fat makes it boost your cholesterol more than margarine will. If you insist on butter, at least get a light whipped brand (some of its fat will be replaced by water and air). As for margarine, a tub always beats a stick, but a light tub or spread has the least cholesterol-raising *trans* and saturated fat of all.

3. c. In a recent study from Harvard Medical School, women who drank a little over a cup of cranberry juice cocktail a day were twice as likely to be cured of their urinary tract infections as women who drank a look-alike, taste-alike beverage with no cranberry juice.

4. b. When women of all ages are combined, heart disease kills four times as many women as breast cancer.

5. d. The saturated fat and cholesterol in red meat—especially ground beef—raise the risk of heart disease.

6. a. A few animal studies suggest that something in fruits or vegetables may reduce the risk of breast cancer. But in humans, other cancers are more strongly linked to a lack of fruits and vegetables.

7. e. A true Mediterranean diet is very low in saturated fat. That means very little cheese (and meat, poultry, and butter).

8. b. In the United States, blood pressure rises with age for most people.

9. d. There's convincing evidence for all but the vitamin C. Limiting alcohol to no more than two drinks a day should also keep your blood pressure from rising.

10. c. Most grains aren't rich in potassium. A serving of any of the other four foods will give you at least 500 mg. Most fruits, vegetables, beans, fish, poultry, and milk (but not cheese) are good sources.

Continued

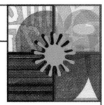
ANSWERS

11. d. A high-salt diet is most clearly linked to the risk of stroke. But the more salt you eat, the more calcium your body excretes, which can lead to osteoporosis, or brittle bones. While stomach cancer is deadly, the kind that's linked to salty foods is on the decline in the United States.

12. e.

13. a. The best places to get folic acid are fruits, vegetables, beans, fortified cereals, and vitamin supplements.

14. c. Most people think that vitamin C prevents colds, but the research always seems to come up empty. In several studies, though, one to three grams (1,000 to 3,000 mg) a day reduced the average duration of volunteers' colds from 6 days to $4\frac{1}{2}$ days.

15. b. A high dose of B_{12} (500 micrograms a day) can prevent B_{12} deficiency. And it's safe. A high dose of B_6 (possibly as little as 200 mg a day), on the other hand, can cause (reversible) nerve damage. Niacin (about 500 mg a day or more) is considered a drug. While it lowers cholesterol, it can cause side effects, such as flushing and liver damage. Vitamin D may cause side effects at levels as low as 1,200 IU a day.

16. d. If you want to get close to 100% of the U.S. Recommended Daily Allowance from a supplement, you'll need to take calcium separately.

17. d. You should also see a physician if any milder food poisoning symptom lasts for more than three days.

18. e. Despite its reputation for spoiling easily, mayonnaise is not as risky as undercooked poultry, rare hamburger, the raw egg in Caesar salad dressing, or raw shellfish.

19. a. Other low-fat seafood, such as cod, haddock, Pacific halibut, ocean perch, pollock, sole, and cooked shellfish, are also likely to be safe. Ditto for salmon and canned tuna.

20. c. Since 1986, more than 110,000 children have been poisoned by taking an overdose of their parents' (often brightly colored) iron supplements or iron-containing multivitamins, some after swallowing as few as five pills.

Source: Copyright 1995, CSPI. Excerpted from Bonnie Liebman, "What's Your EQ (Eating Quotient)?" *Nutrition Action Healthletter* (October 1995): 9–10. (1875 Connecticut Ave., NW, Suite 300, Washington, DC 20009-5728. $24.00 for 10 issues).

the foods we eat. With our country's overabundance of food and vast array of choices, media that "prime" us to want the tasty morsels shown on advertisements, and easy access to almost every type of **nutrient** (proteins, carbohydrates, fats, vitamins, minerals, and water), Americans should have few nutritional problems. However, these "diets of affluence" contribute to several major diseases, including obesity-related problems with heart disease, certain types of cancer, diabetes, hypertension (high blood pressure), cirrhosis of the liver, sleep apnea, varicose veins, gout, gallbladder disease, respiratory problems, abdominal hernias, flat feet, complications in pregnancy and surgery, and even higher accident rates, to name but a few.[5]

Nutrients The constituents of food that sustain us physiologically: proteins, carbohydrates, fats, vitamins, minerals, and water.

Calorie A unit of measure that indicates the amount of energy obtained from a particular food.

Eating for Health

Americans consume more calories per person than any other group of people in the world and have the highest rates of obesity. A **calorie** is a unit of measure that indicates the amount of energy we obtain from a particular food. Calories are eaten in the form of *proteins, fats,* and *carbohydrates,* three of the basic nutrients necessary for life. Three other nutrients, *vitamins, minerals,* and *water,* are necessary for bodily function but do not contribute any calories to our diets.

Excess calorie consumption is a major factor in our tendency to be overweight. However, it is not so much the quantity of food we eat that is likely to cause weight problems and resultant diseases as it is the relative proportion of nutrients in our diets and lack of physical activity. Americans typically get approximately 38 percent of their calories from fat, 15 percent from proteins, 22 percent from complex carbohydrates, and 24 percent from simple sugars.[6] Nutritionists recommend increasing complex carbohydrates to make up 48 percent of our total calories and reducing proteins to 12 percent, simple sugars to 10 percent, and fats to no more than 30 percent of our total diets.

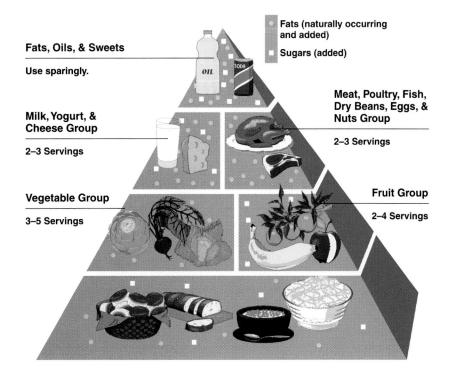

Figure 9.1
Food Guide Pyramid: A Guide to Daily Food Choices
Source: Walter C. Willett, M.D., *Eat, Drink, and Be Healthy,* © 2001. Reprinted with permission from The Harvard Medical School Guide to Healthy Eating. Simon & Schuster.

It is the high concentration of fats in the American diet, particularly saturated fats (largely animal fats), that appears to increase risk for heart disease. Although excessive consumption of sugar has been implicated in the development of many diseases, much of this information is inaccurate. Contrary to popular opinion, American consumption of sugar has not changed dramatically in recent years. In addition, the only disease associated with long-term excessive sugar intake is dental cavities. Most diet-related diseases result from excess calories and increased consumption of fat. Over the years, several federal agencies have worked to modify the average American's diet through a series of dietary goals and guidelines. How healthy are your eating habits? Find out by completing the questionnaire in the accompanying Assess Yourself box.

The Food Guide Pyramid

The Food Guide Pyramid, promoted by the United States Department of Agriculture (USDA) since 1993, illustrates graphically the importance of grains, cereals, vegetables, and fruits compared to meat, fish, poultry, dairy products, and other foods. Figure 9.1 shows the Food Guide Pyramid with recommended servings. The following examples show the equivalent of one serving from each of the major food groups.

Breads, Cereals, Rice, and Pasta Group (6–11 servings)
- 1 slice of bread or medium dinner roll
- $\frac{1}{2}$ hamburger bun, hot dog bun, bagel, or English muffin
- $\frac{1}{2}$ cup cooked rice, pasta, or other grains
- 6 saltines (the small squares) or snack crackers, or 3 ring pretzels
- 1 ounce ready-to-eat cereal
- $\frac{1}{2}$ cup cooked cereal
- 3 cups popped popcorn
- 1 tortilla, pancake, or waffle square
- 3 graham cracker squares or small, unfrosted cookies

Fruit Group (2–4 servings)
- Whole fruit, such as 1 medium apple, banana, or orange
- $\frac{1}{2}$ cup of raw, cooked, or canned fruit
- $\frac{3}{4}$ cup of fruit juice
- $\frac{1}{2}$ cup canned fruit
- $\frac{1}{4}$ cup dried fruit

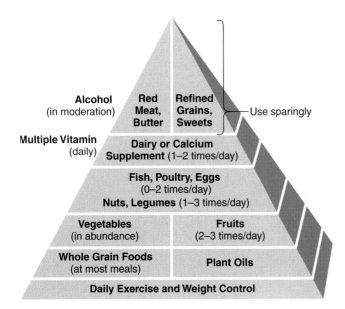

Figure 9.2
Proposed New Food Guide Pyramid
Source: W. C. Willett, *Eat, Drink, and Be Healthy* (New York: Simon and Schuster, 2001).

Vegetable Group (3–5 servings)
- 1 cup leafy raw vegetables
- $\frac{1}{2}$ cup chopped fresh, frozen, or canned vegetables
- $\frac{3}{4}$ cup fresh, frozen, or canned juice
- $\frac{3}{4}$ cup dried vegetables

Meat, Poultry, Fish, Dry Beans, Eggs, and Nuts Group (2–3 servings)
- 2–3 ounces lean, trimmed, and baked or roasted meat, fish, or poultry

The following can substitute for 1 ounce of meat:

- 2 tablespoons peanut butter or other nut or seed butter
- $\frac{1}{4}$ cup nuts
- $\frac{1}{2}$ cup cooked legumes
- 3 ounces tofu
- 1 egg

Milk, Yogurt, and Cheese (2 servings; 3 servings for pregnant and breast-feeding women and teens; 4 servings for teens who are pregnant or breast-feeding)
- 1 cup milk or yogurt
- $1\frac{1}{2}$ ounces natural cheese
- 2 ounces processed cheese
- $\frac{1}{2}$ cup cottage cheese
- $1\frac{1}{2}$ cups ice cream, ice milk, or frozen yogurt
- 1 cup sauces or puddings made with milk

A Call for a New Pyramid

After being asked to follow the USDA's Food Guide Pyramid for nearly a decade, researchers have begun a collective movement to significantly "up-end" the current pyramid.

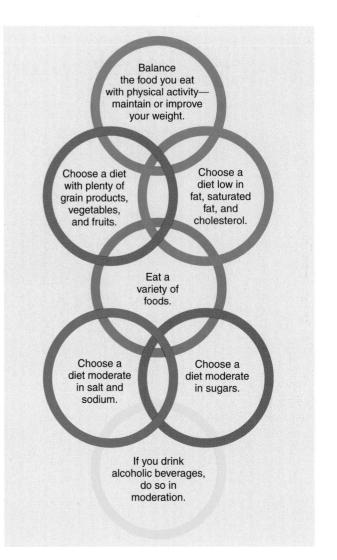

Figure 9.3
Dietary Guidelines for Americans
Source: U.S. Department of Agriculture, 1998.

They favor a pyramid that downplays meat and dairy products and moves whole-grain foods and plant oils to the top of the list of foods that should make up your daily intake of nutrients. Experts at a recent conference on diet and optimum health have proposed a pyramid that looks much like that in Figure 9.2 and will be the topic of much debate in the coming years.[7]

Today's Dietary Guidelines

With so many changes in the field of nutrition science, the federal government revised its Dietary Guidelines for Americans in 1998 (Figure 9.3) as follows:

- *Alcohol, in moderation, has health benefits. Moderation* refers to one drink per day for women, two drinks per day for men, preferably with a meal. This dose of alcohol has been consistently linked to higher levels of HDL, or "good" cholesterol, and fewer heart attacks than those among people who never drink. However, drinking beyond this magic limit increases the risk for several serious health problems.

- *Vegetarianism is healthful.* The USDA acknowledges for the first time that a vegetarian diet is beneficial. It advocates avoiding organ meat and high-fat processed meats, such as hot dogs and cold cuts.
- *Limit hydrogenated polyunsaturated fats.* The USDA strongly suggests cutting back on foods containing *trans*-fatty acids, such as margarines and shortenings, which are found in many snack foods.
- *Vitamin and mineral supplements are no substitute for a variety of foods.* In general, it is better to obtain nutrients from foods than to obtain them from supplements. The exceptions include calcium, folate, and vitamin D, which are believed to be okay in supplement form, particularly for those at risk of deficiency.
- *Use sugar and salt sparingly.* Although much of the information about ill-health effects, hyperactivity, and other problems associated with excess sugar is not true, sugar is a major source of excess calories in the average American's diet. While the negative effects of salt may be overexaggerated, some individuals react hypertensively to excess sodium. Because we don't know who will be affected, and because sodium levels are so high in most of our foods, everyone is advised to reduce salt intake.
- *Weight should* not *increase with age.* Because of increasing levels of information about the relationship between weight gain and premature health risks, maintaining a stable weight throughout life is recommended.

Making the Pyramid Work for You

Many people are overwhelmed by their first glance at the pyramid. However, take a look at what the USDA considers to be a serving: an ounce of ready-to-eat cereal, half a small hamburger bun or bagel, four to five potato chips, or one slice of bread. A normal bowl of cereal has three to four ounces of cereal. When was the last time you ate a quarter bowl of cereal? Or only half a hamburger bun? When you consider breakfast, lunch, dinner, and snacks in between, it is really quite easy to get all the servings in each food group that you need.

With any bread, cereal, or grain product, consider the amount of fat. Many people are duped into thinking that granola is a health food and bran muffins are better than bagels or bread. Sometimes these products are loaded with fat, sugar, and calories. Read the package labels and opt for reduced-fat, whole-grain products. When eating out, abiding by the guidelines may be challenging.

Eating "Nutrient-Dense" Foods

Although eating the proper number of servings from the food pyramid is important, it is also important to recognize that there are large caloric, fat, and energy differences between food categories within pyramid groups. For example, you might get the same number of calories from a glass of beer as you would a glass of milk. However, you would get many more nutrients from the milk than from the beer. Likewise, fish and hot dogs provide vastly different fat and energy levels ounce per ounce, with fish providing better energy and calorie value per serving. Nutrient density is even more important for someone who is ill and unable to keep food down. That is why nutrient supplements, such as Ensure and others, are often provided for cancer patients who need a nutrient "hit" in a small package.

The Digestive Process

Food provides the chemicals we need for energy and body maintenance. Because our bodies cannot synthesize or produce certain essential nutrients, we must obtain them from the foods we eat. Even though we may take in adequate amounts of foods and nutrients, if our body systems are not functioning properly, much of the nutrient value in our food may be lost. Before foods can be utilized properly, the digestive system must break the larger food particles down into smaller, more usable forms. The process by which foods are broken down and either absorbed or excreted by the body is known as the **digestive process.**

Even before you take your first bite of pizza, your body has already begun a series of complex digestive responses. Your mouth prepares for the food by increasing production of **saliva.** Saliva contains mostly water, which aids in chewing and swallowing, but it also contains important enzymes that begin the process of food breakdown, including amylase, which breaks down carbohydrates. *Enzymes* are protein compounds that facilitate chemical reactions but are not altered in the process. From the mouth, the food passes

Digestive process   The process by which foods are broken down and either absorbed or excreted by the body.

Saliva   Fluid secreted by the salivary glands; enzymes in the fluid aid in the breakdown of certain foods for digestion.

down the **esophagus,** a 9- to 10-inch tube that connects the mouth and stomach. A series of contractions and relaxations by the muscles lining the esophagus gently move food to the next digestive organ, the **stomach.** Here food mixes with enzymes and stomach acids. Hydrochloric acid begins to work in combination with pepsin, an enzyme, to break down proteins. In most people, the stomach secretes enough mucus to protect the stomach lining from these harsh digestive juices.

Further digestive activity takes place in the **small intestine,** a 20-foot coiled tube containing three sections: the *duodenum, jejunum,* and *ileum.* Each section secretes digestive enzymes that, when combined with enzymes from the liver and the pancreas, further contribute to the breakdown of proteins, fats, and carbohydrates. These nutrients are absorbed into the bloodstream to supply body cells with energy. The liver is the major organ that determines whether nutrients are stored, sent to cells or organs, or excreted. Solid wastes consisting of fiber, water, and salts are dumped into the large intestine, where most of the water and salts are reabsorbed into the system and the fiber is passed out through the anus. The entire digestive process may take anywhere from 24 hours to 80 hours.

Obtaining Essential Nutrients

Water: A Crucial Nutrient

If you were to go on a survival trip, which would you take with you—food or water? You may be surprised to learn that you could survive for much longer without food than you could without water. Even in severe conditions, the average person can go for weeks without certain vitamins and minerals before experiencing serious deficiency symptoms. **Dehydration,** however, can cause serious problems within a matter of hours; after a few days without water, death is likely.

Just what function does water serve in the body? Between 50 and 60 percent of our total body weight is water. The water in our system bathes cells, aids in fluid and electrolyte balance, maintains pH balance, and transports molecules and cells throughout the body. Water is the major component of the blood, which carries oxygen and nutrients to the tissues and is responsible for maintaining cells in working order.

How much water do you need? Most experts believe that six to eight glasses of water per day are necessary. Because of high concentrations of water in most of the foods we consume, however, the actual number of glasses needed each day is somewhat less than this. Individual needs vary drastically according to dietary factors, age, size, environmental temperature and humidity levels, exercise, and the effectiveness of the individual's system. Certain diseases, such as diabetes and cystic fibrosis, cause people to lose fluids at a rate necessitating a higher volume of fluid intake.

Is bottled water healthier than city water? In most instances, expensive "spring" and bottled waters are no healthier than chlorinated and fluoride-containing city water. Have your current water source tested if you are in doubt. Otherwise, be careful not to spend your money needlessly.

Proteins

Next to water, **proteins** are the most abundant substances in the human body. Proteins are major components of nearly every cell and have been called the "body builders" because of their role in developing and repairing bone, muscle, skin, and blood cells. Proteins are also the key elements of the antibodies that protect us from disease, of enzymes that control chemical activities in the body, and of hormones that regulate body functions. Moreover, proteins aid in the transport of iron, oxygen, and nutrients to all body cells and supply another source of energy to cells when fats and carbohydrates are not readily available. In short, adequate amounts of protein in the diet are vital to many body functions and ultimately to survival.

Whenever you consume proteins, your body breaks them down into smaller molecules known as **amino acids,** which link together like beads in a necklace to form 20 different combinations. Nine of these combinations are termed **essential,** meaning that the body must obtain them from the diet.

Dietary protein that supplies all of the essential amino acids is called **complete (high-quality) protein.** Typically, protein from animal products is complete. When we consume foods that are deficient in some of the essential amino

---

Esophagus   Tube that transports food from the mouth to the stomach.

Stomach   Large muscular organ that temporarily stores, mixes, and digests foods.

Small intestine   Muscular, coiled digestive organ; consists of the duodenum, jejunum, and ileum.

Dehydration   Abnormal depletion of body fluids; a result of lack of water.

Proteins   The essential constituents of nearly all body cells; necessary for the development and repair of bone, muscle, skin, and blood; the key elements of antibodies, enzymes, and hormones.

Amino acids   The building blocks of protein.

Essential amino acids   The nine basic nitrogen-containing building blocks of protein that must be obtained from foods to ensure health.

Complete (high-quality) proteins   Proteins that contain all of the nine essential amino acids.

acids, the total amount of protein that can be synthesized from the other amino acids is decreased. For proteins to be complete, they must also be present in digestible form and in amounts proportional to body requirements.

What about plant sources of protein? Proteins from plant sources are often **incomplete proteins** in that they are missing one or two of the essential amino acids. Nevertheless, it is relatively easy for the non–meat-eater to combine plant foods effectively and eat complementary sources of plant protein. An excellent example of this mutual supplementation process is eating peanut butter on whole-grain bread. Although each of these foods lacks certain essential amino acids, eating them together provides high-quality protein.

Plant sources of protein fall into three general categories: *legumes* (beans, peas, peanuts, and soy products), *grains* (whole grains, corn, and pasta products), and *nuts* and seeds. Certain vegetables, such as leafy green vegetables and broccoli, also contribute valuable plant proteins. Mixing two or more foods from each of these categories during the same meal will provide all of the essential amino acids necessary to ensure adequate protein absorption. People who are not interested in obtaining all of their protein from plants can combine incomplete plant proteins with complete low-fat animal proteins, such as chicken, fish, turkey, and lean red meat. Low-fat or nonfat cottage cheese, skim milk, egg whites, and nonfat dry milk all provide high-quality proteins and have few calories and little dietary fat.

You need to eat enough protein, but make sure you don't consume too much. Eating too much protein, particularly animal protein, can place added stress on the liver and kidneys. It also may increase calcium excretion in urine, which can elevate the risk of osteoporosis and bone fractures.[8]

Recently, several low-calorie diets that practically eliminate carbohydrates and focus on eating large quantities of protein have reemerged in the popular press. Although diets that deviate from a balanced nutritional approach are almost certainly flawed, most won't cause major health threats in otherwise healthy people when used for short periods of time. However, people who have kidney or liver problems or suffer from fluid imbalances or problems should avoid high-protein diets.

A person might need to eat extra protein if he or she is fighting off a serious infection, recovering from surgery or blood loss, or recovering from burns. In these instances, proteins that are lost to cellular repair need to be replaced. There is considerable controversy over whether someone in high-level physical training needs additional protein to build and repair muscle fibers or whether normal daily requirements should suffice.

Although protein deficiency continues to pose a threat to the global population, few Americans suffer from protein deficiencies. In fact, the average American consumes more than 100 grams of protein daily, and about 70 percent of this comes from high-fat animal flesh and dairy products.[9] The recommended protein intake for the average man is only 63 grams, and the average woman needs only 50 grams. The typical recommendation is that in a 2,000-calorie diet, about 10 percent of calories should come from protein, 60 percent from carbohydrates, and less than 30 percent from fat. The excess is stored as extra calories, leading to extra fat.

Carbohydrates

Although the importance of proteins in the body should not be underestimated, it is **carbohydrates** that supply us with the energy needed to sustain normal daily activity. Long maligned by weight-conscious people, carbohydrates can actually be metabolized more quickly and efficiently than proteins. Carbohydrates are a quick source of energy for the body, being easily converted to glucose, the fuel for the body's cells. These foods also play an important role in the functioning of internal organs, the nervous system, and the muscles. They are the best fuel for endurance athletics because they provide both an immediate and a time-released energy source as they are digested easily and then consistently metabolized in the bloodstream. For many people, a plate of pasta represents an attractive, healthy alternative to a fatty steak.

There are two major types of carbohydrates: **simple sugars,** which are found primarily in fruits, and **complex carbohydrates,** which are found in grains, cereals, dark green leafy vegetables, yellow fruits and vegetables (carrots, yams), *cruciferous* vegetables (such as broccoli, cabbage, and cauliflower), and certain root vegetables, such as potatoes. Most of us do not get enough complex carbohydrates in our daily diets.

A typical American diet contains large amounts of simple sugars. The most common form is *glucose.* Eventually, the human body converts all types of simple sugars to glucose to provide energy to cells. In its natural form, glucose is sweet and is obtained from substances such as corn syrup, honey, molasses, vegetables, and fruits. *Fructose* is another simple sugar found in fruits and berries. Glucose and fructose are **monosaccharides;** that is, contain only one molecule of sugar.

Incomplete proteins   Proteins that are lacking in one or more of the essential amino acids.

Carbohydrates   Basic nutrients that supply the body with the energy needed to sustain normal activity.

Simple sugar   A major type of carbohydrate, which provides short-term energy.

Complex carbohydrates   A major type of carbohydrate, which provides sustained energy.

Monosaccharide   A simple sugar that contains only one molecule of sugar.

Disaccharides are combinations of two monosaccharides. Perhaps the best-known example is common granulated table sugar (known as sucrose), which consists of a molecule of fructose chemically bonded to a molecule of glucose. Lactose, found in milk and milk products, is another form of disaccharide, formed by the combination of glucose and galactose (another simple sugar). Disaccharides must be broken down into simple sugars before they can be used by the body.

Controlling the amount of sugar in your diet can be difficult because sugar, like sodium, is often present in food products that you might not expect to contain it. Such diverse items as ketchup, Russian dressing, Coffee-Mate, and Shake 'n' Bake derive between 30 and 65 percent of their calories from sugar. Read food labels carefully before purchasing.

Polysaccharides are complex carbohydrates formed by long chains of saccharides. Like disaccharides, they must be broken down into simple sugars before they can be utilized by the body. There are two major forms of complex carbohydrates: *starches* and *fiber,* or **cellulose.**

Starches make up the majority of the complex carbohydrate group. Starches in our diets come from flours, breads, pasta, potatoes, and related foods. They are stored in body muscles and the liver in a polysaccharide form called **glycogen.** When the body requires a sudden burst of energy, it breaks down glycogen into glucose.

Carbohydrates and Athletic Performance

In the past decade, carbohydrates have become the "health foods" of many athletes. Some fitness enthusiasts consume concentrated sugary foods or drinks before or during athletic activity, thinking that the sugars will provide extra energy. This may actually be counterproductive.

One possible problem involves the gastrointestinal tract. If your intestines react to activity (or the nervousness before competition) by moving material through the small intestine more rapidly than usual, undigested disaccharides and/or unabsorbed monosaccharides will reach the colon, which can result in a very inopportune bout of diarrhea.

Consuming large amounts of sugar during exercise can also have a negative effect on hydration. Concentrations exceeding 24 grams of sugar per 8 ounces of fluid can delay stomach emptying and hence absorption of water. Some fruit juices, fruit drinks, and other sugar-sweetened beverages have more than this amount of sugar. If you use these products, dilute them with ice cubes or water.

Marathon runners and other people who require reserves of energy for demanding tasks often attempt to increase stores of glycogen in the body by *carbohydrate loading.* This process involves modifying the nature of both workouts and diet, usually during the week or so before competition. The athletes train very hard early in the week while eating small amounts of carbohydrates. Right before competition, they dramatically increase their intake of carbohydrates to force the body to store more glycogen, to be used during endurance activities (such as the last miles of a marathon).

The Myth of Sugar and Hyperactivity

Contrary to early media reports, extensive research in recent years indicates that sugars do *not* cause hyperactivity.[10] In well-controlled dietary challenge studies, consumption of sugar has not been shown to have negative effects on motor activity, spontaneous behavior, performance in psychological tests, learning, memory, attention span, or problem-solving ability. In addition, sugar intake is not related to violence or criminal activity.

Fiber

Fiber, often referred to as "bulk" or "roughage," is the indigestible portion of plant foods that helps move foods through the digestive system and softens stools by absorbing water. Fiber also helps to control weight by creating a feeling of fullness without adding extra calories. Although nutritionists have been very vocal in advocating increased fiber intake, the average American consumes only about 12 grams of fiber a day, about half the recommended daily amount of 25 grams.[11]

Insoluble fiber, which is found in bran, whole-grain breads and cereals, and most fruits and vegetables, is associated with these gastrointestinal benefits and has also been found to reduce the risk for several forms of cancer. *Soluble fiber* appears to be a factor in lowering blood cholesterol levels, thereby reducing risk for cardiovascular disease. Major sources of soluble fiber in the diet include oat bran, dried beans (such as kidney, garbanzo, pinto, and navy beans), and some fruits and vegetables.

The best way to increase intake of dietary fiber is to eat more complex carbohydrates, such as whole grains, fruits, vegetables, dried peas and beans, nuts, and seeds. As with most nutritional advice, however, too much of a good thing can pose problems. Sudden increases in dietary fiber may cause flatulence (intestinal gas), cramping, or a bloated feeling. Consuming plenty of water or other liquids may reduce such side effects.

A few years ago, fiber was thought by some to be the remedy for just about everything. Much of this hope was exaggerated. However, current research does support many benefits of fiber, such as the following:[12]

- *Protection against colon and rectal cancer.* One of the leading causes of cancer deaths in the United States, colorectal cancer is much rarer in countries having diets high in fiber

---

Disaccharide   A combination of two monosaccharides.

Polysaccharide   A complex carbohydrate formed by the combination of long chains of saccharides.

Cellulose   Fiber; a major form of complex carbohydrates.

Glycogen   The polysaccharide form in which glucose is stored in the liver.

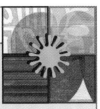

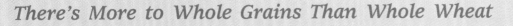

There's More to Whole Grains Than Whole Wheat

It's hard to beat whole grains. They are packed with vitamins, minerals and fiber that you just don't find in plain white bread, processed cereals or white rice or even in many healthful-looking enriched "multi-grain" breads, for that matter. Plus, whole grains have a new health cachet, now that researchers have uncovered disease-fighting properties from the phytonutrients they contain (see *Environmental Nutrition*, February 2001).

Besides nutrition, whole grains are loaded with flavor and texture, adding interest to meals. Here is *Environmental Nutrition* magazine's guide to some less traditional whole grains and how and why to give them a try.

If you can't find these grains or flours in your supermarket or local health food store, try these mail-order sources:

- **Get Healthy Shop**—(800) 420-4726; www.gethealthyshop.com

- **King Arthur Flour**—(800) 827-6836; www.kingarthurflour.com

- **True Foods Market**—(877) 274-5914; www.truefoodsmarket.com

Whole Grain Alternatives

GRAIN	WHAT IT IS & NUTRIENTS	FLAVOR BASICS & SHOPPING TIPS	PREPARATION & SERVING SUGGESTIONS
Amaranth	A high-protein grain that's a good source of fiber and vitamin E. Rich in lysine, an amino acid often missing in grain foods. Tolerated by people sensitive to wheat or gluten-intolerant.	Amaranth seeds have a pleasant peppery flavor.	• Amaranth flour is higher in fat than wheat, resulting in moister bread; replace no more than $\frac{1}{4}$ of the flour in bread recipes. • Boil and eat as a cereal or use in soups and granolas. The seeds of some varieties can be popped like popcorn. • To prepare: Cook 1 cup amaranth in 3 cups water for $\frac{1}{2}$ hour.
Kasha (Buckwheat groats)	Technically, a fruit (the roasted seed of the buckwheat plant), but the food world classifies it as a grain. It's an excellent source of magnesium and a good source of copper and fiber. Like amaranth, it is rich in lysine. Tolerated by people sensitive to wheat or gluten-intolerant, though be careful of mixes that also contain wheat.	Kasha has a hearty, nutty flavor and chewy texture. Kasha comes in whole, coarse, medium and fine consistencies. Also available as flour. Or make your own by pulverizing whole groats in a food processor or blender until the consistency of flour.	• Great when served as a hot cereal. Or as a hearty salad with vegetables and paired with a light soup. • Kasha makes an exceptionally flavorful pilaf; prepare with caramelized or browned onions and mushrooms. • Kasha flour makes flavorful, hearty pancakes and pasta. • You can replace up to half the wheat flour in many recipes with kasha flour, but replace only $\frac{1}{5}$ the flour in breads. • To prepare: Simmer 1 part groats in 2 parts water for 15 minutes (medium and fine grades cook more quickly).
Quinoa (KEEN-wah)	A staple of ancient Incan culture. It is an excellent source of B vitamins, copper, iron, magnesium and lysine. It provides a more complete protein than many other grains. A popular alternative for people sensitive to wheat or gluten-intolerant.	Quinoa has a mild flavor and a slightly crunchy texture. It comes in different colors, ranging from a pale yellow to red and black. Health food stores sell a variety of pasta and other products made from it.	• Quinoa flakes are seeds that have been steamed, rolled, then flaked to make an oatmeal-like hot cereal. • Quinoa flour is higher in fat than traditional bread flours, so it tends to make bread moister. Replace up to $\frac{1}{4}$ of the flour in a bread recipe with it. • Rinse quinoa before cooking to remove bitter natural coating. • To prepare: Cook 1 cup quinoa in 2 cups water for 20 minutes.

Continued

GRAIN	WHAT IT IS & NUTRIENTS	FLAVOR BASICS & SHOPPING TIPS	PREPARATION & SERVING SUGGESTIONS
Spelt	Spelt, a distant cousin to wheat, is hearty and grows well without chemical fertilizers, pesticides, and herbicides and, therefore, is a commonly available organic grain. It is a good source of fiber and B vitamins.	Available as whole berries and whole or refined flour. Also found in breads and pastas in natural food stores.	• Use whole spelt berries as you would rice and barley, in hearty grain salads, pilafs, and fillings. • Use spelt flour to make breads and pastas. Spelt tends to make bread heavier. Experiment by adding a little extra yeast to help bread rise or look for commercial bread mixes. • To prepare: Cook 1 cup berries in 4 cups water for 30–40 minutes.
Teff	This Ethiopian staple is the world's smallest grain and is less refined than many common grains. As a result, it's a nutritional powerhouse, especially rich in protein and calcium. Tolerated by people sensitive to wheat or gluten-intolerant.	Teff has a sweet, nutty flavor and comes in different colors, ranging from creamy white to reddish-brown.	• Serve as a hot breakfast cereal, sprinkled with cinnamon and brown sugar, maple syrup, raisins or sliced fruit. • To prepare: Cook 1 cup teff in 3 cups water for 15–20 minutes: to add flavor, roast teff with cornmeal for 5 minutes before boiling.
Triticale (Tri-ti-CAY-lee)	This relatively young (only 200 years old) grain is a cross between wheat and rye. It is an excellent source of fiber, B vitamins, and magnesium, plus a good source of iron.	Triticale berries are gray-brown and oval shaped, similar to wheat berries but with a subtle rye flavor. Available as flour, flakes (for cereal), berries, and as part of muesli, granola, or whole-grain cereal combinations.	• Triticale makes wonderful sandwich bread, similar in taste to honey wheat bread. • When making bread, replace no more than half the flour in recipes. Knead gently and let rise only once. • Use triticale flakes like rolled oats to make a hot breakfast cereal. They cook in about 15 minutes. • To prepare: Cook 1 cup berries in 4 cups water for 1 hour.

Source: Reprinted by permission of *Environmental Nutrition* magazine, from L. Hughes, "There's More to Whole Grains Than Whole Wheat," *Environmental Nutrition* (October 2001). © Copyright 2001 by Environmental Nutrition. Inc., 52 Riverside Drive, New York, NY 10024.

and low in animal fat. Several studies have supported the theory that fiber-rich diets, particularly those including insoluble fiber, prevent the development of precancerous growths. Whether this is because consuming more fiber helps to move foods through the colon faster, thereby reducing the colon's contact time with cancer-causing substances, or because insoluble fiber reduces bile acids and certain bacterial enzymes that may promote cancer, has remained in question. Research exploring the importance of fiber in colon cancer prevention continues today.

• *Protection against breast cancer.* Research into the effects of fiber on breast cancer risks is inconclusive. However, some studies have indicated that wheat bran (rich in insoluble fiber) reduces blood estrogen levels, which may affect the risk for breast cancer. Another theory is that people who eat more fiber have proportionally less fat in their diets and this is what reduces overall risk. The jury is still very much out in this area.

• *Protection against constipation.* Insoluble fiber, consumed with adequate fluids, is the safest, most effective way to prevent or treat constipation. The fiber acts like a sponge, absorbing moisture and producing softer, bulkier stools that are easily passed. Fiber also helps produce gas, which in turn may initiate a bowel movement.

• *Protection against diverticulosis.* About one American in ten over the age of 40 and at least one in three over 50 suffers from *diverticulosis,* a condition in which tiny bulges or pouches form on the large intestinal wall. These bulges become irritated and cause chronic pain if under strain from constipation. Insoluble fiber helps to reduce constipation and discomfort.

• *Protection against heart disease.* Many studies have indicated that soluble fiber (as in oat bran, barley, and fruit pectin) helps reduce blood cholesterol, primarily by lowering LDL ("bad") cholesterol. Whether this reduction is a direct effect or occurs instead through the displacement of fat calories by fiber calories or through intake of other nutrients, such as iron, remains in question.

- *Protection against diabetes.* Some studies have suggested that soluble fiber improves control of blood sugar and can reduce the need for insulin or medication in people with diabetes. Exactly why isn't clear, but soluble fiber seems to delay the emptying of the stomach and slow the absorption of glucose by the intestine.
- *Protection against obesity.* Because most high-fiber foods are high in carbohydrates and low in fat, they help control caloric intake. Many take longer to chew, which slows you down at the table and makes you feel full sooner.

Most experts believe that Americans should double their current consumption of dietary fiber—to 20 to 30 grams per day for most people and perhaps to 40 to 50 grams for others. Here are some tips for increasing your fiber intake:

1. Eat a variety of foods. Aim for at least five servings of fruits and vegetables and three to six servings of whole-grain breads, cereals, and legumes per day throughout the day.
2. Consume less processed food.
3. Eat the skins of fruits and vegetables.
4. Get your fiber from foods rather than pills or powders. Pills and powders do not supply enough essential nutrients.
5. Spread out your fiber intake.
6. Drink plenty of liquids—at least 64 ounces of water daily.

Fats

Fats (or *lipids*), another group of basic nutrients, are perhaps the most misunderstood of the body's required energy sources. Fats play a vital role in maintaining healthy skin and hair, insulating body organs against shock, maintaining body temperature, and promoting healthy cell function. Fats make foods taste better and carry the fat-soluble vitamins A, D, E, and K to the cells. They also provide a concentrated form of energy in the absence of sufficient amounts of carbohydrates. If fats perform all these functions, why are we constantly urged to cut back on them?

Although moderate consumption of fats is essential to health, overconsumption can be dangerous. The most common form of fat circulating in the blood is the **triglyceride,** which makes up about 95 percent of total body fat. When we consume too many calories, the liver converts the excess into triglycerides, which are stored throughout our bodies.

The remaining 5 percent of body fat is composed of substances such as **cholesterol,** which can accumulate on the inner walls of arteries, causing a narrowing of the channel through which blood flows. This buildup, called **plaque,** is a major cause of *atherosclerosis* (hardening of the arteries). At one time, the amount of circulating cholesterol in the blood was thought to be crucial. Current thinking is that the actual amount of circulating cholesterol itself is not as important as the ratio of total cholesterol to a group of compounds called **high-density lipoproteins (HDLs).** Lipoproteins are the transport facilitators for cholesterol in the blood. High-

density lipoproteins are capable of transporting more cholesterol than are **low-density lipoproteins (LDLs).** Whereas LDLs transport cholesterol to the body's cells, HDLs apparently transport circulating cholesterol to the liver for metabolism and elimination from the body. People with a high percentage of HDLs therefore appear to be at lower risk for developing cholesterol-clogged arteries. Regular vigorous exercise plays a part in reducing cholesterol by increasing high-density lipoproteins.

Fat cells consist of chains of carbon and hydrogen atoms. Those that are unable to hold any more hydrogen in their chemical structure are labeled **saturated fats.** They generally come from animal sources, such as meats and dairy products, and are solid at room temperature. **Unsaturated fats,** which come from plants and include most vegetable oils, are generally liquid at room temperature and have room for additional hydrogen atoms in their chemical structure. The terms *monounsaturated fat* and *polyunsaturated fat* refer to the relative number of hydrogen atoms that are missing. Peanut and olive oils are high in monounsaturated fats, whereas corn, sunflower, and safflower oils are high in polyunsaturated fats. There is currently a great deal of controversy about which type of unsaturated fat is most beneficial. Although nutritional researchers in the 1980s favored polyunsaturated fats, today many believe that polyunsaturates may decrease beneficial HDL levels while reducing LDL

Fats Basic nutrients composed of carbon and hydrogen atoms; needed for the proper functioning of cells, insulation of body organs against shock, maintenance of body temperature, and healthy skin and hair.

Triglyceride The most common form of fat in the body; excess calories consumed are converted into triglycerides and stored as body fat.

Cholesterol A form of fat circulating in the blood that can accumulate on the inner walls of arteries.

Plaque Cholesterol buildup on the inner walls of arteries, causing a narrowing of the channel through which blood flows; a major cause of atherosclerosis.

High-density lipoproteins (HDLs) Compounds that facilitate the transport of cholesterol in the blood to the liver for metabolism and elimination from the body.

Low-density lipoproteins (LDLs) Compounds that facilitate the transport of cholesterol in the blood to the body's cells.

Saturated fats Fats that are unable to hold any more hydrogen in their chemical structure; derived mostly from animal sources; solid at room temperature.

Unsaturated fats Fats that do have room for more hydrogen in their chemical structure; derived mostly from plants; liquid at room temperature.

Table 9.1
A Guide to Vitamins

VITAMIN	BEST SOURCES	CHIEF ROLES
Water-Soluble Vitamins		
Thiamin 1.5 mg (RDA + RDI)	Meat, pork, liver, fish, poultry, whole-grain and enriched breads, cereals, pasta, nuts, legumes, wheat germ, oats	Helps enzymes release energy from carbohydrate; supports normal appetite and nervous system function
Riboflavin 1.7 mg (RDA + RDI)	Milk, dark green vegetables, yogurt, cottage cheese, liver, meat, whole-grain or enriched breads and cereals	Helps enzymes release energy from carbohydrate, fat, and protein; promotes healthy skin and normal vision
Niacin 20 mg NE (RDA + RDI)	Meat, eggs, poultry, fish, milk, whole-grain and enriched breads and cereals, nuts, legumes, peanuts, nutritional yeast, all protein foods	Helps enzymes release energy from energy nutrients; promotes health of skin, nerves, and digestive system
Vitamin B_6 2.0 mg (RDA + RDI)	Meat, poultry, fish, shellfish, legumes, whole-grain products, green, leafy vegetables, bananas	Protein and fat metabolism, formation of antibodies and red blood cells; helps convert tryptophan to niacin
Folate 400 μg (DFE + RDA)	Green, leafy vegetables, liver, legumes, seeds	Red blood cell formation; protein metabolism; new cell division; prevents neural tube defects
Vitamin B_{12} 2.4 mg (RDA)	Meat, fish, poultry, shellfish, milk, cheese, eggs, nutritional yeast	Helps maintain nerve cells; red blood cell formation; synthesis of genetic material
Pantothenic acid 5–7 mg (AI)	Widespread in foods	Coenzyme in energy metabolism
Biotin 30 μg (AI)	Widespread in foods	Coenzyme in energy metabolism; fat synthesis; glycogen formation
Vitamin C (ascorbic acid) (RDI + RDA) = 60 mg	Citrus fruits, cabbage-type vegetables, tomatoes, potatoes, dark green vegetables, peppers, lettuce, cantaloupe, strawberries, mangos, papayas	Synthesis of collagen (helps heal wounds, maintains bone and teeth, strengthens blood vessels); antioxidant; strengthens resistance to infection; helps body's absorption of iron
Fat-Soluble Vitamins		
Vitamin A 5,000 I.U.	*Retinal:* fortified milk and margarine, cream, cheese, butter, eggs, liver *Carotene:* spinach and other dark leafy greens, broccoli, deep orange fruits (apricots, peaches, cantaloupe) and vegetables (squash, carrots, sweet potatoes, pumpkin)	Vision; growth and repair of body tissues; reproduction; bone and tooth formation; immunity; cancer protection; hormone synthesis
Vitamin D 400–600 I.U. (RDA + RDI)	Self-synthesis with sunlight, fortified milk, fortified margarine, eggs, liver, fish	Calcium and phosphorus metabolism (bone and tooth formation); aids body's absorption of calcium
Vitamin E 30 I.U. (RDA + RDI)	Vegetable oils, green leafy vegetables, wheat germ, whole-grain products, butter, liver, egg yolk, milk fat, nuts, seeds	Protects red blood cells; antioxidant; stabilization of cell membranes
Vitamin K 70–140 μg	Liver, green, leafy, and cabbage-type vegetables, milk	Bacterial synthesis in digestive tract. Synthesis of blood-clotting proteins and a blood protein that regulates blood calcium

levels. Monounsaturated fats seem to lower only LDL levels and thus are currently the "preferred" fats.

Reducing Fat in Your Diet   Want to cut the fat? These guidelines offer a good place to start:

- *Know what you are putting in your mouth.* Read food labels. Remember that no more than 10 percent of your total calories should come from saturated fat, and no more than 30 percent should come from all forms of fat.

- *Choose fat-free or low-fat versions of cakes, cookies, crackers, or chips.* Remember, though, that calories still count. Don't eat *more* chips just because they're lower in fat.

- *Use olive oil for baking and sautéing.* Animal studies have shown that it doesn't raise cholesterol or promote the growth of tumors.

- *Whenever possible, use liquid, diet, or whipped margarine.* These products have far less *trans*-fatty acid than solid fat.

- *Choose lean meats, fish, or poultry.* Remove skin. Broil or bake whenever possible. In general, the more well-done the meat, the fewer the calories. Drain off fat after cooking.

Table 9.1
A Guide to Vitamins

DEFICIENCY SYMPTOMS	TOXICITY SYMPTOMS
Beriberi, edema, heart irregularity, mental confusion, muscle weakness, low morale, impaired growth	Rapid pulse, weakness, headaches, insomnia, irritability
Eye problems, skin disorders around nose and mouth	None reported, but an excess of any of the B vitamins can cause a deficiency of the others
Pellagra: skin rash on parts exposed to sun, loss of appetite, dizziness, weakness, irritability, fatigue, mental confusion, indigestion	Flushing, nausea, headaches, cramps, ulcer irritation, heartburn, abnormal liver function, low blood pressure
Nervous disorders, skin rash, muscle weakness, anemia, convulsions, kidney stones	Depression, fatigue, irritability, headaches, numbness, damage to nerves, difficulty walking
Anemia, heartburn, diarrhea, smooth tongue depression, poor growth	Diarrhea, insomnia, irritability, may mask a vitamin B_{12} deficiency
Anemia, smooth tongue, fatigue, nerve degeneration progressing to paralysis	None reported
Rare; sleep disturbances, nausea, fatigue	Occasional diarrhea
Loss of appetite, nausea, depression, muscle pain, weakness, fatigue, rash	None reported
Scurvy, anemia, atherosclerotic plaques, depression, frequent infections, bleeding gums, loosened teeth, pinpoint hemorrhages, muscle degeneration, rough skin, bone fragility, poor wound healing, hysteria	Nausea, abdominal cramps, diarrhea, breakdown of red blood cells in persons with certain genetic disorders, deficiency symptoms may appear at first on withdrawal of high doses
Night blindness, rough skin, susceptibility to infection, impaired bone growth, abnormal tooth and jaw alignment, eye problems leading to blindness, impaired growth	Red blood cell breakage, nosebleeds, abdominal cramps, nausea, diarrhea, weight loss, blurred vision, irritability, loss of appetite, bone pain, dry skin, rashes, hair loss, cessation of menstruation, growth retardation
Rickets in children; osteomalacia in adults; abnormal growth, joint pain, soft bones	Raised blood calcium, constipation, weight loss, irritability, weakness, nausea, kidney stones, mental and physical retardation
Muscle wasting, weakness, red blood cell breakage, anemia, hemorrhaging, fibrocystic breast disease	Interference with anticlotting medication, general discomfort
Hemorrhaging	Interference with anticlotting medication; may cause jaundice

Values vary (increase) among women who are pregnant or lactating.

Sources: Adapted by permission of Wadsworth Publishing Company from pp. 152–153 of *Personal Nutrition,* 2d ed., by Marie Boyle and Gail Zyla. Copyright 1991 by West Publishing Company. All rights reserved; National Academy Press Website under "Reading Room," at http://www.Nap.edu (1999).

- *Choose fewer cold cuts, bacon, sausages, hot dogs, and organ meats.* Be careful of those products claiming to be "95 percent fat-free," because they may still have high levels of fat.
- *Select nonfat dairy products whenever possible.* Part-skim-milk cheeses, such as mozzarella, farmer's, lappi, and ricotta, are good choices.
- *When cooking, use substitutes for butter, margarine, oils, sour cream, mayonnaise, and salad dressings.* Chicken broths, wine, vinegar, and low-calorie dressings provide flavor with less fat.
- *Think of your food intake as an average over a day or a couple of days.* If you have a high-fat breakfast or lunch, balance it with a low-fat dinner.

Table 9.2
A Guide to Minerals

MINERAL	SIGNIFICANT SOURCES	CHIEF FUNCTIONS IN THE BODY
Calcium RDA = 800–1,200 mg+ RDI = 1,000 mg	Milk and milk products, small fish (with bones), tofu, greens, legumes	Principal mineral of bones and teeth; involved in muscle contraction and relaxation, nerve function, blood clotting, blood pressure
Phosphorus RDA = 1,000 mg	All animal tissues	Part of every cell; involved in acid–base balance
Magnesium RDA = 400 mg	Nuts, legumes, whole grains, dark green vegetables, seafood, chocolate, cocoa	Involved in bone mineralization, protein synthesis, enzyme action, normal muscular contraction, nerve transmission
Sodium RDA = 500 mg DRV = 2,400 mg	Salt, soy sauce; processed foods; cured, canned, pickled, and many boxed foods	Helps maintain normal fluid and acid-base balance
Chloride RDA = 750 mg	Salt, soy sauce; processed foods	Part of stomach acid, necessary for proper digestion, fluid balance
Potassium RDA = 2,000 mg DRV = 3,500 mg	All whole foods: meats, milk, fruits, vegetables, grains, legumes	Facilitates many reactions including protein synthesis, fluid balance, nerve transmission, and contraction of muscles
Iodine RDA = 150 μg RDI = 150 μg	Iodized salt, seafood	Part of thyroxine, which regulates metabolism
Iron RDA = 18 mg RDI = 18 mg	Beef, fish, poultry, shellfish, eggs, legumes, dried fruits	Hemoglobin formation; part of myoglobin; energy utilization
Zinc RDA = 15 mg RDI = 15 mg	Protein-containing foods: meats, fish, poultry, grains, vegetables	Part of many enzymes; present in insulin; involved in making genetic material and proteins, immunity, vitamin A transport, taste, wound healing, making sperm, normal fetal development
Copper RDA = 2 mg RDI = 2 mg	Meats, drinking water	Absorption of iron; part of several enzymes
Fluoride 1.5–4.0 mg	Drinking water (if naturally fluoride-containing or fluoridated), tea, seafood	Formation of bones and teeth; helps make teeth resistant to decay and bones resistant to mineral loss
Selenium 50–70 μg	Seafood, meats, grains	Helps protect body compounds from oxidation
Chromium 50–200 μg	Meats, unrefined foods, fats, vegetable oils	Associated with insulin and required for the release of energy from glucose
Molybdenum 75–250 μg	Legumes, cereals, organ meats	Facilitates, with enzymes, many cell processes
Manganese 2.0–5.0 mg	Widely distributed in foods	Facilitates, with enzymes, many cell processes

Trans-*Fatty Acids: Still Bad?* Since 1961, Americans have decreased their intake of butter by over 43 percent. Instead, they have substituted margarine, which became known as the "better butter" after reports labeled unsaturated fats the "heart-healthy" alternative. But a widely publicized landmark study in 1990 questioned the benefits of margarine; it indicated that margarine contains fats that raise blood choles-terol at least as much as the saturated fat in butter does.[13] The culprits? ***Trans*-fatty acids**, fatty acids having unusual shapes, are produced when polyunsaturated oils are *hydrogenated*, a process in which hydrogen is added to unsaturated fats to make them more solid and resistant to chemical change.[14] Besides raising cholesterol levels, *trans*-fatty acids have been implicated in certain types of cancer.[15]

A more recent study found that the *trans*-fatty acids found in margarine may in fact pose an even greater risk for heart disease than the saturated fat in butter and lard.[16] But before you dash out and fill your refrigerator with butter, be aware that this research is controversial.

***Trans*-fatty acids** Fatty acids that are produced when polyunsaturated oils are hydrogenated to make them more solid.

Table 9.2
A Guide to Minerals

DEFICIENCY SYMPTOMS	TOXICITY SYMPTOMS
Stunted growth in children; bone loss (osteoporosis) in adults	Excess calcium is excreted except in hormonal imbalance states
Unknown	Can create relative deficiency of calcium
Weakness, confusion, depressed pancreatic hormone secretion, growth failure, behavioral disturbances, muscle spasms	Not known
Muscle cramps, mental apathy, loss of appetite	Hypertension (in salt-sensitive persons)
Growth failure in children, muscle cramps, mental apathy, loss of appetite	Normally harmless (the gas chlorine is a poison but evaporates from water); disturbed acid-base balance; vomiting
Muscle weakness, paralysis, confusion; can cause death, accompanies dehydration	Causes muscular weakness; triggers vomiting; if given into a vein, can stop the heart
Goiter, cretinism	Very high intakes depress thyroid activity
Anemia: weakness, pallor, headaches, reduced resistance to infection, inability to concentrate	Iron overload: infections, liver injury
Growth failure in children, delayed development of sexual organs, loss of taste, poor wound healing	Fever, nausea, vomiting, diarrhea
Anemia, bone changes (rare in human beings)	Unknown except as part of a rare hereditary disease (Wilson's disease)
Susceptibility to tooth decay and bone loss	Fluorosis (discoloration of teeth)
Anemia (rare)	Digestive system disorders
Diabetes-like condition marked by inability to use glucose normally	Unknown as a nutrition disorder. Occupational exposures damage skin and kidneys
Unknown	Enzyme inhibition
In animals: poor growth, nervous system disorders, abnormal reproduction	Poisoning, nervous system disorders

Because we have less information about minerals than about vitamins, RDA recommendations are estimates of minimum requirements.

Source: Adapted by permission of Wadsworth Publishing Company from pp. 178–179 of Personal Nutrition, 2d ed., by Marie Boyle and Gail Zyla; and pp. 298–300 of Nutrition Concepts and Controversies, 5th ed., by Eva Hamilton, Eleanor Whitney, and Frances Sizer. Copyright 1994 by West Publishing Company. All rights reserved.

Keep in mind that *trans*-fatty acids, even monounsaturated acids, alter blood cholesterol the same way as some saturated fats; they raise LDL and lower HDL cholesterol.[17] The American Heart Association has steadfastly stated that because butter is rich in both saturated fat and cholesterol, whereas margarine is made from vegetable fat with no dietary cholesterol, margarine is still preferable to butter.[18] Others disagree, claiming that the occasional use of butter is preferable to margarine.[19] The majority of experts claims that the whole area of *trans*-fatty acids needs much more research. As a result, they advise that moderation in all fat intake is probably the best rule of thumb.[20] Whenever possible, opt for other condiments on your bread, using jams, fat-free cream cheese, garlic, or other toppings. Some experts advocate using low-fat salad dressings as toppings for bread and pasta, or using olive oil in moderation to add a bit of flavor. If you have high cholesterol, reducing all types of fat and cholesterol in the diet is still sound advice.

Vitamins

Vitamins are potent, essential, organic compounds that promote growth and help maintain life and health. Every minute of every day, vitamins help maintain nerves and skin, produce blood cells, build bones and teeth, heal wounds, and convert food energy to body energy. And they do all of this without adding any calories to your diet.

Age, heat, and other environmental conditions can destroy vitamins in food. Vitamins can be classified as either *fat soluble,* meaning that they are absorbed through the intestinal tract with the help of fats, or *water soluble,* meaning that they are easily dissolved in water. Vitamins A, D, E, and K are fat soluble; B complex vitamins and vitamin C are water soluble. Fat-soluble vitamins tend to be stored in the body, and toxic accumulations in the liver may cause cirrhosis-like symptoms. Water-soluble vitamins are generally excreted and cause few toxicity problems (see Table 9.1).

Despite many media suggestions to the contrary, few Americans suffer from true vitamin deficiencies if they eat a diet containing all of the food groups at least part of the time. Nevertheless, Americans continue to purchase large quantities of vitamin supplements. For the most part, vitamin supplements are unnecessary and, in certain instances, may even be harmful. Overusing them can even lead to a toxic condition known as **hypervitaminosis.**

Minerals

Minerals (see Table 9.2) are the inorganic, indestructible elements that aid physiological processes within the body. Without minerals, vitamins could not be absorbed. Minerals are readily excreted and are usually not toxic. **Macrominerals** are those minerals that the body needs in fairly large amounts: sodium, calcium, phosphorus, magnesium, potassium, sulfur, and chloride. **Trace minerals** include iron, zinc, manganese, copper, iodine, and cobalt. Only trace amounts of these minerals are needed, and serious problems may result if excesses or deficiencies occur.

Vitamins   Essential organic compounds that promote growth and reproduction and help maintain life and health.

Hypervitaminosis   A toxic condition caused by overuse of vitamin supplements.

Trace minerals   Minerals that the body needs in only very small amounts.

Minerals   Inorganic, indestructible elements that aid physiological processes.

Macrominerals   Minerals that the body needs in fairly large amounts.

Although minerals are necessary for body function, there are limits on the amounts we should consume. Americans tend to overuse or underuse certain minerals.

Sodium   Sodium is necessary for the regulation of blood and body fluids, transmission of nerve impulses, heart activity, and certain metabolic functions. However, we consume much more than we need. It is estimated that the average adult who does not sweat profusely needs only 500 milligrams of sodium (about 1/4 teaspoon) per day, yet the average American consumes 6,000 to 12,000 milligrams. The RDA Subcommittee recommends restricting sodium to no more than 2,400 milligrams per day; less is better.

The most common form of sodium in the American diet comes from table salt. However, table salt accounts for only 15 percent of sodium intake. The remainder comes from water and from highly processed foods that are infused with sodium to enhance flavor. Pickles, salty snack foods, processed cheeses, many breads and bakery products, and smoked meats and sausages often contain several hundred milligrams of sodium per serving. Many fast-food entrees and convenience entrees pack 500 to 1,000 milligrams of sodium per serving.

Many experts believe that there is a link between excessive sodium intake and hypertension (high blood pressure). Although this theory is controversial, researchers recommend that hypertensive Americans cut back on sodium to reduce their risk for cardiovascular disorders.[21] Osteoporosis researchers are confirming that high sodium intake may increase calcium loss in urine, increasing your risk for debilitating fractures as you age.

Calcium   The issue of calcium consumption has gained national attention with the rising incidence of osteoporosis among elderly women. Although calcium plays a vital role in building strong bones and teeth, muscle contraction, blood clotting, nerve impulse transmission, regulating heartbeat, and fluid balance within cells, most Americans do not consume the 1,200 milligrams of calcium per day established by the RDA.

Because calcium intake is so important throughout life for maintaining a strong bone structure, it is critical to consume the minimum required amounts each day. Over half of our calcium intake usually comes from milk, one of the highest sources of dietary calcium. New, calcium-fortified orange juice provides a good way to get calcium if you are not a milk drinker. Many green, leafy vegetables are good sources of calcium, but some contain oxalic acid, which makes their calcium harder to absorb. Spinach, chard, and beet greens are not particularly good sources of calcium, whereas broccoli, cauliflower, and many peas and beans offer good supplies (pinto beans and soybeans are among the best). Many nuts, particularly almonds, Brazil nuts, and hazelnuts, and seeds, such as sunflower and sesame, contain good amounts of calcium. Molasses is fairly high in calcium. Some fruits—such as citrus fruits, figs, raisins, and dried apricots—have moderate amounts. Bone meal is not a recommended calcium source because of possible contamination.

Do you consume carbonated soft drinks? Be aware that the added phosphoric acid (phosphate) in these drinks can cause you to excrete extra calcium, which may result in calcium being pulled out of your bones. Calcium/phosphorus imbalance may lead to kidney stones and other calcification problems as well as to increased atherosclerotic plaque.

We also know that sunlight increases the manufacture of vitamin D in the body and is therefore like having an extra calcium source because vitamin D improves absorption of calcium. Stress, however, contributes to calcium depletion. It is generally best to take calcium throughout the day, consuming it with foods containing protein, vitamin D, and vitamin C for optimum absorption. Experts vary on which type of supplemental calcium is most readily and efficiently absorbed, although aspartate and citrate salts of calcium are often recommended. The best way to obtain calcium, like all nutrients, is to consume it as part of a balanced diet.

Iron   Worldwide, iron deficiency is the most common nutrient deficiency, affecting more than 1 billion people. In developing countries, more than one third of the children and women of childbearing age suffer from *iron-deficiency anemia*.[22] **Anemia** is a problem resulting from the body's inability to produce hemoglobin, the bright red, oxygen-carrying component of the blood. In the United States iron deficiency anemia is less prevalent, but it still affects 10 percent of toddlers, adolescent girls, and women of childbearing age, making prevention a high priority.[23] People with iron-deficiency anemia may also develop a condition known as **pica,** an appetite for ice, clay, paste, and other nonfood substances that do not actually contain iron and, in fact, may inhibit iron absorption.

How much iron do adults need? Females aged 19–50 need about 18 milligrams per day, and males aged 19–50 need about 10 milligrams.

When iron deficiency occurs, body cells receive less oxygen, and carbon dioxide wastes are removed less efficiently. As a result, the iron-deficient person feels tired and run down. While iron deficiency in the diet is a common cause of anemia, anemia can also result from blood loss, cancers, ulcers, and other conditions. Generally, women are more likely to develop iron-deficiency problems because they typically eat less than men and their diets contain less iron. Women having heavy menstrual flow may be at greater risk. To date, considerable research has linked iron to a host of problems. Iron deficiency may tax the immune system, causing it to function less effectively. Research suggesting a link between cardiovascular disease and elevated iron stores is inconclusive.[24] Likewise, there appears to be a slight association between iron deficiency and cancer, but the mechanism remains inconclusive.[25]

Iron overload (known as **hemochromatosis**), or iron toxicity due to ingesting too many iron-containing supplements, remains the leading cause of accidental poisoning in small children in the United States. Symptoms of toxicity include nausea, vomiting, diarrhea, rapid heartbeat, weak pulse, dizziness, shock, and confusion. Overdoses of as few as five iron tablets containing as little as 200 milligrams of iron have killed dozens of children.

The Medicinal Value of Food

The old adage "You are what you eat" is indeed a motto to live by. Beneficial foods are now often called functional foods. This terminology is based on the ancient belief that eating the right foods may not only prevent disease, but also actually cure it. This perspective is gaining credibility among the scientific community.

Two major studies, the *Dietary Approaches to Stop Hypertension (DASH) Study* and the *Dietary Intervention Study (DIS)* provide compelling evidence that diet may be as effective as drugs in bringing borderline hypertension back to the normal range. Diet may also play a role in reducing cholesterol and controlling insulin-dependent diabetes.[26] In these clinically controlled trials, subjects were assigned to two groups: treatment and control. In the treatment group, subjects had to follow recommended diets, which were low in fats and high in fiber and fruits. The control group followed typical American dietary intervention. In each study, subjects in the treatment groups showed significantly improved health indicators (blood pressure, cholesterol, and blood glucose in the DIS study), which reflected the potential benefits of diet in improving health and treating disease.

Antioxidants: Finding the Right Balance

Antioxidants have been touted as doing everything from protecting DNA to preventing some cancers. The public, responding to these reports, has been consuming these products in droves, a trend that has many health experts alarmed. The beneficial effects of moderate doses of vitamin C appear to be well substantiated.[27] A recent British study of 30 healthy men and women showed that taking a daily 500-milligram supplement of vitamin C had both positive and negative effects on DNA. Similarly, a widely cited Finnish study of 29,000 men reported that for those who smoked a pack of cigarettes a day and took daily beta-carotene supplements, the risk of lung cancer actually increased by 18 percent over those who took no supplement.[28] Newer research on the benefits of the antioxidant compound *lycopene,* found in tomatoes and tomato-based products, indicates a possible beneficial effect as a prostate and lung cancer protector. If this conflicting information leaves you confused, you are not alone.

According to the experts, the answer is moderation. "Antioxidants should always be taken as part of a well-balanced mixture, either as a diet or as a supplement, and not singly," says Dr. John R. Smythies, a researcher at the

Anemia   Iron deficiency disease that results from the body's inability to produce hemoglobin.

Pica   Iron deficiency disease characterized by craving for certain foods and substances.

Hemochromatosis   Iron toxicity due to excess consumption.

News from the World of Nutrition Research

In May 2001, nutritional experts from the international community met for a conference titled Diet and Optimum Health, held in Portland, Oregon. Below is a synopsis of nutritional research from the last decade and summary opinion conclusions from large clinical trials or longitudinal dietary studies.

- When considered together, genetics, sedentary lifestyle, and consumption of too much dietary fat are probably not as responsible for our steep increases in obesity in the United States as the recommendation to eat less saturated fat and to eat more carbohydrates. When these recommendations hit the public media, Americans shifted to nonfat or low-fat diets and consumed more refined carbohydrates. One need only look at the ingredients of many nonfat or low-fat foods to see the hefty doses of sugars and refined starches that tempt our palates. Experts believe that in our attempts to reduce saturated fats, we may have actually increased prevalence of CVD and obesity.
- There is little support for the theory that increasing your consumption of dietary fat will increase your risk of breast or colon cancer. In fact, the highest rates of these cancers appear to be among those with the lowest overall fat intake. Experts are focusing on the type of fat we consume—not the total amount consumed—and are recommending higher rates of consumption of monounsaturated, vegetable-based fats, such as olive and canola oil. As a result of these studies, the American Heart Association is likely to move away from recommending nonfat/low-fat products, because they may actually cause people to eat more. Instead, they will focus on encouraging more olive oil and vegetable-based fats in the diet.
- Diets focusing on the glycemic index (a measure of rate of carbohydrate absorption after a meal) seem to be the most effective. Low-glycemic-index foods (which contain more complex carbohydrates, normal levels of monounsaturated fats, and reasonable amounts of proteins) suppress appetite longer, raise HDL cholesterol levels, and seem to protect against disease (hence the call for more olive oil indicated above). The new U.S. Dietary Guidelines are likely to be modified to reflect this body of work. Bad news: Potatoes don't fare well on this index. Good news: Pasta remains on the positive side of the index.
- There is dramatic new evidence that eating olive oil and other monounsaturated fats found in certain salad dressings may be protective for CVD and cancer, but if you want super protection, eating olive oil and similar fats with green, leafy vegetables (which contain nutrients that are abundant in chlorophyll) may reduce risk sevenfold.
- Increases in obesity, CVD risks, and certain cancers and diabetes may in fact be attributable in large part to displacing monounsaturated fats (e.g., olive and canola oils) with refined carbohydrates and processed sugars, as well as hydrogenated fat versions found in low-fat and nonfat foods. (Check your labels when purchasing low-fat and nonfat items at the store.)
- White tea is the hottest new food/beverage surfacing as a possible protective mechanism for cancer, particularly colon cancer. Preliminary research is indicating a sevenfold reduction in colon cancer risks and other cancers from two to three servings of white tea per day.
- Lipoic acid and acetyl carnitine (natural, not synthetic forms) have shown amazing results in mice and pig studies. (Natural forms of acetyl carnitine are currently available in health food stores, but natural forms of lipoic acid are not yet available.) When these substances are combined and given in modest doses to older animals, their brain function reverts to that of younger animals within five to six weeks. The combination of these two seems to have significant effects on the wear-and-tear of aging. Animals fed these substances regenerate brain cells as well as repairing damaged ones. Human trials will begin soon. Doses for effectiveness are not known.
- There seems to be little evidence that supplementing with chromium or selenium is of any benefit.
- Are you using vitamin E as a health aid? You may want to rethink this practice. According to antioxidant experts at this conference, newer research implicates vitamin E supplementation with reducing HDL levels and a variety of other potential risks, rather than benefits.
- Folic acid has shown promising results in reducing CVD and cancer risks. Deficiencies in folate also lead to chromosome damage.
- Researchers are gaining new information on the importance of iron. Too much or too little iron can cause damage to mitochondria and oxidative stress damage to cells.

Source: Linus Pauling Institute, Public Sessions, International Conference on Diet and Optimum Health, May 2001, Portland, Oregon.

University of California at San Diego and author of *Every Person's Guide to Antioxidants.*[29] Smythies, like many other experts, advocates balance in intake and advises that adults take 500 milligrams daily of vitamin C and 400 to 800 I.U. of vitamin E, plus 10 milligrams of beta-carotene. Other antioxidant researchers recommend 1,000 milligrams of vitamin C for the general population and more vitamin E for anyone who exercises intensely for more than an hour each day.[30] Other experts, such as Dr. Balz Frei at the Linus Pauling Institute, indicate that the "200 rule" might be the best option. This recommendation calls for fruits and vegetables in the diet and a supplement of 200 milligrams of vitamin C, 200 I.U. of vitamin E, and 200 micrograms of selenium, along with 400 micrograms of folate and 3 milligrams of

Table 9.3
Antioxidant Options for Your Daily Diet

Beta-carotene	Apricots, cantaloupe, carrots, collard greens, fennel, kale, mustard greens, peaches, pumpkin, red pepper, romaine lettuce, spinach, sweet potatoes, Swiss chard, winter squash
Vitamin C	Broccoli, Brussels sprouts, cantaloupe, cauliflower, citrus fruits, green pepper, kiwi, papaya, peaches, red cabbage, red pepper, strawberries, potatoes
Vitamin E	Wheat germ, seeds, nuts, dark green leafy vegetables, avocados, peanuts, sweet potatoes
Lycopene	Tomatoes, apricots, guava, pink grapefruit, mango, oranges, peaches, papaya, watermelon
Lutein/zexanthin	Dark leafy green vegetables, especially spinach and broccoli
Flavonoids	Apples, citrus fruits, flaxseed, lentils, onions, peanuts, rice, soybeans, blueberries, cranberries, currants, olive oil, red wine, green tea, chamomile tea, black tea
Polyphenols	Chocolate, coffee, grapes, nuts, oranges, strawberries, green tea, black tea, red wine

vitamin B_6.[31] It is believed that these combinations will reduce the body's overproduction of free radicals, those unstable molecules that can damage healthy cells and turn low-density lipoproteins into artery-clogging compounds.[32] However, even the lowering of free radicals is controversial. Many believe that free radicals are beneficial and work to kill germs in the same way they kill other cells. From this standpoint, killing off free radicals may lower resistance to harmful pathogens.[33] See Table 9.3 for suggested sources of various antioxidants. To find the right balance, keep in mind the following:

- Adults should keep their daily vitamin C intake from both food and supplements below 2,000 milligrams because anything higher may cause diarrhea.
- The upper limit for vitamin E, based only on supplements, is 1,000 milligrams. That's roughly equivalent to 1,500 I.U. of D-alpha-tocopherol, sometimes labeled *natural vitamin E*. More than these amounts could increase the risk of stroke and uncontrolled bleeding. Additionally, new research indicates that the purported benefits of vitamin E may be grossly overexaggerated.[34]
- The maximum intake level for selenium from both food and supplements is 400 micrograms per day. More than this amount could cause *selenosis,* a toxic reaction marked by hair loss and brittle nails.

Folate

In 1998, the Food and Drug Administration (FDA) took a major dietary plunge by mandating *folate* fortification of all bread, cereal, rice, and macaroni products sold in the United States. This practice, which will boost folate intake by an average of about 100 micrograms daily, is expected to decrease the number of infants born with spina bifida and other neural tube defects.

Folate is a form of vitamin B that is believed to be protective for cardiovascular disease and decreases blood levels of *homocysteine,* an amino acid that has been linked to vascular diseases.[35] Homocysteine results from the breakdown of methionine, an amino acid found in meat and other protein-laden foods. Two B vitamins—folate and B_6—are believed to control homocysteine levels.[36] When intake of folate and B_6 is low, homocysteine levels rise in the blood. Recent studies indicate that when the level of homocysteine rises, arterial walls and blood platelets become sticky, which encourages clotting. (Note: Homocysteine levels tend to rise with age, smoking, and menopause.) When clots develop in areas already narrowed by atherosclerosis, a heart attack or stroke is likely.

Although the amount of folate needed to protect the heart has not been determined, many adults have jumped on the folate bandwagon, taking daily folate supplements of up to 800 micrograms. Recently, a new *dietary folate equivalent (DFE)* was established to distinguish folate in food from its synthetic counterpart, *folic acid.* As a food additive or a supplement, folic acid is absorbed about twice as efficiently as folate. The DFE for folate in women age 19 or over is approximately 400 micrograms, with higher levels for pregnant or lactating women. (See Table 9.1 for daily recommended amounts of other B vitamins.) Potential dangers of taking too much folate include a masking of B_{12} deficiencies and resulting problems, ranging from nerve damage, immunodeficiency problems, anemia, fatigue, and headache, to constipation, diarrhea, weight loss, gastrointestinal disturbances, and a host of neurological symptoms.[37]

> **Folate** A type of vitamin B that is believed to decrease levels of homocysteine, an amino acid that has been linked to vascular diseases.

Gender and Nutrition

Men and women differ in body size, body composition, and overall metabolic rates. They therefore have differing needs for most nutrients throughout the life cycle (see Tables 9.1 and 9.2 on vitamin and mineral requirements) and face unique difficulties in keeping on track with their dietary goals. Some of these differences have already been discussed. However, there are some factors that need further consideration. Have you ever wondered why men can eat more than women without gaining weight? Although there are many possible reasons, one factor is that women have a lower ratio of lean body mass to adipose (fatty) tissue at all ages and stages of life. Also, after sexual maturation, the rate of metabolism is higher in men, meaning that they will burn more calories doing the same things women do.

Different Cycles, Different Needs

In addition to these differences, women have many more "landmark" times in life when their nutritional needs vary significantly from requirements at other times. From menarche to menopause, women undergo cyclical physiological changes that can exert dramatic effects on metabolism and nutritional needs. For example, during pregnancy and lactation, women's nutritional requirements increase substantially. Those who are unable to follow the strict dietary recommendations of their doctors may find themselves gaining much more weight during pregnancy and retaining it afterwards. During the menstrual cycle, many women report significant food cravings. Later in life, with the advent of menopause, nutritional needs again change rather dramatically. With depletion of the hormone estrogen, the body's need for calcium to ward off bone deterioration becomes pronounced. Women must pay closer attention to exercise patterns and to getting enough calcium through diet or dietary supplements, or they run the risk of osteoporosis.

Changing the "Meat and Potatoes Man"

Although men do not have the same cyclical patterns and dietary needs as women, they do suffer from a heritage of dietary excesses that are difficult to change. Since our earliest agrarian years, many Americans have relied on a "meat and potatoes" diet. What's wrong with all those hot dogs, steaks, and hamburgers? Heart disease, stroke, and cancer are probably the greatest threats. Add increased risks for colon and prostate cancers, and the rationale for dietary change becomes even more compelling. Consider the following points:

- Men who eat red meat as a main dish five or more times a week have four times the risk of colon cancer of men who eat red meat less than once a month.
- Heavy red meat eaters are more than twice as likely to get prostate cancer and nearly five times more likely to get colon cancer.

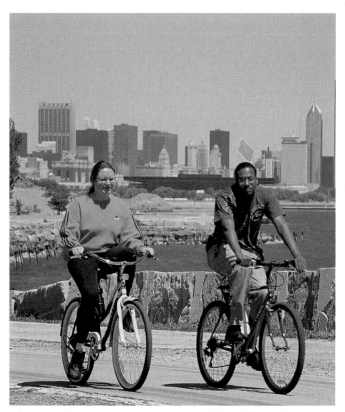

Because men and women metabolize food differently, particularly during certain periods in life, their nutritional needs also differ. Regular exercise can help both men and women manage their weight and maximize their energy.

- For every three servings of fruits or vegetables they consume per day, men can expect a 22 percent lower risk of stroke.
- Diets high in fruit and vegetables may lower the risk of lung cancer in smokers from 20 times the risk of nonsmokers to "only" ten times the risk. They may also protect against oral, throat, pancreatic, and bladder cancers, all of which are more common among smokers.
- The fastest-rising malignancy in the United States is cancer of the lower esophagus, particularly among white men. Though obesity seems to be a factor, fruits and vegetables are the protectors. (The average American male eats fewer than three servings per day, although five to nine servings are recommended. Women average three to seven servings per day.)

Does something in meat make it inherently bad? The fat content of meat and fried potatoes and the potential carcinogenic substances produced through cooking have been implicated. Probably something more basic is also involved. By eating so much protein, a person fills up sooner and never gets around to the fruits and vegetables. Thus, the potential protective value of consuming these foods is lost.

Determining Nutritional Needs

Determining the right amount of a nutrient that people of different ages, sex, activity levels, or physical conditions must obtain daily is no easy task. Since the early 1940s, various committees have devised several standards for nutritional needs.

Recommended Dietary Allowances—Adequate Intake For more than 50 years, a document called the **Recommended Dietary Allowances (RDAs)** has been the gold standard for nutrient intake in the United States.[38] Established by the Committee on Dietary Allowances, the RDAs are the average daily intakes of energy and nutrients considered adequate to meet the needs of most healthy people in the United States under usual conditions. Revised every five years, the RDAs reflect the fact that a person's need for a nutrient can be influenced by age, sex, body size, growth, and reproductive status. Thus, pregnant and lactating women have their own set of RDAs. Today, RDAs are based on the quantity necessary to provide health benefits. When evidence doesn't support an RDA, **Adequate Intakes (AIs)** are used as the best estimates of nutritional needs.

Daily Values, RDIs, and DRVs From the RDAs came the more familiar U.S. RDA (U.S. Recommended Daily Allowances) established by the Food and Drug Administration (FDA). The U.S. RDAs were set as maximum values to account for potential nutrient loss during absorption, cooking, and storage of food. People followed the U.S. RDAs for years until the entire system was overhauled and made even more specific for consumers. In 1993, the FDA supplemented most U.S. RDAs with "% Daily Values," a set of standard values that represents the nutrient needs of the typical consumer. Daily Values consist of two reference values. The first, the Reference Daily Intake (RDI), reflects the average daily allowances for proteins, vitamins, and minerals based on the RDA. The second, the Daily Reference Values (DRV), covers nutrients and food components, such as fat and fiber, that do not have an established RDA but are highly correlated with health. At the same time the new Daily Values were issued, the FDA also issued a new food label that is now familiar to most consumers. Some of the RDIs and DRVs are included with the Daily Value information now found on food labels.

> ### What do you think?
> *Of all of the nutrients discussed in this section, which one is most lacking in your diet?* ✳ *Why should this lack concern you?* ✳ *What actions can you take to make sure your daily intake is adequate?*

Vegetarianism: Eating for Health

For aesthetic, animal rights, economic, personal, health, cultural, or religious reasons, some people choose specialized diets. Between 5 and 15 percent of all Americans today claim to be vegetarians. Normally, vegetarianism provides a

Reading food labels before you purchase food will help you make smart nutritional choices.

superb alternative to our high-fat, high-calorie, meat-based cuisine, but without proper information and food choices, vegetarians can also develop dietary problems.

The term **vegetarian** means different things to different people. Strict vegetarians, or *vegans,* avoid all foods of

---

Recommended Dietary Allowances (RDAs) The average daily intakes of energy and nutrients considered adequate to meet the needs of most healthy people in the United States under usual conditions.

Adequate Intakes (AIs) Best estimates of nutritional needs.

Vegetarian A term with a variety of meanings: *vegans* avoid all foods of animal origin; *lacto-vegetarians* avoid flesh foods but eat dairy products; *ovo-vegetarians* avoid flesh foods but eat eggs; *lacto-ovo-vegetarians* avoid flesh foods but eat both dairy products and eggs; *pesco-vegetarians* avoid meat but eat fish, dairy products, and eggs; *semivegetarians* eat chicken, fish, dairy products, and eggs.

animal origin, including dairy products and eggs. Vegans must be careful to obtain all of the necessary nutrients. Far more common are *lacto-vegetarians*, who eat dairy products but avoid flesh foods. Their diet can be low in fat and cholesterol, but only if they consume skim milk and other low-fat or nonfat products. *Ovo-vegetarians* add eggs to their diet, while *lacto-ovo-vegetarians* eat both dairy products and eggs. *Pesco-vegetarians* eat fish, dairy products, and eggs, while *semivegetarians* eat chicken, fish, dairy products, and eggs. Some people in the semivegetarian category prefer to call themselves "non–red meat eaters."

Generally, people who follow a balanced vegetarian diet weigh less and have better cholesterol levels, fewer problems with irregular bowel movements (constipation and diarrhea), and a lower risk of heart disease than do nonvegetarians. Some preliminary evidence suggests that vegetarians may also have a reduced risk for colon and breast cancer.[39] Whether these lower risks are due to the vegetarian diet per se or to some combination of lifestyle variables remains unclear.[40]

Although in the past vegetarians often suffered from vitamin deficiencies, the vegetarian of the new millennium is usually extremely adept at combining the right types of foods to ensure proper nutrient intake. People who eat dairy products and small amounts of chicken or fish are seldom nutrient-deficient; in fact, while vegans typically get 50 to 60 grams of protein per day, lacto-ovo-vegetarians normally consume between 70 and 90 grams per day, well beyond the RDA. Vegan diets may be deficient in vitamins B_2 (riboflavin), B_{12}, and D. Riboflavin is found mainly in meat, eggs, and dairy products; however, broccoli, asparagus, almonds, and fortified cereals are also good sources. Vitamins B_{12} and D are found only in dairy products and fortified products such as soy milk. Vegans are also at risk for deficiencies of calcium, iron, zinc, and other minerals, but they can obtain these nutrients from supplements. Strict vegans have to pay much more attention to what they eat than the average person does, but by eating complementary combinations of plant products, they can receive adequate amounts of essential amino acids. Examples of complementary combinations are corn and beans, and peanut butter and whole-grain bread. Eating a full variety of grains, legumes, fruits, vegetables, and seeds each day will help to keep even the strictest vegetarian in excellent health. Pregnant women, the elderly, the sick, and children who are vegans need to take special care to ensure that their diets are adequate. People who take part in heavy aerobic exercise programs (over three hours per week) may need to increase their protein consumption. In all cases, seek advice from a health care professional if you have questions.

The Vegetarian Pyramid

Dr. Arlene Spark, a nutritionist at New York Medical College, has devised a food guide pyramid that conveys the essentials of a vegetarian diet. Modeled after the USDA Food Guide Pyramid discussed earlier in this chapter, the vegetarian version clarifies what people who don't eat meat need to do to stay healthy. The vegetarian pyramid defines the fol-

lowing categories. We include examples of single servings in each category:

Grains and Starchy Vegetables Group (6–11 servings/day)
- 1 slice bread
- $\frac{1}{2}$ roll or bagel
- 1 tortilla (6-inch)
- 1 ounce cold cereal
- $\frac{1}{2}$ cup cooked cereal, rice, or pasta
- 3–4 crackers
- 3 cups popcorn
- $\frac{1}{2}$ cup corn
- 1 medium potato
- $\frac{1}{2}$ cup green peas

Vegetable Group (3 + servings/day)
- $\frac{1}{2}$ cup cooked or chopped raw vegetables
- 1 cup raw leafy vegetables
- $\frac{3}{4}$ cup vegetable juice

Fruit Group (2–4 servings/day)
- 1 medium whole piece of fruit
- $\frac{1}{2}$ cup canned, chopped, or cooked fruit
- $\frac{3}{4}$ cup fruit juice

Milk and Milk Substitutes Group (3 servings/day for preteens and 4 for teens; 2–4 servings/day for adults)
- 1 cup milk or yogurt
- 1 cup calcium- and vitamin B_{12}-fortified soy milk
- $1\frac{1}{2}$ ounces hard cheese
- $1\frac{1}{2}$ ounces calcium- and vitamin B_{12}-fortified soy cheese

Meat/Fish Substitutes Group (2–3 servings/day)
- 1 cup cooked dry beans, peas, or lentils
- 2 eggs
- 8 ounces bean curd or tofu
- $\frac{1}{2}$ cup shelled nuts
- 3–4 tablespoons peanut butter
- 3–4 tablespoons tahini
- $\frac{1}{3}$ to $\frac{1}{2}$ cup seeds

Vegans Must Consume Daily
- 3–5 teaspoons vegetable oil + 1 tablespoon blackstrap molasses + 1 tablespoon brewer's yeast

> **What do you think?**
> *Why are so many people today becoming vegetarians?* ✳ *How easy is it to be a vegetarian on your campus?* ✳ *What concerns about vegetarianism would you have, if any?* ✳ *What difficulties might you face in adjusting your lifestyle to a vegan lifestyle?*

Improved Eating for the College Student

College students often face a challenge when trying to eat healthy foods. Some students live in dorms and do not have their own cooking or refrigeration facilities. Others live in crowded apartments where everyone forages in the refrigerator for everyone else's food. Still others eat at university food services where food choices may be limited. Most students have financial and time constraints that make buying, preparing, and eating healthy food a difficult task. What's a student to do?

Eating on the Run

If your campus is like many others, you've probably noticed a distinct move toward fast-food restaurants in your student unions, so that they now resemble the food courts found in most major shopping malls. These new eating centers fit student's needs for a fast bite of food at a reasonable price between classes and also bring in money to your school. Many fast foods are high in fat and sodium. But are all fast foods unhealthy? Not all fast foods are created equal and not all are bad for you. Even at the often-maligned burger chains, menus are healthier than ever before and offer excellent choices for the discriminating eater. The key word here is *discriminating*. It really is possible to eat healthy food if you follow these suggestions:

- Ask for nutritional analyses of items. Most fast-food chains now have them. For your convenience, we have included a summary of many of these analyses in Appendix C at the end of this book.
- Avoid mayonnaise, sauces, and other add-ons. Some places even have fat-free mayonnaise if you ask. Put a hold on extra ketchup.
- Hold the cheese. This extra contributes substantially to total fat while not adding a lot to taste.
- Order single, small burgers rather than large, high-calorie, bacon- or cheese-topped choices. Put on your own ketchup, and keep portions small.
- Order salads and be careful how much dressing you put on. Many people think they are being health-smart by eating salad, only to load it with calorie- and fat-rich dressing. Try the vinegar and oil or low-fat alternative dressings. Stay away from eggs and other high-fat add-ons, such as bacon bits.
- When ordering a chicken sandwich, order the skinless broiled version rather than the deep-fried version. Many people think that the deep-fried chicken sandwich is a more healthy choice when it really has more fat than the loaded double burger.
- Check to see what type of oil is used to cook fries, if you must have them. Avoid lard-based or other saturated fat products.
- Order the wheat buns or bread, and ask them to hold the butter.
- Avoid fried foods in general, including hot apple pies and other crust-based fried foods.
- Opt for places where foods tend to be broiled rather than fried.

When Funds Are Short

Maintaining a nutritious diet within the confines of student life can be challenging. However, if you take the time to plan healthy meals, you will find that you are eating better, enjoying your food more, and actually saving money. Follow these steps to ensure a healthy but affordable diet:

- Buy fruits and vegetables in season whenever possible for their lower cost, higher nutrient quality, and greater variety.
- Use coupons and specials to get price reductions.
- Shop at discount warehouse food chains; capitalize on volume discounts and no-frills products.
- Plan ahead to get the most for your dollar and avoid extra trips to the store; extra trips usually mean extra purchases. Make a list, and stick to it.
- Purchase meats and other products in volume, freezing portions for future needs. Or purchase small amounts of meats and other expensive proteins and combine them with beans and plant proteins for lower cost, calories, and fat.
- Cook large meals, and freeze small portions for later use.
- Drain off extra fat after cooking. Save juices to use in soups and other dishes.
- If you find that you have no money for food, talk to staff at your county or city health department. They may know of ways for you to get assistance.

What do you think?

*What problems cause you the most difficulty when you try to eat more healthful foods? * Are these problems typical in your family, or are they unique to your situation as a student? * What actions can you take to improve your current eating practices?*

Food Safety: A Growing Concern

As we become increasingly worried that the food we put in our mouths may be contaminated with bacteria, insects, worms, or other substances, the food industry has come under fire. To convince us that their products are safe, some manufacturers have come up with "new and improved" ways of protecting our foods. How well do they work?

Food-Borne Illnesses

Are you concerned that the chicken you are buying doesn't look pleasingly pink, or that your "fresh" fish smells a little *too* fishy or has a grayish tinge? Are you *sure* that your apple juice is free of animal wastes? You may have good reason to be worried. In increasing numbers, Americans are becoming sick from what they eat, and many of these illnesses are life threatening. Scientists estimate, based on several studies conducted over the past 10 years, that food-borne pathogens sicken between 6.5 and 81 million people and cause some 9,000 deaths in the United States annually.[41] Because most of us don't go to the doctor every time we are sick, we may not make a connection between what we eat and later symptoms.

Signs of food-borne illnesses vary tremendously and usually include one or several symptoms: diarrhea, nausea, cramping, and vomiting. Depending on the amount and virulence of the pathogen, symptoms may appear as early as 30 minutes after eating contaminated food, or as long as several days or weeks. Most of the time, symptoms occur five to eight hours after eating and last only a day or two. For certain populations, however, such as the very young or very old or persons with AIDS or other severe illnesses, food-borne diseases can be fatal.

Several factors may be contributing to the increase in food-borne illnesses. According to Michael T. Osterholm, Ph.D., state epidemiologist in Minneapolis,[42] the movement away from a traditional meat-and-potato American diet to "heart-healthy" eating—increasing consumption of fruits, vegetables, and grains—has spurred demand for fresh foods that are not in season most of the year. This means that we must import fresh fruits and vegetables, thus putting ourselves at risk for ingesting exotic pathogens. Depending on the season, up to 70 percent of the fruits and vegetables consumed in the United States come from Mexico alone. The upshot is that a visit to developing countries isn't necessary to be stricken with food-borne "traveler's diarrhea" because the produce does the traveling.[43] Although when we travel to developing countries, we are told to "boil it, peel it, or don't eat it," we bring these foods into our kitchens and eat them often without even basic washing.[44] Food can become contaminated by being watered with contaminated water, fertilized with "organic" fertilizers (animal manure), and not subjected to the same rigorous pesticide regulations as American-raised produce. To give you an idea of the implications, studies have shown that *Escherichia coli* (a lethal bacterial pathogen) can survive in cow manure for up to 70 days and can multiply in foods grown with manure unless heat or additives such as salt or preservatives are used to kill the microbes.[45] There are essentially no regulations that say farmers can't use animal manure in growing their crops. Turkey manure, pig manure, and other agribusiness by-products are often sprayed on fields that ultimately grow foods for consumers.

Key factors associated with the increasing spread of food-borne diseases include the following:[46]

- *Globalization of the food supply.* Because the food supply is distributed worldwide, the possibility of exposure to pathogens native to remote regions of the world is greater. For example, a large outbreak of *Shigella* occurred in Norway, Sweden, and the United Kingdom from lettuce that originated in southern Europe.
- *Inadvertent introduction of pathogens into new geographic regions.* One theory is that cholera was introduced into waters off the coast of the southern United States when a

cargo ship discharged contaminated ballast as it came into harbor. Other pathogens may enter into aquatic life in a similar manner.
- *Exposure to unfamiliar food-borne hazards.* Travelers, refugees, and immigrants who move through foreign countries are exposed to food-borne hazards and bring them home with them.
- *Changes in microbial populations.* Changing microbial populations can lead to the evolution of new pathogens. As a result, old pathogens develop new virulence factors or become resistant to antibiotics, making diseases more difficult to treat.
- *Increased susceptibility of varying populations.* People are becoming more vulnerable to disease. The numbers of highly susceptible persons are expanding worldwide because of aging populations, HIV infection, and other underlying medical conditions, such as malnutrition and the compromised health status that results from the use of immunosuppressive drugs. High birth rates and increased longevity have increased the numbers of vulnerable populations at the margins.
- *Insufficient education about food safety.* Increased urbanization, industrialization, and travel, combined with more people eating out, raise the risk of unsafe food handling and illness.

Responsible Use: Avoiding Risks in the Home

Part of the responsibility for preventing food-borne illness lies with consumers—over 30 percent of all such illnesses result from unsafe handling of food at home.

- When shopping, pick up packaged and canned foods first, and save frozen foods and perishables such as meat, poultry, and fish for last.
- Check for cleanliness at the salad bar and meat and fish counters.
- When shopping for fish, buy from markets that get their supplies from state-approved sources.
- Most cuts of meat, fish, and poultry should be kept in the refrigerator no more than one or two days.
- Eat leftovers within three days.
- Keep hot foods hot and cold foods cold.
- Use a thermometer to ensure that meats are completely cooked. Beef and lamb should be cooked to at least 140°F, pork to 150°F, and poultry to 165°F. Don't eat poultry that is pink inside.
- Fish is done when the thickest part becomes opaque and the fish flakes easily when poked with a fork.
- Never leave cooked food standing on the stove or table for more than two hours.
- Never thaw frozen foods at room temperature.
- Wash your hands and countertop with soap and water when preparing food, particularly after handling meat, fish, or poultry.

- When freezing foods like chicken, make sure juices can't spill over into ice cubes or into other areas of the refrigerator.

Food Irradiation: How Safe Is It?

Each year, thousands of people get sick from largely preventable diseases such as that caused by *E. coli* as well as other bacteria such as *Salmonella* and *Listeria*. In response to these illnesses, in February 2000 the USDA approved large-scale irradiation of beef, lamb, poultry, pork, and other raw animal foods. **Food irradiation** is a process that involves treating foods with gamma radiation from radioactive cobalt, cesium, or other sources of x-rays. When foods are irradiated, they are exposed to low doses of radiation, or ionizing energy, which breaks chemical bonds in the DNA of harmful bacteria, destroying the pathogens and keeping them from replicating. The rays essentially pass through the food without leaving any radioactive residue.[47]

Some companies use cobalt 60, a radioactive substance, for irradiation, but others are beginning to use a new kind of irradiation that dispenses with radioactive compounds and uses electricity as the energy source instead. Thus, as foods pass along a conveyor belt, the energy used to kill bacteria comes from electron beams rather than gamma rays.[48] Irradiation lengthens food products' shelf life and prevents the spread of deadly microorganisms, particularly in high-risk foods such as ground beef and pork. Thus, the minimal costs of irradiation should result in lower overall costs to consumers, in addition to reducing the need for toxic chemicals now used to preserve foods and prevent contamination from external pathogens.

Food irradiation has been approved for potatoes, spices, pork carcasses, and fruits and vegetables since the mid-1980s. Some environmentalists and consumer groups have raised concerns, so irradiated products are not common fare. However, the facts appear to support the use of irradiation.

Food Additives

Additives generally reduce the risk of food-borne illness (i.e., nitrates added to cured meats), prevent spoilage, and enhance the ways foods look and taste. Additives can also enhance nutrient value, especially to benefit the general public. A deficiency can be a terrible public health problem, and a solution is relatively easy to administer. The fortification of milk with vitamin D serves as a perfect example. Many other such examples exist. One of the newest additives to our daily food is folate, one of the B vitamins. Produced by plants and yeasts, folate is believed to offer many health benefits, reducing the risk of neural tube defects, certain anemias, cervical dysplasia, and heart attacks. According to the FDA and the U.S. Public Health Service, folate's benefits have been proved again and again in observational and clinical trials. In 1992, the U.S. Public Health Service recommended folate for all women who might become pregnant. All women should get 180 micrograms per day, and if pregnant, 400 micrograms per day. The best sources of folate are fruits and vegetables, particularly beans, spinach, and broccoli. Many multivitamin supplements also supply this amount. Recently, the Public Health Service took the recommendation one step further by approving the addition of folate to flour.

Although the FDA regulates additives according to effectiveness, safety, and ability to detect them in foods, questions have been raised about those additives put into foods intentionally and those that get in unintentionally before or after processing.

Intentional Food Additives
- Antimicrobial agents: substances such as salt, sugar, nitrates, and others that tend to make foods less hospitable for microbes.
- Antioxidants: substances that preserve color and flavor by reducing loss due to exposure to oxygen. Vitamins C and E are among those antioxidants believed to play a role in reducing the risk of cancer and cardiovascular disease. BHA and BHT are additives that also are antioxidant in action.
- Artificial colors.
- Nutrient additives.

Indirect Food Additives
- Substances that inadvertently get into food products from packaging and/or handling.
- Dioxins: found in coffee filters, milk containers, and frozen foods.
- Methylene chloride: found in decaffeinated coffee.
- Hormones: bovine growth hormone (BGH) found in animal meat.

Whenever such products are added, consumers should take the time to determine what the substances are and whether there are alternatives. As a general rule of thumb, the fewer chemicals, colorants, and preservatives, the better. Also, certain foods and additives have an effect on medications. Being aware of these potential dietary interactions is a key to wise consumerism. See Table 9.4 for specific information on common food-medication interactions.

Food Allergies: On the Increase

Once believed to be a rare event, approximately 5 percent of all children in the United States and more than 10 percent of all adults may have an allergic reaction to something they eat. Typical culprits include milk, eggs, peanuts, soybeans, tree nuts, fish and shellfish, and wheat. Reactions can range from minor rashes to severe swelling in the mouth, tongue, and

---

Food irradiation Treating foods with gamma radiation from radioactive cobalt, cesium, or some other source of x-rays to kill microorganisms.

Table 9.4
Common Food–Medication Interactions

Interactions are listed by drug category, followed by examples of specific medications (with generic and brand names). As always, alert your physician and pharmacist to any over-the-counter medications, herbal remedies and supplements you are taking.

MEDICATIONS	INTERACTIONS WITH FOODS/NUTRIENTS	WHAT TO DO
Antibiotics ciprofloxacin (*Cipro*) doxycycline (*Vibramycin*) minocycline (*Minocin*) tetracycline (*Achromycin-V, surrycin*) penicillin (*Ledercillin*)	• Calcium and iron bind with these drugs, inhibiting absorption of the drug plus the calcium and iron. Results in less antibiotic effect, risking the possibility that the bacteria causing the infection will not be killed. • Food slows down absorption of the drug.	• Do not take within three hours of taking calcium-containing antacids, iron supplements or multivitamin/minerals. • Do not take ciprofloxacin or tetracycline with foods rich in calcium, such as milk and other dairy products. • Take an hour before or two hours after eating.
Cardiovascular Medications **ACE Inhibitors:** captopril (*Capoten*) enalapril (*Vasotec*) lisinopril (*Prinivil, Zestril*) moexipril (*Univasc*)	• Some ACE inhibitors cause hyperkalemia (elevated blood potassium). • Licorice can disrupt potassium balance. • Chili pepper worsens persistent cough side effect. • Food decreases absorption of captopril and moexipril.	• Limit potassium-rich foods (see above) and salt substitutes containing potassium. • Avoid natural licorice. • Avoid chili pepper. • Take captopril, moexipril an hour before or two hours after eating.
Blood Thinners: warfarin (*Coumadin*)	• Vitamin K reduces the effectiveness of anticoagulants. If you maintain a consistent intake of vitamin K, your doctor can adjust your medication level accordingly.	• Keep a consistent intake of vitamin K-rich foods: broccoli, spinach, kale, turnip greens, Swiss chard, cauliflower, Brussels sprouts, asparagus, beet and chicken liver.
Calcium Channel Blockers: amlodipine (*Norvasc*) felodipine (*Plendil*) nifedipine (*Adalat, Procardia*)	• Licorice can increase potassium excretion, sodium reabsorption and raise blood pressure. • Grapefruit can increase blood levels of these drugs up to twofold, causing blood pressure to drop dangerously low.	• Avoid natural licorice. • Avoid grapefruit, grapefruit juice and Seville oranges.
HMG-CoA Reductase Inhibitors ("statins"): atorvastatin (*Lipitor*) lovastatin (*Mevacor*) simvastatin (*Zocor*)	• Grapefruit significantly increases blood levels of the drug, causing more side effects or toxicity. • Soluble fiber inhibits absorption of lovastatin. • Lovastatin best absorbed with a big meal containing fat. Works best when asleep.	• Avoid grapefruit, grapefruit juice and Seville oranges. • Don't eat foods rich in fiber, oat bran or pectin within several hours of taking lovastatin. • If taken once a day, take lovastatin with the evening meal.
Diuretics **Potassium-Losing Diuretics:** lurosumide (*Lasix*) hydrochlorothiazide (*HydroDIURIL*)	• Cause a loss of potassium and magnesium, requiring extra potassium and magnesium in the diet or supplements. A potassium deficiency can trigger a heart attack. • Licorice can cause a loss of potassium.	• Eat plenty of potassium-rich foods; apricots, bananas, cantaloupe, dairy foods, dried beans, lentils, oranges, tomatoes. • Eat magnesium-rich foods: bananas, dried beans, lentils, nuts. • Avoid natural licorice.
Potassium-Sparing Diuretics: spironolactone (*Aldactone*)	• Prevent kidneys from excreting potassium. Taking in too much potassium can cause irregular heartbeat. • Licorice can disrupt potassium balance.	• Don't overdo foods rich in potassium (see above). • Avoid salt substitutes that contain potassium. • Avoid natural licorice.
Psychotherapeutic Medications buspirone (*Buspar*)—treats anxiety	• Grapefruit significantly increases blood levels of the drug.	• Avoid grapefruit, grapefruit juice and Seville oranges.

Table 9.4
Common Food–Medication Interactions

MEDICATIONS	INTERACTIONS WITH FOODS/NUTRIENTS	WHAT TO DO
Mononamine Oxidase Inhibitors (MAOIs): isocarboxazid (*Marplan*) phenelzine (*Nardil*) tranylcypromine (*Parmate*)	• Combining with too much caffeine, beer or wine (even alcohol-free) or foods rich in tyramine can lead to a dangerous increase in blood pressure.	• Avoid excessive caffeine; use with caution. Avoid foods rich in tyramine: aged cheeses and meats, beer, fava beans, sauerkraut, soy sauce, wine. Use small amounts of beer (one or two 12-oz. bottles a day) and wine (2 to 4 oz. a day) with caution.
Other Medications cilostazol (*Pletal*)— treats circulatory conditions	• Grapefruit significantly increases blood levels of the drug, causing increased side effects or drug toxicity.	• Avoid grapefruit, grapefruit juice and Seville oranges.
colchicine—treats gout	• Grapefruit significantly increases blood levels of the drug.	• Avoid grapefruit, grapefruit juice and Seville oranges.
levodopa (*Dopar, Larodopa, Sinernet*)— treats Parkinson's disease	• Pyridoxine decreases effectiveness of the drug. Keep pyridoxine (vitamin B_6) intake to less than 5 mg a day.	• Limit foods rich in pyridoxine: chicken, fish, pork, liver and kidney. Go easy on legumes, nuts and whole grains.
theophylline (*Slo-bid, Theobid, Elixophyllin, Theo-Dur, Uniphyl*)— treats asthma and other pulmonary disorders.	• Caffeine increases theophylline's side effects: dizziness, nausea, vomiting convulsions or coma.	• Avoid excessive caffeine (e.g. coffee, tea, cola).
	• Black pepper and chili pepper increase drug blood levels.	• Avoid excessive black pepper or chili pepper.
	• Amount of protein and carbohydrate in diet can alter enzyme levels that affect theophylline breakdown.	• Keep intake of protein and carbohydrate consistent to keep drug levels consistent.

oz = ounces   mg = milligrams

Source: Reprinted by permission of *Environmental Nutrition* magazine, from K. Neville, "Foods, Too, Can Interfere with Medications, If You're Not Careful," *Environmental Nutrition* (November 2001). Data from *Food Medication Interactions—12th edition* (2002: available at 800-746-2324); *Food & Drug Interactions* (Food and Drug Administration with National Consumers League. 1998, online updated 2000; available at http:// ~irdilfainter.html): interviews with Zaneta Pronsky, M.S., R.D., F.A.D.A., Sr. Jeanne Crowe, Pharm D., R.Ph. and Dean Elbe, B.Sc. © Copyright, 2001 by Environmental Nutrition, Inc., New York, NY: www.environmentalnutrition.com

throat to violent vomiting and diarrhea, and, occasionally, death. Emergency rooms throughout the country report rapid increases in the number of incidents tied to food allergies.

Food allergies occur when a person's body treats a specific food, usually a protein, as an invader or a threat. The body's immune system kicks into high gear and tries to rid the body of the problem by using typical immune system responses. The first signs are typically rapid breathing or wheezing, hives, rash, eczema, or a chronic runny nose. More dramatic symptoms include facial swelling or respiratory problems related to *anaphylactic reaction,* which require a shot of epinephrine, a hormone that stimulates the heart and relieves overt symptoms.

If you have been diagnosed with a food allergy, look for a nutrition specialist (with a degree or academic training in nutrition) who can help with necessary dietary adjustments. Also, many apparent reactions to foods are really not allergic reactions per se, but may instead point to one of the following problems:

• **Food intolerance** occurs in people who lack certain digestive chemicals and suffer adverse effects when they consume substances that their bodies have difficulty in breaking down. A common example is lactose intolerance, experienced by people who do not have the digestive chemicals needed to break down the lactose in milk.
• Reactions to food additives, such as sulfites and MSG.

Food allergies   Overreaction by the body to normally harmless proteins, which are perceived as allergens. In response, the body produces antibodies, triggering allergic symptoms.

Food intolerance   Adverse effects resulting when people who lack the digestive chemicals needed to break down certain substances eat those substances.

- Reactions to substances occurring naturally in some foods, such as tyramine in cheese, phenylethylamine in chocolate, caffeine in coffee, and some compounds in alcoholic beverages.
- Food-borne illnesses.
- Unknown reactions in people who have adverse symptoms that they attribute to foods. The symptoms may subside when treated as allergies, but there is no evidence of a physiological basis for them.

Organic Foods

Mounting concerns about food safety have led many people to refuse to buy processed foods and mass-produced agricultural products. Instead, they purchase foods that are **organically grown**—foods reported to be pesticide- and chemical-free. Though they are sold at premium prices, many of these products are of only average quality. When purchasing these products, consumers must consider cost, in light of several factors.

First, whether food has been exposed to pesticides at some time in the production cycle is not as important as the residual pesticides in the food at the time you consume it. Obviously, too much of anything is potentially harmful, but if a "nonorganic" food has been sprayed and the poison has since evaporated, changed into a nontoxic compound, or been diluted below the point at which it can do any harm, the food may be no more harmful than a product labeled as "organic."

Second, even though so-called organic foods generally claim to be pesticide-free, tests indicate that many contain the same amount of pesticide residues as nonorganic foods. These traces may be the result of pesticide drift from neighboring farms and water supplies, sneak sprays by unscrupulous producers, or soils that have residue from previous growers. Fortunately by October 21, 2002, the USDA mandates that all truly organic products must bear a USDA seal. To display the USDA organic seal, organically produced products must have been produced and handled by operations certified by a USDA-accredited certifying agent.

Until uniform standards are in place to guarantee the growing practices of foods labeled "organic," consumers must act with care. Check on products labeled organic. At farmers markets, ask questions of growers. Unless you see a USDA label, beware. In fact, these labels are often placed on foods that are far from healthy and may actually be of very low quality. Although the ideals on which the organic foods movement was founded are sound, more testing and regulation are needed before people can be assured that what they are paying high prices for is a truly pesticide-free product.

> **Organically grown** Foods that are grown without use of pesticides or chemicals.

Taking Charge

Managing Eating Behavior

By paying attention, reading, seeking help from reputable trained professionals, and planning ahead, you can increase your own nutritional health.

Checklist for Change

Making Personal Choices

✓ *Eat lower on the food chain.* Substitute fruits, vegetables, nuts, or grains for animal products at least once a day.

✓ *Eat seasonal foods whenever possible.* By eating foods at the peak of harvest, you are most apt to avoid nutrient losses incurred by storage, freezing, canning, and so on.

✓ *Eat lean.* Pay attention to labels, assess your food intake, and balance high-fat meals with low-fat meals. Choose leaner cuts, and bake, grill, boil, or broil whenever possible.

✓ *Consume more fruits and vegetables.* Eat the real thing instead of just drinking the juices.

✓ *Combine foods for optimum nutrition.* Identify the best ways to combine grains, beans, fruits, vegetables, nuts, and other foods. You will then be able to optimize the nutrition you receive from your food. Call your local home economics extension office for recommendations.

✓ *Practice responsible consumer safety.* Avoid unnecessary chemicals, and buy, prepare, and store foods prudently to avoid food-borne illness.

✓ *Eat in moderation.* Learn to separate true hunger feelings from the food cravings that come from boredom. Don't undereat or overeat. Reduce your consumption of sugars and other dietary "extras."

✓ *Keep your systems functioning well*. Even the best diets are doomed to failure if stress, drugs, lack of exercise, sleep deprivation, and other life problems are dragging your body down, particularly your digestive system.

✓ *Keep dietary foods in balance*. Consume appropriate amounts of fats, carbohydrates, proteins, vitamins, minerals, amino acids, fatty acids, and water.

✓ *Pay attention to changing nutrient needs*. Various factors in life may require that you adjust your nutritional intake. Remain informed about new information from reputable sources concerning specific nutrient benefits and hazards.

Making Community Choices

✓ Pay attention to the types of eating establishments available on your campus. If you don't have the options you think you should, take action. Involve your student newspaper and student organizations, talk with food service representatives, involve your student health service, and solicit the support of key people on campus.

✓ Assess your elected officials' priorities regarding nutrition as it pertains to schools, the elderly, pregnant women, and the homeless. Do they support adequate nutrition for high-risk groups? If not, write letters asking for clarification of their positions.

✓ If you patronize certain food establishments, review the food choices. Tell them when they are doing a good job, and request other options when they are not.

✓ Be informed about key nutritional concepts. Demand accuracy in reported claims. Speak only from an informed perspective.

Summary

✳ Recognizing that we eat for more reasons than just survival is the first step toward changing our health.

✳ The Food Guide Pyramid provides guidelines for healthy eating.

✳ The major nutrients that are essential for life and health include water, proteins, carbohydrates, fiber, fats, vitamins, and minerals.

✳ Experts are interested in the role of food as medicine and in the benefits of "functional foods." These foods may play an important role in improving certain conditions, such as hypertension.

✳ Men and women have differing needs for most nutrients throughout the life cycle because of different body size and composition.

✳ Vegetarianism can provide a healthy alternative for those wishing to cut fat from their diets or to reduce animal consumption. The vegetarian pyramid provides dietary guidelines to help vegetarians obtain needed nutrients.

✳ College students face unique challenges in eating healthfully. Learning to make better choices at fast-food restaurants, eat healthfully when funds are short, and eat nutritionally in the dorm are all possible when you use the information contained in this chapter.

✳ Food-borne illnesses, food irradiation, food allergies, and other food safety and health concerns are becoming increasingly important to health-wise consumers. Recognizing potential risks and taking steps to prevent problems are part of a sound nutritional plan.

Discussion Questions

1. What factors influence the dietary patterns and behaviors of the typical college student? What factors have been the greatest influences on your eating behaviors? Why is it important to recognize influences on your diet as you think about changing eating behaviors?

2. What are the six major food groups in the USDA Food Guide Pyramid? From which groups do you eat too few servings? What can you do to increase or decrease your intake of selected food groups to improve your health? How can you remember the six groups? What possible changes are being recommended in a new pyramid?

3. What are the major types of nutrients that you need to obtain from the foods you eat? What happens if you fail to get enough of some of them? Are there significant differences between the sexes in particular areas of nutrition?

4. Distinguish between the different types of vegetarianism. Which types are most likely to lead to nutrient deficiencies? What can be done to ensure that even the most strict vegetarian receives enough of the major nutrients?

5. What are functional foods? What are the major functional foods discussed in this chapter? What are their reported benefits, if any?

6. What are the major problems that many college students face when trying to eat the right foods? List five actions that you and your classmates could take immediately to improve your eating.

7. What are the potential benefits and risks of food irradiation? Why is it being used? What are the major risks for food-borne illnesses, and what can you do to protect yourself? How are food illnesses and food allergies different?

Application Exercise

Reread the What Do You Think? scenario at the beginning of the chapter and answer the following questions.

1. Critique Roberto's eating and fitness habits.
2. What suggestions could you make to help Roberto? How could you make these suggestions in a way that won't offend him?

3. Why is it often difficult to talk with friends or family members about their eating behaviors? How do you feel when other people criticize your own eating patterns?

Accessing Your Health on the Internet http

Visit the following Internet sites to explore further topics and issues related to personal health. To visit an organization's website, go to the Companion Website for *Health: The Basics, Fifth Edition* at www.aw.com/donatelle, click on the book image, and select "Accessing Your Health on the Internet" from the navigation menu on the left.

1. *U.S. Department of Agriculture (USDA).* Offers a full discussion of the USDA Dietary Guidelines for Americans.
2. *Food and Drug Administration (FDA).* Provides information for consumers and professionals in the areas of food safety, supplements, and medical devices. Links to other sources of information about nutrition and food.

3. *American Heart Association (AHA).* Includes information about a heart-healthy eating plan and an easy-to-follow guide to healthy eating.
4. *American Dietetic Association (ADA).* Provides information on a full range of dietary topics, including sports nutrition, healthful cooking, and nutritional eating; also links to scientific publications and information on scholarships and public meetings.
5. *Food and Nutrition Information Center.* Offers a wide variety of information related to food and nutrition.

Further Reading

Nutrition Action Healthletter.
> *This newsletter, published ten times a year, contains up-to-date information on diet and nutritional claims and current research issues. The newsletter can be obtained by writing to the Center for Science in the Public Interest, 1501 16th St. NW, Washington, DC 20036.*

Nutrition Today.
> *An excellent magazine for the interested nonspecialist. Covers controversial issues and provides a forum for conflicting opinions. Six issues per year. Order from Williams and Wilkins, 351 West Camden Street, Baltimore, MD 21201-2436.*

Tufts University Health and Nutrition Letter.
> *An excellent source for quick "fixes" on current nutritional topics. Reputable sources and information. E-mail tufts@tiac.net, or phone 1-800-274-7581.*

U.S. Department of Agriculture.
> *For information on the proper handling of meat and poultry and other information, call the USDA's Meat and Poultry Hot Line at the toll-free number 1-800-535-4555 between 10:00 A.M. and 4:00 P.M. on weekdays. Write to the Meat and Poultry Hot Line, USDA-FSIS, Room 1165-S, Washington, DC, 20250 for a new booklet,* A Quick Consumer's Guide to Safe Food Handling.

Whitney, E., and S. Rolfes. *Understanding Nutrition.*
> San Francisco: Wadsworth Publishing, 2002.
> *An introductory college health text that provides an outstanding overview of nutritional information in a highly accessible, easy-to-read format.*

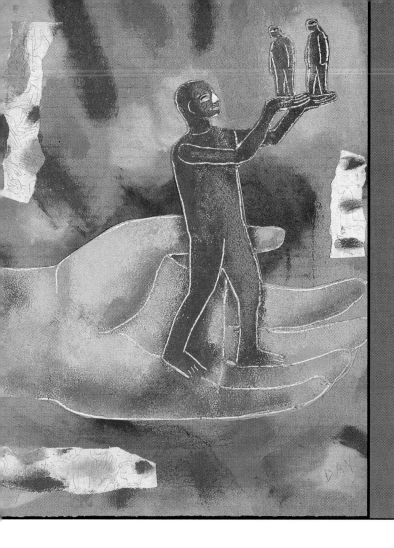

10
Managing Your Weight
FINDING A HEALTHY BALANCE

objectives

* Explain why so many people are obsessed with thinness and how to determine the right weight for you. Define obesity.

* Describe the options available for determining body content. Indicate which are the most reliable.

* Describe those factors that place people at risk for problems with obesity. Indicate which factors a person can control and those that cannot be controlled.

* Discuss the roles of exercise, dieting, nutrition, lifestyle modification, fad diets, and other strategies of weight control. Describe the most effective methods of weight management.

* Describe the three major eating disorders, and explain the health risks related to these conditions.

What do you think?

Angela, a college freshman, is worried about losing the "freshman 15," which she has gained from eating junk food and drinking too much on weekends. She decides to stop eating altogether and has consumed nothing for the past two days except water.

Nick, a senior, weighs 365 pounds, eats three large meals per day, and snacks on junk food between meals. A defensive lineman for the football team, he would like to gain even more weight. He is sure he'll be able to lose what he has gained after the season.

How typical are the eating behaviors of these students? ⁕ *What do you think is motivating them to eat as they do?* ⁕ *What risks does each face?* ⁕ *What advice might you give to each individual?*

In spite of society's messages about diet and exercise, numerous studies on eating patterns suggest that Americans are doing worse with each successive decade. In fact, the most recent National Health and Nutrition Examination Survey (NHANES III), conducted by the Centers for Disease Control and Prevention, shows that 61 percent of U.S. adults are either overweight or obese—an increase of more than 5 percent over the NHANES III 1988–94 data set.[1]

Clearly, obesity is a major public health problem that needs to be addressed. The threats to life and overall health and happiness are staggering. In fact, officials estimate that more than 500,000 lives are lost each year to conditions directly related to obesity, and perhaps many more deaths are indirectly related to a history of obesity throughout a person's life.[2] Associated health risks include coronary heart disease, hypertension, dyslipidemias, diabetes, gallstones, sleep apnea, osteoarthritis, and several cancers. In addition, the re-

lationship between obesity and psychosocial development, including self-esteem, is believed to be quite close. See the accompanying box. The estimated annual health care cost due to obesity in the United States exceeds $100 billion in medical expenses and lost productivity.[3] U.S. agriculture secretary Dan Glickman predicts that obesity will soon rival smoking as a cause of preventable death.[4] This chapter will help you understand what *underweight, normal weight, overweight,* and *obesity* really mean, and why managing your weight is essential to overall health and well-being.

Body Image

Most of us think of the obsession with thinness as a recent phenomenon. Beginning with supermodel Twiggy in the 1960s and continuing with supermodel Kate Moss, the thin look has dominated fashion and the media.

Health Risks from Overweight and Obesity

Overweight and obesity are known risk factors for:

* Diabetes
* Heart disease
* Stroke
* Hypertension
* Gallbladder disease

* Osteoarthritis (degeneration of cartilage and bone of joints)
* Sleep apnea and other breathing problems

* Some forms of cancer (uterine, breast, colorectal, kidney, and gallbladder)

Obesity is associated with:

* High blood cholesterol
* Complications of pregnancy
* Menstrual irregularities
* Hirsutism (presence of excess body and facial hair)

* Stress incontinence (urine leakage caused by weak pelvic-floor muscles)
* Psychological disorders such as depression

* Increased surgical risk

Source: http://www.niddk.nih.gov/health/nutrit/pubs/statobes.htm

---

But the thin look has been around for a long time. Anorexia nervosa, an eating disorder, has been defined as a psychiatric illness since 1873. During the Victorian era, women wore corsets to achieve unrealistically tiny waists. By the 1920s, it was common knowledge that obesity was linked to poor health. The American Tobacco Company coined the phrase "Reach for a Lucky instead of a sweet" to promote the idea that cigarettes dulled appetite. American Tobacco even formed the Moderation League to promote the virtues of moderation in, among other things, eating.

Today, underweight models, actresses, and Miss Americas exemplify desirability and success, delivering the subtle message that thin is in. In addition, public health warnings that being overweight increases risk for heart disease, certain cancers, and a number of other disorders can send a panic through people when their weight isn't what they think it should be. Some of these distorted views of self-image arise from misinterpreting height–weight charts, making some people strive for the lower readings stipulated for a light-boned person when determining their own normal weight.

Sadly, increasing numbers of adolescents, teens, and adults are so preoccupied with trying to be like the size 4 models that they make themselves ill in their quest to be thin.

Determining the Right Weight for You

What weight is right for you? This depends on a wide range of variables, including your body structure, height, the distribution of the weight that you carry, and the ratio of fat to lean tissue. In fact, your weight can be a deceptive indicator. Many extremely muscular athletes would be considered overweight based on traditional height–weight charts. Many young women think that they are the right weight based on charts but are shocked to discover that 35 to 40 percent of their weight is body fat!

The United States Department of Agriculture and the Department of Health and Human Services devised one weight table for both men and women that allows for variations in body structure, distribution of weight, and weight gains in middle age (Table 10.1). Weights at the lower end of the range are recommended for individuals with a low ratio of muscle and bone to fat; those at the upper end are advised for people with more muscular builds.

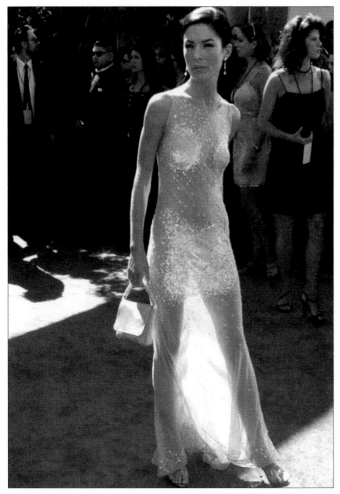

Images in the media, such as this photo of ultra-slim Lara Flynn Boyle, convey the message that a thin body is the ideal body.

Table 10.1
Healthy Weight Ranges*

HEIGHT WITHOUT SHOES	WEIGHT† WITHOUT CLOTHES
4'10"	91–119
4'11"	94–124
5'0"	97–128
5'1"	101–132
5'2"	104–137
5'3"	107–141
5'4"	111–146
5'5"	114–150
5'6"	118–155
5'7"	121–160
5'8"	125–164
5'9"	129–169
5'10"	132–174
5'11"	136–179
6'0"	140–184
6'1"	144–189
6'2"	148–195
6'3"	152–200
6'4"	156–205
6'5"	160–211
6'6"	164–216

*Each data entry applies to both men and women.
†In pounds

Source: Dietary Guidelines for Americans, 1995, USDA.

Readiness for Weight Loss

To see how well your attitudes equip you for a weight loss program, answer the questions that follow. For each question, circle the answer that best describes your attitude. As you complete each of the six sections, tally your score and analyze it according to the scoring guide.

I. GOALS, ATTITUDES, AND READINESS

1. Compared to previous attempts, how motivated are you to lose weight this time?

1	2	3	4	5
Not at all motivated	Slightly motivated	Somewhat motivated	Quite motivated	Extremely motivated

2. How certain are you that you will stay committed to a weight loss program for the time it will take to reach your goal?

1	2	3	4	5
Not at all certain	Slightly certain	Somewhat certain	Quite certain	Extremely certain

3. Considering all outside factors at this time in your life—stress at work, family obligations, and so on—to what extent can you tolerate the effort required to stick to a diet?

1	2	3	4	5
Cannot tolerate	Can tolerate somewhat	Uncertain	Can tolerate well	Can tolerate easily

4. Think honestly about how much weight you hope to lose and how quickly you hope to lose it. Figuring a weight loss of 1 to 2 pounds per week, how realistic is your expectation?

1	2	3	4	5
Very unrealistic	Somewhat unrealistic	Moderately unrealistic	Somewhat realistic	Very realistic

5. While dieting, do you fantasize about eating a lot of your favorite foods?

1	2	3	4	5
Always	Frequently	Occasionally	Rarely	Never

6. While dieting, do you feel deprived, angry, and/or upset?

1	2	3	4	5
Always	Frequently	Occasionally	Rarely	Never

IF YOU SCORED:

6 to 16: This may not be a good time for you to start a diet. Inadequate motivation and commitment and unrealistic goals could block your progress. Think about what contributes to your unreadiness and consider changing these factors before undertaking a diet.

17 to 23: You may be close to being ready to begin a program but should think about ways to boost your readiness.

24 to 30: The path is clear: you can decide how to lose weight in a safe, effective way.

II. HUNGER AND EATING CUES

7. When food comes up in conversation or in something you read, do you want to eat, even if you are not hungry?

1	2	3	4	5
Never	Rarely	Occasionally	Frequently	Always

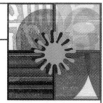

II. HUNGER AND EATING CUES

8. How often do you eat because of physical hunger?

1	2	3	4	5
Never	Rarely	Occasionally	Frequently	Always

9. Do you have trouble controlling your eating when your favorite foods are around the house?

1	2	3	4	5
Never	Rarely	Occasionally	Frequently	Always

IF YOU SCORED:

3 to 6: You might occasionally eat more than you should, but it does not appear to be due to high responsiveness to environmental cues. Controlling the attitudes that make you eat may be especially helpful.

7 to 9: You may have a moderate tendency to eat just because food is available. Losing weight may be easier for you if you try to resist external cues and eat only when you are physically hungry.

10 to 15: Some or much of your eating may be in response to thinking about food or exposing yourself to temptations to eat. Think of ways to minimize your exposure to temptations so you eat only in response to physical hunger.

III. CONTROL OVER EATING

If the following situations occurred while you were on a diet, would you be likely to eat more or less immediately afterward and for the rest of the day?

10. Although you planned on skipping lunch, a friend talks you into going out for a midday meal.

1	2	3	4	5
Would eat much less	Would eat somewhat less	Would make no difference	Would eat somewhat more	Would eat much more

11. You "break" your plan by eating a fattening, "forbidden" food.

1	2	3	4	5
Would eat much less	Would eat somewhat less	Would make no difference	Would eat somewhat more	Would eat much more

12. You have been following your diet faithfully and decide to test yourself by eating something you consider a treat.

1	2	3	4	5
Would eat much less	Would eat somewhat less	Would make no difference	Would eat somewhat more	Would eat much more

IF YOU SCORED:

3 to 7: You recover rapidly from mistakes. However, if you frequently alternate between eating that is out of control and dieting very strictly, you may have a serious eating problem and should get professional help.

8 to 11: You do not seem to let unplanned eating disrupt your program. This is a flexible, balanced approach.

12 to 15: You may be prone to overeat after an event breaks your control or throws you off the track. Your reaction to these problem-causing events can be improved.

Continued

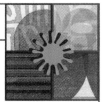

IV. BINGE EATING AND PURGING

13. Aside from holiday feasts, have you ever eaten a large amount of food rapidly and felt afterward that this eating incident was excessive and out of control?

2	0
Yes	No

14. If yes to question 13, how often have you engaged in this behavior during the past year?

1	2	3	4	5	6
Less than once a month	About once a month	A few times a month	About once a week	About three times a week	Daily

15. Have you purged (used laxatives or diuretics, or induced vomiting) to control your weight?

5	0
Yes	No

16. If you answered yes to question 15, how often have you engaged in this behavior during the past year?

1	2	3	4	5	6
Less than once a month	About once a month	A few times a month	About once a week	About three times a week	Daily

IF YOU SCORED:

0: It appears that binge eating and purging are not problems for you.

2 to 11: Pay attention to these eating patterns. Should they arise more frequently, get professional help.

12 to 19: You show signs of having a potentially serious eating problem. See a counselor experienced in evaluating eating disorders right away.

V. EMOTIONAL EATING

17. Do you eat more than you would like to when you have negative feelings such as anxiety, depression, anger, or loneliness?

1	2	3	4	5
Never	Rarely	Occasionally	Frequently	Always

18. Do you have trouble controlling your eating when you have positive feelings—do you celebrate feeling good by eating?

1	2	3	4	5
Never	Rarely	Occasionally	Frequently	Always

19. When you have unpleasant interactions with others in your life, or after a difficult day at work, do you eat more than you'd like?

1	2	3	4	5
Never	Rarely	Occasionally	Frequently	Always

IF YOU SCORED:

3 to 8: You do not appear to let your emotions affect your eating.

9 to 11: You sometimes eat in response to emotional highs and lows. Monitor this behavior to learn when and why it occurs, and be prepared to find alternate activities.

12 to 15: Emotional ups and downs can stimulate your eating. Try to deal with the feelings that trigger the eating and find other ways to express them.

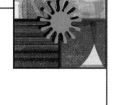

VI. EXERCISE PATTERNS AND ATTITUDES

20. How often do you exercise?

1	2	3	4	5
Never	Rarely	Occasionally	Somewhat frequently	Frequently

21. How confident are you that you can exercise regularly?

1	2	3	4	5
Not at all confident	Slightly confident	Somewhat confident	Highly confident	Completely confident

22. When you think about exercise, do you develop a positive or negative picture in your mind?

1	2	3	4	5
Completely negative	Somewhat negative	Neutral	Somewhat positive	Completely positive

23. How certain are you that you can work regular exercise into your daily schedule?

1	2	3	4	5
Not at all certain	Slightly certain	Somewhat certain	Quite certain	Extremely certain

IF YOU SCORED:

4 to 10: You're probably not exercising as regularly as you should. Determine whether attitudes about exercise or your lifestyle is blocking your way, then change what you must and put on those walking shoes!

11 to 16: You need to feel more positive about exercise so you can do it more often. Think of ways to be more active that are fun and fit your lifestyle.

17 to 20: It looks as if the path is clear for you to be active. Now think of ways to get motivated.

After scoring yourself in each section of this questionnaire, you should be able to better judge your dieting strengths and weaknesses. Remember that the first step in changing eating behavior is to understand the conditions that influence your eating habits.

Source: Reprinted from Kelly D. Brownell, "The Diet Readiness Test," in "When and How to Diet," *Psychology Today* (June 1989): 41–46. Reprinted with permission from *Psychology Today* magazine, copyright ©1989 (Sussex Publishers, Inc.).

Redefining Obesity: Past Scales

Obesity generally is defined as an accumulation of fat (*adipose tissue*) beyond what is considered normal for a person's age, sex, and body type. Historically, nutritionists have defined *overweight* as being 1 to 19 percent above one's ideal weight, based on height–weight tables. A person who slipped over 19 percent was labeled *obese.* Today, most experts define obesity in terms of fat content rather than in terms of weight content alone.

Experts label people who are 20 to 40 percent above their ideal weight as *mildly obese* (90 percent of the obese fit into this category). Those 41 to 99 percent above their ideal weight are described as *moderately obese* (about 9 percent to 10 percent of the obese), and those who are 100 percent or

more above their ideal weight are identified as *severely, morbidly,* or *grossly overweight* (about 1 percent). Even the terminology (e.g., *gross obesity*) speaks volumes about the way society views these individuals.[5]

The difficulty with defining obesity lies in determining what is normal. To date, there are no universally accepted standards for the most "desirable" or "ideal" body weight or *body composition* (the ratio of lean body mass to fat body mass). Although sources vary slightly, men's bodies should contain between 11 and 15 percent total body fat, and women should be within the range of 18 to 22 percent body fat. At various ages and stages of life, these ranges also vary, but

> **Obesity** A weight disorder generally defined as an accumulation of fat beyond that considered normal for a person based on age, sex, and body type.

generally, when men exceed 20 percent body fat and women exceed 30 percent body fat, they have slipped into obesity.

Why the difference between men and women? Much of it may be attributed to the normal structure of the female body and to sex hormones. Lean body mass consists of the structural and functional elements in cells, body water, muscle, bones, and other body organs such as the heart, liver, and kidneys. Body fat is composed of two types: essential and storage fat. Essential fat is necessary for normal physiological functioning, such as nerve conduction. Essential fat makes up approximately 3 to 7 percent of total body weight in men and approximately 15 percent of total body weight in women. Storage fat, the part that many of us are always trying to shed, makes up the remainder of our fat reserves. It accounts for only a small percentage of total body weight for very lean people and between 5 and 25 percent of body weight of most American adults. Female bodybuilders, who are among the leanest of female athletes, may have body fat percentages ranging from 8 to 13 percent, nearly all of which is essential fat.

Too Little Fat?

A certain amount of body fat is necessary for insulating the body, cushioning parts of the body and vital organs, and maintaining body functions. In men, this lower limit is approximately 3 to 4 percent. Women should generally not go below 8 percent. Excessively low body fat in females may lead to amenorrhea, a disruption of the normal menstrual cycle. The critical level of body fat necessary to maintain normal menstrual flow is believed to be between 8 and 13 percent, but there are many additional factors that affect the menstrual cycle. Under extreme circumstances, such as starvation diets and certain diseases, the body utilizes all available fat reserves and begins to break down muscle tissue as a last-ditch effort to obtain nourishment.

The fact is that too much fat and too little fat are both potentially harmful. The key is to find a healthy level at which you are comfortable with your appearance and your ability to be as active as possible. Many options are available for determining your body fat and weight.

Assessing Fat Levels

Weight-For-Height Charts

One age-old method for determining whether you are within an acceptable weight range has been to look at your height on a particular chart and then try to determine what your weight

should be, based on gender, build, or other variables. These measures give a good idea of how much you weigh, but they do not account for the proportion of muscle to fat mass in your body. You could be a power weightlifter with heavy muscle mass and be deemed unfit by such charts. There are many varieties of these tables, and health professionals often disagree on which are best. The 2000 Dietary Guidelines for Americans, published jointly by the U.S. Department of Agriculture and Health and Human Services, provide the most up-to-date weight-for-height chart. (See Table 10.1 on page 255.)

Body Mass Index

Body Mass Index (BMI) can be used to measure both overweight and obesity in adults. It is an index of the relationship of height and weight and is the measurement of choice for obesity researchers and other health professionals. It is not gender specific, and although it does not directly measure percentage of body fat, it does provide a more accurate measure of overweight and obesity than relying on weight alone.[6]

BMI is found by dividing a person's weight in kilograms by height in meters squared. The mathematical formula is:

Weight (kg) ÷ height squared (m^2)

To determine BMI using pounds and inches, multiply your weight in pounds by 704.5, then divide the result by your height in inches, and divide that result by your height in inches a second time. (The multiplier 704.5 is used by the National Institutes of Health. Other organizations, such as the American Dietetic Association, suggest multiplying by 700. The variation in outcomes between the two is insignificant, and 700 is easier for most people to remember.)

Healthy weights have been defined as those associated with BMIs of 19 to 25, the range of lowest statistical health risk.[7] The desirable range for females falls between 21 and 23; for males, between 22 and 24.[8] A BMI greater than 25 indicates overweight and potentially significant health risks. A body mass index over 30 is considered obese.[9] Many experts believe that this number is too high, particularly for younger adults.

Calculating BMI is simple, quick, and inexpensive—but it does have limitations. One problem with using BMI as a measurement is that very muscular people may fall into the "overweight" category when they are actually healthy and fit. Another problem with using BMI is that people who have lost muscle mass, such as the elderly, may be in the "healthy weight" category according to BMI, when they actually have reduced nutritional reserves.[10] Many people may also look at these numbers and have difficulty conceptualizing what they really mean.

These standards may seem almost impossible for people who consistently exceed the target weights and who have difficulty keeping off any lost weight. Constant failure may lead them to stop trying. The secret lies in establishing a healthful weight at a young age and maintaining it—a task easier said than done. The U.S. Dietary Guidelines for Americans encourages a weight gain of no more than 10

Body mass index (BMI) A technique of weight assessment based on the relationship of weight to height.

	Normal						Overweight					Obese										Extreme Obesity														
BMI	19	20	21	22	23	24	25	26	27	28	29	30	31	32	33	34	35	36	37	38	39	40	41	42	43	44	45	46	47	48	49	50	51	52	53	54
Height (inches)												Body Weight (pounds)																								
58	91	96	100	105	110	115	119	124	129	134	138	143	148	153	158	162	167	172	177	181	186	191	196	201	205	210	215	220	224	229	234	239	244	248	253	258
59	94	99	104	109	114	119	124	128	133	138	143	148	153	158	163	168	173	178	183	188	193	198	203	208	212	217	222	227	232	237	242	247	252	257	262	267
60	97	102	107	112	118	123	128	133	138	143	148	153	158	163	168	174	179	184	189	194	199	204	209	215	220	225	230	235	240	245	250	255	261	266	271	276
61	100	106	111	116	122	127	132	137	143	148	153	158	164	169	174	180	185	190	195	201	206	211	217	222	227	232	238	243	248	254	259	264	269	275	280	285
62	104	109	115	120	126	131	136	142	147	153	158	164	169	175	180	186	191	196	202	207	213	218	224	229	235	240	246	251	256	262	267	273	278	284	289	295
63	107	113	118	124	130	135	141	146	152	158	163	169	175	180	186	191	197	203	208	214	220	225	231	237	242	248	254	259	265	270	278	282	287	293	299	304
64	110	116	122	128	134	140	145	151	157	163	169	174	180	186	192	197	204	209	215	221	227	232	238	244	250	256	262	267	273	279	285	291	296	302	308	314
65	114	120	126	132	138	144	150	156	162	168	174	180	186	192	198	204	210	216	222	228	234	240	246	252	258	264	270	276	282	288	294	300	306	312	318	324
66	118	124	130	136	142	148	155	161	167	173	179	186	192	198	204	210	216	223	229	235	241	247	253	260	266	272	278	284	291	297	303	309	315	322	328	334
67	121	127	134	140	146	153	159	166	172	178	185	191	198	204	211	217	223	230	236	242	249	255	261	268	274	280	287	293	299	306	312	319	325	331	338	344
68	125	131	138	144	151	158	164	171	177	184	190	197	203	210	216	223	230	236	243	249	256	262	269	276	282	289	295	302	308	315	322	328	335	341	348	354
69	128	135	142	149	155	162	169	176	182	189	196	203	209	216	223	230	236	243	250	257	263	270	277	284	291	297	304	311	318	324	331	338	345	351	358	365
70	132	139	146	153	160	167	174	181	188	195	202	209	216	222	229	236	243	250	257	264	271	278	285	292	299	306	313	320	327	334	341	348	355	362	369	376
71	136	143	150	157	165	172	179	186	193	200	208	215	222	229	236	243	250	257	265	272	279	286	293	301	308	315	322	329	338	343	351	358	365	372	379	386
72	140	147	154	162	169	177	184	191	199	206	213	221	228	235	242	250	258	265	272	279	287	294	302	309	316	324	331	338	346	353	361	368	375	383	390	397
73	144	151	159	166	174	182	189	197	204	212	219	227	235	242	250	257	265	272	280	288	295	302	310	318	325	333	340	348	355	363	371	378	386	393	401	408
74	148	155	163	171	179	186	194	202	210	218	225	233	241	249	256	264	272	280	287	295	303	311	319	326	334	342	350	358	365	373	381	389	396	404	412	420
75	152	160	168	176	184	192	200	208	216	224	232	240	248	256	264	272	279	287	295	303	311	319	327	335	343	351	359	367	375	383	391	399	407	415	423	431
76	156	164	172	180	189	197	205	213	221	230	238	246	254	263	271	279	287	295	304	312	320	328	336	344	353	361	369	377	385	394	402	410	418	426	435	443

Figure 10.1 Body Mass Index Table

Source: Adapted from Clinical Guidelines on the Identification, Evaluation, and Treatment of Overweight and Obesity in Adults: The Evidence Report.

pounds after reaching adult height and endorses small weight losses of one-half to one pound per week, if needed, as well as smaller weight losses of 5 to 10 percent to make a difference toward health.[11]

Waist-to-Hip Ratio

Another useful measure is the *waist-to-hip ratio,* a measure of regional fat distribution. Research has shown that excess fat in the abdominal area poses a greater health risk than excess fat in the hips and thighs and is associated with a number of disorders, including high blood pressure, diabetes, heart disease, and certain cancers. A waist-to-hip ratio greater than 1.0 in men and 0.8 in women indicates increased health risks.[12] Therefore, knowing where your fat is carried may be more important than knowing your total fat content.

Men and postmenopausal women tend to store fat in the upper regions of their body, particularly in the abdominal area. Premenopausal women usually store their fat in lower regions of their bodies, particularly the hips, buttocks, and thighs.[13] In fact, waist measurement alone may be a viable way to assess fat distribution. Some research suggests that a waistline greater than 40 inches (102 cm) in men and 35 inches (88 cm) in women may indicate greater health risk.[14]

Measures of Body Fat

Hydrostatic Weighing Techniques From a clinical perspective, **hydrostatic weighing techniques** offer the most accurate method of measuring body fat. This method measures the amount of water a person displaces when completely submerged. Because fat tissue is less dense than muscle or bone tissue, a relatively accurate indication of actual body fat can be computed by comparing a person's underwater and out-of-water weights. Although this method may be subject to errors, it is one of the most sophisticated techniques currently available.

Pinch and Skinfold Measures Perhaps the most commonly used method of determining body fat is the **pinch test.**

Hydrostatic weighing techniques Methods of determining body fat by measuring the amount of water displaced when a person is completely submerged.

Pinch test A method of determining body fat whereby a fold of skin just behind the triceps is pinched between the thumb and index finger to determine the relative amount of fat.

Numerous studies have determined that the triceps area (the back of the upper arm) is one of the most reliable regions of the body for assessing the amount of fat in the subcutaneous (just under the surface) layer of the skin. In making this assessment, a person pinches a fold of skin just behind the triceps with the thumb and index finger and assesses the distance between thumb and finger. It is important to pinch only the fat layer and not the triceps muscle. If the size of the pinch is thicker than 1 inch, the person is generally considered overweight.

Another technique, the **skinfold caliper test,** resembles the pinch test but is much more accurate. This procedure involves pinching folds of skin at various points on the body with the thumb and index finger. A specially calibrated instrument called a *skinfold caliper* is used to measure the fat layer. Besides the triceps, the areas most often measured are the biceps (front of the arm), the subscapular (upper back), and the iliac crest (hip). Special formulas are employed to arrive at a combined prediction of total body fat.

Girth and Circumference Measures   Another common method of body fat assessment is the use of **girth and circumference measures.** Diagnosticians use a measuring tape to take girth, or circumference, measurements at various body sites. These measurements are then converted into constants, and a formula is used to determine relative percentages of body fat. Although this technique is inexpensive, easy to use, and commonly performed, it is not as accurate as many of the other techniques listed here.

Soft-Tissue Roentgenogram   A relatively new technique for determining body fat, the **soft-tissue roentgenogram,** involves injecting a radioactive substance into the body and allowing this substance to penetrate muscle (lean) tissue, so that fat and lean tissue can be distinguished by means of imaging.

Bioelectrical Impedance Analysis   Another method of determining body fat levels, **bioelectrical impedance analysis (BIA),** involves sending a small electrical current through the subject's body. The body's ability to conduct an electrical current reflects the total amount of water in the body. Generally, the more water, the more muscle and lean tissue. The amount of resistance to the current and the person's age, sex, and other physical characteristics are fed into a computer that uses special formulas to determine the total amount of lean and fat tissue. To obtain the most accurate readings, fasting for four hours prior to testing is recommended. BIA may not be as accurate for severely obese individuals.

Total Body Electrical Conductivity   One of the newest (and most expensive) assessment techniques is **total body electrical conductivity (TOBEC),** which uses an electromagnetic force field to assess relative body fat. Although based on the same principle as impedance, this assessment requires much more elaborate, expensive equipment, and therefore is not practical for most people.

Although all of these methods can be useful, they can also be inaccurate and even harmful unless the testers are skillful and well trained. Before undergoing any procedure, make sure you understand the expense, potential for accuracy, risks, and training of the tester.

> **What do you think?**
>
> *Calculate your BMI using the formula provided. If possible, try to have your percentage of body fat tested with calipers or one of the other methods listed. Which value is most important to you? ✳ Why? ✳ How are they similar?*

Risk Factors for Obesity

In spite of massive efforts to keep Americans fit and in good health, obesity is the most common nutritional disorder in the United States, with rates that have increased dramatically among children and adults in recent decades.[15] Minority populations, particularly African Americans, Hispanic and Native American women, are disproportionately affected.[16] Why is this happening?

The majority of research supports the idea that environmental factors may play an even greater role. In particular, those environmental factors that favor increased energy intake (eating too much) while engaging in decreasing energy expenditures (too little physical activity) are in the spotlight.

Key Environmental Factors

Although there is a long list of potential environmental contributors, the following are currently receiving the greatest amounts of attention as influences on energy intake:

Skinfold caliper test   A method of determining body fat whereby folds of skin and fat at various points on the body are grasped between thumb and forefinger and measured with calipers.

Girth and circumference measures   A method of assessing body fat that employs a formula based on girth measurements of various body sites.

Soft-tissue roentgenogram   A technique of body fat assessment in which radioactive substances are used to determine relative fat.

Bioelectrical impedance analysis (BIA)   A technique of body fat assessment in which electrical currents are passed through fat and lean tissue.

Total body electrical conductivity (TOBEC)   Technique using an electromagnetic force field to assess relative body fat.

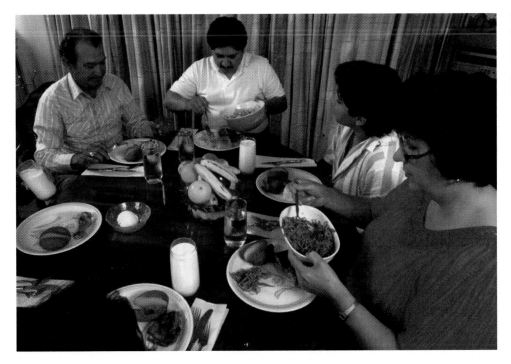

Many factors help determine body type, including heredity and genetic makeup, environmental factors, and learned eating patterns, many of which are connected to habits learned from family.

- Bombardment with advertising designed to increase energy intake—ads for high-calorie foods at a low price, marketing larger portion sizes[17]
- Changes in the number of working women, leading to greater frequency of restaurant meals and the use of more fast foods and convenience foods[18]
- Bottle feeding of infants, which may increase energy intake relative to breast feeding[19]

Factors contributing to decreased energy expenditure are often cited as follows:

- The increasingly sedentary nature of many jobs.[20]
- Universal use of automated equipment and electronic communications, such as cell phones, remote controls, other labor-saving devices[21]
- Spending more time in front of the computer and TV and playing video games[22]
- Fear of playing or being outside based on threat of violence
- Decline in physical education requirements in schools[23]
- Lack of community resources for exercise

What do you think?

Based on the lists provided, can you think of other environmental factors that contribute to obesity? ☀ *What actions could you take to reduce your risk of each of these factors?*

Heredity

Are some people born to be fat? Several factors appear to influence why one person becomes obese and another remains thin; genes seem to interact with many of these factors.

Body Type and Genes   In some animal species, the shape and size of the individual's body are largely determined by its parents' shape and size. Many scientists have explored the role of heredity in determining human body shapes. You need only look at your parents and then glance in the mirror to see where you got your own body type. Children whose parents are obese also tend to be overweight. In fact, a family history of obesity increases one's chances of becoming obese by 25 to 30 percent.[24] Some researchers argue that obesity has a strong genetic determinant—it tends to run in families. They cite statistics that 80 percent of children who have two obese parents are also obese.[25] Genes play a significant role in how the body balances calories and energy. Also, by influencing the amount of body fat and fat distribution, genes can make a person more susceptible to gaining weight.

Twin Studies   Studies of identical twins who were separated at birth and raised in different environments provide the strongest evidence yet that the genes a person inherits are the major factor determining overweight, leanness, or average weight. Whether raised in family environments with fat or thin family members, twins with obese natural parents tend to be obese in later life.[26] According to another study, sets of identical twins who were separated and raised in different families and who ate widely different diets still grew up to weigh about the same.[27]

Although the exact mechanism remains unknown, it is believed that genes set metabolic rates, influencing how the body handles calories. Other experts believe that this genetic tendency may contribute as much as 25 to 40 percent of the reason for being overweight.[28]

Specific Obesity Genes?   In the past decade, more and more research has pointed to the existence of a "fat gene." The most promising candidate is the *Ob* gene (for obesity), which is believed to disrupt the body's "I've had enough to eat" signaling system and may prompt individuals to keep eating past the point of being comfortably full. Research on Pima Indians, who have an estimated 75 percent obesity rate (nine out of ten are overweight), seems to point to an Ob gene that is a "thrifty gene." It is theorized that because their ancestors struggled through centuries of famine, their ancestors' basal metabolic rates slowed, allowing them to store precious fat for survival. Survivors may have passed these genes on to their children, which would explain the lower metabolic rates found in Pimas today and their tendency toward obesity.[29] Scientists have found that they can manipulate mice genes and construct an Ob gene that invariably leads to fatness in mice and the development of type II diabetes. Many suspect a human counterpart to this gene, but an actual gene formation has yet to be found. In addition, the (beta)-3 adrenergic-receptor gene has been identified and found in human beings and mice. When mutated, it is thought to impede the body's ability to burn fat.[30]

Although the 1994 discovery of the Ob gene in mice has provided fertile ground for speculation, researchers have further refined their theories to focus on a protein that the Ob gene may produce, known as leptin, and a new leptin receptor in the brain. According to these studies, leptin is the chemical that signals the brain when you are full and need to stop eating.[31] Although obese people have adequate

amounts of leptin and leptin receptors, they do not seem to work properly.

Other scientists have isolated a more direct route to appetite suppression, a protein called *GLP-1,* which is known to slow down the passage of food through the intestines to allow the absorption of nutrients. When scientists injected GLP-1 into the brains of hungry rats, the rats stopped eating immediately.[32] Are leptin and GLP-1 key factors in appetite suppression? It is speculated that leptin and GLP-1 might play complementary roles in weight control. Leptin and its receptors may regulate body weight over the long term, calling on fast-acting appetite suppressants such as GLP-1 when necessary.

Hunger, Appetite, and Satiety

Theories abound concerning the mechanisms that regulate food intake. Some sources indicate that the hypothalamus (the part of the brain that regulates appetite) closely monitors levels of certain nutrients in the blood. When these levels fall, the brain signals us to eat. In the obese person, it is possible that the monitoring system does not work properly and the cues to eat are more frequent and intense than they are in people of normal weight.

Other sources indicate that thin people may send more effective messages to the hypothalamus. This concept, known as **adaptive thermogenesis,** states that thin people can consume large amounts of food without gaining weight because the appetite center of their brains speeds up metabolic activity to compensate for the increased consumption. Older studies have indicated that specialized types of fat cells, called **brown fat cells,** may send signals to the brain, which controls the thermogenesis response.

The hypothesis that food tastes better to obese people, thus causing them to eat more, has largely been refuted. Scientists do distinguish, however, between **hunger,** an inborn physiological response to nutritional needs, and **appetite,** a learned response to food that is tied to an emotional or psychological craving often unrelated to nutritional need. Obese people may be more likely than thin people to satisfy their appetite and eat for reasons other than nutrition.

In some instances, the problem with overconsumption may be more related to **satiety** than to appetite or hunger. People generally feel satiated, or full, when they have satisfied their nutritional needs and their stomach signals "no more." For undetermined reasons, obese people may not feel full until much later than thin people. The leptin and GLP-1 studies seem to support this theory.

Developmental Factors

Some obese people may have excessive numbers of fat cells. This type of obesity, **hyperplasia,** usually appears in early childhood and perhaps, because of the mother's dietary habits, even prior to birth. The most critical periods for the

---

Adaptive thermogenesis   Theoretical mechanism by which the brain regulates metabolic activity according to caloric intake.

Brown fat cells   Specialized type of fat cell that affects the ability to regulate fat metabolism.

Hunger   An inborn physiological response to nutritional needs.

Appetite   A learned response that is tied to an emotional or psychological craving for food often unrelated to nutritional need.

Satiety   The feeling of fullness or satisfaction at the end of a meal.

Hyperplasia   A condition characterized by an excessive number of fat cells.

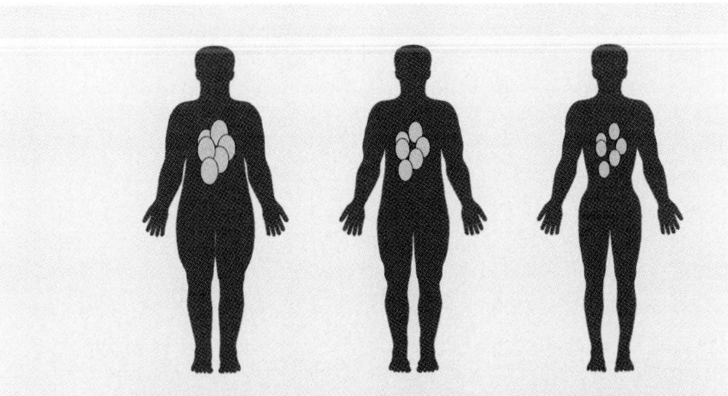

Figure 10.2
One Person at Various Stages of Weight Loss
Note that, according to theories of hyperplasia, the number of fat cells remains constant, but their size decreases when a person loses weight.

	Before body weight reduction	Initial weight reduction	Second weight reduction
Body weight	328 lb	227 lb	165 lb
Fat cell size	0.9 µg/cell	0.6 µg/cell	0.2 µg/cell
Fat cell number	75 billion	75 billion	75 billion

development of hyperplasia seem to be the last two to three months of fetal development, the first year of life, and between the ages of 9 and 13. Parents who allow their children to eat without restrictions and become overweight may be setting them up for a lifelong excess of fat cells. Central to this theory is the belief that the number of fat cells in a person's body does not increase appreciably during adulthood. However, the ability of each of these cells to swell and shrink, known as **hypertrophy,** does carry over into adulthood. Weight gain may be tied to both the number of fat cells in the body and the capacity of individual cells to enlarge.

An adult of average weight has approximately 25 billion to 30 billion fat cells, a moderately obese adult about 60 billion to 100 billion, and an extremely obese adult as many as 200 billion.[33] People who add large numbers of fat cells to their bodies in childhood may be able to lose weight by decreasing the size of each cell in adulthood, but the total number of cells will remain the same. With the next calorie binge, the cells swell and sabotage weight loss efforts (Figure 10.2).

Setpoint Theory

In 1982, nutritional researchers William Bennett and Joel Gurin presented the **setpoint theory,** which stated that a person's body has a setpoint of weight at which it is pro-

grammed to be comfortable. If your setpoint is around 160 pounds, you will gain and lose weight fairly easily within a given range of that point. For example, if you gain five to ten pounds on vacation, it will be fairly easy to lose that weight and remain around the 160-pound mark for a long period of time. Through a process of *adaptive thermogenesis,* the body actually tries to maintain this weight. Some people have equated this point with the **plateau** that dieters sometimes reach after losing a certain amount of weight. The setpoint theory proposes that after losing a predetermined amount of weight, the body will actually sabotage additional weight loss by slowing down metabolism. In extreme cases, the metabolic rate will decrease to a point at which the body will maintain its weight on as little as 1,000 calories per day.

Can a person change this predetermined setpoint? Proponents of this theory argue that it is possible to raise one's setpoint over time by continually gaining weight and failing to exercise. Conversely, reducing caloric intake and exercising regularly can slowly decrease one's setpoint. Exercise may be the most critical factor in readjusting setpoint, although diet may also be important.

The setpoint theory remains controversial. Perhaps its greatest impact was the sense of relief it provided for people who have lost weight, plateaued, and regained weight time and time again. It told them that their failure was not due to lack of willpower alone. The setpoint theory also prompted nutritional experts to look more carefully at popular methods of weight loss. If it is correct, an extremely low calorie diet isn't just dangerous; it may also cause the body to protect the dieter from "starvation" by slowing down metabolism, making weight loss even more difficult.

Endocrine Influence

Over the years, many people have attributed obesity to problems with their **thyroid gland.** They believed that an underactive thyroid impeded their ability to burn calories. However, most authorities agree that less than 2 percent of the obese population have a thyroid problem and can trace their weight problems to a metabolic or hormone imbalance.[34]

Hypertrophy   The ability of fat cells to swell and shrink.

Setpoint theory   A theory of obesity causation that suggests that fat storage is determined by a thermostatic mechanism in the body that acts to maintain a specific amount of body fat.

Plateau   That point in a weight loss program at which the dieter finds it difficult to lose more weight.

Thyroid gland   A two-lobed endocrine gland located in the throat region that produces a hormone that regulates metabolism.

Are Super-Sized Meals Super-Sizing Americans?

Today, super-sized meals are the norm at many restaurants. Biscuits and gravy, huge steaks, and plate-filling meals are popular fare. Across the country, restaurants and food companies are piling it on as customers seek "comfort food" in large portions. Consider the 25-ounce prime rib for cowboys served at a local steak chain. At nearly 3,000 calories and 150 grams of fat for the meat alone, these dinners serve the dual purpose of slamming shut arteries while adding on pounds. Add a baked potato with sour cream and/or butter, a salad loaded with creamy salad dressing, fresh bread with real butter, and the meal may surpass the 5,000-calorie mark and ring in at close to 300 grams of fat. This scale-tipping dinner exceeds what most adults should eat in two days!

And this is just the beginning. Soft drinks, once commonly served in 12-ounce sizes, now come in big gulps and 1-liter bottles. Cinnamon buns at local chains now come in giant, butter-laden, 700-calorie portions. What is the result? Super-sized portions consumed by super-sized Americans. A quick glance at the fattening of Americans provides growing evidence of a significant health problem. According to Donna Skoda, a dietitian and chair of the Ohio State University Extension Service, "People are eating a ton of extra calories. For the first time in history, more people are overweight in America [55%] than are underweight. Ironically, although the U.S. fat intake has dropped in the past 20 years from an average of 40 to 33 percent of calories, the daily calorie intake has risen from 1,852 calories per day to over 2,000 per day. In theory, this translates into a

weight gain of 15 pounds a year." Skoda and others say that the main reason that Americans are gaining weight is that people no longer know what a normal serving size is. In a recent U.S. Department of Agriculture survey, only 1 percent of the respondents could correctly identify the serving sizes recommended in the Food Guide Pyramid, the visual dietary aid developed by the USDA.

McDonald's super-sized fries weigh 7 ounces and contain 540 calories and 26 grams of fat. Compare that to the 1950s versions your parents and grandparents enjoyed with 220 calories and 12 grams of fat. "Blooming onions" weigh in at over 2,000 calories for a relatively small size onion. Grand-sized tacos, huge bagels and muffins, and giant pizzas top off a short list of typical dietary splurging. According to Carrie Wiatt, a Los Angeles dietitian and author of the recently released book *Portion Savvy*, one telling marker of the big-food trend is that restaurant plates have grown from an average of 9 to 13 inches in the past decade. Studies show that people eat 40 to 50 percent more than they normally would now that large portions are available.

These statistics alone are alarming; however, they are made worse by a growing trend toward sedentary lifestyles, increased use of technology and gadgetry, and computer-gazing among far too many Americans. The relationship between energy input and output is being knocked out of balance on both sides. Americans are taking in more calories and doing less to burn them off. Hence, an epidemic of obesity prevails and is getting worse. Younger and younger kids are eating more and more and picking up lifetime habits that will be hard to change. To reduce your own risk of super-sizing, follow these simple strategies:

- Avoid super-sizing anything. Order the smallest size available when dining out.

Focus on taste, not quantity. Get used to eating less and enjoying what you are eating.

- Chew your food, and avoid the urge to wash it down with high-calorie drinks. Take time, and let your fullness indicator have a chance to kick in while there is still time to quit.
- Serve food on a small or medium plate. Put those big platter-size dinner plates on the top shelf of your cupboard, and leave them there.
- Always order dressings, gravies, and sauces on the side. Sprinkle these added calories on carefully, rather than washing your foods down with them. Remember that a tablespoon of gravy could mean an hour on the treadmill to burn off its 200+ calories!
- If you order large muffins or bagels, share them with a friend, or bring only half with you and wrap up the rest. Carry a small zip-lock bag, and use it to take home part of those big portions for another day.
- Avoid appetizers in restaurants. Often they cost a lot, in terms of money, calories, and fat content.
- Share your dinner with a friend, and order a side salad for each of you. Alternatively, eat only half of your dinner, and save the rest for another day.
- Measure portions. Before ordering, ask for the size of servings, and always order a size smaller than you really want. When the server tells you it is a "rich dish" or "a lot of food," avoid it.
- Avoid buffets and all-you-can-eat establishments. Most of us can eat two to three times what we need—or more.

Source: Some statistics from J. Snow, "Are Super-Sized Meals Super-Sizing Americans?" *Corvallis Gazette Times,* May 24, 2000, Section C8.

Psychosocial Factors

The relationship of weight problems to deeply rooted emotional insecurities, needs, and wants remains uncertain. Food is often used as a reward for good behavior in childhood. As adults face unemployment, broken relationships, financial uncertainty, fears about health and other problems, the bright spot in the day is often "what's on the table for dinner" or "we're going to that restaurant tonight." Again, the research underlying this theory is controversial. What is certain is that eating tends to be a focal point of people's lives, and the comfort foods of childhood may provide a salve for painful social pressures, hence the label "comfort food" for foods that taste good, and are both warm and filling. Eating is essentially a social ritual associated with companionship, celebration, and enjoyment. For many people, the social emphasis on the eating experience is a major obstacle to successful dieting. Although some restaurants offer menu items designed to aid dieters, many people have difficulty choosing responsibly when confronted with an entire menu of delicious, fattening foods.

Metabolic Changes

Even when completely at rest, the body consumes a certain amount of energy. The amount of energy your body uses at complete rest is your **basal metabolic rate (BMR).** About 60 to 70 percent of all the calories you consume on a given day go to support your basal metabolism: heartbeat, breathing, maintaining body temperature, and so on. So if you consume 2,000 calories per day, between 1,200 and 1,400 of those calories are burned without your doing any significant physical activity. But unless you exert yourself enough to burn the remaining 600 to 800 calories, you will gain weight. Your BMR can fluctuate considerably, with several factors influencing whether it slows down or speeds up. In general, the younger you are, the higher your BMR, partly because in young people cells undergo rapid subdivision, which consumes a good deal of energy. BMR is highest during infancy, puberty, and pregnancy, when bodily changes are most rapid. BMR is also influenced by body composition. Muscle tissue is highly active—even at rest—compared to fat tissue. In essence, the more lean tissue you have, the greater your BMR, and the more fat tissue you have, the lower your BMR. Men have a higher BMR than women do, at least partly because of their greater proportion of lean tissue.

Age is another factor that affects BMR. After age 30, BMR slows down by about 1 to 2 percent a year. Therefore, people over 30 commonly find that they must work harder to burn off an extra helping of ice cream than they did when in their teens. "Middle-aged spread," a reference to the tendency to put on weight later in life, is partly related to this change. A slower BMR, coupled with less activity and shifting priorities (family and career become more important than fitness), puts the weight of many middle-aged people in jeopardy.

In addition, the body has a number of self-protective mechanisms that signal BMR to speed up or slow down. For example, when you have a fever, the energy needs of your cells increase, which generates heat and speeds up your BMR. In starvation situations, the body protects itself by slowing down BMR to conserve precious energy. Thus, when people repeatedly resort to extreme diets, it is believed that their bodies "reset" their BMRs at lower rates. **Yo-yo diets,** in which people repeatedly gain weight and then starve themselves to lose it, are doomed to failure. When they resume eating after their weight loss, they have a BMR that is set lower, making it almost certain that they will regain the pounds they just lost. After repeated cycles of dieting and regaining weight, these people find it increasingly hard to lose weight and increasingly easy to regain it, so they become heavier and heavier.

According to a recent study by Kelly Brownell of Yale University, middle-aged men who maintained a steady weight (even if they were overweight) had a lower risk of heart attack than men whose weight cycled up and down in a yo-yo pattern. Brownell found that smaller, well-maintained weight losses are more beneficial for reducing cardiovascular risk than larger, poorly maintained weight losses.[35]

Lifestyle

Of all the factors affecting obesity, perhaps the most critical is the relationship between activity levels and calorie intake. Obesity rates are rising. But how can this be happening? Aren't more people exercising than ever before? Though the many advertisements for sports equipment and the popularity of athletes may give the impression that Americans love a good workout, the facts are not so positive. Data from a newly released National Health Interview Survey show that four in ten adults in the United States never engage in any exercise, sports, or physically active hobbies in their leisure time.[36] Women (43.2 percent) were somewhat more likely than men (36.5 percent) to be sedentary, a finding that was consistent across all age groups. Among both men and women, African American and Hispanic adults were more sedentary than white adults.[37] Leisure-time physical activity was also strongly associated with level of education. About 72 percent of adults who never attended high school were sedentary, declining steadily to 45 percent among high school graduates and about 24 percent among adults with graduate-level college degrees.[38]

Do you know people who seemingly can eat whatever they want without gaining weight? With few exceptions, if you were to follow them around for a typical day and monitor the level and intensity of activity, you would discover the reason. Even if their schedule does not include jogging or intense exercise, it probably includes a high level of activity.

Basal metabolic rate (BMR)   The energy expenditure of the body under resting conditions at normal room temperature.

Yo-yo diet   Cycles in which people repeatedly gain weight, then starve themselves to lose weight. This lowers their BMR, which makes regaining weight even more likely.

Smoking   Women who smoke tend to weigh six to ten pounds less than nonsmokers. After they quit, their weight generally increases to the level found among nonsmokers. Weight gain after smoking cessation may be partly due to nicotine's ability to raise metabolic rate. When smokers stop, they burn fewer calories. Another reason former smokers often gain weight is that they generally eat more to satisfy free-floating cravings.[39]

> **What do you think?**
>
> *Why do you think men and women differ in their physical activity patterns?* ✳ *Why are certain minority groups less likely to exercise than other groups?* ✳ *What might be done in terms of policies, programs, and services to change these statistics?*

Gender and Obesity

Throughout a woman's life, issues of appearance and beauty are constantly in the foreground. Only recently have researchers begun to understand just how significant the quest for beauty and the perfect body really is.

Of increasing interest is another emerging problem seen in both young men and women, known as **social physique anxiety (SPA),** in which the desire to "look good" has a destructive and sometimes disabling effect on one's ability to function effectively in relationships and interactions with others. People suffering from SPA may spend a disproportionate amount of time "fixating" on their bodies, working out, and performing tasks that are ego centered and self-directed, rather than focusing on interpersonal relationships and general tasks.[40] Incessant worry about their bodies and their appearance permeates their lives. Overweight and obesity are clear risks for these people, and experts speculate that this anxiety may contribute to eating-disordered behaviors.

Researchers have determined that being severely overweight in adolescence may predetermine one's social and economic future—particularly for females. Researchers found that obese women complete about half a year less schooling, are 20 percent less likely to get married, and earn $6,710 on average less per year than their slimmer counterparts. Obese women also have rates of household poverty 10 percent higher than those of women who are not overweight. In contrast, the study found that overweight men are 11 percent less likely to be married than thinner men but suffer few adverse economic consequences.

Social physique anxiety (SPA)   A desire to look good that has a destructive effect on a person's ability to function effectively socially.

It is more likely that women will suffer such consequences of obesity simply because they are more likely than men to be overweight. Compared to men, women have a lower ratio of lean body mass to fatty mass, in part due to differences in bone size and mass, muscle size, and other variables. Muscle uses more energy than fat does. Because men have more muscle, they burn 10 to 20 percent more calories than women do during rest.[41] For all ages after sexual maturity, men have higher metabolic rates, making it easier for them to burn off excess calories than it is for women. Women also face greater potential for weight fluctuation due to hormonal changes, pregnancy, and other conditions that increase the likelihood of weight gain. Also, as a group, men are more socialized into physical activity from birth. Strenuous activity in both work and play are encouraged for men, whereas women's roles have typically been more sedentary and required a lower level of caloric expenditure.

Not only are women more vulnerable to weight gain, but also pressures to maintain and/or lose weight make them more likely to take dramatic measures. For example, eating disorders are more prevalent among women, and more women then men take diet pills. However, men experience these pressures too. The male image is becoming more associated with the bodybuilder shape and size, and men are becoming more preoccupied with their own physical form. Thus eating disorders, exercise addictions, and other maladaptive responses are on the increase among men.

Managing Your Weight

At some point in our lives, almost all of us will decide to go on a diet, and many will meet with mixed success. The problem is probably related to the fact that we think about losing weight in terms of "dieting" rather than adjusting lifestyle and eating behaviors. It is well documented that hypocaloric (low-calorie) diets produce only temporary losses and may actually lead to disordered binge eating or related problems.[42] While repeated bouts of restrictive dieting may be physiologically harmful, the sense of failure that we get each time we try and fail can also exact far-reaching psychological costs.[43] Drugs and intensive counseling have contributed to positive weight loss, but even then, weight is often regained after treatment.

Keeping Weight Control in Perspective

Although experts say that losing weight simply requires burning more calories than are consumed, putting this principle into practice is far from simple. According to William W. Hardy, M.D., president of the Michigan-based Rochester Center for Obesity,

> to say weight control is simply a matter of pushing away from the table is ludicrous. Nature is a cheat. Sure, calories in minus calories out equals weight, but

people of the same age, sex, height, and weight can have differences of as much as 1,000 calories a day in "resting metabolic rate"—this may explain why one person's gluttony is another's starvation, even if it results in the same readout on the scale. And while people of normal weight average 25–35 billion fat cells, obese people can inherit a billowing 135 billion. A roll of the genetic dice adds more variety: at least 240 genes affect weight.[44]

To lose weight is more difficult for some people, and it may require more supportive friends and relatives plus extraordinary efforts to prime the body for burning extra calories. Being overweight does not mean people are weak-willed or lazy. As scientists unlock the many secrets of genetic messengers that influence body weight and learn more about the role of certain foods in the weight loss equation, dieting may not be the same villain in the future that it is today.

Setting Realistic Goals

Rather than focusing on weight loss per se, some health professionals emphasize the importance of psychological and physical health.[45] Modern weight-management programs incorporate the following goals:

- Helping people establish tolerable, enjoyable, and stable eating and exercise patterns
- Focusing on small gains and benefits to health and well-being initially; later focusing on long-term functional improvements, improvements in energy, and reduced risk from disease
- Establishing maintainable goals
- Making a lifetime commitment to a healthful lifestyle that includes exercise, prudent food choices, and stress management
- Seeking continued support from professionals and loved ones
- Improving access to low-cost, healthful foods and broadening one's perspective on food possibilities, such as eating more grains and fewer processed foods
- Deemphasizing food as a central focus and learning to enjoy other activities that bring joy
- Becoming a wise food consumer

Develop a program of exercise and healthy eating behaviors that will work for you now and in the long term. To become a wise food consumer, you need to become familiar with important concepts in weight control.

What Is a Calorie?

A *calorie* is a unit of measure that indicates the amount of energy we obtain from a particular food. One pound of body fat contains approximately 3,500 calories. So each time you consume 3,500 calories more than your body needs to maintain weight, you gain a pound. Conversely, each time your body expends an extra 3,500 calories, you lose a pound. So if you add a can of Coca-Cola (140 calories) to your daily diet and make no other changes in diet or activity, you would gain a pound in 25 days (3,500 calories ÷ 140 calories/day = 25 days). Conversely, if you walked for half an hour each day at a pace of 15 minutes per mile (172 calories burned), you would lose a pound in approximately 20 days (3,500 calories ÷ 172 calories/day = 20.3 days). The two ways to lose weight, then, are to lower calorie intake (through improved eating habits) and to increase exercise (thereby expending more calories).

Exercise

Approximately 90 percent of the daily calorie expenditures of most people occurs as a result of the **resting metabolic rate (RMR).** The RMR is slightly higher than the BMR; it includes the BMR plus any additional energy expended through daily sedentary activities, such as food digestion, sitting, studying, or standing. The **exercise metabolic rate (EMR)** accounts for the remaining 10 percent of all daily calorie expenditures; it refers to the energy expenditure that occurs during physical exercise. For most of us, these calories come from light daily activities, such as walking, climbing stairs, and mowing the lawn. If we increase the level of physical activity to moderate or heavy, however, our EMR may be 10 to 20 times greater than typical resting metabolic rates and can contribute substantially to weight loss.

Increasing BMR, RMR, or EMR levels will help burn calories. An increase in the intensity, frequency, and duration of daily exercise levels can have significant impact on total calorie expenditure.

Physical activity makes a greater contribution to BMR when large muscle groups are used. The energy spent on physical activity is the energy used to move the body's muscles—the muscles of the arms, back, abdomen, legs, and so on—and the extra energy used to speed up heartbeat and respiration rate. The number of calories spent depends on three factors:

1. The amount of muscle mass moved
2. The amount of weight moved
3. The amount of time the activity takes

An activity involving both the arms and legs burns more calories than one involving only the legs, an activity performed by a heavy person burns more calories than one

---

Resting metabolic rate (RMR)   The energy expenditure of the body under BMR conditions plus other daily sedentary activities.

Exercise metabolic rate (EMR)   The energy expenditure that occurs during exercise.

performed by a lighter person, and an activity performed for 40 minutes requires twice as much energy than one performed for only 20 minutes. Thus, obese persons walking for 1 mile burn more calories than slim people walking the same distance. It may also take overweight people longer to walk the mile, which means that they are burning energy for a longer time and therefore expending more overall calories than the thin walkers.

> ### What do you think?
> *If you were going to try to lose weight, what strategies would you most likely use? ✳ What aspects of your weight loss strategies would offer the lowest health risk and the greatest chances for success? ✳ What factors might serve to sabotage your weight loss efforts?*

Changing Your Eating Habits

At any given time, many Americans are trying to lose weight. Given the hundreds of different diets and endless expert advice available, why do we find it so difficult?

Determining What Triggers an Eating Behavior Before you can change a behavior, you must first determine what causes it. Many people have found it helpful to keep a chart of their eating patterns: when they feel like eating, where they are when they decide to eat, the amount of time they spend eating, other activities they engage in during the meal (watching television or reading), whether they eat alone or with others, what and how much they consume, and how they felt before they took their first bite. If you keep a detailed daily log of eating triggers for at least a week, you will discover useful clues about what in your environment or your emotional makeup causes you to want food. Typically, these dietary "triggers" center on problems in everyday living rather than on real hunger pangs. Many people find that they eat compulsively when stressed or when they have problems in their relationships. For other people, the same circumstances diminish their appetite, causing them to lose weight.

Changing Your Triggers Once you recognize the factors that cause you to eat, removing the triggers or substituting other activities for them will help you develop more sensible eating patterns. Below are some examples of substitute behaviors. More weight management tips are offered in the accompanying Skills for Behavior Change box.

1. When eating dinner, turn off all distractions, including the television and radio.
2. Replace snack breaks or coffee breaks with exercise breaks.

3. Instead of gulping your food, force yourself to chew each bite slowly.
4. Vary the time of day when you eat. Instead of eating by the clock, do not eat until you are truly hungry and allow yourself only a designated amount of time for eating.
5. If you find that you generally eat all that you can cram on a plate, use smaller plates.
6. Stop buying high-calorie foods that tempt you to snack, or store them in an inconvenient place.

> ### What do you think?
> *Do you eat because it's time to eat, or because you are really hungry? ✳ Do you know what real hunger feels like? ✳ Chart your eating behaviors for the next two to three days. Each time you find yourself "grazing" for food or drink, ask yourself (1) whether you are really hungry and (2) what triggered you to eat.*

Selecting a Nutritional Plan

Once you have discovered what factors tend to sabotage your weight loss efforts, you will be well on your way to healthy weight control. To succeed, however, you must plan for success. By setting goals that are unrealistic or too far in the future, you will doom yourself to failure. Do not try to lose 40 pounds in two months. Try, instead, to lose a healthy one to two pounds during the first week, and stay with this slow and easy regimen. Reward yourself when you lose pounds, and if you binge and go off your nutrition plan, get right back on it the next day. Remember that you did not gain 40 pounds in eight weeks, so it is unrealistic to punish your body by trying to lose that amount of weight in such a short time.

Seek assistance from reputable sources in selecting a dietary plan that is nutritious and easy to follow. Registered dietitians, some physicians (not all physicians have a strong background in nutrition), health educators and exercise physiologists with nutritional training, and other health professionals can provide reliable information. Beware of people who call themselves "nutritionists." There is no such official designation, leaving the door open for just about anyone to call himself or herself a nutritional expert. Avoid weight loss programs that promise quick miracle results.

For any weight loss program, ask about the credentials of the adviser, assess the nutrient value of the prescribed diet, verify that dietary guidelines are consistent with reliable nutrition research, and analyze the suitability of the diet to your tastes, budget, and lifestyle. Any diet that requires radical behavior changes is doomed to failure. The most successful plans allow you to make food choices and do not ask you to sacrifice everything you enjoy.

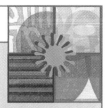

New Tips for Weight Control

This chapter presents many ideas for achieving and maintaining a healthy weight. In addition, here are several new strategies that are gaining credibility in the scientific community:

- *Eat breakfast.* According to new Mayo Clinic research, you'll be more likely to burn fat if you eat this meal. People who chronically skip breakfast burn an average of 150 fewer calories per day than regular breakfast eaters. The proposed reason? Breakfast eaters awake with a souped-up metabolism; breakfast skippers greet each day cold and tired with the "metabolic furnace" set on low until lunch.

- *Eat wet foods.* Try a juicy apple or cup of soup instead of a dry granola bar or bag of popcorn. Recent experiments show that the water content within foods plays a critical role in weight control. Dehydration stimulates the appetite, and eating foods with high water content will make you feel even more full than drinking water to wash down dry foods with the same calorie count.

- *Eat large servings of low-calorie foods rather than small amounts of calorie-dense foods.* You'll feel fuller on fewer calories.

- *Don't eliminate fat.* It adds flavor, and if fat levels get too low, biochemical systems trigger intense pig-out cravings. Keep fat calories to 20–30 percent of your total, and boost your fiber intake.

- *Eat more monounsaturated fats.* New research seems to indicate that eating monounsaturated fats, such as olive oil, works better in delaying hunger cravings than eating other fats.

- *Eat nuts.* Studies show that a well-timed handful of nuts satisfies the appetite and prevents overeating.

- *Narrow your choices.* If it's not there, you won't eat it. Don't stock your kitchen with foods you'd best avoid. If you don't have all kinds of choices, you won't be so intrigued by food options, and you'll eat less.

- *Eat a well-rounded diet.* Never eat fewer than 1,000 calories per day.

- *Burn calories rather than cutting them.* If you eat fewer calories, your body compensates by slowing its metabolic rate, leaving you sluggish, cold, and craving more. Exercising boosts metabolism and counteracts any fat-guarding legacy you may have inherited.

- *Lift weights.* A Tufts study of women who took up moderate weight lifting found that they increased their strength by an average of 35 percent to 76 percent, improved their balance by 14 percent, and boosted bone density by 1 percent. The greater your muscle mass, the greater your basal metabolic rate and, hence, the more calories you burn.

- *Start fidgeting.* A recent study suggests that constantly repeated mini-movements, such as those you make when fidgeting, may play a tremendous role in weight control. Walk around while talking on that cordless phone. Keep walking while brushing your teeth. Every little motion adds up.

Source: Adapted from J. Thornton, "Cheat and Run," *USA Today Weekend,* July 14–16, 2000.

"Miracle" Diets

Fasting, starvation diets, and other forms of **very low calorie diets (VLCDs)** have been shown to cause significant health risks. Typically, depriving the body of food for prolonged periods forces it to make adjustments to prevent the shutdown of organs. The body depletes its energy reserves to obtain necessary fuels. One of the first reserves the body turns to in order to maintain its supply of glucose is lean, protein tissue. As this occurs, weight is lost rapidly because protein contains only half as many calories per pound as fat. At the same time, significant water stores are lost. Over time, the body begins to run out of liver tissue, heart muscle, blood, and so on, as these readily available substances are burned to supply energy. Only after depleting the readily available proteins from these sources does the body begin to burn fat reserves. In this process, known as **ketosis,** the body adapts to prolonged fasting or carbohydrate deprivation by converting body fat to ketones, which can be used as fuel for some brain cells. Within about ten days after the typical adult begins a complete fast, the body will have used many of its energy stores and death may occur.

In very low calorie diets, powdered formulas are usually given to patients under medical supervision. These formulas have daily values of 400 to 700 calories plus vitamin and mineral supplements. Although these diets may be beneficial for people who have failed at all conventional weight-loss methods and who face severe health risks due to

Very low calorie diets (VLCDs)   Diets with caloric value of 400 to 700 calories per day.

Ketosis   A condition in which the body adapts to prolonged fasting or carbohydrate deprivation by converting body fat to ketones, which can be used as fuel for some brain activity.

obesity, they should never be undertaken without strict medical supervision. Problems associated with fasting, VLCDs, and other forms of severe calorie deprivation include blood sugar imbalances, cold intolerance, constipation, decreased BMR, dehydration, diarrhea, emotional problems, fatigue, headaches, heart irregularity, ketosis, kidney infections and failure, loss of lean body tissue, weakness, and eventual weight gain due to the yo-yo effect and other variables.

Trying to Gain Weight

Although trying to lose weight poses a major challenge for many people, a smaller group of Americans, for metabolic, hereditary, psychological, and other reasons, can't seem to gain weight no matter how hard they try. If you are one of these individuals, determining the reasons for your difficulty in gaining weight is a must. Once you know what is causing a daily caloric deficit, there are steps you can take to gain extra weight:

- *Control your exercise.* Cut back if you are doing too much, slow down, and keep a careful record of calories burned.
- *Eat more.* Obviously, you are not taking in enough calories to support whatever is happening in your body. Eat more frequently, spend more time eating, eat the high-calorie foods first if you fill up fast, and always start with the main course. Take time to shop, to cook, to eat slowly. Put extra spreads such as peanut butter, cream cheese, or cheese on your foods. Make your sandwiches with extra-thick slices of bread, and add more filling. Take seconds whenever possible, and eat high-calorie snacks during the day.
- *Supplement your diet.* Add high-calorie drinks that have a healthy balance of nutrients.
- *Relax.* Many people who are underweight operate at high gear most of the time. Slow down, get more rest, and control stress.

Eating Disorders

On occasion, over one-third of all Americans fit the descriptions of obesity and diet obsessiveness. For an increasing number of people, particularly young women, this obsessive

relationship with food develops into **anorexia nervosa,** a persistent, chronic eating disorder characterized by deliberate food restriction and severe, life-threatening weight loss. **Bulimia nervosa,** or a variation known as **binge eating disorder (BED),** involves frequent bouts of binge eating followed by purging (self-induced vomiting), laxative abuse, or excessive exercise. In the United States more than 10 million people, 90 percent of whom are women, meet the established criteria for one of these disorders, and their numbers appear to be increasing.[46] Many more suffer from minor forms of these conditions—not enough for a true diagnosis, but dangerously close to the precipice that will ultimately lead to life-threatening results (Table 10.2).

Anorexia Nervosa

Anorexia involves self-starvation motivated by an intense fear of gaining weight along with an extremely distorted body image. When anorexia occurs in childhood, failure to gain weight in a normal growth pattern may be the key indicator; later, this typically results in actual weight loss. Nearly 1 percent of girls in late adolescence meet the full criteria for anorexia; many others suffer from significant symptoms.

Usually people with anorexia achieve their weight loss through initial reduction in total food intake, particularly of high-calorie foods, eventually leading to restricted intake of almost all foods. What they do eat, they often purge through vomiting or using laxatives. Although they lose weight, people with anorexia never seem to feel "thin enough" and constantly identify body parts that are "too fat."

Bulimia Nervosa

People with bulimia often binge and then take inappropriate measures, such as secret vomiting, to lose the calories they have just acquired. Up to 3 percent of adolescents and young female adults are bulimic, with male rates being about 10 percent of the female rate. People with bulimia are also obsessed with their bodies, weight gain, and how they appear to others. Unlike those with anorexia, people with bulimia are often "hidden" from the public eye because their weight may vary only slightly or fall within a normal range. Also, treatment for bulimia appears to be more effective than for anorexia.

Binge Eating Disorder (BED)

Individuals with binge eating disorder (BED) also binge like their bulimic counterparts, but they do not take excessive measures to lose the weight that they gain. Often they are clinically obese, and they tend to binge much more often than the typical obese person who may consume too many calories but spaces his or her eating over a more normal daily eating pattern. To date, binge eating disorder is still under consideration as a psychiatric disorder.

Anorexia nervosa   Eating disorder characterized by excessive preoccupation with food, self-starvation, and/or extreme exercising to achieve weight loss.

Bulimia nervosa   Eating disorder characterized by binge eating followed by inappropriate measures to prevent weight gain.

Binge eating disorder (BED)   Eating disorder characterized by recurrent binge eating, without excessive measures to prevent weight gain.

Table 10.2
DSM-IV Eating Disorder Criteria

ANOREXIA

According to the American Psychiatric Association's *Diagnostic and Statistical Manual of Mental Disorders,* 4th edition (*DSM-IV*), people who meet the criteria for anorexia nervosa experience all of the following symptoms:

- Refusal to maintain the minimum body weight for one's height and age
- Intense fear of gaining weight even though underweight
- Disturbed perception of one's body weight or size
- In post-pubescent women, the absence of at least three consecutive menstrual cycles (In some women, the loss of periods precedes any significant weight loss.)

BULIMIA

People with bulimia experience all of the following:

- Recurrent episodes of consuming a much larger amount of food than most people would during a similar time period (this is usually about two hours) and a sense of loss of control over eating during each episode
- Accompanying attempts to compensate for eating binges by vomiting, abusing laxatives or other drugs, or by fasting or excessive exercise
- Both the binge eating and purging occur at least twice a week for three months
- A negative perception of one's shape and weight

Source: From *DSM-IV,* reported in "Treating Eating Disorders," *Harvard Women's Health Watch,* May 1996, 4–5. Reprinted with permission from the *Diagnostic and Statistical Manual of Mental Disorders,* Fourth Edition, Copyright 1994 American Psychiatric Association.

Who's at Risk?

There's no simple explanation for why intelligent, often highly accomplished young people spiral downward into the destructive behaviors associated with eating disorders. Obsessive-compulsive disorder, depression, and anxiety can all play a role, as can a desperate need to win social approval or gain control of their lives through food.

Sufferers tend to be women from white middle-class or upper-class families in which there is undue emphasis on achievement, body weight, and appearance. Contrary to popular thinking, however, eating disorders span social class, gender, race, and ethnic backgrounds and are present in countries throughout the world. In addition, increasing numbers of males suffer from various forms of eating disorders.

Treatment for Eating Disorders

Because eating disorders result from many factors, spanning many years of development, there are no quick or simple solutions. Treatment often focuses on reducing the threat to life; once the patient is stabilized, long-term therapy involves family, friends, and other significant people in the individual's life. Therapy focuses on the psychological, social, environmental, and physiological factors that have led to the problem. Finding a therapist who really understands the multidimensional aspects of the problem is a must. Therapy allows the patient to focus on building new eating behaviors, recognizing threats, building self-confidence, and finding other ways of dealing with life's problems. Support groups often help the family and the individual gain understanding and emotional support and learn self-development techniques designed to foster positive reactions and actions. Treatment of underlying depression may also be a focus.

What do you think?

Which groups or individuals on your campus appear to be at greatest risk for eating disorders? ✳ What social factors might encourage this? ✳ Why do you think society tends to overlook eating disorders in males? ✳ What programs or services on your campus are available for someone with an eating disorder?

Taking Control of Your Weight

Controlling your weight involves gaining control over food, modifying behaviors, and making exercise a priority. To ensure success, look at weight control as a lifelong commitment rather than a temporary diet. The first step in managing weight is an honest self-assessment of where you are. What did you find out about yourself as you read this chapter? Are you satisfied with your weight? If not, what can you do to make a change? Next, set a realistic goal. Ask yourself, why do I want to meet this goal? What will I do when I reach it? Then develop a plan to reach your goal. Each person must find his or her own best strategy, recognize potential difficulties, and work to modify behaviors to help bring weight under control. Your school and community have resources to help. If you are in doubt, ask your instructor or your student health center. Here are some suggestions to help you get started.

Checklist for Change

Making Personal Choices

✓ Design your plan based on your needs. It must fit your personality, your priorities, and your work and recreation schedules.

Allow for sufficient rest and relaxation.

✓ Include nutrient-dense foods. Get the most from the foods you eat by selecting foods with high nutritional value.

✓ Balance food intake throughout the day. Rather than gorging yourself at one main meal, you are probably better off eating several smaller meals throughout the day.

✓ Plan for plateaus. If you prepare yourself psychologically for plateaus, you will be less likely to become discouraged. Exercise is probably the critical factor in getting past a plateau.

✓ Chart your progress. Weigh yourself weekly, not daily, to avoid frustration. After all, it is long-range success you are after.

✓ Chart your setbacks. Rather than thinking in terms of failure and punishment, think in terms of temporary setbacks and how to accommodate them. By carefully recording your emotional states when eating, eating habits, environmental cues, and feelings, you may determine why you needed that ice cream cone or why you chose a pizza instead of a salad. Women may need to take into account weight fluctuations due to hormonal changes over the course of the monthly cycle.

✓ Become aware of your feelings of hunger and fullness. For many of us, eating is time dependent, and we stop eating only when the food is gone (the "clean your plate" syndrome). Long years of eating when it is time to eat instead of eating when we need to has cost us the ability to tell when we are really hungry and when we are really full. By training yourself to become more aware of the eating process, by learning to recognize true hunger pangs and the first signals that you have eaten enough, you will be able to change your eating patterns.

✓ Accept yourself. For many people, this is the most important aspect of successful weight management. It is important to keep weight in perspective. Unless you feel good about who you are inside, exterior changes will not help you very much.

✓ Exercise, exercise, exercise. Although we would all like to wish away our extra pounds, losing weight requires hard work and concentration. Different people benefit from different types of activities. Select an exercise program that you consider fun, not a daily form of punishment for overeating. Remember, every little effort contributes toward long-term results.

Summary

* Overweight, obesity, and weight-related problems appear to be on the rise in the United States. Obesity is now defined in terms of fat content rather than in terms of weight alone.
* There are many different methods of assessing body fat. Body Mass Index (BMI) is one of the most commonly accepted measures of weight based on height. Body fat percentages more accurately indicate how fat or lean a person is.

* Many factors contribute to one's risk for obesity, including genetics, developmental factors, setpoint, endocrine influences, psychosocial factors, eating cues, lack of awareness, metabolic changes, lifestyle, and gender. Women often have considerably more difficulty in achieving weight loss.
* Exercise, dieting, diet pills, and other strategies are used to maintain or lose weight. However, sensible eating behavior and adequate exercise probably offer the best options.

✳ Eating disorders consist of severe disturbances in eating behaviors, unhealthy efforts to control body weight, and abnormal attitudes about body and shape. Anorexia nervosa, bulimia nervosa, and binge eating disorder are the three main eating disorders. Though prevalent among white women of upper- and middle-class families, eating disorders affect women of all backgrounds as well as a number of men.

Discussion Questions

1. Discuss the pressures, if any, you feel to improve your personal body image. Do these pressures come from media, family, friends, and other external sources, or from concern for your personal health? Do you have friends or family members who you believe have body image problems? What makes you think this?
2. What type of measurement would you choose in order to assess your fat levels? Why?
3. List the risk factors for obesity. Evaluate which seem to be most important in determining whether you will be obese in middle age.
4. Create a plan to help someone lose the "freshman 15" over the summer vacation. Assume that the person is male, 180 pounds, and has 15 weeks to lose the excess weight.
5. Differentiate among the three eating disorders. Then give reasons why females might be more prone to anorexia and bulimia than males are.

Application Exercises

Reread the What Do You Think? scenarios at the beginning of the chapter, and answer the following questions:

1. What factors have contributed to Angela's and Nick's weight gain? Do you know people in similar situations?
2. What advice would you give Angela and Nick? Describe practical solutions to their problems.

Accessing Your Health on the Internet http

Visit the following Internet sites to explore further topics and issues related to personal health. To visit an organization's website, go to the Companion Website for *Health: The Basics, Fifth Edition* at www.aw.com/donatelle, click on the book image, and select "Accessing Your Health on the Internet" from the navigation menu on the left.

1. *Helping to End Eating Disorders (HEED).* The website of an organization dedicated to fighting eating disorders and helping individuals through the ordeal. Includes a chatroom for people to exchange thoughts and share support.
2. *American Dietetic Association.* Recommended dietary guidelines and other current information about weight control.
3. *Shape Up America.* Strategies and ideas for getting in shape and losing those extra pounds.
4. *Mayo Health O@sis.* Summary of many weight control issues and concerns.
5. *Duke University Diet and Fitness Center.* Information about one of the best programs in the country focused on helping people live healthier, fuller lives through weight control and lifestyle change.

Further Reading

Gaesser, G. *Big Fat Lies.* New York: Fawcett Columbine Press, 1997.
   Excellent overview of leading theories on fat, obesity, and a host of related problems and issues. Also discusses potential weight loss strategies that are "keepers" for life.
Piscatella, J. *The Fat-Gram Guide to Restaurant Food,* 3rd ed. New York: Workman Press, 2000.
   Excellent guide to fast foods and restaurant fat content.

Price, D. *Healing the Hungry Self: The Diet-Free Solution to Lifelong Weight Management.* New York: Plume, 1998.
   Interestingly written, realistic approach to weight control.

11

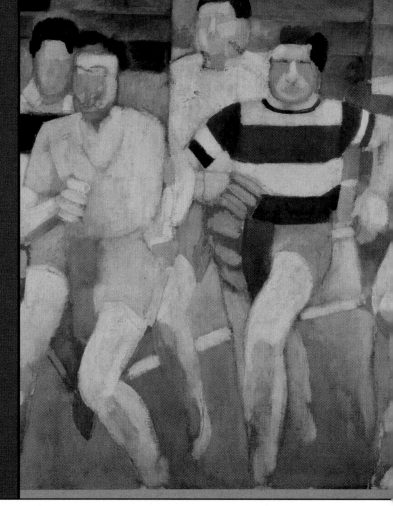

11
Personal Fitness
IMPROVING HEALTH THROUGH EXERCISE

11

11

11

11

objectives

* Describe physical fitness and the benefits of regular physical activity, including improvements in cardiorespiratory fitness, muscular fitness, bone mass, weight control, stress management, mental health, and life span.

* Describe the components of an aerobic exercise program and how to determine proper frequency, intensity, and duration of exercise.

* Describe different stretching exercises designed to improve flexibility.

* Compare the various types and benefits of resistance exercise programs.

* Describe common fitness injuries, suggest ways to prevent injuries, and list the treatment process.

* Summarize the key components of a personal fitness program.

A century ago in the United States, simple survival required performing physical labor on a daily basis. However, science and technology have transformed our lives. Today most adults in our country lead sedentary lifestyles and perform little physical labor or exercise.[1]

The growing percentage of Americans who live sedentary lives has been linked to dramatic increases in the incidence of chronic disease. Heart disease is a cause of death almost 30 times more frequently today than it was in 1900.[2] Between 1958 and 1993, the incidence of type 2 (non–insulin-dependent) diabetes increased sixfold, and over the past 20 years the incidence of obesity has doubled in the United States.

Especially when combined with a healthy diet, regular physical activity combats obesity and reduces risk of heart disease, high blood pressure, type 2 diabetes, and colon cancer.[3] In fact, regular physical activity improves more than 50 different physiological, metabolic, and psychological aspects of human life.[4] Now is an excellent time to develop exercise habits that will increase the quality and duration of your life.

What Is Physical Fitness?

Physical fitness is the ability to perform moderate to vigorous physical activity on a regular basis without excessive fatigue. **Exercise training** is the systematic performance of exercise at a specified frequency, intensity, and duration to achieve a desired level of physical fitness.[5] Major health-related components of physical fitness include cardiorespiratory fitness, muscular strength and endurance, flexibility, and body composition. These components play a vital role in overall health (Table 11.1).

To be considered physically fit, you generally need to attain (and then maintain) certain minimum standards for each component that have been established by exercise physiologists and other fitness experts. Some people have

Table 11.1
Major Components of Physical Fitness

Cardiorespiratory fitness	Ability to sustain moderate-intensity whole-body activity for extended time periods
Muscular strength and endurance	Maximum force applied with a single muscle contraction; ability to perform repeated high-intensity muscle contractions
Flexibility	Range of motion at a joint or series of joints
Body composition	A composite of total body mass, fat mass, fat-free mass, and fat distribution

Source: From the American College of Sports Medicine, "ACSM Position Stand on the Recommended Quantity and Quality of Exercise for Developing and Maintaining Cardiorespiratory and Muscular Fitness and Flexibility in Adults," *Medicine and Science in Sports and Exercise* 30 (1998): 975–991.

physical limitations that make achieving one or more of these standards difficult. That doesn't mean they can't become physically fit. For example, a woman with limited flexibility due to arthritis in the knee and hip joints may be unable to jog without extreme pain. Yet by exercising in a swimming pool, where the buoyancy of the water will relieve

Physical fitness The ability to perform regular moderate to rigorous physical activity without great fatigue.

Exercise training The systematic performance of exercise at a specified frequency, intensity, and duration to achieve a desired level of physical fitness.

much of the stress on her joints, she can improve her range of motion. She can also develop muscular strength and cardiovascular fitness by "jogging" at the deep end of a swimming pool while wearing a flotation device. Similarly, a man who needs to use a wheelchair may be unable to run or walk a mile, as is required in some fitness tests, but can achieve physical fitness by playing wheelchair basketball.

Athletic skill is not a requirement for physical fitness—you do not have to possess the talents of an Olympic athlete to achieve health benefits from regular physical activity and exercise. Many activities that create health benefits, such as walking, running, swimming, and cycling, require no special skill to be performed and enjoyed. Our definition of physical fitness should be adapted to address individual differences in capabilities.

Benefits of Regular Physical Activity

Physical activity is any force exerted by skeletal muscles that results in energy usage above the level used when the body's systems are at rest.[6] Higher levels of physical activity are associated with a lower risk of coronary heart disease (the leading cause of death in the United States for both men and women), diabetes, osteoporosis,[7] high blood pressure (hypertension), cancers of the colon and reproductive organs,[8] and psychological disorders such as depression and anxiety.[9] A recent study reported that regular exercise (4 hours a week or more) beginning in adolescence and continuing into adulthood can significantly reduce the risk of breast cancer in women age 40 and younger.[10] The recent Surgeon General's report on physical activity and health[11] indicates that physical activity need not be strenuous in order to achieve health benefits and that women and men of all ages benefit from a moderate amount of *daily* physical activity.

Improved Cardiorespiratory Fitness

Cardiorespiratory fitness refers to the ability of the circulatory and respiratory systems to supply oxygen to the body during sustained physical activity.[12] Regular exercise will make these systems more efficient by enlarging the heart muscle, thereby enabling more blood to be pumped with each stroke, and increasing the number of *capillaries* (small arteries) in trained skeletal muscles, which supply more blood to working muscles. Exercise improves the respiratory system by increasing the amount of oxygen that is inhaled and distributed to body tissues.[13]

Reduced Risk of Heart Disease   Your heart is a muscle made up of highly specialized tissue. Because muscles become stronger and more efficient with use, regular exercise strengthens the heart, enabling it to pump more blood with each beat. This increased efficiency means that the heart requires fewer beats per minute to circulate blood throughout the body. A stronger, more efficient heart is better able to meet the ordinary demands of life.

Prevention of Hypertension   *Blood pressure* refers to the force exerted by blood against blood vessel walls, generated by the pumping action of the heart. Hypertension, the medical term for abnormally high blood pressure, is a significant risk factor for cardiovascular disease and stroke. Regular physical activity can reduce blood pressure in people with normal blood pressure and in those with high blood pressure.[14]

Improved Blood Lipid and Lipoprotein Profile   Lipids are fats that circulate in the bloodstream and are stored in various places in the body. Regular exercise is known to reduce the levels of low-density lipoproteins (LDLs—"bad cholesterol") while increasing the number of high-density lipoproteins (HDLs—"good cholesterol") in the blood. Higher HDL levels are associated with lower risk for artery disease because they remove some of the "bad cholesterol" from artery walls and hence prevent clogging. The bottom line: Regular exercise lowers the risk of cardiovascular disease. (For more on cholesterol and blood pressure, see Chapter 12).

Improved Bone Mass

A common affliction among older adults is **osteoporosis,** a disease characterized by low bone mass and deterioration of bone tissue, which increase fracture risk. Osteoporosis is more common among women than among men for at least three reasons: Women live longer than men; they have lower peak bone mass than men; and women lose bone mass at an accelerated rate after menopause as their estrogen levels decrease. Thus, the incidence of osteoporosis and fractures increases substantially with age in both women and men. In the United States alone, nearly 1.5 million osteoporosis-related fractures occur every year.[15]

Bone, like other human tissues, responds to the demands placed on it. Women (and men) have much to gain by remaining physically active as they age—bone mass levels are significantly higher among active than among sedentary women.[16] Regular weight-bearing exercise, when combined with a balanced diet containing adequate calcium, will help maintain bone mass.

Cardiorespiratory fitness   The ability of the heart, lungs, and blood vessels to supply oxygen to skeletal muscles during sustained physical activity.

Osteoporosis   A disease characterized by low bone mass and deterioration of bone tissue, which increase risk of fracture.

Improved Weight Control

Many people start exercising because they want to lose weight. Level of physical activity does have a direct effect on metabolic rate, even raising it for several hours following a vigorous workout. According to the American College of Sports Medicine (ACSM), if you are planning to lose weight through exercise alone, without decreasing the amount of food you eat, you'll have to exercise frequently (at least four days a week) for extended time periods (at least 50 minutes per workout).[17] A more effective method for losing weight combines regular endurance-type exercises with a moderate decrease in food intake. Decreasing daily caloric intake beyond this range ("severe dieting") appears to decrease metabolic rate by up to 20 percent, making weight loss more difficult.

A recent meta-analysis challenges the commonly held view that exercise alone is not a useful strategy for obesity reduction. Moderately obese white men who participated in daily exercise of moderate intensity (brisk walking) for 45 to 60 minutes per day, without decreasing their caloric intake, made rapid improvements in cardiovascular fitness and lost weight.[18] Regular exercise also reduced the incidence of heart disease and type 2 diabetes in these participants and reduced the overall death rate.[19]

Improved Health and Life Span

Prevention of Diabetes Non–insulin-dependent diabetes (type 2 diabetes) is a complex disorder that affects millions of Americans, many of whom have no idea that they have the disease. (See Chapter 14.) Risk factors for diabetes include obesity, high blood pressure, and high cholesterol, as well as a family history of the disease.[20] Physicians suggest exercise combined with weight loss and proper diet to manage diabetes. A recent large study found that for every 2,000 calories of energy expended during leisure-time activities, the incidence of diabetes was reduced by 24 percent. Perhaps the most encouraging finding was that the protective effect of exercise was greatest among those individuals who were at the highest risk.[21]

Increased Longevity A landmark study conducted at the Institute for Aerobics Research in Texas found that exercise does increase longevity. More than 13,000 white men and women of ages 20 to 80 were followed for eight years. Participants were assigned fitness levels based on their age, sex, and results of exercise tests. The death rate in the least physically fit group was more than three times higher than that of the most fit group. How much physical activity was required to produce a difference? Sedentary participants who started taking a brisk 30- to 60-minute walk each day experienced significant increases in life expectancy.[22]

Increased Immunity to Disease Recent research suggests that regular moderate exercise makes people less susceptible to disease, but that this potential benefit may depend on whether the person perceives exercise as pleasurable or stressful.[23] However, extreme exercise may actually be detrimental. For example, athletes engaging in marathon-type events or very intense physical training have an increased risk of colds and flu.[24] In a recent study of 2,300 marathon runners, those who ran more than 60 miles per week suffered twice as many upper respiratory tract infections as those who ran fewer than 20 miles per week.[25]

Just how exercise alters immunity is not well understood. We do know that brisk exercise temporarily increases the number of white blood cells (WBCs), the blood cells responsible for fighting infection. Generally speaking, the less fit the person and the more intense the exercise, the greater the increase in WBCs.[26] After brief periods of exercise (without injury), the number of WBCs typically returns to normal levels within one to two hours. After exercise bouts lasting longer than 30 minutes, WBCs may be elevated for 24 hours or more before returning to normal levels.[27] An increased number of WBCs suggests greater immunity to disease and infection.

Improved Mental Health and Stress Management

People who engage in regular physical activity also notice psychological benefits. Regular vigorous exercise has been shown to "burn off" the chemical by-products released by the nervous system during normal response to stress. This reduces stress levels by accelerating the body's return to a balanced state. Regular exercise improves a person's physical appearance by toning and developing muscles and reducing body fat. Feeling good about personal appearance boosts self-esteem. At the same time, as people come to appreciate the improved strength, conditioning, and flexibility that accompany fitness, they often become less obsessed with physical appearance.[28] They learn new skills and develop increased abilities in favorite recreational activities, which also help improve self-esteem.

> **What do you think?**
> Which of the key aspects of physical fitness do you currently possess? ✳ Which ones would you like to improve or develop? ✳ What types of activities could you do to improve your fitness level?

Improving Cardiorespiratory Fitness

The number of walkers, joggers, bicyclists, step aerobics classes, and swimmers is tangible evidence of Americans' increased interest in cardiorespiratory fitness. The primary category of physical activity known to improve cardiorespiratory

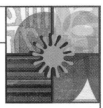

Self-Assessment of Cardiorespiratory Endurance

Once you've been exercising regularly for several weeks, you might want to assess your cardiorespiratory endurance level. Find a local track, typically one-quarter mile per lap, to perform your test. You may either run or walk for 1.5 miles and measure how long it takes to reach that distance, or run or walk for 12 minutes and determine the distance you covered in that time. Use the chart below to estimate your cardiorespiratory fitness level based upon your age and sex. Note that women have lower standards for each fitness category because they have higher levels of essential fat than men do. If you are now at the Good level, your emphasis should be on maintaining this level for the rest of your life. If you are now at lower levels, you should set realistic goals for improvement.

AGE*	1.5-Mile Run (min:sec)		12-Minute Run (miles)	
	WOMEN (MIN:SEC)	MEN (MIN:SEC)	WOMEN (MILES)	MEN (MILES)
Good				
15–30	<12:00	<10:00	>1.5	>1.7
35–50	<13:30	<11:30	>1.4	>1.5
55–70	<16:00	<14:00	>1.2	>1.3
Adequate for most activities				
15–30	<13:30	<11:50	>1.4	>1.5
35–50	<15:00	<13:00	>1.3	>1.4
55–70	<17:30	<15:30	>1.1	>1.3
Borderline				
15–30	<15:00	<13:00	>1.3	>1.4
35–50	<16:30	<14:30	>1.2	>1.3
55–70	<19:00	<17:00	>1.0	>1.2
Need extra work on cardiovascular fitness				
15–30	>17:00	>15:00	<1.2	<1.3
35–50	>18:30	>16:30	<1.1	<1.2
55–70	>21:00	>19:00	<0.9	<1.0

*Cardiorespiratory fitness declines with age.

Source: Reprinted by permission from Edward T. Howley and B. Don Franks, 1992, *Health/Fitness Instructor's Handbook*, 2nd ed. (Champaign, Ill.: Human Kinetics Publishers), 85.

Aerobic exercise Any type of exercise, typically performed at moderate levels of intensity for extended periods of time (typically 20 to 30 minutes or longer), that increases heart rate.

Aerobic capacity The current functional status of a person's cardiovascular system; measured as $VO_{2\,max}$.

Graded exercise test A test of aerobic capacity administered by a physician, exercise physiologist, or other trained professional; two common forms are the treadmill running test and the stationary bike test.

endurance is **aerobic exercise.** The term *aerobic* means "with oxygen" and describes any type of exercise, typically performed at moderate levels of intensity for extended periods of time, that increases your heart rate. A person said to be in "good shape" has an above-average **aerobic capacity**—a term used to describe the functional status of the cardiorespiratory system (i.e., heart, lungs, blood vessels). Aerobic capacity (commonly written as $VO_{2\,max}$) is defined as the maximum volume of oxygen consumed by the muscles during exercise.

To measure your maximal aerobic capacity, an exercise physiologist or physician will typically have you exercise on a treadmill. He or she will initially ask you to walk at an easy pace, and then, at set time intervals during this **graded -exercise test,** will gradually increase the workload

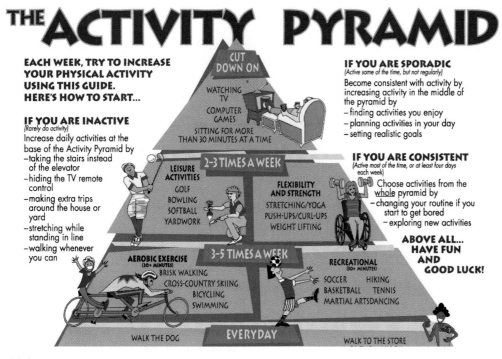

THE ACTIVITY PYRAMID

EACH WEEK, TRY TO INCREASE YOUR PHYSICAL ACTIVITY USING THIS GUIDE. HERE'S HOW TO START...

IF YOU ARE INACTIVE
(Rarely do activity)
Increase daily activities at the base of the Activity Pyramid by
– taking the stairs instead of the elevator
– hiding the TV remote control
– making extra trips around the house or yard
– stretching while standing in line
– walking whenever you can

CUT DOWN ON
WATCHING TV
COMPUTER GAMES
SITTING FOR MORE THAN 30 MINUTES AT A TIME

IF YOU ARE SPORADIC
(Active some of the time, but not regularly)
Become consistent with activity by increasing activity in the middle of the pyramid by
– finding activities you enjoy
– planning activities in your day
– setting realistic goals

2-3 TIMES A WEEK

LEISURE ACTIVITIES
GOLF
BOWLING
SOFTBALL
YARDWORK

FLEXIBILITY AND STRENGTH
STRETCHING/YOGA
PUSH-UPS/CURL-UPS
WEIGHT LIFTING

IF YOU ARE CONSISTENT
(Active most of the time, or at least four days each week)
Choose activities from the whole pyramid by
– changing your routine if you start to get bored
– exploring new activities

ABOVE ALL... HAVE FUN AND GOOD LUCK!

3-5 TIMES A WEEK

AEROBIC EXERCISE *(20+ MINUTES)*
BRISK WALKING
CROSS-COUNTRY SKIING
BICYCLING
SWIMMING

RECREATIONAL *(30+ MINUTES)*
SOCCER   HIKING
BASKETBALL   TENNIS
MARTIAL ARTS DANCING

EVERYDAY

WALK THE DOG

WALK TO THE STORE

Figure 11.1
Guidelines for Various Activity Levels
Source: Copyright © 1996. Institute for Research and Education, HealthSystem Minnesota.

(i.e., a combination of running speed and the angle of incline of the treadmill). Generally, the higher your cardiorespiratory endurance level, the more oxygen you can transport to exercising muscles and the longer you can exercise without becoming exhausted. In other words, the higher the $VO_{2 \, max}$ value, the higher your level of aerobic fitness.

You can test your own aerobic capacity by using either the 1.5-mile run or the 12-minute run endurance test described in the accompanying Assess Yourself box. However, you should not use these endurance-run tests if you are just starting to exercise.[29] Progress slowly through a walking/jogging program at low intensities before measuring your aerobic capacity with one of these tests. If you have any medical conditions, such as asthma, diabetes, heart disease, or obesity, consult your physician before beginning an exercise program.

Aerobic Fitness Programs

The most beneficial aerobic exercises are total body activities, for example, swimming, cross-country skiing, and rowing, that involve all the large muscle groups of your body. If you have been sedentary for quite a while, simply initiating a physical activity program may be the hardest task you'll face. Don't be put off by the next-day soreness you are likely to feel. The key is to begin at a very low intensity, progress slowly . . . and stay with it! For example, if you want to start jogging, you'll need several weeks of workouts combining walking and jogging before you will reach a fitness level that enables you to jog continuously for 15 to 20 minutes. Adjust the frequency, intensity, and duration of your aerobic activity program to accommodate your cardiorespiratory fitness.

Determining Exercise Frequency If you are a newcomer to regular physical activity, try to exercise at least three times per week. If you exercise less frequently, you will achieve fewer health benefits. The Surgeon General recommends moderate amounts of *daily* physical activity.[30] As your fitness level improves, your goal should be to exercise 20 to 30 minutes per day, five days a week. Figure 11.1 provides guidelines for various activity levels.

Determining Exercise Intensity Your aerobic exercise program should employ activities of moderate intensity that use large muscle groups and can be maintained for prolonged periods of time. The measure of such a workout is your

target heart rate, which is a percentage of your maximum heart rate. To calculate target heart rate, subtract your age from 220 for females or from 226 for males. The result is your maximum heart rate. You determine your target heart rate by calculating a desired percentage of maximum heart rate, often 60 percent. Thus, if you are a 20-year-old female, your 60 percent target heart rate would be 120 [(220 − 20) × 0.60].

People in poor physical condition should set a target heart rate between 40 and 50 percent of maximum. As your condition improves, you can gradually increase your target heart rate. Increases should be made in small increments, from 40 to 45 percent, then from 45 to 50 percent.

Once you know your target heart rate, you can take your pulse to determine how close you are to this value during your workout. As you exercise, lightly place your index and middle fingers (don't use your thumb) on your radial artery (inside your wrist, on the thumb side). Using a watch or clock, take your pulse for six seconds and multiply this number by 10 (just add a zero to your count) to get the number of beats per minute (bpm). Your pulse should be within a range of 5 bpm above or below your target heart rate. If necessary, adjust the pace or intensity of your workout to achieve your target heart rate.

A target heart rate of 70 percent of maximum is sometimes called the "conversational level of exercise" because you are able to talk with a partner while exercising.[31] If you are breathing so hard that talking is difficult, your intensity of exercise is too high. If you can sustain a conversational level of aerobic exercise for 20 to 30 minutes, you will improve your cardiorespiratory fitness.

Determining Exercise Duration   Duration refers to the number of minutes of activity performed during any one session. The Centers for Disease Control and Prevention (CDC) and the American College of Sports Medicine (ACSM) suggest that every adult engage in 20 to 60 minutes of continuous or intermittent (if intermittent, bouts of at least 10-minutes' duration) moderate-intensity physical activity most days of the week.[32] Activities that can contribute to this total include dancing, walking up stairs (instead of taking the elevator), gardening, and raking leaves, as well as planned physical activities such as jogging, swimming, and cycling. One way to meet the CDC/ACSM recommendation is to walk 2 miles briskly.

The lower the intensity of your activity, the longer the duration you'll need to get the same caloric expenditure. For example, a 120-pound woman will burn 180 calories walking for one hour at 2.0 miles per hour, but will burn 330 calories if she walks for an hour at a pace of 4.5 miles per hour. A 180-pound man will expend 288 calories per hour of playing golf if he carries his clubs, but he will burn 805 calories per hour if he is cross-country skiing.[33] Your goal should be to expend 300 to 500 calories per exercise session, with an eventual weekly goal of 1,500 to 2,000 calories. As you progress, add to your exercise load by increasing duration or intensity, but not both at the same time. From week to week, don't increase duration or intensity by more than 10 percent.

A program of repeated sessions of exercise over several months or years—exercise training—changes the way your cardiovascular system meets your body's oxygen requirements at rest and during exercise. Because many of the health benefits associated with cardiorespiratory fitness activities take about one year of regular exercise to achieve, don't expect improvements overnight.[34] However, any physical activity of low to moderate intensity will benefit your overall health almost from the start.

What do you think?

Calculate your maximum heart rate. Pick an intensity of exercise that suits your fitness level, for example, 60 percent of your maximum heart rate. Using a familiar physical activity and monitoring your pulse, experiment by exercising at three different intensities. Do you notice any difference in the way you feel while exercising? Afterward?

Why Flexibility and Strength Exercise?

Stretching Exercises and Well-Being

Who would guess that improved flexibility has much, if anything, to do with a better sense of well-being, with being able to deal with stress better, or with the fact that your joints don't hurt as much as they used to? But that's just what people who have improved their flexibility through stretching exercises are saying. Stretching exercises have become the main highway to improved flexibility. Today, they are extremely popular, especially in the forms of *Yoga* and *Tai chi*. And, an exercise program called *Pilates,* which includes many stretching exercises, has been growing in popularity as well. This popularity seems to be the result of people responding to exercise programs that work and the fact that someone can begin at virtually any age and enjoy them for a lifetime.

One main objective of stretching exercises is improving flexibility, but what exactly is flexibility? **Flexibility** is a measure of the range of motion, or the amount of movement possible, at a particular joint. Improving the range of motion through stretching exercises enhances efficiency, extent of movement, and improves posture. In addition, flexibility exercises have been shown to be effective in reducing the incidence and severity of lower back problems and muscle or

---

Target heart rate   Calculated as a percentage of maximum heart rate (220 [females] or 226 [males] minus age); heart rate (pulse) is taken during aerobic exercise to check whether exercise intensity is at the desired level (e.g., 70 percent of maximum heart rate).

Flexibility   The measure of the range of motion, or the amount of movement possible, at a particular joint.

tendon injuries that can occur during sports or everyday physical activities.[35] Improved flexibility can also mean less tension and pressure on joints resulting in less joint pain and reduced joint deterioration.

Flexibility is enhanced by the controlled stretching of muscles and muscle attachments that act on a particular joint. Each muscle involved in a stretching exercise is attached to our skeleton by tendons. An example of the connection between muscle, bone, and tendons is offered in Figure 11.2. The goal of stretching is to decrease the resistance of a muscle and its tendons to tension, that is, to reduce resistance to being stretched. Stretching exercises gradually result in greater flexibility. In stretching exercises a muscle or group of muscles is stretched to a point of slight discomfort and that position is held for 20 to 30 seconds, or more. For many people a regular program of stretching exercises enhances psychological as well as physical well-being.

Types of Stretching Exercises

In the language of exercise science all of the commonly practiced stretching exercises fall into two major categories: static and proprioceptive neuromuscular facilitation (PNF).[36] **Static** techniques involve the slow, gradual stretching of muscles and their tendons, then holding them at a point. During this holding period—the stretch—participants may feel a mild discomfort and a warm sensation in the muscles that are being stretched. Static stretching exercises involve specialized tension receptors that are found in our muscles. When done properly, static stretching slightly lessens the sensitivity of tension receptors, which allows the muscle to relax and be stretched to greater length.[37] The stretch is followed by a slow return to the starting position. The physical aspect of yoga and tai chi is largely composed of static techniques as are some of the exercises in Pilates programs. (See next section.)

The second major type of stretching exercise, **proprioceptive neuromuscular facilitation (PNF),** is relatively new. While PNF techniques have been shown to be superior to other stretching techniques for improving flexibility, they are, unfortunately, quite complex in their original form. A certified athletic trainer or physical therapist may be required to help in performing PNF exercises correctly; however, several PNF techniques have been simplified to the point that they can be performed with an exercise partner or even alone. PNF techniques involve contraction of a muscle followed by a stretch.

Yoga, Tai Chi, and Pilates

Three major styles of exercise that include stretching have recently become widely practiced in the United States and other Western countries. **Yoga** originated in India about 5,000 years ago. **Tai chi** is an ancient Chinese form of exercise that, like yoga, combines stretching, balance, coordination, and meditation. Yoga and tai chi are excellent activities for

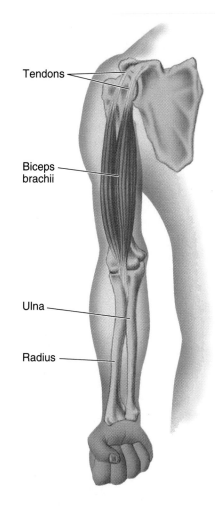

Figure 11.2
Muscles, Bones, and Tendons
Source: From *Exercise Physiology for Health, Fitness, and Performance, second edition* by Sharon A. Plowman and Denise L. Smith, 2003.

Static stretching   Techniques that gradually lengthen a muscle to an elongated position (to the point of discomfort) and hold that position for 10 to 30 seconds.

Proprioceptive neuromuscular facilitation (PNF) stretching   Techniques that involve the skillful use of alternating muscle contractions and static stretching in the same muscle.

Yoga   A variety of Indian traditions geared toward self-discipline and the realization of unity; includes forms: of exercise widely practiced in the West today that promote balance, coordination, flexibility, and meditation.

Tai chi   An ancient Chinese form of exercise widely practiced in the West today that promotes balance, coordination, stretching, and meditation.

improving flexibility and muscular coordination. **Pilates** exercise programs combine stretching with movement against resistance, which is aided by devices such as tension springs or heavy rubber bands. All three of these currently popular approaches include a joining of mind and body as a result of intense concentration on breathing and on body position.

Yoga has burst upon the scene as one of the most popular fitness and static stretching activities. Yoga blends the mental and physical aspects of exercise, a kind of joining of mind and body that participants find rewarding and satisfying. Its combination of mental focus and physical effort regularly results in more vitality, improved posture, greater agility, and improved coordination.

The practice of yoga focuses attention on controlled breathing as well as the purely physical exercise. In addition to its mental dimensions, yoga incorporates a complex array of static stretching exercises expressed as postures (*asanas*). Over 200 postures exist, but only about 50 are commonly practiced postures. During a session participants move to different asanas and hold them for 30 seconds or more. Yoga not only improves flexibility, it has the great advantage of being flexible itself. Asanas and combinations of asanas can be changed and adjusted for young and old and to accommodate people with physical limitations or disabilities. Combinations of asanas can also be linked together in ways that provide even conditioned athletes with challenging sessions.

A typical yoga session will move the spine and joints through their full range of motion. Yoga postures lengthen, strengthen, and balance musculature leading to increased flexibility, stamina, and strength—and many people report a psychological sense of general well-being.

There are many styles of yoga. Three of the most popular are:

- *Iyengar yoga* emphasizes focusing attention on precision and alignment in the poses. Standing poses are basic to this style, and poses are often held longer than in other styles.
- *Ashtanga yoga* in its pure form is based on a specific flow of poses that creates internal heat. The copious sweating that results is said to have a cleansing effect. Power yoga, a style growing in popularity, is a derivative of Ashtanga yoga.
- *Bikram's yoga* is similar to power yoga but does not incorporate a specific flow of poses. It is literally the hottest yoga going; it is performed in temperatures of 100° Fahrenheit, or even a bit higher.

Tai chi is an exercise regimen that is designed to increase the range of motion, flexibility, and to reduce muscular tension. Developed about 1000 AD from a Taoist philosophy dedicated to spiritual growth and good health called Chi Kung, tai chi emerged from monks to defend themselves from bandits and warlords. Tai chi involves a series of positions called *forms* that are performed continuously.

Pilates is a popular technique that includes both flexibility and strength training. Compared to yoga and tai chi, Pilates is the new kid on the exercise block. It was developed by Joseph Pilates who came from Germany to New York City in 1926. Shortly after his arrival, he introduced his exercise methodology, which emphasizes flexibility, coordination, strength, and tone. Pilates differs in part from yoga and tai chi in that it includes a component designed to increase strength. The method consists of a sequence of carefully performed movements. Some are carried out on specially designed equipment, while others are performed on mats. Each exercise stretches and strengthens the muscles involved and has a specific breathing pattern associated with it. A class will focus on strengthening specific muscle groups, using equipment that provides resistance.

> **What do you think?**
>
> *Why is it so important to have good flexibility throughout life?* ❋ *What are some situations in which improved flexibility would help you perform daily activities with less effort?* ❋ *What specific actions can you take to improve your flexibility?*

Designing Your Own Stretching Exercise Program: General Guidelines

If participation in formal exercise classes isn't for you, you can easily design your own stretching exercise program. Figure 11.3 shows a selection of exercises that will stretch the major muscle groups of your body, and can be used as a warm-up for other physical activities and exercise programs such as jogging and tennis.

A program of regular stretching exercise doesn't need to take up a great deal of time and doesn't require buying expensive equipment. You can reap the benefits of stretching with just two or three 10-minute sessions per week. Start off slowly with a five-minute session for the first week, then add a five-minute session each week, until you reach a schedule and comfort level that suit you. A hefty program would consist of five 30-minute sessions each week. Sessions get longer as you slowly increase the time you hold a particular stretch and how many times you repeat each type of stretch.

Improving Muscular Strength and Endurance

To get a sense of what resistance training is about, do a resistance exercise. Start by holding your right arm straight down by your side, then turn your hand palm up and bring it

---

Pilates   Exercise programs that combine stretching with movement against resistance, aided by devices such as tension springs and heavy bands.

Use these general-purpose stretching techniques as part of your warm-up and cool-down. Hold each stretch for at least 10 seconds, and repeat four times on each limb.

After only a few weeks of regular stretching, you'll begin to see improvements.

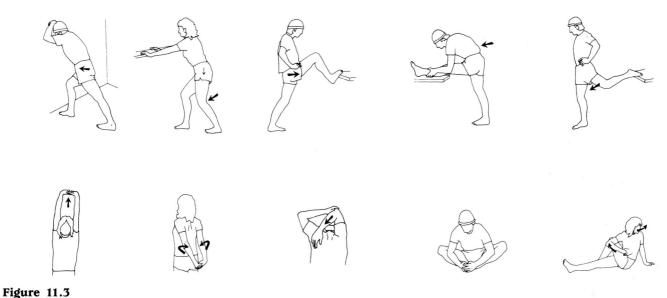

Figure 11.3
Stretching Exercises to Improve Flexibility
Source: Drawings excerpted from *Stretching,* revised edition © 2000 by Bob Anderson. Shelter Publications. Reprinted by permission.

up toward your shoulder. That's a resistance exercise, using a muscle, your biceps, to move a resistance, in this case, just the weight of your hand—not very much resistance. (See Figure 11.2 on page 283.) Much more weight or tension is usually involved in resistance training exercises, but unlike our simple exercise and unlike flexibility training, resistance training is usually equipment intense. You don't get to look like Arnold Schwarzenegger doing these exercises empty handed. Free weights such as dumbbells and barbells and all sorts of tension producing machines are usually part and parcel of resistance training. It's not just bodybuilding that uses this type of training either. Fitness programs and many sports employ resistance training to improve strength and endurance, and many rehabilitation programs for recovery from injuries to muscles and joints are designed around resistance exercises.

Strength and Endurance

We all have a general sense of what strength and endurance are, but to explore the world of resistance training, more formal definitions are needed. **Muscular strength** is the amount of force a muscle or group of muscles is capable of exerting. The most common way to assess strength in a resistance exercise program is to measure the **one repetition maximum (1 RM),** which is the maximum amount of weight a person can move one time in a particular exercise. For example,

1 RM for the simple exercise done at the beginning of this section is the maximum weight you lift to your shoulder one time. **Muscular endurance** is the ability of muscle to exert force repeatedly without fatiguing. If you can perform the exercise described earlier holding a 5-pound weight in your hand and lifting ten times, you will have greater endurance than someone who attempts that same exercise but is only able to lift the weight seven times.

Some resistance programs are designed primarily for increasing strength; others are aimed more at increasing endurance. Winning an Olympic weight lifting event depends on the amount of weight that is lifted in just a few seconds. Endurance doesn't play a large role. Conversely, a soccer event lasts much longer and requires enormous endurance but not as much instantaneous brute strength as weight

Muscular strength   The amount of force that a muscle is capable of exerting.

One repetition maximum (1RM)   The amount of weight/resistance that can be lifted or moved once, but not twice; a common measure of strength.

Muscular endurance   A muscle's ability to exert force repeatedly without fatiguing.

lifting. In football, strength and endurance are both important. Training for endurance uses smaller weights, but repeats an exercise more times than training for strength. If you were endurance training for performing the hand to shoulder exercise used as an example (called a curl in weight-training circles), you might hold a 5-pound weight in each hand and curl 15 times per exercise segment. In training for strength, 40-pound weights might be used for a five-time curl.

Principles of Strength Development

An effective **resistance exercise program** involves three key principles: tension, overload, and specificity of training.[38]

The Tension Principle   The key to developing strength is to create tension within a muscle or group of muscles. Tension is created by resistance provided by weights such as barbells or dumbbells, specially designed machines, or the weight of the body.

The Overload Principle   The overload principle is the most important of our three key principles. Overload doesn't mean forcing a muscle or group of muscles to do too much, which could result in injuries. Overload in resistance training requires muscles to do more than they are used to. Everyone begins a resistance training program with an initial level of strength. To become stronger, you must regularly create a degree of tension in your muscles that is greater than you are accustomed to. This overload will cause your muscles to adapt to a new level. As your muscles respond to a regular program of overloading by getting larger, they become stronger. Figure 11.4 illustrates how a continual process of overload and adaptation to the overload improves strength. Remember that resistance training exercises cause microscopic damage (tears) to muscle fibers, and the rebuilding process that increases the size and capacity of the muscle takes about 24 to 48 hours. Thus resistance training exercise programs should include at least one day of rest and recovery between workouts before overloading the same muscles again.

The Specificity of Training Principle   The specificity of training principle refers to the fact that only the muscle or muscle group that you exercise responds to the demands placed upon it. According to the specificity principle, the effects of resistance exercise training are specific to the

---

Resistance exercise program   A regular program of exercises designed to improve muscular strength and endurance in the major muscle groups.

Hypertrophy   Increased size (girth) of a muscle.

Isometric muscle action   Force produced without any resulting joint movement.

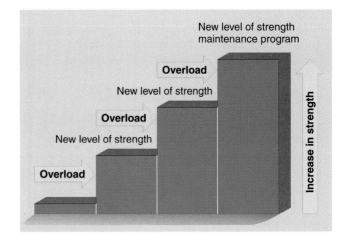

Figure 11.4
The Overload Principle
The overload principle contributes to an increase in strength. Notice that once the muscle has adapted to the original overload, a new overload must be placed on the muscle for subsequent strength gains to occur.
Source: From Philip A. Sienna, *One Rep Max: A Guide to Beginning Weight Training*, Fig. 2.1, 8. Copyright © 1989. Wm. C. Brown Communications, Inc., Dubuque, Iowa. Reprinted by permission of Times Mirror Higher Education Group, Inc., Dubuque, Iowa. All rights reserved.

muscles being exercised. If you regularly do curls, the muscles involved, your biceps, will become larger and stronger; however, the other muscles in your body won't change.

Gender Differences in Weight Training

The results of resistance training in men and women are quite different. Women don't normally develop the muscle to the same extent that men do. The main reason for the difference between the sexes is that men and women have different levels of the hormone testosterone in their blood. Before puberty, testosterone levels in blood are similar for both boys and girls. During adolescence, testerone levels in boys increase dramatically, about ten-fold, but, testosterone levels in girls are unchanged. Women's muscles will become larger (**hypertrophy**) as a result of resistance training exercise but typically not to the same degree as in adult males. To enhance muscle bulk, some bodybuilders (both men and women) take synthetic hormones (anabolic steroids) that mimic the effects of testosterone. Use of anabolic steroids is a dangerous and illegal practice. (See Chapter 7.)

Types of Muscle Activity

Your skeletal muscles act in three different ways: isometric, concentric, and eccentric.[39] (See Figure 11.5.) In **Isometric muscle action,** force is produced through tension and muscle contraction, not movement. Figure 11.5 shows an isometric contraction. A **concentric muscle action** causes joint movement and a production of force while the muscle shortens. (See Figure 11.5b.) The empty-hand curl we did at the beginning of this section is a concentric exercise, with joint movement occurring at the elbow. In general, concentric muscle actions produce movement in a direction opposite of the downward pull of gravity.

Eccentric muscle action describes the ability of a muscle to produce force while lengthening. Typically, eccentric muscle actions occur when movement is in the same direction as the pull of gravity. Once you've brought a weight up during a curl, an eccentric muscle action would be lowering your hands and the weights back to their original position. Figure 11.5c demonstrates an eccentric muscle action.

Methods of Providing Resistance

There are four commonly used resistance exercise methods.

- **Body Weight Resistance (Calisthenics)** Strength and endurance training doesn't always have to rely on equipment. Your own body weight can be used to develop skeletal muscle fitness without relying on resistance equipment. Calisthenics use part or all of your body weight to offer resistance during exercise. While calisthenics are not as effective as other resistance methods in developing large muscle mass and strength, they are quite adequate for improving general muscular fitness and are generally sufficient to improve muscle tone and maintain a level of muscular strength.
- **Fixed Resistance** Fixed resistance exercises provide a constant amount of resistance throughout the full range of movement. Barbells, dumbbells, and some types of machines provide fixed resistance because their weight, or the amount of resistance, does not change during an exercise. Fixed resistance equipment has the potential to strengthen all the major muscle groups in the body.

  One advantage of dumbbells and barbells is that they are relatively inexpensive. Fixed resistance exercise machines are commonly available at college recreation/fitness facilities, health clubs, and many resorts and hotels.
- **Variable Resistance** Variable resistance equipment alters the resistance encountered by a muscle during a movement, so that the effort by the muscle is more consistent throughout the full range of motion. Variable resistance machines, such as Nautilius™ and Hammer Strength™, are typically single-station devices; a person stays on the same machine throughout the whole series of exercises. Other types of machines, such as Soloflex™, have multiple stations; the person using them moves from one machine to another. While some of these machines are expensive and too big to move easily, others are affordable and more portable. Many forms of variable resistance devices are sold for home use.
- **Accommodating Resistance Devices** These devices adjust the resistance according to the amount of force generated by the person using the equipment. The exerciser performs at maximal level of effort, while the exercise ma-

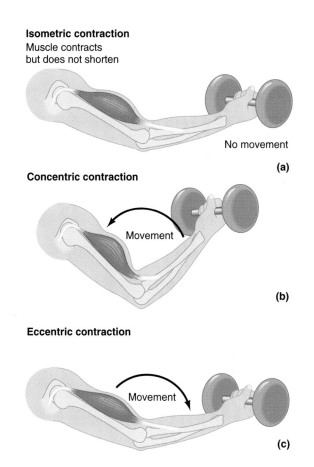

Figure 11.5
Isometric, Concentric, and Eccentric Muscle Actions.
Source: Powers, S. and E. Howley. *Exercise Physiology: Theory and Application to Fitness and Performance*. Madison, WI: Brown and Benchmark, 1997.

chine controls the speed of the exercise. The machine is set to a particular speed, and muscles being exercised must move at a rate faster than or equal to that speed in order to encounter resistance.[40]

The Benefits of Strength Training

You may wonder about the benefits associated with strength training beyond that of simple strength gain. It turns out that strength type of training can reduce the occurrence of lower back pain and joint and muscle injuries. It can postpone loss of muscle tissue due to the otherwise sedentary habits associated with aging. Strength training may contribute to

Concentric muscle action   Force produced while the muscle is shortening.

Eccentric muscle action   Force produced while the muscle is lengthening.

prevention of osteoporosis, a bone wasting disease associated with aging. (See Chapter 17.)

Strength training leads to an improvement in muscle definition and tone and an improvement in personal appearance that, in turn, leads to enhanced self-esteem. Surprisingly, strength training has a hidden benefit. Muscle tissue burns calories faster than most other tissues, even when it is resting. So, increased muscle mass can play a role in weight loss and maintaining weight loss.

Getting Started

When beginning a resistance exercise program, always consider your age, fitness level, and personal goals. Injuries can easily result from overestimating your state of readiness or strength, so it's a good idea to seek expert advice before starting out. Strength training involves a series of exercises done in sets. For example, 1 set of curls could be 15 repetitions using 10-pound dumbells, which means three sets would consist of doing 15 repetitions three times during an exercise session. Typically, a strength training session includes several strength and resistance types of exercises performed in cycles. A set of each exercise in the series is completed before another set is begun. A full workout would usually include three sets of each exercise. The American College of Sports Medicine[41] recommends resistance programs of up to 15 repetitions per exercise, performed at least two days per week. Each workout session should include 8 to 10 different resistance exercises that involve the major muscle groups of the upper and lower extremities and the trunk. Experts suggest allowing at least one day of rest and recovery between workouts.

> ### What do you think?
> *What types of resistance equipment can you currently access?* ✳ *Based on what you've read, what actions can you take to increase your muscular strength? Your muscular endurance?* ✳ *How would you measure your improvement?*

Body Composition

Body composition is the fifth and final component of a comprehensive fitness program. Body composition parameters that can be influenced by regular physical activity include to-

tal body mass, fat mass, fat-free mass, and regional fat distribution.[42] Body composition is significantly different between women and men. Women have a higher percentage of body fat and a significantly lower percentage of fat-free mass (such as muscle and bone) and bone mineral density.[43]

The most successful weight loss programs combine diet and exercise effectively; when a person participates in endurance training programs for the purpose of losing weight, total body mass and fat mass are generally reduced while fat-free mass remains constant. If your main reason for participating in a regular exercise program is to lose weight, then you'll need to combine diet with at least three workouts per week that expend 250 to 300 kcal per session (at least 30 to 45 minutes of continuous low-to-moderate intensity activity, depending on your body weight) in order to see significant reductions in your total body mass and fat mass.[44]

Fitness Injuries

Overtraining is the most frequent cause of injuries associated with fitness activities. Enthusiastic but out-of-shape beginners often injure themselves by doing too much too soon. Overtraining injuries occur most often in repetitive activities, such as swimming, running, bicycling, and step aerobics. However, use common sense and you're likely to remain injury free. Pay attention to your body's warning signs. To avoid injuring a particular muscle group or body part, vary your fitness activities throughout the week to give muscles and joints a rest. Set appropriate short-term and long-term training goals. Establishing realistic but challenging fitness goals can help you stay motivated without overdoing it.

Causes of Fitness-Related Injuries

There are two basic types of injuries stemming from participation in fitness-related activities: overuse injuries and traumatic injuries. **Overuse injuries** result from cumulative, day-after-day stresses placed on tendons, bones, and ligaments during exercise. The forces that occur normally during a session of physical activity are not enough to cause a ligament sprain or muscle strain, but when these forces are applied on a daily basis for weeks or months, they can result in an injury. Common sites of overuse injuries are the leg, knee, shoulder, and elbow joints.

Traumatic injuries occur suddenly and violently, typically by accident. Typical traumatic injuries are broken bones, torn ligaments and muscles, contusions, and lacerations. Most traumatic injuries occur quickly and are difficult to avoid—for example, spraining your ankle by landing on another person's foot after jumping up for a rebound in basketball. If your traumatic injury causes a noticeable loss of function and immediate pain or pain that does not go away after 30 minutes, you should have a physician examine it.

Overuse injuries Injuries that result from the cumulative effects of day-after-day stresses placed on tendons, muscles, and joints.

Traumatic injuries Injuries that occur suddenly and violently and, usually, by accident (e.g., fractured bones, ruptured tendons, and sprained ligaments).

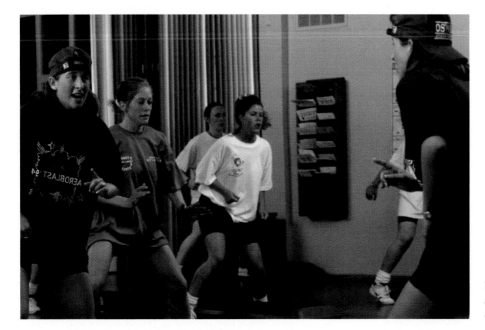

Most college campuses provide a recreation facility so that students and staff can stay fit.

Preventing Fitness-Related Injuries

Your exercise clothing is more than a fashion statement: Smart choices can help you prevent injuries. For some types of physical activity, you will need clothing that allows body heat to dissipate—for example, light-colored nylon shorts and mesh tank top for running in hot weather. For other types, you will need clothing that retains body heat without getting you sweat-soaked—for example, layers of polypropylene and/or wool clothing for cross-country skiing.

Appropriate Footwear When you purchase running shoes, look for several key components. Biomechanics research has revealed that running is a "collision" sport—that is, with each stride, the runner's foot collides with the ground with a force three to five times the runner's body weight.[45] The 150-pound runner who takes 1,000 strides per mile applies a cumulative force to his or her body of 450,000 pounds per mile. The force not absorbed by the running shoe is transmitted upward into the foot, leg, thigh, and back. The body is able to absorb forces such as these, but it may be injured by the cumulative effects of repetitive impacts (e.g., running 40 miles per week). Therefore, the ability of running shoes to absorb shock is critical.

The midsole of a running shoe must absorb impact forces but must also be flexible. To evaluate the flexibility of the midsole, hold the shoe between the index fingers of your right and left hand. When you push on both ends of the shoe with your fingers, the shoe should bend easily at the midsole. If the force exerted by your index fingers cannot bend the shoe, its midsole is probably too rigid and may irritate your Achilles tendon, among other problems.[46] Other basic characteristics of running shoes include a rigid plastic insert within the heel of the shoe (known as a heel counter) to control the movement of your heel; a cushioned foam pad surrounding the heel of the shoe to prevent Achilles tendon irritation; and a removable thermoplastic innersole that customizes the fit of the shoe by using your body heat to mold it to the shape of your foot. Shoes are the runner's most essential piece of equipment, so carefully select appropriate footwear before you start a running program.

Shoe companies also sell cross-training shoes to help combat the high cost of having to buy separate pairs of running shoes, tennis shoes, weight-training shoes, and so on. Although the cross-training shoe can be used for participation in several different fitness activities by the novice or recreational athlete, a distance runner who runs 25 or more miles per week needs a pair of specialty running shoes to prevent injury.

Appropriate Exercise Equipment Some activities require special protective equipment to reduce chances of injury. Eye injuries can occur in virtually all fitness-related activities, although some activities are more risky than others. As many as 90 percent of the eye injuries resulting from racquetball and squash could be prevented by wearing appropriate eye protection—for example, goggles with polycarbonate lenses.[47] Nearly 100 million people in the United States ride bikes for pleasure, fitness, or competition. Head injuries used to account for 85 percent of all deaths attributable to bicycle accidents; however, bike helmets have significantly reduced the numer of skull fractures and facial injuries.[48] Look for helmets that meet the standards established by the American National Standards Institute (ANSI) and the Snell Memorial Foundation (SNELL).

> **What do you think?**
> *Given your activity level, what injury risks are you exposed to on a regular basis?* ❋ *What changes can you make in your equipment or clothing to reduce these risks?*

Common Overuse Injuries

Body movements in physical activities such as running, swimming, and bicycling are highly repetitive, so participants are susceptible to overuse injuries. In fitness activities, the joints of the lower extremities (foot, ankle, knee, and hip) tend to be injured more frequently than the upper-extremity joints (shoulder, elbow, wrist, and hand). Three of the most common overuse injuries are plantar fasciitis, shin splints, and runner's knee.

Plantar Fasciitis   Plantar fasciitis is an inflammation of the plantar fascia, a broad band of dense, inelastic tissue (fascia) that runs from the heel to the toe on the bottom of the foot. The main function of the plantar fascia is to protect the nerves, blood vessels, and muscles of the foot from injury. Repetitive weight-bearing fitness activities such as walking and running can inflame the plantar fascia. Common symptoms are pain and tenderness under the ball of the foot, at the heel, or at both locations.[49] The pain of plantar fasciitis is particularly noticeable during the first steps out of bed in the morning. If not treated properly, this injury may progress to the point that weight-bearing exercise is too painful to endure. Uphill running is not advised, because each uphill stride severely stretches (and thus irritates) the already inflamed plantar fascia. This injury can often be prevented by regularly stretching the plantar fascia prior to exercise and by wearing athletic shoes with good arch support and shock absorbency. Stretch the plantar fascia by slowly pulling all five toes upward toward your head, holding for 10 to 15 seconds, and repeating this three to five times on each foot prior to exercise.

Shin Splints   A general term for any pain that occurs below the knee and above the ankle is shin splints. This broad description includes more than 20 different medical conditions. Problems range from stress fractures of the tibia (shin bone) to severe inflammation in the muscles of the lower leg, which can interrupt the flow of blood and nerve supply to the foot. The most common type of shin splints occurs along the inner side of the tibia and is usually a combination of a muscle irritation and irritation of the tissues that attach the muscles to the bone in this region. Sedentary people who start a new weight-bearing exercise program are at the greatest risk for shin splints, though well-conditioned aerobic exercisers who rapidly increase their distance or pace may also develop them.[50] Running is the most frequent cause of shin splints, but people who do a great deal of walking (e.g., mail carriers, servers in restaurants) may also develop this injury.

To help prevent shin splints, wear athletic shoes that have good arch support and shock absorbency. If the pain continues, see your physician. You may be advised to substitute a non–weight-bearing activity, such as swimming, during your recovery period.

Runner's Knee   Runner's knee describes a series of problems involving the muscles, tendons, and ligaments about the knee. The most common problem identified as runner's knee is abnormal movement of the kneecap, which irritates the cartilage on the back side of the kneecap as well as nearby tendons and ligaments.[51] Women experience this problem more often than men. (See the accompanying Women's Health, Men's Health box.)

The main symptom of this kind of runner's knee is the pain experienced when downward pressure is applied to the kneecap after the knee is straightened fully. Additional symptoms may include swelling, redness, tenderness around the kneecap, and a dull, aching pain in the center of the knee.[52] If you have these symptoms, your physician will probably recommend that you stop running for a few weeks and reduce daily activities that compress the kneecap (e.g., exercise on a stair-climbing machine or doing squats with heavy resistance) until you no longer feel any pain.

Treating Fitness-Related Injuries

First-aid treatment for virtually all personal fitness injuries involves **RICE: r**est, **i**ce, **c**ompression, and **e**levation. *Rest,* the first component of this treatment, is required to avoid further irritation of the injured body part. *Ice* is applied to relieve pain and constrict the blood vessels in order to stop any internal or external bleeding. Never apply ice cubes, reusable gel ice packs, chemical cold packs, or other forms of cold directly to your skin. Instead, place a layer of wet toweling or elastic bandage between the ice and your skin. Ice should be applied to a new injury for approximately 20 minutes every hour for the first 24 to 72 hours. *Compression* of the injured body part can be accomplished with a 4- or 6-inch-wide elastic bandage; this applies indirect pressure to damaged blood vessels to help stop bleeding. Be careful, though, that the compression wrap does not interfere with normal blood flow. A throbbing, painful hand or foot is an indication that the compression wrap should be loosened. *Elevation* of the injured extremity above the level of your heart also helps to control internal or external bleeding by making the blood flow uphill to reach the injured area.

Exercising in the Heat

Heat stress includes several potentially fatal illnesses resulting from excessive core body temperatures. Be aware of the potential for heat stress whenever you exercise in warm, humid weather. In these conditions, your body's rate of heat production can exceed its ability to cool itself.

You can help prevent heat stress by following certain precautions. First, proper acclimatization to hot and/or humid climates is essential. Heat acclimatization increases your body's cooling efficiency; in this process; you increase activity gradually over 10 to 14 days in the hot environment. Second, avoid dehydration by replacing the fluids

---

RICE   Acronym for the standard first-aid treatment for virtually all traumatic and overuse injuries: rest, ice, compression, and elevation.

Women Athletes and Knee Injuries

As women continue to raise the bar in the world of sports, we learn more and more about their potential. At the same time, however, we also learn more about their tendencies toward injury. Although medical experts are unsure of the reasons, female athletes appear to be more susceptible to knee injuries, particularly injuries to the anterior cruciate ligaments (ACLs). Recent studies indicate that women are anywhere from five to eight times more likely than men to suffer painful, disabling ACL injuries at some point in their lives.

The ACL is a strand of soft tissue that, along with other ligaments, muscles, and tendons, helps stabilize the knee joint. Its role in pivoting, jumping, and sudden changes of direction is critical. Once it is damaged, mobility is often reduced. This ligament is most severely compromised when women partake in contact sports, such as soccer, basketball, and volleyball, although injuries have occurred in non-contact activities as well.

Once injured, the ACL must be repaired surgically and requires months of painful rehabilitation for any chance of a return to normal athletic levels. Even with therapy, ACL injuries can predispose people to later bouts of immobility, injuries due to lingering instability, and various forms of arthritis.

Why are we seeing this trend? Is it because more women are participating in sports, or are female athletes truly more susceptible to these injuries? According to the American Academy of Orthopedic Surgeons, the answer lies in physiological differences between males and females. Female athletes are thought to be at a disadvantage because of an imbalance in strength between the hamstring muscles behind the thigh and the quadriceps muscles in front of the thigh. When these two muscle groups work together, they act antagonistically to protect each other and supporting ligature, including that around the knee, from damage. Some researchers suggest that women tend to have underdeveloped or weak hamstrings, which increases the stress placed on the ACL, particularly during unusual movements. In addition, it is thought that during actions such as jumping and landing, women tend to land more straight-legged and flat-footed, a tendency related to weaker thigh muscles. In contrast, men often have much stronger quadriceps and hamstrings and tend to bend their knees and cushion the shock when jumping, causing less stress on supporting structures. Thus, women who are underexercised or have a severe imbalance between their quadriceps and hamstrings face a greater risk of ACL injury. In addition to weaker muscles, sports medicine officials speculate that structural characteristics of females, such as wider hips, put greater pressure on the inside of the knee and less on the leg muscle.

Another hypothesis is that women are more prone to ACL injuries during ovulation, when increased estrogen reduces the production of collagen, the body's connective tissue. Orthopedic surgeon Dr. Edward M. Wojtys put this theory to the test by evaluating the injuries of 40 young women with acute ACL injuries. He discovered that a majority of these women did in fact sustain their injuries during ovulation, pointing to the need for further investigation.

So what can women do to protect themselves from ACL injuries? At this point, Dr. Wojtys says that there is no evidence that hormone supplements will protect women against ACL injuries. Doctors advise women to get involved in sports at an early age and perform weight training and other types of conditioning that will build the hamstring muscles. When knee injuries do occur, they must be taken seriously and treated with rest, ice, compression, and elevation (RICE). If pain doesn't subside, a visit to an orthopedic surgeon may be necessary.

Sources: Johns Hopkins Health website, Health News Zone, http://www.intelihealth. com, "Keeping in the Game: Young Women and Their Knees"; *The Doctor's Guide to Medical and Other News,* "Link Found Between Menstrual Cycle and Knee Injuries," June 25, 1997.

---

you lose during and after exercise. Third, wear clothing appropriate for your activity and the environment. And finally, use common sense—for example, on a day when the temperature is 85 degrees and the humidity is 80 percent, postpone your usual lunchtime run until the cool of evening.

There are three different heat stress illnesses, which are progressive in severity: heat cramps, heat exhaustion, and heat stroke. **Heat cramps** (heat-related muscle cramps), the least serious problem, can be easily prevented by adequate fluid replacement and a diet that includes the electrolytes lost during sweating (sodium and potassium). **Heat exhaustion** is caused by excessive water loss resulting from prolonged exercise or work. Symptoms of heat exhaustion include nausea, headache, fatigue, dizziness and faintness,

and, paradoxically, "goosebumps" and chills. If you are suffering from heat exhaustion, your skin will be cool and moist. Heat exhaustion is actually a mild form of shock, in which the blood pools in the arms and legs away from the brain and major organs of the body, causing nausea and

Heat cramps   Muscle cramps that occur during or following exercise in warm or hot weather.

Heat exhaustion   A heat stress illness caused by significant dehydration resulting from exercise in warm or hot conditions; frequent precursor to heat stroke.

fainting. **Heat stroke,** often called sunstroke, is a life-threatening emergency condition having a 20 to 70 percent death rate.[53] Heat stroke occurs during vigorous exercise when the body's heat production significantly exceeds its cooling capacities. Body core temperature can rise from normal (99.6°F) to 105°F to 110°F within minutes after the body's cooling mechanism shuts down. If no cooling takes place, the rapid increase in core temperatures can cause brain damage, permanent disability, and death. Common signs of heat stroke are dry, hot, and usually red skin; very high body temperature; and a very rapid heart rate.

If you experience any of the symptoms mentioned here, stop exercising immediately, move to the shade or a cool spot to rest, and drink large amounts of cool fluids. Be aware that heat stress illnesses can strike in situations in which the danger is not obvious. Serious or fatal heat strokes may result from prolonged sauna or steam baths, prolonged total immersion in a hot tub or spa, or by exercising in a plastic or rubber head-to-toe "sauna suit."[54]

What are the best fluids to drink? In comparing participants' performance during exercise sessions lasting less than one hour, the American College of Sports Medicine (ACSM) found little difference between plain water versus "sports drinks" (drinks containing carbohydrates and electrolytes).[55] However, a recent study suggests otherwise. In a laboratory study requiring intense stationary bicycling (50 minutes of high-level activity followed by a 9- to 12-minute "sprint to the finish"), subjects' cycling performance improved by 6 percent when they drank enough water to replace 80 percent of the fluid they lost as sweat—and by 12 percent when they consumed a similar amount of a sports drink.[56]

Dehydration of "only" 1 to 2 percent of body weight quickly affects physiological function and performance. Dehydration of greater than 3 percent of body weight increases the risk of heat cramps, heat exhaustion, and heat stroke.[57] During intense exercise lasting longer than one hour, the ACSM recommends drinking fluids that contain 4 percent to 8 percent carbohydrates (to delay muscular fatigue) and a small amount of sodium (to improve taste and promote fluid retention). Fluid intake *following* physical activity is also very important to prevent dehydration—be sure to drink at least a pint of fluid (your choice!) for every pound of body weight lost during your exercise session.

Exercising in the Cold

When you exercise in cool weather, especially in windy conditions, your body's rate of heat loss is frequently greater than its rate of heat production. Under these conditions, **hypothermia**—a potentially fatal condition resulting from abnormally low body core temperature, which occurs when body heat is lost faster than it is produced—may result. Hypothermia can occur as a result of prolonged, vigorous exercise (e.g., snowboarding or rugby) in 40°F to 50°F temperatures, particularly if there is rain, snow, or a strong wind.

In mild cases of hypothermia, as body core temperature drops from the normal 99.6°F to about 93.2°F, you will begin to shiver. Shivering—the involuntary contraction of nearly every muscle in the body—increases body temperature by using the heat given off by muscle activity. During this first stage of hypothermia, you may also experience cold hands and feet, poor judgment, apathy, and amnesia.[58] Shivering ceases in most hypothermia victims as body core temperatures drop to between 87°F and 90°F, a sign that the body has lost its ability to generate heat. Death usually occurs at body core temperatures between 75°F and 80°F.

To prevent hypothermia, follow these commonsense guidelines:

- Analyze weather conditions and your risk of hypothermia before you undertake a planned outdoor physical activity, remembering that wind and humidity are as significant as temperature.
- Use the "buddy system"—that is, have a friend join you for cold weather outdoor activities.
- Wear layers of appropriate clothing to prevent excessive heat loss (e.g., polypropylene or woolen undergarments, a windproof outer garment, and wool hat and gloves).
- Finally, don't allow yourself to become dehydrated.[59]

> **What do you think?**
> *Given what you've read about the symptoms of common fitness injuries, are you currently developing any overuse injuries? ✳ If so, what specific actions can you take to prevent these problems from becoming more serious?*

Planning a Fitness Program

Identify Your Fitness Goals

Before you initiate a fitness program, analyze your personal needs, limitations, physical activity likes and dislikes, and daily schedule. Do you want to improve your quality of life? Lose weight? Lower your risk of health problems? Your specific goal may be to achieve (or maintain) healthy levels of body fat, cardiovascular fitness, muscular strength and endurance, or flexibility and mobility.

Once you become committed to regular physical activity and exercise, you will observe gradual improvements in your functional abilities and note progress toward your goals. Perhaps your most vital goal will be to become committed to fitness for the long haul—to establish a realistic schedule of

---

Heat stroke   A deadly heat stress illness resulting from dehydration and overexertion in warm or hot conditions; can cause body core temperature to rise from normal to 105°F to 110°F in just a few minutes.

Hypothermia   Potentially fatal condition caused by abnormally low body core temperature.

diverse exercise activities that you can maintain and enjoy throughout your life.

Design Your Program

Once you commit yourself to becoming physically active, decide what type of fitness program is best suited to your needs. The amount and type of exercise required to yield beneficial results vary with the age and physical condition of the exerciser. Men over age 40 and women over age 50 should consult their physicians before beginning any fitness program.

Good fitness programs are designed to improve or maintain cardiorespiratory fitness, flexibility, muscular strength and endurance, and body composition. A comprehensive program might include a warm-up period of easy walking followed by stretching activities to improve flexibility, then selected strength development exercises, followed by an aerobic activity for 20 minutes or more, and concluding with a cool-down period of gentle flexibility exercises.

The greatest proportion of exercise time should be spent developing cardiovascular fitness, but you should not exclude the other components. Choose an aerobic activity you think you will like. Many people find cross training—alternate-day participation in two or more aerobic activities (i.e., jogging and swimming)—less monotonous and more enjoyable than long-term participation in only one aerobic activity. Cross training is also beneficial because it strengthens a variety of muscles, thus helping you avoid overuse injuries to muscles and joints.

Jogging, walking, cycling, rowing, step aerobics, and cross-country skiing are all excellent activities for developing cardiovascular fitness. Most colleges and universities have recreation centers where students can use stair-climbing machines, stationary bicycles, treadmills, rowing machines, and ski-simulators. Table 11.2 describes various workout machines and provides tips for their use.

What do you think?

You now have the ability to design your own fitness program. Which two activities would you select for a cross-training program? ✳ *Do the activities you selected exercise different major muscle groups?* ✳ *How can you supplement them with other forms of exercise?*

Table 11.2
Picking Your Workout Machine

Exercise Rider

Workout: Upper body   Fair
Lower body   Fair
Learning curve   Easy

For the best workout: Experiment with seat heights until you find one that's comfortable. Make sure your legs don't bend more than 90 degrees at the bottom phase of the motion, which can be hard on the knees. Then, as you straighten, don't arch your spine backward; that stresses your lower back.

Rowing Machine

Workout: Upper body   Excellent
Lower body   Excellent
Learning curve   Hard

For the best workout: Don't hyperextend your back as you finish your stroke. Keep your elbows tight to your body to best strengthen your arms.

Ski Machine

Workout: Upper body   Excellent
Lower body   Excellent
Learning curve   Hard

For the best workout: Perfect arm movements first, then the leg actions, then put it all together; it usually takes a few sessions. One habit to avoid: constantly leaning against the hop pad to hold yourself upright.

Stair-Climber

Workout: Upper body   Poor
Lower body   Excellent
Learning curve   Hard

For the best workout: Keep your posture upright, your steps shallow (no deeper than 6 inches), and your weight off your arms.

Treadmill

Workout: Upper body   Poor
Lower body   Excellent
Learning curve   Easy

For the best workout: Start on the flat as a warm-up, gradually increase speed and incline (to 10 percent), then wind down to a slow, flat walk.

Stationary Bike

Workout: Upper body   Poor
Lower body   Excellent
Learning curve   Easy

For the best workout: Adjust the seat so your leg is almost fully extended when the pedal is at its lowest. Then just start pumping.

Source: Adapted by permission of Time Inc. Health from Karmen Butterer, "Picking Your Dream Machine," *Health* (September 1995): 48. © 1995.

Taking Charge

Managing Your Fitness Behaviors

Do you want to improve your fitness level? Begin by making a list of your favorite physical activities that can increase strength, flexibility, and cardiorespiratory fitness. Choose which you would like to make part of a regular routine. Then identify specific times to exercise. Consider how exercise could become part of your daily activities. Then do it!

Checklist for Change

Making Community Choices

✓ Does your college have facilities for exercise? Are there special student rates? What hours are those facilities available?

✓ What community facilities for exercise are available in your hometown? Have you ever considered using these facilities?

✓ Are opportunities available for you to volunteer at a local exercise facility? Have you considered volunteering to help low-income individuals? Children? Why or why not?

Summary

* The physiological benefits of regular physical activity include reduced risk of heart attack, hypertension, and diabetes; and improved blood lipid profile, skeletal mass, weight control, immunity to disease, mental health and stress management, and physical fitness. Regular activity can also increase life span.
* An aerobic exercise program improves cardiorespiratory fitness. Exercise frequency begins with three days per week and eventually moves up to five. Exercise intensity involves working out at target heart rate. Exercise duration should increase to 30 to 45 minutes; the longer the exercise period, the more calories burned, and the greater the improvement in cardiovascular fitness.
* Flexibility exercises should involve static stretching exercises performed in sets of four or more repetitions held for 10 to 30 seconds on at least two to three days a week.

* The key principles for developing muscular strength and endurance are the tension principle, the overload principle, and the specificity of training principle. The different types of muscle actions include isometric, concentric, and eccentric. Resistance training programs include fixed resistance, variable resistance, and accommodating resistance.
* Fitness injuries are generally caused by overuse or trauma; the most common ones are plantar fasciitis, shin splints, and runner's knee. Proper footwear and equipment can help prevent injuries. Exercise in the heat or cold requires special precautions.
* Planning a fitness program involves setting goals and designing a program to achieve these goals.

Discussion Questions

1. How do you define physical fitness? What are the key components of a physical fitness program? What might you need to consider when beginning a fitness program?
2. How would you determine the proper intensity and duration of an exercise program? How often should exercise sessions be scheduled?
3. Why is stretching vital to improving physical flexibility?
4. Identify at least four physiological and psychological benefits of physical fitness. What is the significance of the latest fitness report from the Surgeon General's Office? How might it help more people realize the benefits of physical fitness?
5. Describe the different types of resistance employed in an exercise program. What are the benefits of each type of resistance?
6. Your roommate has decided to start running first thing in the morning in an effort to lose weight, tone muscles, and improve cardiorespiratory fitness. What advice would you give to make sure your roommate begins properly and doesn't get injured?
7. What key components would you include in a fitness program for yourself?

Application Exercise

Reread the What Do You Think? scenario at the beginning of the chapter, and answer the following questions.

1. Assume for a moment that you are Marta, thinking about starting an exercise program after a period of inactivity. Create an outline for a three-month program that starts slowly and gradually progresses.

2. One of the hardest obstacles for Marta will be breaking old habits: driving instead of walking, watching TV, and eating unhealthy foods. What advice would you give to Marta to help her change these habits?

Accessing Your Health on the Internet

Visit the following Internet sites to explore further topics and issues related to personal health. To visit an organization's website, go to the Companion Website for *Health: The Basics, Fifth Edition* at www.aw.com/donatelle, click on the book image, and select "Accessing Your Health on the Internet" from the navigation menu on the left.

1. ***ACSM Online.*** A link with the American College of Sports Medicine and all their resources.
2. ***American Council on Exercise.*** Information on exercise and disease prevention.

3. ***The American Medical Association's Health Insight.*** Provides a fitness assessment and guidelines to help you develop your own fitness program.
4. ***Just Move.*** The American Heart Association's fitness website has the latest information on heart disease and exercise, plus a guide to local, regional, and national fitness events.
5. ***National Institute on Health, Osteoporosis, and Related Bone Disease—National Resource Center.*** Outstanding, reputable source for the latest information on bone and joint disorders.

Further Reading

Fahey, T. D. *Super Fitness for Sports, Conditioning, and Health.* Boston: Allyn & Bacon, 2000.
   A brief guide to developing fitness that emphasizes training techniques for improving sports performance.
Getchell, B., et al. *Physical Fitness: A Way of Life.* 5th ed. Boston: Allyn & Bacon, 1998.
   A practical guide for improving all areas of fitness, complying with the latest standards of the ACSM.

Schlosberg, S. *The Ultimate Workout Log: An Exercise Diary and Fitness Guide.* Boston: Houghton Mifflin, 1999.
   A 6-month log that also provides fitness definitions, training tips, and motivational quotes.

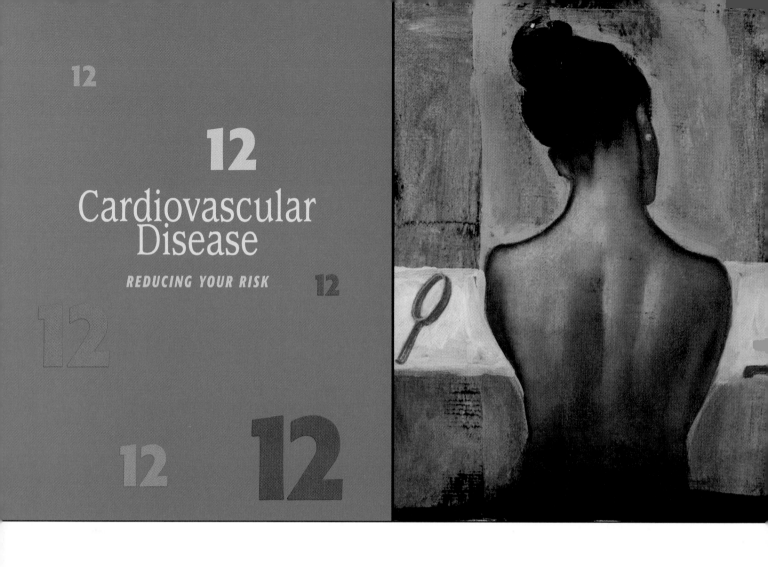

12
Cardiovascular Disease

REDUCING YOUR RISK

12 12 12 12 12

objectives

* Discuss the incidence, prevalence, and outcomes of cardiovascular disease in the United States, including its impact on society.

* Describe the anatomy and physiology of the heart and circulatory system and the importance of healthy heart functioning.

* Review the various types of heart disease, factors that contribute to their develop-

ment, current diagnostic and treatment options, and the importance of fundamental lifestyle modifications aimed at prevention.

* Discuss the controllable risk factors for cardiovascular disease, including smoking, cholesterol and triglycerides, certain infectious organisms, diet and obesity, exercise, hypertension, diabetes mellitus, and stress. Examine your

own risk profile, and determine which risk factors you can and cannot control.

* Discuss the issues surrounding cardiovascular disease risk and disease burden in women.

* Discuss some of the newer methods of diagnosing and treating cardiovascular disease, and evaluate the importance of being a wise health care consumer.

Despite the many medical advances we enjoy, diseases of the heart and cardiovascular system continue to be a significant health threat in the United States (Figure 12.1). In fact, cardiovascular disease (CVD) remains the leading single cause of death around the world.

An Epidemiological Overview

In 2000, CVD accounted for over 41 percent of all deaths in the United States, nearly 1 out of every 2.5. This is nearly three times the rate of the second leading killer, cancer, and more than the number of deaths caused by all other diseases combined. Nearly 2 million deaths occur per year in the United States; CVD was listed as a primary or contributing cause of death on about 1.4 million death certificates.[1] To realize just how serious CVD is, consider the following points:[2]

- More than 2,600 Americans die of CVD each day, an average of one death every 33 seconds. That's more than 950,000 deaths per year.
- Many of these fatalities are **sudden cardiac deaths,** meaning that these Americans die from sudden, abrupt

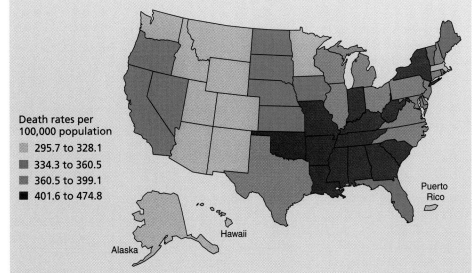

Death rates per 100,000 population
- 295.7 to 328.1
- 334.3 to 360.5
- 360.5 to 399.1
- 401.6 to 474.8

Figure 12.1
1995–1997 Total Cardiovascular Disease Age-Adjusted Death Rates (2000 Standard) by State
Source: American Heart Association, *2001 Heart and Stroke Facts—Statistical Update.*

Cardiovascular disease (CVD)   Term encompassing a variety of diseases of the heart and blood vessels.

Sudden cardiac death   Death that occurs as a result of sudden, abrupt loss of heart function.

loss of heart function (cardiac arrest), either instantly or shortly after symptoms occur. Most of these deaths result from coronary heart disease (CHD); in fact, over 220,000 people—nearly half of all victims of heart attack—die from CHD before they get to a hospital. People who attempt to save such victims through cardiac resuscitation are sometimes riddled with guilt when they fail to save a life. However, many such deaths are due to sudden heart stoppage or slowing that even the most heroic efforts cannot prevent.

- CVD claims nearly 11,000 more lives each year than the next six leading causes of death combined.
- More than 150,000 Americans killed by CVD are under age 65.
- The 2000 death rates from CVD were 419.3 for white males and 532.0 for African American males; for white females, 294.9; and for African American females, 400.7. (The rate is per 110,000 of population.)
- From 1988 to 1998, death rates from CVD declined by 20.4 percent. However, because of increases in the total population, the decline in actual numbers of deaths was only about 3 percent.
- If all forms of major CVD were eliminated, life expectancy would rise by almost 7 years.
- The probability at birth of eventually dying of CVD is 47 percent; of dying from cancer, 22 percent; from accidents, 3 percent; from diabetes, 2 percent; and from HIV, 0.7 percent.

Though these statistics seem grave enough, they do not include the effects of CVD experienced by the untold numbers who live with the ravages of the disease. Today, nearly 61 million Americans live with one of the major categories of CVD. Many do not know they have a serious problem.[3] Nearly 13 million of them have a history of heart attack, angina pectoris (chest pain), or both.[4] In spite of major improvements in medication, surgery, and other health care procedures, the prognosis for many of these individuals is not good:[5]

- Twenty-five percent of women and 38 percent of men will die within one year after having an initial heart attack.
- People who survive the acute stages of a heart attack have a chance of illness and death that is 1.5 to 15 times higher than that of the general population, depending on their sex and clinical outcomes. The risk of another heart attack, sudden death, angina pectoris, heart failure, and stroke—for both men and women—is substantial.
- Within six years after a recognized heart attack, 18 percent of men and 35 percent of women will have another heart attack, 7 percent of men and 6 percent of women will experience sudden death, about 22 percent of men and 46 percent of women will be disabled with heart failure, about two-thirds of heart attack patients won't make a complete recovery, but 88 percent of those under age 65 will be able to return to their usual work.
- CHD will permanently disable 19 percent of the U.S. labor force.

Although it is impossible to place a monetary value on human life, the economic burden of cardiovascular disease on

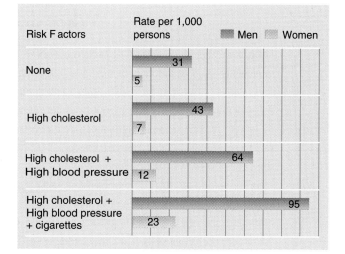

Figure 12.2
Heart Attacks: Compounded Risks
This graph shows how the risk of heart disease rises dramatically in people who have high cholesterol, who have high blood pressure, and/or who smoke cigarettes. In the graph, "high cholesterol" is 260 or above and "high blood pressure" is 150 or above (that is systolic pressure—the higher number).
Source: Copyright 1995, CSPI. Reprinted from Nutrition Action Healthletter, October 1995, 4 (1875 Connecticut Ave., NW Suite 300, Washington, DC 20009-5728. $24.00 for 10 issues.). Data from Framingham Heart Study. Personal communication, Thomas Thorn, National Heart, Lung and Blood Institute.

our society is staggering—more than $298 billion estimated in 2001.[6] This figure includes the cost of physician and nursing services, hospital and nursing home services, medications, and lost productivity resulting from disability. To keep this dollar amount in perspective, consider that between 1979 and 1998, the number of cardiovascular operations and procedures increased by nearly 400 percent.[7] As Americans live longer, these numbers will continue to increase, resulting in a tremendous burden on the health care system. The many Americans who think that CVD can be cured with a bypass or other surgical procedure, after which life simply returns to normal, are wrong. The effects of CVD are far reaching and take a toll on quality of life.

The best line of defense against CVD is to prevent its occurrence and reduce your risk throughout your life span. How can you cut your risk? Take steps now to change certain behaviors. For example, controlling high blood pressure and reducing intake of saturated fats and cholesterol are two things you can do to lower your chances of heart attack. By maintaining your weight, decreasing your intake of sodium, exercising, not smoking, and changing your lifestyle to reduce stress, you can lower your blood pressure. You can also monitor the levels of fat and cholesterol in your blood and adjust your diet to prevent arteries from becoming clogged. Having combinations of risk factors seems to increase overall risk by a factor greater than those of the combined risks (Figure 12.2). Happily, the converse is also true: reducing several risk factors can have a dramatic effect. Understanding how your cardiovascular system works will help you understand risks to cardiovascular health and reduce them.

> ### What do you think?
> *Consider what happens when people who suffer a heart attack survive. What unique challenges do they face? * What difficulties might they encounter at home, at work, and in leisure time? * What might it be like to live "in fear" that the heart might give out or that a problem could crop up at any time? * What support services are available for coping with the unique fears and anxieties faced by CVD survivors and their families?*

Understanding the Cardiovascular System

The **cardiovascular system** is the network of elastic tubes through which blood flows as it carries oxygen and nutrients to all parts of the body. It includes the *heart, lungs, arteries, arterioles* (small arteries), and *capillaries* (minute blood vessels). It also includes *venules* (small veins) and *veins,* the blood vessels though which blood flows as it returns to the heart and lungs.

The Heart: A Mighty Machine

The heart is a muscular, four-chambered pump, roughly the size of your fist. It is a highly efficient, extremely flexible organ that manages to contract 100,000 times each day, pumping the equivalent of 2,000 gallons of blood to all areas of the body. In a 70-year lifetime, an average human heart beats 2.5 billion times. This number is significantly higher for hearts that must fight to keep people moving who are out of shape and overweight.

Under normal circumstances, the human body contains approximately six quarts of blood. This blood transports nutrients, oxygen, waste products, hormones, and enzymes throughout the body. Blood also regulates body temperature, cellular water levels, and acidity levels of body components, and it helps the body defend itself against toxins and harmful microorganisms. An adequate blood supply is essential to health and well-being.

The heart has four chambers that work together to recirculate blood constantly throughout the body (Figure 12.3). The two upper chambers of the heart, called **atria,** or *auricles,* are large collecting chambers that receive blood from the rest of the body. The two lower chambers, known as **ventricles,** pump the blood out again. Small valves regulate the steady, rhythmic flow of blood between chambers and prevent inappropriate backwash. The *tricuspid valve* (located between the right atrium and the right ventricle), the *pulmonary (pulmonic)*

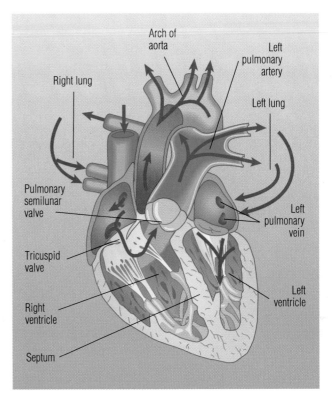

Figure 12.3
Anatomy of the Heart

valve (between the right ventricle and the pulmonary artery), the *mitral valve* (between the left atrium and left ventricle), and the *aortic valve* (between the left ventricle and the aorta) permit blood to flow in only one direction.[8]

Heart Function Heart activity depends on a complex interaction of biochemical, physical, and neurological signals. The following is a simplified version of the steps involved in heart function:

1. Deoxygenated blood enters the right atrium after having been circulated through the body.
2. From the right atrium, blood moves to the right ventricle and is pumped through the pulmonary artery to the lungs, where it receives oxygen.

> **Cardiovascular system** A complex system consisting of the heart and blood vessels. It transports nutrients, oxygen, hormones, and enzymes throughout the body and regulates temperature, the water levels of cells, and the acidity levels of body components.
>
> **Atria** The two upper chambers of the heart, which receive blood.
>
> **Ventricles** The two lower chambers of the heart, which pump blood through the blood vessels.

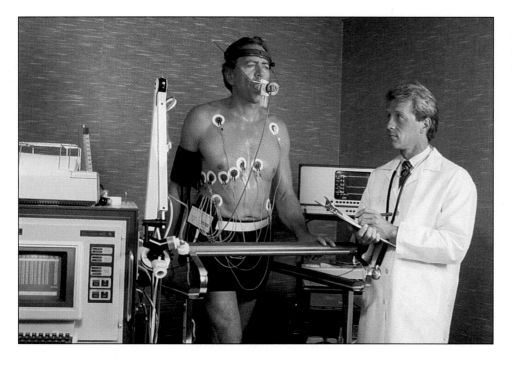

Extensive research on the heart's functioning and capacity has revealed a great deal about how to keep it healthy and what puts it at risk.

3. Oxygenated blood from the lungs then returns to the left atrium of the heart.
4. Blood from the left atrium is forced into the left ventricle.
5. The left ventricle pumps blood through the aorta to all body parts.

Different types of blood vessels are required for different parts of this process. **Arteries** carry blood away from the heart—except for pulmonary arteries, which carry deoxygenated blood to the lungs, where it picks up oxygen and gives off carbon dioxide. As they branch off from the heart, the arteries divide into smaller blood vessels called **arterioles,** and then into even smaller blood vessels called **capillaries.** Capillaries have thin walls that permit the ex-

change of oxygen, carbon dioxide, nutrients, and waste products with body cells. The carbon dioxide and waste products are transported to the lungs and kidneys through **veins** and venules (small veins).

For the heart to function properly, the four chambers must beat in an organized manner. Your heartbeat is governed by an electrical impulse that directs the heart muscle to move when the impulse moves across it, which results in a sequential contraction of the four chambers. This signal starts in a small bundle of highly specialized cells, the **sinoatrial node (SA node),** located in the right atrium. The SA node serves as a form of natural pacemaker for the heart.[9] People with a damaged SA node must often have a mechanical pacemaker implanted to ensure the smooth passage of blood through the sequential phases of the heartbeat.

The average adult heart at rest beats 70 to 80 times per minute, although a well-conditioned heart may beat only 50 to 60 times per minute to achieve the same results. When overly stressed, a heart may beat over 200 times per minute, particularly in an individual who is overweight or out of shape. A healthy heart functions more efficiently and is less likely to suffer damage from overwork.

Types of Cardiovascular Disease

There are several different types of cardiovascular disease:

- Atherosclerosis (fatty plaque buildup in the arteries)
- Coronary heart disease (CHD)
- Chest pain (angina pectoris)

Arteries   Vessels that carry blood away from the heart to other regions of the body.

Arterioles   Branches of the arteries.

Capillaries   Minute blood vessels that branch out from the arterioles; their thin walls allow for the exchange of oxygen, carbon dioxide, nutrients, and waste products among body cells.

Veins   Vessels that carry blood back to the heart from other regions of the body.

Sinoatrial node (SA node)   Node serving as a form of natural pacemaker for the heart.

- Irregular heartbeat (arrhythmia)
- Congestive heart failure (CHF)
- Congenital and rheumatic heart disease
- Stroke (cerebrovascular accident)

These diseases may be prevented or treated by a variety of methods, ranging from changes in diet and lifestyle to medications and surgery.

Atherosclerosis

Atherosclerosis is a general term for thickening and hardening of the arteries, a condition that underlies many cardiovascular health problems. Atherosclerosis is actually a type of **arteriosclerosis** and is characterized by deposits of fatty substances, cholesterol, cellular waste products, calcium, and *fibrin* (a clotting material in the blood) in the inner lining of the artery. The resulting buildup is referred to as **plaque.**[10] Often, atherosclerosis is called *coronary artery disease (CAD)* because of the resultant damage done to coronary arteries.

Atherosclerotic plaque appears primarily in large and medium-sized elastic and muscular arteries and can block blood flow to the heart, brain, or extremities. Plaque may be present throughout a person's lifetime. The earliest formation, known as a "fatty streak," is fairly common in infants and young children.[11]

Early Theories Initially, it was thought that plaque developed in response to injury and tended to collect at sites of injury. Many scientists believed that the process of plaque buildup begins when the protective inner lining of the artery (*endothelium*) becomes damaged and fats, cholesterol, and other substances in the blood tend to aggregate in these damaged areas. High blood pressure surges, elevated cholesterol and triglyceride levels in the blood, and cigarette smoking were the main suspects in having caused this injury to artery walls. As a result of national campaigns aimed at reducing dietary fats, millions of people cut down on animal fat and dairy products. However, despite massive lifestyle changes and the use of cholesterol-lowering drugs, cardiovascular diseases continue to be the leading cause of death in the United States, Europe, and most of Asia.[12]

Inflammatory Risks Today, scientists are beginning to view the formation of atherosclerotic lesions in a new way, with a vastly expanded list of possible causes. Many experts believe that atherosclerosis is an *inflammatory* disease, with numerous factors contributing to plaque formation.[13] Among these culprits are elevated and modified levels of low-density lipoprotein, free radicals caused by cigarette smoking, high blood pressure, diabetes mellitus, and certain infectious microorganisms, such as herpesviruses or *Chlamydia pneumoniae,* and a combination of these and other factors.[14] The bottom line is that although elevated cholesterol levels continue to be significant in approximately 50 percent of patients with cardiovascular disease,[15] other factors need to be taken into consideration, particularly those that inflame and injure the interior of artery walls.[16]

Syndrome X According to Gerald Reaven, an endocrinologist at Stanford University, when people consume too many calories, particularly carbohydrates, their bodies eventually become insulin resistant, meaning that their cells resist (or don't work properly in) handling blood glucose levels. Consequently, insulin and blood sugar levels remain high over time. According to Reaven's new book, *Syndrome X: Overcoming the Silent Killer That Can Give You a Heart Attack,* these dynamics can cause a cluster of metabolic problems that raise the risk of heart disease.[17]

> **What do you think?**
> *What risk factors for plaque formation might typical college-aged students have?* ✴ *If the new theories discussed in this section prove true, what information should new CVD prevention guidelines include?*

Coronary Heart Disease (CHD)

Of all the major cardiovascular diseases, coronary heart disease (CHD) is the greatest killer. In fact, this year well over 1,100,000 people will suffer from a heart attack, and over 40 percent of them will die.[18] Those of you raised on a weekly dose of TV doctor programs will recognize *code blue* as the term for a **myocardial infarction (MI),** or **heart attack.** A heart attack involves an area of the heart that suffers permanent damage because its normal blood supply has been interrupted. This condition is often brought on by a **coronary thrombosis,** or blood clot in the coronary artery, or through an atherosclerotic narrowing that blocks an artery. When blood does not flow readily, there is a corresponding decrease in oxygen flow. If the heart blockage is extremely

---

Atherosclerosis   A general term for thickening and hardening of the arteries.

Arteriosclerosis   Condition characterized by deposits of fatty substances, cholesterol, cellular waste products, calcium, and fibrin in the inner lining of an artery.

Plaque   Buildup of deposits in the arteries.

Myocardial infarction (MI)   Heart attack.

Heart attack   A blockage of normal blood supply to an area in the heart.

Coronary thrombosis   A blood clot occurring in the coronary artery.

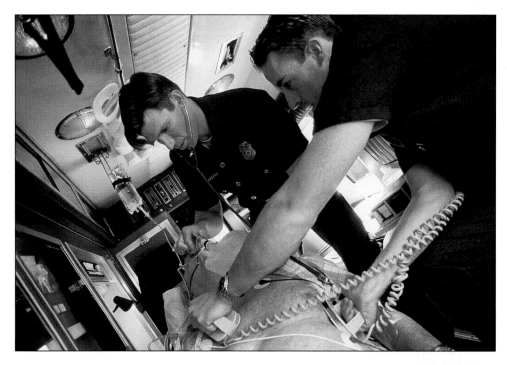

Because 40 percent of heart attack victims die within the first hour, immediate attention is vital to the patient's survival.

minor, the otherwise healthy heart will adapt over time by utilizing small unused or underused blood vessels to reroute needed blood through other areas. This system, known as **collateral circulation,** is a form of self-preservation that allows a damaged heart muscle to cope and in some cases to heal without additional stress.

When heart blockage is more severe, however, the body is unable to adapt on its own, and outside lifesaving support is critical. The hour following a heart attack is the most critical period—over 40 percent of heart attack victims die within this time. These sudden deaths are caused by cardiac arrest, usually resulting from *ventricular fibrillation,* or irregular, inefficient heartbeats.

Angina Pectoris

As a result of atherosclerosis and other circulatory impairments, the heart's oxygen supply is often reduced, a condition known as **ischemia.** Individuals with ischemia often

suffer from varying degrees of **angina pectoris,** or chest pains. In fact, an estimated 2.3 million men and 4 million women suffer mild to crushing forms of chest pain each day.[19] Many people experience short episodes of angina whenever they exert themselves physically. Symptoms may range from a slight feeling of indigestion to a feeling that the heart is being crushed. Generally, the more serious the oxygen deprivation, the more severe the pain. Although angina pectoris is not a heart attack, it does indicate underlying heart disease.

Currently, there are several methods of treating angina. In mild cases, rest is critical. The most common treatments for more severe cases involve using drugs that affect (1) the supply of blood to the heart muscle or (2) the heart's demand for oxygen. Pain and discomfort are often relieved with *nitroglycerin,* a drug used to relax (dilate) veins, thereby reducing the amount of blood returning to the heart and thus lessening its workload. Patients whose angina is caused by spasms of the coronary arteries are often given drugs called *calcium channel blockers.* These drugs prevent calcium atoms from passing through coronary arteries and causing heart contractions. They also appear to reduce blood pressure and slow heart rates. *Beta blockers* are the other major type of drugs used to treat angina. Beta blockers control potential overactivity of the heart muscle.

Arrhythmias

Over 4 million Americans experience some type of **arrhythmia,** an irregularity in heart rhythm. A person who complains of a racing heart in the absence of exercise or anxiety may be experiencing *tachycardia,* the medical term for

---

Collateral circulation   Adaptation of the heart to partial damage; accomplished by rerouting needed blood through unused or underused blood vessels while the damaged heart muscle heals.

Ischemia   Reduced oxygen supply to the heart.

Angina pectoris   Severe chest pain occurring as a result of reduced oxygen flow to the heart.

Arrhythmia   An irregularity in heartbeat.

abnormally fast heartbeat. On the other end of the continuum is *bradycardia,* or abnormally slow heartbeat. When a heart goes into **fibrillation,** it beats in a sporadic, quivering pattern resulting in extreme inefficiency in moving blood through the cardiovascular system. If untreated, fibrillation may be fatal.

Not all arrhythmias are life threatening. In many instances, excessive caffeine or nicotine consumption can trigger an arrhythmia episode. However, severe cases may require drug therapy or external electrical stimulus to prevent serious complications.

Congestive Heart Failure (CHF)

When the heart muscle is damaged or overworked and lacks the strength to keep blood circulating normally through the body, its chambers are often taxed to the limit. **Congestive heart failure (CHF)** affects over 5 million Americans and dramatically increases risk of premature death.[20] The heart muscle may be injured by a number of health conditions, including rheumatic fever, pneumonia, heart attack, or other cardiovascular problems. In some cases, the damage is due to radiation or chemotherapy treatments for cancer. These weakened muscles respond poorly, impairing blood flow out of the heart through the arteries. The return flow of blood through the veins begins to back up, causing congestion in body tissues. This pooling of blood causes the heart to enlarge and decreases the amount of blood that can be circulated. Fluid begins to accumulate in other body areas, such as in the vessels in the legs and ankles or the lungs, causing swelling or difficulty in breathing. Today, CHF is the single most frequent cause of hospitalization in the United States.[21] If untreated, congestive heart failure can be fatal. However, most cases respond well to treatment that includes *diuretics* (water pills) for relief of fluid accumulation; drugs, such as *digitalis,* that increase the pumping action of the heart; and drugs called *vasodilators,* which expand blood vessels and decrease resistance, allowing blood to flow more easily and making the heart's work easier.

Congenital and Rheumatic Heart Disease

Approximately 1 out of every 125 children is born with some form of **congenital heart disease** (disease present at birth). These forms may be relatively minor, such as slight *murmurs* (low-pitched sounds caused by turbulent blood flow through the heart), resulting from valve irregularities, which some children outgrow. Other congenital problems involve serious complications in heart function that can be corrected only with surgery. Their underlying causes are unknown but may be related to hereditary factors; maternal diseases, such as rubella, occurring during fetal development; or chemical intake (particularly alcohol) by the mother during pregnancy. Because of advances in pediatric cardiology, the prognosis for children with congenital heart defects is better than ever before.

Rheumatic heart disease can cause similar heart problems in children. It is attributed to rheumatic fever, an inflammatory disease that may affect many connective tissues of the body, especially those of the heart, joints, brain, or skin, and is caused by an unresolved *streptococcal infection* of the throat (strep throat). In a small number of cases, this infection can lead to an immune response in which antibodies attack the heart as well as the bacteria. Many of the 75,000 annual operations on heart valves in the United States are related to rheumatic heart disease.[22]

Stroke

Like heart muscle, brain cells must have a continuous adequate supply of oxygen in order to survive. A **stroke** (also called a *cerebrovascular accident*) occurs when the blood supply to the brain is interrupted. Strokes may be caused by a **thrombus** (blood clot), an **embolus** (a wandering clot), or an **aneurysm** (a weakening in a blood vessel that causes it to bulge and, in severe cases, burst). Figure 12.4 illustrates these blood vessel disorders. When any of these events occurs, the result is the death of brain cells, which do not have the capacity to heal or regenerate. Some strokes are mild and cause only temporary dizziness or slight weakness or numbness. More serious interruptions in blood flow may cause speech impairments, memory problems, and loss of motor control.

Other strokes affect parts of the brain that regulate heart and lung function and kill within minutes. Stroke killed more than 159,000 Americans in 1999 and accounted for 1 in 14 of our total deaths, surpassed only by CHD and

---

Fibrillation   A sporadic, quivering pattern of heartbeat resulting in extreme inefficiency in moving blood through the cardiovascular system.

Congestive heart failure (CHF)   An abnormal cardiovascular condition that reflects impaired cardiac pumping and blood flow; pooling blood leads to congestion in body tissues.

Congenital heart disease   Heart disease that is present at birth.

Rheumatic heart disease   A heart disease caused by untreated streptococcal infection of the throat.

Stroke   A condition occurring when the brain is damaged by disrupted blood supply.

Thrombus   Blood clot.

Embolus   Blood clot that is forced through the circulatory system.

Aneurysm   A weakened blood vessel that may bulge under pressure and, in severe cases, burst.

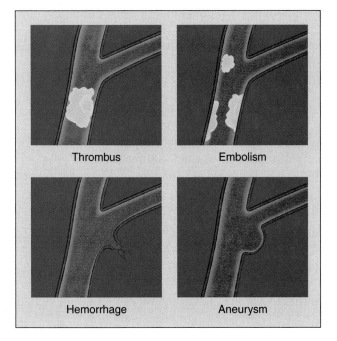

Figure 12.4
Common Blood Vessel Disorders

cancer.[23] On average, someone suffers a stroke every 53 seconds, and someone dies every 3.3 minutes.[24] About one in ten major strokes is preceded (days, weeks, or months before) by **transient ischemic attacks (TIAs),** brief interruptions of the blood supply to the brain that cause only temporary impairment. TIAs are often indications of an impending major stroke. The following are warning signs of stroke:

- Sudden weakness or numbness of the face, arm, or leg on one side of the body
- Sudden dimness or loss of vision, particularly in only one eye
- Loss of speech, or trouble talking or understanding speech
- Sudden, severe headaches with no known cause
- Unexplained dizziness, unsteadiness, or sudden falls, especially with any of the previously listed symptoms

If you experience any of these symptoms, or if you are with someone who does, seek medical help immediately. The earlier treatment starts, the more effective it will be.

One of the greatest medical successes in recent years has been the decline in the fatality rates from strokes, a rate that has dropped by one-third in the United States since the 1980s and continues to decline. Improved diagnostic procedures, better surgical options, clot-busting drugs injected early after a stroke has occurred, and acute care centers specializing in stroke treatment and rehabilitation have all been factors. Increased awareness of risk factors for stroke, especially high

Transient ischemic attack (TIA) Mild form of stroke; often an indicator of impending major stroke.

blood pressure, and an emphasis on prevention also have contributed to the decline in stroke fatality rates. It is estimated that more than half of all remaining strokes could be avoided if more people followed the recommended preventive standards.

Reducing Your Risk for Cardiovascular Diseases

What is your own risk for heart disease? To find out, add up your score in the accompanying Assess Yourself box. Factors that increase the risk for cardiovascular problems fall into two categories: those we can control and those we cannot. Fortunately, we can take steps to minimize many risk factors.

Risks You Can Control

Avoid Tobacco As early as 1984, the Surgeon General of the United States asserted that smoking was the greatest risk factor for heart disease. Today, one in five deaths from CVD are directly related to smoking.[25] Generally, the more a person smokes, the greater the risk for heart attack or stroke. The risk for cardiovascular disease is 70 percent greater for smokers than for nonsmokers. Smokers who have a heart attack are more likely to die suddenly (within one hour) than are nonsmokers. Evidence also indicates that chronic exposure to environmental tobacco smoke (ETS or passive smoking) increases the risk of heart disease by as much as 30 percent.[26]

How does smoking damage the heart? There are two plausible explanations. One theory states that nicotine increases heart rate, heart output, blood pressure, and oxygen use by heart muscles. Because the carbon monoxide in cigarette smoke displaces oxygen in heart tissue, the heart is forced to work harder to obtain sufficient oxygen. The other theory states that chemicals in smoke damage the lining of the coronary arteries, allowing cholesterol and plaque to accumulate more easily. This additional buildup constricts the vessels, increasing blood pressure and causing the heart to work harder.

When people stop smoking, regardless of how long or how much they've smoked, their risk of heart disease declines rapidly.[27] Three years after quitting, the risk of death from heart disease and stroke for people who smoked a pack a day or less is almost the same as for people who never smoked. Quitting today will also raise your high-density lipoprotein (HDL) levels, reducing your risks even further (see the next section).[28]

Cut Back on Fats and Cholesterol How concerned should you be about the amount of fat and cholesterol in your diet? Very concerned. In fact, according to recent evidence, cholesterol risks may be greater than ever for Americans. When dietary experts from the National Heart, Lung and Blood Institute met recently to prepare their *Third Report on Detection, Evaluation, and Treatment of Cholesterol National Guidelines,* they gave Americans a wake-up call by slashing the levels of cholesterol that are considered acceptable. These guidelines not only provide evidence that cholesterol levels

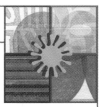

Find Your Cholesterol Plan

The following two-step program will guide you through the National Cholesterol Education Program's new treatment guidelines. The first step helps you establish your overall coronary risk; the second uses that information to determine your LDL treatment goals and how to reach them.

You'll need to know your blood pressure, your total LDL, and HDL cholesterol levels, and your triglyceride and fasting glucose levels. If you're not sure of those numbers, ask your doctor and, if necessary, schedule an exam to get them. (Everyone should have a complete lipid profile every five years, starting at age 20.)

STEP 1: TAKE THE HEART-ATTACK RISK TEST

This test will identify your chance of having a heart attack or dying of coronary disease in the next 10 years. (People with previously diagnosed coronary disease, diabetes, aortic aneurysm, or symptomatic carotid- or peripheral-artery disease already face more than a 20 percent risk; they can skip the test and go straight to Step 2.) The test uses data from the Framingham Heart Study, the world's longest-running study of cardio-vascular risk factors. The test is limited to established, major factors that are easily measured.

Circle the point value for each of the risk factors shown at right and below.

1 Age

YEARS	WOMEN	MEN
20–34	−7	−9
35–39	−3	−4
40–44	0	0
45–49	3	3
50–54	6	6
55–59	8	8
60–64	10	10
65–69	12	11
70–74	14	12
75–79	16	13

2 Total Cholesterol

MG/DL	AGE 20–39 WOMEN	AGE 20–39 MEN	AGE 40–49 WOMEN	AGE 40–49 MEN	AGE 50–59 WOMEN	AGE 50–59 MEN	AGE 60–69 WOMEN	AGE 60–69 MEN	AGE 70–79 WOMEN	AGE 70–79 MEN
<160	0	0	0	0	0	0	0	0	0	0
160–199	4	4	3	3	2	2	1	1	1	0
200–239	8	7	6	5	4	3	2	1	1	0
240–279	11	9	8	6	5	4	3	2	2	1
280+	13	11	10	8	7	5	4	3	2	1

3 High-density Lipo-protein (HDL) Cholesterol

MG/DL	WOMEN AND MEN
60+	−1
50–59	0
40–49	1
<40	2

4 Systolic Blood Pressure (The Higher Number)

MM/HG	UNTREATED WOMEN	UNTREATED MEN	TREATED WOMEN	TREATED MEN
<120	0	0	0	0
120–129	1	0	3	1
130–139	2	1	4	2
140–159	3	1	5	2
>159	4	2	6	3

Continues on page 306

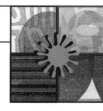

5 Smoking

	AGE 20–39		AGE 40–49		AGE 50–59		AGE 60–69		AGE 70–79	
	WOMEN	MEN	WOMEN	MEN	WOMEN	MEN	WOMEN	MEN	WOMEN	MEN
	9	8	7	5	4	3	2	1	1	1

TOTAL YOUR POINTS:

Now find your total-point score in the men's or women's column at right, then locate your 10-year risk in the far-right column.

WOMEN'S SCORE	MEN'S SCORE	YOUR 10-YEAR RISK
Less than 20	Less than 12	Less than 10%
20–22	12–15	10%–20%
Greater than 22	Greater than 15	Greater than 20%

STEP 2: FIND YOUR LOW DENSITY LIPOPROTEIN (LDL) TREATMENT PLAN

Consult the table below to learn how your overall coronary risk affects whether you need to lower your LDL cholesterol level and, if you do, by how much. First, locate your coronary risk in the left-hand column. (That's based on the 10-year heart-attack risk that you just calculated as well as your coronary risk factors and any heart-threatening diseases you may have.) Then look across that row to see whether you should make lifestyle changes and take cholesterol-lowering medication, based on your current LDL level.

CORONARY-RISK GROUP	START LIFESTYLE CHANGES IF YOUR LDL LEVEL IS . . .[1]	ADD DRUGS IF YOUR LDL LEVEL IS . . .
Very High 1. 10-year heart-attack risk of 20% or more or 2. history of coronary heart disease, diabetes, peripheral-artery disease, carotid-artery disease, or aortic aneurysm.	100 mg/dl or higher. (Aim for an LDL under 100.) Get retested after three months.	130 or higher. (Drugs are optional if your LDL is between 100 and 130.)
High 1. 10-year heart-attack risk of 10% to 20% and 2. two or more major coronary risk factors.[2]	130 or higher. (Aim for an LDL under 130.) Get retested after three months.	130 or higher, and lifestyle changes don't achieve your LDL goal in three months.
Moderately High 1. 10-year heart-attack risk under 10% and 2. two or more major coronary risk factors.[2]	Same as above.	160 or higher, and lifestyle changes don't achieve your LDL goal in three months.[3]

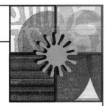

CORONARY-RISK GROUP	START LIFESTYLE CHANGES IF YOUR LDL LEVEL IS . . .[1]	ADD DRUGS IF YOUR LDL LEVEL IS . . .
Low to Moderate 1. One or no major coronary risk factors.[2, 4]	160 or higher. (Aim for an LDL under 160.) Get retested after three months.	190 or higher, and lifestyle changes don't achieve your LDL goal in three months. (Drugs are optional if your LDL is between 160 and 189.)

1. *People who have the metabolic syndrome should make lifestyle changes, even if their LDL level alone doesn't warrant it. You have the metabolic syndrome if you have three or more of these risk factors: HDL under 40 in men, 50 in women; systolic blood pressure of 130 or more or diastolic pressure of 85 or more; fasting glucose level of 110 to 125; triglyceride level of 150 or more; and waist circumference over 40 inches in men, 35 inches in women. People with the syndrome should limit their carbohydrate intake, get up to 30 to 35 percent of their calories from total fat (more than usually recommended), and make the other lifestyle changes, including restriction of saturated fat.*
2. *The major coronary risk factors are cigarette smoking; coronary disease in a father or brother before age 55 or a mother or sister before age 65; systolic blood pressure of 140 or more, a diastolic pressure of 90 or more, or being on drugs for hypertension; and an HDL level under 40. If your HDL is 60 or more, subtract one risk factor. (High LDL is a major factor, of course, but it's already figured into the table.)*
3. *While the goal is to get LDL under 130, the use of drugs in these people usually isn't worthwhile, even if lifestyle steps fail to achieve that goal.*
4. *People in this group usually have less than 10 percent 10-year risk. Those who have higher risk should ask their doctor whether they need more aggressive treatment than shown here.*

are out of control in the United States but also indicate that the numbers of people needing cholesterol-cutting drugs may be three times what we originally thought. In fact, the problem is so severe that nearly 36 million people in the United States, or one-fifth of all adults, are believed to need drugs to provide the degree of risk reduction that is necessary to avoid cardiovascular problems.[29]

Why all of the fuss about fats and cholesterol? Diets high in saturated fats are known to raise cholesterol levels, send the body's blood-clotting system into high gear, and make the blood sludgy in just a few hours, increasing the risk of heart attacks or stroke. Studies indicate that fatty foods apparently trigger production of *factor VII,* a blood-clotting substance. Switching to a low-fat diet promptly eliminates the risk of this clotting.

A fatty diet also increases the amount of cholesterol in the blood, contributing to atherosclerosis. In past years, cholesterol levels between 200 to 240 milligrams per 100 milliliters of blood (mg/dL) were considered normal. Recent research indicates that levels between 180 and 200 mg/dL are more desirable and that 150 mg/dL levels would be even better if you really want to reduce CVD risks.[30] See Table 12.1.

However, it isn't just the total cholesterol level that you should be concerned about. It is important to know that cho-

lesterol comes in two main varieties: **low-density lipoprotein (LDL)** and **high-density lipoprotein (HDL).** Low-density lipoprotein is often referred to as the "bad" kind of cholesterol and is believed to build up or clump on artery walls. In contrast, high-density lipoprotein is known as the "good" cholesterol and is widely believed to sweep cholesterol off of artery walls, thus serving as a great protector. In theory, if LDL levels get too high or HDL levels too low, largely because of too much saturated fat in the diet, a lack of physical exercise, high stress levels, or genetic predisposition, cholesterol will accumulate on artery walls, leading to cardiovascular problems. Scientists now believe that there are other factors that may contribute to increased CVD risk. A specific component

Low-density lipoproteins (LDLs) Compounds that facilitate the transport of cholesterol in the blood to the body's cells.

High-density lipoproteins (HDLs) Compounds that facilitate the transport of cholesterol in the blood to the liver for metabolism and elimination from the body.

Table 12.1
Classification of LDL, Total, and HDL Cholesterol (mg/dL) and Recommended Levels for Adults

LDL Cholesterol
<100	Optimal
100–129	Near optimal/above optimal
130–159	Borderline high
160–189	High
≥190	Very high

Total Cholesterol
<200	Desirable
200–239	Borderline high
≥240	High

HDL Cholesterol
<40	Low
≥60	High

Triglycerides
<200	Normal
200–399	Borderline high
400–1,000	High
1,000>	Very high

Source: National Heart, Lung, and Blood Institute, May 2001.

of HDL known as *LP(a)* may be the most important element of the HDL makeup. The more of this protective protein a person has, the lower the risk for CVD seems to be.[31]

Control the ratio of HDL to total cholesterol by either lowering LDL levels or by raising HDL levels. Dietary reductions of saturated fat and increased exercise continue to be the best methods for maintaining healthy ratios. However, if dietary efforts and exercise do not reduce total cholesterol or LDL levels, several medications are available that may help.

Triglycerides, another type of fat in the blood, also appears to promote clogged arteries. As people get older, fatter, or both, their triglycerides and cholesterol levels tend to rise. Although some CVD patients have elevated triglyceride levels, a causal link between high triglyceride levels and CVD has yet to be established. It may be that high triglyceride levels do not directly cause atherosclerosis but, rather, are among the abnormalities that speed its development. It is also important to remember not to reduce fat consumption too greatly, because some fat is necessary to overall health. Newer research also indicates that consuming too many low-fat or fat-free foods, such as salad dressings and other products may actually contribute to the escalating problem of obesity in America. Current thinking among top researchers is that it would be better to eat foods with olive oil, canola oil, and other mo-

Triglycerides The most common form of fat in the body; excess calories are converted into triglycerides and stored as body fat.

nounsaturated fats than to eat products containing low fat or no fat content. (For a complete discussion of this topic, see Chapter 9.) Of course, all fat intake should be in moderation.

Monitor Your Cholesterol Levels In order to get an accurate assessment of your total cholesterol and LDL and HDL levels, you should have a *lipoprotein analysis.* This analysis requires that you not eat or drink anything for 12 hours prior to the test and that a reputable health provider do the analysis. The LDL level is derived using a standard formula:

$$\text{LDL} = \text{total cholesterol} - \text{HDL} - (\text{triglycerides} \div 5).$$

For example, if the level of total cholesterol is 200, the level of HDL 45, and the level of triglycerides 150, the LDL level would be 125 (200 − 45 − 30).

In general, LDL is more closely associated with cardiovascular risks than is total cholesterol. However, most authorities agree that looking only at LDLs ignores the positive effects of HDL. Perhaps the best method of evaluating risk is to examine the *ratio* of HDL to total cholesterol or the percentage of HDL in total cholesterol. If the percentage of HDL is less than 35, the risk increases dramatically.

Change Lifestyle to Reduce Your Risks Of the over 100 million Americans who need to worry about their cholesterol levels, almost half, particularly those at the low to moderate risk levels, should be able to reach their LDL and HDL goals though lifestyle changes alone. People who are at higher risk or those for whom lifestyle modifications make no difference may need to take cholesterol-lowering drugs while they continue modifying their lifestyle. See Table 12.2 for a list of current cholesterol fighting drugs, their side effects, and factors to consider. Current recommendations to help you reduce risk are not only more aggressive, but also more specific.

Reduce Intake of Saturated Fats Current guidelines suggest that you should reduce intake of saturated fat (obtained mostly from animal products) to *less than 7 percent of your total daily caloric expenditures* and minimize your consumption of *trans*-fat (see Chapter 9) found in partially hydrogenated products such as margarine, many fast foods, and many packaged foods. By cutting your intake of saturated fats and *trans*-fats, experts from the National Heart, Lung and Blood Institute (NHLBI) believe that you can reduce your LDL levels by as much as 10 percent.[32] In addition, NHLBI experts indicate that you should consume fewer than 200 milligrams per day of cholesterol, which is found mainly in eggs and meat. Doing so may result in reductions in LDL by as much as 5 percent.[33]

Lose Weight No question about it—body weight plays a role in CVD. Researchers are not certain whether high-fat, high-sugar, high-calorie diets are a direct risk for CVD or whether they invite risk by causing obesity, which strains the heart, forcing it to push blood though the many miles of capillaries that supply each pound of fat. A heart that has to continuously move blood through an overabundance of vessels may become damaged. People who are overweight are more likely to

Table 12.2
Common Cholesterol-Lowering Drugs

DRUG*	COST†	TYPICAL BENEFIT	SIDE EFFECTS	COMMENTS
Statins			Mild stomach or muscle pain fairly common; severe muscle pain rare, though more common when taken with gemfibrozil, niacin, or certain antifungals and antibiotics. Abnormal liver function in 1% to 2% of patients; to prevent liver damage, liver tests must be done for first 3 months, periodically thereafter.	Best choice for most people with high LDL since it's by far the most effective and generally the best tolerated. However, users must be sure to under go periodic liver testing.
Alorvastatin (*Lipitor*)	$57 to $98	LDL ↓ 20%–60%		
Cerivastatin (*Baycol*)	$46 to $68	HDL ↑5%–15%		
Fluvastatin (*Lescol*)	$41 to $83	Triglycerides ↓		
Lovastatin (*Mevacor*)	$70 to $248	15%–30%		
Pravastatin (*Pravachol*)	$70 to $113			
Simvastatin (*Zocor*)	$113			Proven to reduce total mortality in people with coronary disease, almost certainly has some effect on others as well. In addition to lipid effects, may protect heart by reducing inflammation and stabilizing plaque deposits. May also reduce risk of osteoporosis, stroke, Alzheimer's disease.
Folic acids			Heartburn and stomach pain common; diarrhea, nausea, skin rash, gallstones, and muscle pain less common. Both drugs may increase effect of anticoagulants and certain oral antidiabetic drugs.	Good choice in people who have low HDL, high triglycerides, or both, especially when LDL isn't particularly high.
Gemfibrozil (generic, *Lopid*)	$29 to $85	LDL ↓5%–20%		
Fenofibrate (*Tricor*)	$71	HDL ↑ 10%–70%		Gemfibrozil proven to reduce mortality in people who have coronary disease and low HDL elevated triglycerides, and low LDL (including those with the metabolic syndrome).
		Triglycerides ↓ 20%–50%		Fenofibrate has larger effect on LDL and triglycerides but not yet proven to reduce coronary risk.
Niacin			Skin flushing and itching common; gastrointestinal problems, blurred vision, fatigue, glucose intolerance, gout less common. *Niaspan* may be better tolerated.	Can also be good choice in people with low HDL and high triglycerides.
Immediate release (generic *Niacor*)	$13 to $49	LDL ↓5%–25%		
		HDL ↑15%–35%		Proven to reduce mortality in people with coronary disease.
Extended release (generic *Niaspan*)	$11 to $65	Triglycerides 20%–50%		People with diabetes or stomach ulcers should generally avoid niacin.
				Starting with low dose and pretreating with aspirin or ibuprofen can lessen skin side effects.

* A fourth class of drugs not included in the table—bile-acid resins such as cholestyramine (*Questran*), colestipol (*Colestid*), and colesevelam (*Welchol*)—can also be added when LDL levels don't fall enough.
†Average cost to consumer for 30 days of treatment based on data from retail pharmacies nationwide, provided by Scott-Levin's Source Prescription Audit May 2000 to April 2001. Lower price for statins is initial dose, higher price is maximum dose; lower price for others is generic, higher price is brand. Costs rounded off to nearest whole dollar.

develop heart disease and stroke even if they have no other risk factors. If you're overweight, losing even 5 to 10 pounds can make a significant difference of as much as 5 percent LDL reduction,[34] especially if you're an "apple" (thicker around your upper body and waist) rather than a "pear" (thicker around your hips and thighs). Your waist measurement divided by your hip measurement should be less than 0.9 (for men) and less than 0.8 (for women). (See Chapter 10 on weight control).[35]

Modify Other Dietary Habits The NHLBI guidelines recommend the following dietary modifications to reduce CVD risk:

- Consume 5 to 10 milligrams per day of *soluble fiber* from sources such as psyllium seeds, oat bran, fruits, vegetables, and legumes. (See Chapter 9.) Even this small dietary modification may result in another 5 percent drop in LDL levels.

- Consume about 2 grams per day of *plant sterols* (or sterol derivatives) from substances such as Benecol or Take Control margarine. These are the first widely available sources of sterols, but more will be on the market soon. Modification should reduce LDL levels by another 5 percent.

- Although less widely supported by rigorous research findings, many experts believe that consuming at least 25 grams of soy protein from various soy foods instead of dairy sources may reduce LDLs by 5 percent.

Step Up or Maintain Exercise Behaviors According to all available evidence to date, inactivity is a definite risk factor for CVD.[36] Such evidence continues to mount with NHLBI guidelines, providing yet another endorsement for exercise in the CVD battle. The good news is that it has become increasingly clear that you do not have to be an exercise junkie or fanatic to reduce your risk. Even modest levels of low-intensity physical activity are beneficial if done regularly and over the long term. Exercise can increase HDL, lower triglycerides, and reduce coronary risks in several ways. Such activities include walking, gardening, housework, and dancing. For more information, see Chapter 11 on personal fitness.

Making the above modifications could result in as much as a 35 percent reduction in LDL levels—the same level of risk reduction as taking any of the statin drugs typically prescribed.

Control Diabetes Risks The unique difficulties and risks for CVD among people with diabetes are underscored throughout the NHLBI conference and in their guidelines. Diabetics who have taken insulin for a number of years appear to run an increased risk for CVD. In fact, CVD is the leading cause of death among diabetic patients. Because overweight people have a higher risk for diabetes, distinguishing between the effects of the two conditions is difficult. Diabetics also tend to have elevated blood fat levels, increased atherosclerosis, and a tendency toward deterioration of small blood vessels, particularly in the eyes and extremities. Through a prescribed regimen of diet, exercise and medication, diabetics can control much of their increased risk for CVD.

Control Your Blood Pressure **Hypertension** refers to sustained high blood pressure. If it cannot be attributed to any specific cause, it is known as **essential hypertension.** Approximately 90 percent of all cases of hypertension fit this category. **Secondary hypertension** refers to hypertension caused by specific factors, such as kidney disease, obesity, or tumors of the adrenal glands. In general, the higher your blood pressure, the greater your risk for CVD.

Hypertension is known as the "silent killer" because it usually has no symptoms. Although it affects nearly 61 million Americans, 20 percent of them don't know they have the condition, and only one-third of those who are aware of it have it under control.[37] Common forms of treatment are dietary changes (reducing salt and calorie intake), weight loss (when appropriate), the use of diuretics and other medications (only when prescribed by a physician), regular exercise, and the practice of relaxation techniques and effective coping and communication skills.

Blood pressure is measured in two parts and is expressed as a fraction—for example, 110/80, or 110 over 80. Both values are measured in *millimeters of mercury* (mm Hg). The first number refers to **systolic pressure,** the pressure being applied to the walls of the arteries when the heart contracts, pumping blood to the rest of the body. The second value is **diastolic pressure,** the pressure applied to the walls of the arteries during the heart's relaxation phase. During this phase, blood is reentering the chambers of the heart, preparing for the next heartbeat.

Normal blood pressure varies depending on weight, age, and physical condition. It also varies for different groups of people, such as women and minorities. As a rule, men have a greater risk for high blood pressure than women have until age 55, when their risks become about equal. At age 75 and over, women are more likely to have high blood pressure than men.[38] For the average person, 110 over 80 is a healthy blood pressure level. If your blood pressure exceeds 140 over 90, you probably need to take steps to lower it. See Table 12.3 for a summary of blood pressure values and what they mean.

Manage Stress Some scientists have noted a relationship between CVD risk and a person's stress level, behavior habits, and socioeconomic status. These factors may affect established risk factors. For example, people under stress may start smoking or smoke more than they otherwise would.[39] Other studies have challenged the apparent link

---

Hypertension Sustained elevated blood pressure.

Essential hypertension Hypertension that cannot be attributed to any cause.

Secondary hypertension Hypertension caused by specific factors, such as kidney disease, obesity, or tumors of the adrenal glands.

Systolic pressure The upper number in the fraction that measures blood pressure, indicating pressure on the walls of the arteries when the heart contracts.

Diastolic pressure The lower number in the fraction that measures blood pressure, indicating pressure on the walls of the arteries during the relaxation phase of heart activity.

Table 12.3
Blood Pressure Values and What They Mean

CLASSIFICATION	SYSTOLIC READING	DIASTOLIC READING	ACTIONS
Normal	Below 130	Below 85	Recheck in two years.
High normal	130–139	85–89	Recheck in one year.
Mild hypertension	140–159	90–99	Check in two months.
Moderate hypertension	160–179	100–109	See physician within a month.
Severe hypertension	180 or above	110 or above	See physician immediately.

Note: Systolic and diastolic values are based on an average of two or more readings taken at different times.

Source: Adapted from "Fifth Report of the Joint National Committee on Detection, Evaluation, and Treatment of High Blood Pressure," *Archieves of Internal Medicine* 153 (25 January 1993): 154–183 (published by the American Medical Association); and American Heart Association.

between emotional stress and heart disease. Although it was once widely assumed that the Type A personality, who suffers from high stress levels, was a time bomb ticking toward a heart attack, this theory has not been proven clinically.

> ### What do you think?
> *What is your resting heart rate?* ✳ *You can find out by taking your pulse. Gently press the pads of your first two fingers against the inside of your wrist, just below the base of your thumb. Sit quietly, and count the number of beats that occur during a 10-second period. Multiply the number of beats by 6. Repeat the process.* ✳ *How does your heart rate compare to that of your friends?*

Researcher-physician Robert S. Eliot demonstrated that approximately one of five people has an extreme cardiovascular reaction to stressful stimulation. These people experience alarm and resistance so strongly that when they are under stress, their bodies produce large amounts of stress chemicals, which in turn cause tremendous changes in the cardiovascular system, including remarkable increases in blood pressure. These people are called *hot reactors*. Although their blood pressure may be normal when they are not under stress—for example, in a doctor's office—it increases dramatically in response to even small amounts of everyday stress.

Cold reactors are those who are able to experience stress (even to live as Type A personalities) without showing harmful cardiovascular responses. Cold reactors may internalize stress, but their self-talk and perceptions about the stressful events lead them to a nonresponse state in which their cardiovascular system remains virtually unaffected.[40] Some research indicates that people who have an underlying predisposition toward a toxic core personality (in other words, who are chronically hostile and hateful) may be at greatest risk for a CVD event.

Risks You Cannot Control

There are, unfortunately, some risk factors for CVD that we cannot prevent or control. The most important are the following:

- *Heredity.* Having a family history of heart disease appears to increase risks significantly. Whether the increase is due to genetics or environment is an unresolved question.
- *Age.* Seventy-five percent of all heart attacks occur in people over age 65. The risk for CVD increases with age for both sexes.
- *Gender.* Men are at much greater risk for CVD until old age. Women under 35 have a fairly low risk unless they have high blood pressure, kidney problems, or diabetes. Using oral contraceptives and smoking also increase the risk. Hormonal factors appear to reduce risk for women, although after menopause or after estrogen levels are otherwise reduced (e.g., because of hysterectomy), women's LDL levels tend to go up, increasing their chances for CVD. (For more on the gender factor, see the next section.)
- *Race.* Blacks have a 45 percent greater risk for hypertension and thus are at greater risk for CVD than are whites. In addition, African-Americans have less chance of surviving heart attacks. See the accompanying Health in a Diverse World box.

> ### What do you think?
> *What risk factors for heart disease do you currently have?* ✳ *Do you know what your cholesterol level is?* ✳ *Which of your risk factors are the most critical?* ✳ *What actions can you start taking today to reduce your risk?*

Disparity in CVD Risks

Cardiovascular disease is not an "equal opportunity" disease. In fact, when it comes to risk of attack and eventual mortality, there are huge disparities based on gender, race, and age. Consider the following:

- Higher CVD risks exist among African-American and Mexican-American women than among white women of comparable socioeconomic status (SES). The striking differences by both ethnicity and SES underscore the critical need to improve screening, early detection, and treatment of CVD-related conditions for African-American and Mexican-American women, as well as for women of lower SES in all ethnic groups.

- Among Native Americans and Alaska Natives age 18 and older, 63.7 percent of men and 61.4 percent of women have one or more CVD risk factors (hypertension, current cigarette smoking, high blood cholesterol, obesity, or diabetes). If data on physical activity had been included in this analysis, the prevalence of risk factors would have been much higher.
- In 1999, CHD death rates were 225.4 for white males and 216.4 for African-American males (7% higher) at all ages and stages of life.
- In 1999, CHD death rates were 135.0 for white females and 154.7 for African-American females.
- African-Americans are 60 percent more likely to suffer a stroke than are whites, and 250 percent more likely to die from a stroke.

- A family history of diabetes, gout, high blood pressure, or high cholesterol increases one's risk of heart disease. African-Americans are more likely to have these familial risk factors, increasing their overall chances for CVD.

CHOLESTEROL LEVELS BY RACE, AGE 20 AND OVER

The percentages of the following populations who have a cholesterol level of over 200 mg/dL are listed below:

- 53% of non-Hispanic white females
- 47% of non-Hispanic black females
- 43% of Mexican-Americans
- 27% of Asian/Pacific Islanders
- 28% of Indian/Alaskan Natives

Source: American Heart Association, *Heart and Stroke Facts, 2001.*

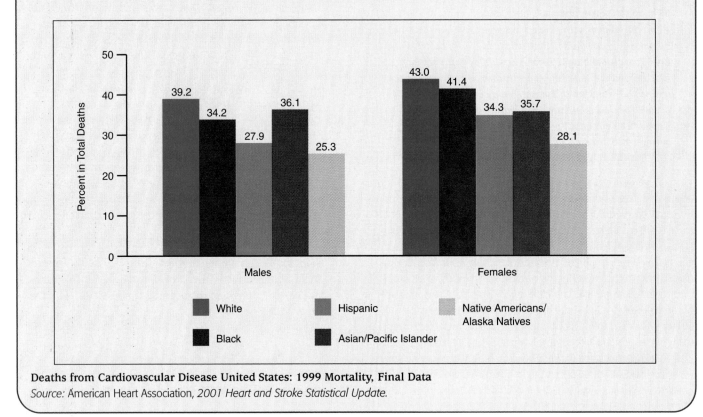

Deaths from Cardiovascular Disease United States: 1999 Mortality, Final Data
Source: American Heart Association, *2001 Heart and Stroke Statistical Update.*

Differences Between the Sexes: Key Factors in Early Detection and Prognosis

As more research is conducted concerning diagnosis and treatment of CVD, it is becoming clear that women sometimes experience different symptoms and benefit from different treatment than men do. Some examples follow below.

FEELING PAIN

Several studies have documented that women experience pain more acutely and more frequently than men, indicating that the sexes may detect and react to pain differently. In a study of dental patients, for example, women responded more favorably than men to a class of pain relievers known as kappa opioids, including pentazocine. This finding suggests that receptors for inhibiting pain may vary by sex. Also, women appear to be less responsive than men to nonsteroidal anti-inflammatory drugs, such as ibuprofen. Women typically need slightly lower doses of aspirin and should be forewarned that taking 325 mg of aspirin per day may result in anticoagulation levels that exceed those of men. Surgical risks, accidents that lead to excessive bleeding, and so on, may be greater for aspirin-using women.

NOTING HEART ATTACK SYMPTOMS

Although we are taught that the classic symptom of a heart attack is chest-crushing pain, this type of pain is not as common in women. Women's heart attacks, by contrast, tend to show up as shortness of breath, fatigue, and jaw pain, stretched out over hours rather than minutes. Women tend to suffer their first heart attack ten years later than men, and in part because they are older when they have these attacks, they are more likely to die.

TREATING CVD

Interestingly, drugs used to break up clots and stabilize erratic heartbeats are less effective in women than in men. Beta blockers, one common form of treatment for reducing blood pressure and migraines, take longer to metabolize in women than in men, meaning that women often have more difficulty regulating dosage and preventing side effects. Hormone replacement therapy—estrogen and progestin—has been shown to help. Currently several studies are investigating the role estrogen plays in CVD and cancer. Recent studies have shown that angiography, a technique in which a small flexible catheter is inserted in coronary vessels to break up plaque and clear blocked arteries, is one of the best techniques for reducing risk of heart attack. However, angiograms are done much less frequently on women than on men.

Source: A. Park, "The Real Truth About Women's Bodies," *Time* (March 16, 1999): 65–73.

Women and Cardiovascular Disease

Although men tend to have more heart attacks and to have them earlier in life than do women, some interesting trends in survivability have emerged. In 1999, CVD claimed the lives of 445,692 men and a surprising 503,927 women. Why do more men have heart attacks and more women die of them? Why do some studies say that women have about the same mortality rates after myocardial infarction and others indicate there are vast differences, supported by actual numbers?[41] Although we understand the mechanisms that cause heart disease in men and women (or at least we think we do!), their experiences in the health care system, their reactions to life-threatening diseases, and a host of other technological and environmental factors may play a role in these statistics.

Risk Factors for Heart Disease in Women

Premenopausal women are unlikely candidates for heart attacks, except for those who suffer from diabetes, high blood pressure, or kidney disease, or who have a genetic predisposition to high cholesterol levels. Family history and smoking can also increase the risk.

The Role of Estrogen Once her estrogen production drops with menopause, a woman's chance of developing CVD rises rapidly. A 60-year-old woman has the same heart attack risk as a 50-year-old man. By her late 70s, a woman has the same heart attack risk as a man her age. To date, much of this changing risk has been attributed to the aging process, but preliminary evidence indicates that hormones may play a bigger role than once thought. Results from the Postmenopausal Estrogen/Progestin Interventions (PEPI) study, a longitudinal study of how various **hormone replacement therapies (HRTs)** affect cardiovascular risk, indicated that HRT may reduce CVD by as much as 12 to 25 percent. In this study, HRT seemed to reduce a woman's risk for CVD by raising HDL and

---

Hormone replacement therapies (HRTs) Therapies that replace estrogen in postmenopausal women.

For decades, the prevailing wisdom has been that hormones are protective for heart disease. After all, it seemed obvious that women's risk for CVD didn't increase substantially until hormone levels decreased after menopause. Thus, it seemed logical to assume that maintaining those hormone levels through hormone replacement therapy (HRT) would nullify those CVD risks for older women. When the **Postmenopausal Estrogen/Progestin Intervention Trial (PEPI)** results were published, indicating that in fact, HRT raised levels of HDL and decreased LDL in the mid-90's, professional organizations, doctors and the lay community promoted Hormone Replacement as a panacea for CVD risk.* Other studies also suggested a link between hormone therapy and lower heart attack rates.

Today, results from three new major studies provide growing evidence that the advice to take HRT for CVD risk reduction, may in fact, be wrong. Consider the following:

* The **1998 Heart and Estrogen/ Progestin Replacement Study (HERS),** a large-scale randomized, controlled clinical trial showed that after 4 years on HRT, there was no difference in heart attack rates and higher rates of coronary death between those on HRT and those taking a placebo. Perhaps more importantly, study results pointed to a 52% **increase** in cardiovascular events in the first year for those in the HRT group.***
* The **2000 Estrogen Replacement and Atherosclerosis (ERA) Trial,** the first trial to use angiographic images to assess the effects of Estrogen Replacement Therapy (ERT) and Estrogen and HRT on women with pre-existing coronary disease, also showed no benefit on angiographic disease progression with hormone replacement.**
* In the spring of 2000, investigators conducting the huge **Women's Health Initiative (WHI)** stirred even more controversy. The WPI trial, similar to the HERS and ERA trial, is a randomized trial comparing HRT with placebo in postmenopausal women. The major differences between WHI trial and the others mentioned above are the WHI's huge size (over 26,000 women enrolled) and the fact that women enrolled in WPI had no preexisting coronary artery disease. Although WHI is scheduled to continue to 2005, investigators stunned the scientific community when they felt compelled to send letters to women in the trial stating that those in the HRT group had experienced an increased risk of heart attacks, strokes, and blood clots during the early portion of the trial.*** They also pointed out that after the first year, these negative outcomes appeared to disappear.

IMPLICATIONS?

As a result of data from the above studies, the American Heart Association, the American College of Obstetricians and Gynecologists, and other organizations promptly reversed their earlier recommendations.

* New Recommendations say that women who've been taking hormones for years without any problems do not need to stop. However, women should not start hormone replacement therapy just to reduce their risk of cardiovascular disease. Instead, the guidelines suggest using hormone replacement therapy to treat common postmenopausal symptoms such as hot flashes and insomnia, and to reduce the risk of brittle bones—in short for the benefits that seem to have withstood the rigors of research over time . . . As far as increased risks for cancer and other problems, there is much that remains unknown. As WHI and other trial data are published, new information may become available. The best rule of thumb is to keep informed and ask questions. The decision to use or not use ERT or HRT is complex and should be made in consultation with knowledgeable health care providers and after checking on the latest information available from reputable sources. A listing of some of these studies and other valuable resources is provided below.

The Postmenopausal Estrogen/Progestin Interventions (PEPI) Trial: The Writing Group for the PEPI Trial. Effects of estrogen or estrogen/progestin regimens on heart disease risk factors in postmenopausal women. *JAMA.* 1995; 273: 199-208.

Hulley, S., Grady, D., Bust, T. et al. Randomized trial of estrogen plus progestin for secondary prevention of coronary heart disease in postmenopausal women: Heart and Estrogen/Progestin Replacement Study (HERS) Research Group. *JAMA,* 1998. 280:605-613.

Mosca, L., Herrington, D., Pasternak, R., Schenck-Gustafsson, K., Smith, S., and N. Wenger. Hormone Replacement Therapy and Cardiovascular Disease. Circulation. 2001. 104:499. (http://circ.ahajournals.org/cgi/content/full/104/4/499.

ADDITIONAL RESOURCES:

National Heart Lung and Blood Institute: Heart Disease and Women: Are you at risk http://www.nhlbi.nih.gov/health/public/heart/other/wmn.htm

American Heart Association: http://www.aha.org

AHA's journal: Circulation: http://circ.ahajournals.org/cgi/content/ful/104/4/499.

* U.S. Department of Health and Human Services, Normal Heart, Lung and Blood Institute (NHLBI) http://www.nhlbi.gov2002

lowering LDL cholesterol levels. The PEPI study results served as the basis for many women opting for HRT because of apparent CVD benefits. However, newer findings appear to throw a huge wrench in what was previously believed to be the CVD-risk-reducing powers of hormone replacement therapy. For more information, see the box *Hormonal Protection from CVD.* Even when their total blood cholesterol levels are higher than men's, women may be at less risk because they typically have a higher percentage of HDL.[42]

But that's only part of the story. It's true that women age 25 and over tend to have lower cholesterol levels than men of the same age. But when they reach 45, things change. Most men's cholesterol levels become more stable, while both LDL and total cholesterol levels in women start to rise. And the gap widens further beyond age 55.[43]

Before age 45, women's total blood cholesterol levels average below 220 mg/dL. By the time she is 45 to 55, the average woman's blood cholesterol rises to between 223 and 246 mg/dL. Studies of men have shown that for every 1 percent drop in cholesterol, there is a 2 percent decrease in CVD risk.[44] If this holds true for women, prevention efforts focusing on dietary interventions and exercise may significantly help postmenopausal women.

Neglect of Heart Disease Symptoms in Women

During the past decade, research has suggested three main reasons for the widespread neglect of the signs of heart disease in women:

1. Physicians may be gender biased in their delivery of health care, tending to concentrate on women's reproductive organs rather than on the whole woman.
2. Physicians tend to view male heart disease as a more severe problem because men have traditionally had a higher incidence of the disease.
3. Women decline major procedures more often than men do.

Other explanations for diagnostic and therapeutic difficulties encountered by women with heart disease include the following:[45]

- Delay in diagnosing a possible heart attack
- The complexity involved in interpreting chest pain in women
- Typically less aggressive treatment of women who are heart attack victims
- Their older age, on average, and greater frequency of other health problems
- The fact that women's coronary arteries are often smaller than men's, making surgical or diagnostic procedures more difficult technically
- Their increased incidence of postinfarction angina and heart failure

In addition, symptoms of heart attack in women often present differently in women from in men, making it more diffi-

cult for a woman to determine whether to go to the doctor or not. Although there is considerable debate over whether inequities between men and women's treatment of CVD exist, at least one study suggests that differences or disparities may reflect overtreatment of men rather than undertreatment of women.[46]

Gender Bias in CVD Research?

The traditional view that heart disease is primarily a male problem has carried over into research as well. A well-publicized example was research suggesting that aspirin could help prevent heart attacks—based entirely on a study of 22,000 male doctors. To address such concerns, the National Institutes of Health has launched a 15-year, $625 million study of 140,000 postmenopausal women (known as the Women's Health Initiative), focusing on the leading causes of death and disease. Researchers hope to determine how a healthy lifestyle and increased medical attention can help prevent women's heart disease, as well as cancer and osteoporosis.

What do you think?

How do men and women differ in their experiences related to CVD? ✳ *Why do you think women's risks were largely ignored until fairly recently?* ✳ *What actions do you think individuals can take to help improve the situation for both men and women?* ✳ *What actions can communities and medical practitioners take?*

New Weapons Against Heart Disease

The victim of a heart attack today has a variety of options that were not available a generation ago. Medications can strengthen heartbeat, control arrhythmias, remove fluids in case of congestive heart failure, and relieve pain. New surgical procedures are saving many lives.

Techniques of Diagnosing Heart Disease

Several techniques are used to diagnose heart disease, including electrocardiogram, angiography, and positron emission tomography scans. An **electrocardiogram (ECG)** is a record of the electrical activity of the heart, measured during a stress test. Patients walk or run on treadmills while their hearts are monitored. A more accurate method of testing for

Electrocardiogram (ECG) A record of the electrical activity of the heart measured during a stress test.

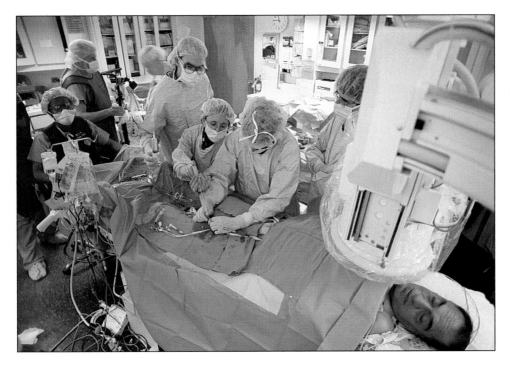

In angioplasty, a catheter with a balloon at the tip is inserted into a blocked artery in the heart. When the balloon is inflated, the fatty deposits within the artery are flattened, increasing blood flow.

heart disease is **angiography** (often referred to as *cardiac catheterization*), in which a needle-thin tube called a *catheter* is threaded through heart arteries, a dye is injected, and an x-ray film is taken to discover which areas are blocked. A more recent and even more effective method of measuring heart activity is **positron emission tomography scan (PET scan),** which produces three-dimensional images of the heart as blood flows through it. During a PET scan, a patient receives an intravenous injection of a radioactive tracer. As the tracer decays, it emits positrons that are picked up by the scanner and transformed by a computer into color images of the heart. Other tests include the following:

- *Radionuclide imaging* (includes tests such as the thallium test, MUGA scan, and acute infarct scintigraphy). These procedures involve injecting substances called radionuclides into the bloodstream. Computer-generated pictures can then show them in the heart. These tests can reveal how well the heart muscle is supplied with blood, how well the heart's chambers are functioning, and which part of the heart has been damaged by a heart attack.

- *Magnetic resonance imaging* (also called MRI or NMR). This test uses powerful magnets to look inside the body. Computer-generated pictures can show the heart muscle and help physicians identify damage from a heart attack, diagnose certain congenital heart defects, and evaluate disease of larger blood vessels, such as the aorta.

- *Digital cardiac angiography* (also called DCA or DSA). This modified form of computer-aided imaging records pictures of the heart and its blood vessels.

Angiography   A technique for examining blockages in heart arteries. A catheter is inserted into the arteries, a dye is injected, and an x-ray film is taken to find the blocked areas. Also called cardiac catheterization.

Positron emission tomography scan (PET scan)
Method for measuring heart activity by injecting a patient with a radioactive tracer that is scanned electronically to produce a three-dimensional image of the heart and arteries.

Coronary bypass surgery   A surgical technique whereby a blood vessel is implanted to bypass a clogged coronary artery.

Angioplasty   A technique in which a catheter with a balloon at the tip is inserted into a clogged artery; the balloon is inflated to flatten fatty deposits against artery walls, allowing blood to flow more freely.

Angioplasty versus Bypass Surgery

Coronary bypass surgery has helped many patients who had coronary blockages or who had suffered heart attacks. In coronary bypass surgery, a blood vessel is taken from another site in the patient's body (usually the *saphenous vein* in the leg or the *internal mammary artery*) and then is implanted to transport blood by bypassing blocked arteries. Bypass patients typically spend between four and seven days in the hospital to recuperate. The average cost of the procedure itself is well over $50,000, and the additional intensive care treatments and follow-ups often result in total medical bills that are closer to $125,000. Death rates are generally much lower at medical centers where surgical teams and intensive care teams see large numbers of patients.[47]

Another procedure called **angioplasty** (sometimes called *balloon angioplasty*) carries fewer risks and may be

New Advances in Heart Disease and Stroke

Although heart disease continues to be the leading cause of death in the United States, actual rates of heart disease have declined substantially in recent decades. Every year we learn more about the functioning of the heart, and this knowledge has helped promote preventive behaviors as well as increases in longevity among those who have experienced a heart or stroke event. As we enter the new millennium, health officials cite major strides in preventing and treating cardiovascular health problems:

- *High blood pressure gene.* Discovery of a gene that produces a special protein receptor that appears to serve as a "master regulator of the body's handling of salt" provides researchers with greater insight into an inherited form of high blood pressure in children. A defective gene makes the receptor stick in the "on" position, which causes the kidneys to retain salt, leading to increases in blood pressure.
- *Congenital heart defects.* A genetic defect has been identified as the cause of DiGeorge syndrome, a condition marked by malformations of the heart and face. Identification of this missing gene, called UFD1, may provide clues to the prevention and treatment of congenital heart defects.
- *New diagnostic testing.* A special process called microarray analysis can detect missing or defective genes more quickly than ever before. Using this process, researchers found a genetic defect in people with Tangier disease, a blood-fat disorder caused by a short-

age of HDL, the "good" cholesterol that carries fat from tissues. This knowledge may help researchers learn more about raising HDL levels for millions of individuals.
- *Reducing "stunning."* Scientists have found the cause of "stunning," a condition in which the heart's pumping action is severely weakened and which often strikes after heart attacks or heart surgery. The problem has been traced to a genetic flaw that affects a protein, troponin I, needed for normal heart contractions.
- *Tissue growth.* Remarkable advances in tissue engineering have enabled scientists to successfully grow heart valves in the laboratory. These new valves may eventually replace the mechanical valves and preserved pig valves commonly used now.
- *Diabetes link.* A link between diabetes and CVD has resulted in diabetes joining smoking, high blood pressure, high cholesterol, and lack of exercise as a risk factor for heart disease and stroke. It is now believed that diabetes increases the risk of dying of heart attack, stroke, heart failure, or kidney failure threefold.
- *New uses for an old drug.* A study of 10,000 heart and diabetes patients found that a standard high blood pressure drug, ramipril, can reduce the risk of death from a wide range of circulatory problems and may help prevent atherosclerosis.
- *New clot busters.* Experimental blood clot busters were shown to prevent brain damage and disability from stroke if given within three to six hours after the attack.
- *New imaging procedures.* New ultrafast CT imaging and magnetic reso-

nance angiography (MRA), which uses magnets and radio waves to view the inside of arteries, offer exciting new means of noninvasive diagnosis of artery blockage.
- *Robotic surgery.* Preliminary studies on the use of robotics in bypass surgery provide hope for safer options. Operating through three small holes in the chest, robotic arms mimic the actions of a surgeon working the controls. The use of robotics provides greater steadiness, eliminates human error, and increases the potential for microsurgery.

Special Note: In 1999, the federal government released its first *Clinical Guidelines on the Identification, Evaluation, and Treatment of Overweight and Obesity in Adults.* Key recommendations from this report are that physicians should use three main measures in evaluating weight and risk: (1) body mass index (BMI), (2) the presence of risk factors for disease and conditions associated with obesity, and (3) waist circumference. For more details on this information, see *Heart Memo* (2001), National Institutes of Health, National Heart, Lung, and Blood Institute, or refer to the Live Healthier, Live Longer website (see sources below).

Sources: Dr. Claude Lenfant and Dr. Phillip Gorden, "Diabetes Mellitus: A Major Risk Factor for Cardiovascular Disease," National Institutes of Health, National Heart, Lung, and Blood Institute News Release (September 1, 1999); Live Healthier, Live Longer; American Heart Association, "Gene Discoveries Among Top 10 Research Advances in Heart Disease and Stroke for 1999," *AHA News Release* (December 30, 1999).

more effective than bypass surgery in selected cases. As in angiography, a needle-thin catheter is threaded through blocked heart arteries. The catheter has a balloon at the tip, which is inflated to flatten fatty deposits against the artery walls, allowing blood to flow more freely. Angioplasty patients are generally awake but sedated during the procedure and spend only one or two days in the hospital after treatment. Most people can return to work within five days. In about 30 percent of patients, the treated arteries become clogged again within six months. Some patients may undergo the procedure as many as three times within a five-year period. Some surgeons argue that given angioplasty's high rate of recurrence, bypass may be a more effective method of treatment.

Research suggests that in many instances, drug treatments may be just as effective in prolonging life as the invasive surgical techniques, but it is critical that doctors follow an aggressive drug treatment program and that patients comply with it.

Aspirin for Heart Disease: Can It Help?

Research has indicated that low doses of aspirin (325 milligrams or less daily or every other day) is beneficial to heart patients because of its blood-thinning properties. Aspirin has even been advised as a preventive strategy for individuals with no current heart disease symptoms. However, major problems associated with aspirin use are gastrointestinal intolerance and a tendency for some people to have difficulty with blood clotting, and these factors may outweigh aspirin's benefits in some cases. People taking aspirin face additional risks from emergency surgery or if accidental bleeding occurs. Although the findings concerning aspirin and heart disease are still inconclusive, the research seems promising.[48]

Thrombolysis

Whenever a heart attack occurs, prompt action is vital. When a coronary artery gets blocked, the heart muscle doesn't die immediately, but time determines how much damage occurs. If a victim gets to an emergency room and is diagnosed fast enough, a form of reperfusion therapy called **thrombolysis** can be performed. Thrombolysis involves injecting an agent such as tissue plasminogen activator, or TPA, to dissolve the clot and restore some blood flow, thereby reducing the amount of tissue that dies from ischemia.[49] These drugs must be used within one to three hours after a heart attack for best results.

Cardiac Rehabilitation

Every year, nearly 1 million people survive heart attacks. Over 7 million more have unstable angina, and about 650,000 undergo bypass surgery or angioplasty. Heart failure is the most common discharge diagnosis for hospitalized Medicare patients and the fourth most common diagnosis among all patients hospitalized in the United States. Most of these patients are eligible for cardiac rehabilitation (including exercise training and health education classes on good nutri-

tion and CVD risk management), needing only a doctor's prescription for these services. However, many Americans do not have access to these programs. Even larger numbers are finding it difficult to afford such programs in light of skyrocketing costs for prescription drugs to treat CVD. While some patients must choose between home health care and cardiac rehabilitation, others stay away from such programs because of cost, transportation, or other factors. Perhaps the biggest deterrent is fear of having another attack resulting from exercise exertion. The benefits of cardiac rehabilitation (including increased stamina and strength and faster recovery), however, far outweigh the risks when these programs are run by certified health professionals.[50]

Personal Advocacy and Heart-Smart Behaviors

People who suspect they have cardiovascular disease are often overwhelmed and frightened. Where should they go for diagnosis? What are the best treatments? Answering these questions becomes even more difficult if they are upset, scared, or tend to listen unquestioningly to doctors' orders. If you or a loved one must face a CVD crisis, it is important to act with knowledge, strength, and assertiveness. These suggestions will help:

1. *Know your rights as a patient.* Ask about the risks and costs of various diagnostic tests. Some procedures, particularly angiography, may pose significant risks for the elderly, those who have had a history of minor stroke, or those who have had chemotherapy or other treatments that could have damaged their blood vessels. Ask for test results and an explanation of any abnormalities.
2. *Find out about informed consent procedures, living wills, durable power of attorney, organ donation, and other legal issues before you become sick.* Having someone shove a clipboard in your face and ask you whether life support can be terminated in case of a problem is one of the great horrors of many people's hospital experiences. Be prepared.
3. *Ask about alternative procedures.* If possible, seek a second opinion at a different health care facility (in other words, get at least two opinions from doctors who are not in the same group and who cannot read each other's diagnoses). New research indicates that doctors may not use drug treatments as aggressively as they could and that medications may be as effective as major bypass or open heart surgeries. Ask, ask, and ask again. Remember, it is your life, and there is always the possibility that another treatment will be better for you.
4. *Remain with your loved one as a "personal advocate."* If your loved one is weak and unable to ask questions, ask the questions yourself. Inquire about new medications, new tests, and other potentially risky procedures that may be undertaken during the course of treatment or recovery. If you feel your loved one is being removed from intensive care or other closely monitored areas prematurely, ask

Thrombolysis Injection of an agent to dissolve clots and restore some blood flow, thereby reducing the amount of tissue that dies from ischemia.

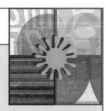
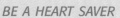

What to Do in the Event of a Heart Attack

Because heart attacks are so serious and frightening, we would prefer not to think about them. However, knowing how to act in an emergency could save your life or that of somebody else.

KNOW THE WARNING SIGNS OF A HEART ATTACK

- Uncomfortable pressure, fullness, squeezing, or pain in the center of the chest, lasting two minutes or longer
- Jaw pain and/or shortness of breath
- Pain spreading to the shoulders, neck, or arms
- Dizziness, fatigue, fainting, sweating, and/or nausea

Not all these warning signs occur in every heart attack. If some of these symptoms do start to occur, however, don't wait. Get help immediately!

KNOW WHAT TO DO IN AN EMERGENCY

- Find out which hospitals in your area have 24-hour emergency cardiac care.
- Determine (in advance) the hospital or medical facility that's nearest your home and office, and tell your family and friends to call this facility in an emergency.
- Keep a list of emergency rescue service numbers next to your telephone and in your pocket, wallet, or purse.
- If you have chest or jaw discomfort that lasts more than two minutes, call the emergency rescue service.
- If you can get to a hospital faster by not waiting for an ambulance, have someone drive you there. Do not drive yourself.

BE A HEART SAVER

- If you're with someone who is showing signs of a heart attack and the warning signs last for two minutes or longer, act immediately.
- Expect a denial. It's normal for a person with chest discomfort to deny the possibility of anything as serious as a heart attack. Don't take no for an answer, however. Insist on taking prompt action.
- Call the emergency rescue service; or
- Get to the nearest hospital emergency room that offers 24-hour emergency cardiac care.
- Give CPR (mouth-to-mouth breathing and chest compression) if it's necessary and if you're properly trained.

Source: American Heart Association.

---

whether the hospital is taking this action to comply with DRGs (diagnosis-related groups, which are established limits of treatment for certain conditions) and whether this action is warranted. Most hospitals have waiting areas or special rooms so family members can stay close to a patient. Exercise your right to this option.

5. *Monitor the actions of health care providers.* To control costs, some hospitals are hiring nursing aides and other untrained personnel to handle duties previously performed by registered nurses. Ask about the patient-to-nurse ratio, and make sure that people monitoring you or your loved ones have appropriate credentials.

6. *Be considerate of your care provider.* One of the most stressful jobs any person can be entrusted with is care of a critically ill person after a major cardiac event. Although questions are appropriate and your emotions are running high, be as tactful and considerate as possible. Nurses often carry a disproportionate responsibility for the care of patients during critical times. They are often forced to carry a higher than necessary patient load. Try to remain out of their way, ask questions as necessary, and report any irregularities in care to the supervisor.

7. *Be patient with the patient.* The pain, suffering, and fears associated with a cardiac event often cause otherwise nice people to act in not-so-nice ways. Be patient and helpful, and allow time for the person to rest. Talk with the patient about his or her feelings, concerns, and fears. Do not ignore these concerns in order to ease your own anxieties.

We still have much to learn about CVD and its causes, treatments, and risk factors. Staying informed is an important fact of staying healthy. Overall, choices in dietary habits, exercise patterns, management of stress, prompt attention to suspicious symptoms, and other behaviors can greatly enhance your chances of remaining CVD-free. Other factors also influence risk. These include the degree of priority our health care systems place on access to health care for all underserved populations, education about risks, and other community-based interventions for those at high risk. Action on both community and individual levels can help address the challenge of CVD.

What do you think?

With all the new diagnostic procedures, treatments, and differing philosophies about various prevention and intervention techniques, how can the typical health consumer ensure that he or she will get the best treatment? ✴ *Where can you go for information?* ✴ *Why might women, members of certain minority groups, and the elderly need a "health advocate" who can help them get through the system?*

Taking Charge

Reducing Risks of Cardiovascular Disease

Although it is easy to read about what we should be doing to keep our hearts and circulatory systems healthy, few of us ever really make a healthy heart one of our priorities. Other issues often take precedence over long-term commitment to cardiovascular wellness. Cardiovascular disease rarely occurs overnight. In some cases, a person is predisposed to it, but in most cases, it is the result of poor health behaviors. What is your risk? Are you taking precautions to prevent the development of a CVD? Although cardiovascular disease continues to plague persons of all ages, races, and socioeconomic statuses, many believe that we are winning the war against this dreaded killer. Medical advances in technology, pharmaceutical agents that control symptoms and lower risk, as well as major lifestyle adjustments can help you remain healthy well into your later years. Are you motivated to change your health behaviors and take action to reduce risks of cardiovasular disease?

Checklist for Change

Making Personal Choices

✓ Determine your hereditary risk. If it is high, outline the steps that you can take to reduce your overall risk.

✓ Regardless of your sex, take actions to reduce your risk factors.

✓ Become familiar with the normal changes in CVD risk that occur with age. Take the extra steps needed to minimize your risks as you age.

✓ If you smoke, quit. If you don't smoke, don't start.

✓ Find out what your cholesterol level is, including your HDL and LDL levels.

✓ Reduce saturated fat in your diet, and take steps to reduce your triglyceride and cholesterol levels.

✓ Get out and exercise. Even a relaxing walk every day is a good CVD risk reducer. Nobody says you have to run and exercise until you drop. Take it easy, but keep it up.

✓ Control your blood pressure. Monitor it regularly, and see your doctor if you are hypertensive.

✓ Lose weight if you are overweight. Obesity is a significant risk factor for both men and women.

✓ Control your stress levels.

Making Community Choices

✓ Take a class in cardiopulmonary resuscitation (CPR). Your local Red Cross likely offers them; even your college may. Be prepared to offer bystander CPR.

✓ Consider becoming an emergency medical technician (EMT). You don't have to make a career of it. But you could be prepared to save people in your dorm, your office building, and your community.

✓ Volunteer for the local chapter of the American Heart Association. Give a few hours of your time answering phone calls and mailing information.

Summary

* The incidence and prevalence rates of cardiovascular disease have changed considerably in the past 50 years. Certain segments of the population have disproportionate levels of risk.

* The cardiovascular system consists of the heart and circulatory system and is a carefully regulated, integrated network of vessels that supply the body with the nutrients and oxygen necessary to perform daily functions.

* Cardiovascular diseases include atherosclerosis (hardening of the arteries), heart attack, angina pectoris, arrhythmias, congestive heart failure, congenital and rheumatic heart disease, and stroke. These combine to be the leading cause of death in the United States today.

* Some factors for cardiovascular disease can be controlled. Controllable risk factors include cigarette smoking, high blood fat and cholesterol levels, hypertension, lack of exercise, high-fat diet, obesity, diabetes, and emotional stress. Other risk factors, such as age, gender, and heredity, cannot be controlled. Many of these factors have a compounded effect when combined. Dietary changes, exercise, weight reduction, and attention to lifestyle risks can reduce susceptibility to cardiovascular disease.

* Women have a unique challenge in controlling their risk for CVD, particularly after menopause, when estrogen levels are no longer sufficient to be protective.

* New methods developed for treating heart blockages include coronary bypass surgery and angioplasty. Also, drugs such as beta blockers and calcium channel blockers can reduce high blood pressure and treat other symptoms. Research has provided important clues on how to best prevent or reduce risk of CVD today. Recognizing your own risks and acting now to reduce risk are important elements of lifelong cardiovascular health.

Discussion Questions

1. Trace the path of a drop of blood from the time it enters the heart until it reaches the extremities.
2. List the different types of CVD. Compare and contrast their symptoms, risk factors, prevention, and treatment.
3. What are the major indicators that CVD poses a particularly significant risk to people of your age? To the elderly? To people from selected minority groups?
4. Discuss the role that exercise, stress management, dietary changes, medical checkups, sodium reduction, and other factors can play in reducing risk for CVD. What role may chronic infections play in CVD risk?
5. Discuss why age is such an important factor in women's risk for CVD. What can be done to decrease women's risks in later life?
6. Describe some of the diagnostic and treatment alternatives for CVD. If you had a heart attack today, which treatment would you prefer? Explain why.

Application Exercise

Reread the What Do You Think? scenarios at the beginning of the chapter, and answer the following questions.

1. Do you know any college athletes like Jim? Do certain sports seem particularly associated with this mentality? Why do you think so many young Americans deny their risk for CVD?
2. Is Jennifer's situation similar to that of anyone you know? Could she have done anything to prevent her heart attack? Explain your answer.
3. Consider the behavior of coaches and doctors in the scenarios. What suggestions would you have for them? What role should colleges play in such situations?

Accessing Your Health on the Internet http

Visit the following Internet sites to explore further topics and issues related to personal health. To visit an organization's website, go to the Companion Website for *Health: The Basics, Fifth Edition* at www.aw.com/donatelle, click on the book image, and select "Accessing Your Health on the Internet" from the navigation menu on the left.

1. *American Heart Association.* Home page for the leading private organization dedicated to heart health. This site provides information, statistics, and resources regarding cardiovascular care, including an opportunity to test your own risk for CVD.
2. *Johns Hopkins Cardiac Rehabilitation Homepage.* Information about prevention of heart disease and rehabilitation from CVD from one of the best cardiac care centers in the United States. Includes information about programs to help individuals stop smoking, lose weight, lower blood pressure and blood cholesterol, and reduce emotional stress.
3. *U.S. National Library of Medicine: Health Services/ Technology Assessment Text.* Access to numerous databases of health care documents outlining procedures for clinicians and patients. Choose the database for the Agency for Health Care Policy and Research (AHCPR) to review various guidelines regarding all forms of cardiac care.

Further Reading

American Heart Association. *Heart and Stroke Facts.* Dallas, TX: American Heart Association.
An annual overview providing facts and figures concerning cardiovascular disease in the United States. Supplement provides key statistics about current trends and future directions in treatment and prevention.

Hales, D. *Just Like a Woman.* New York: Bantam Books, 1999.
An exploration, based on biological and physiological research, of the ways in which women are unique and have certain risk and protection factors for selected health problems.

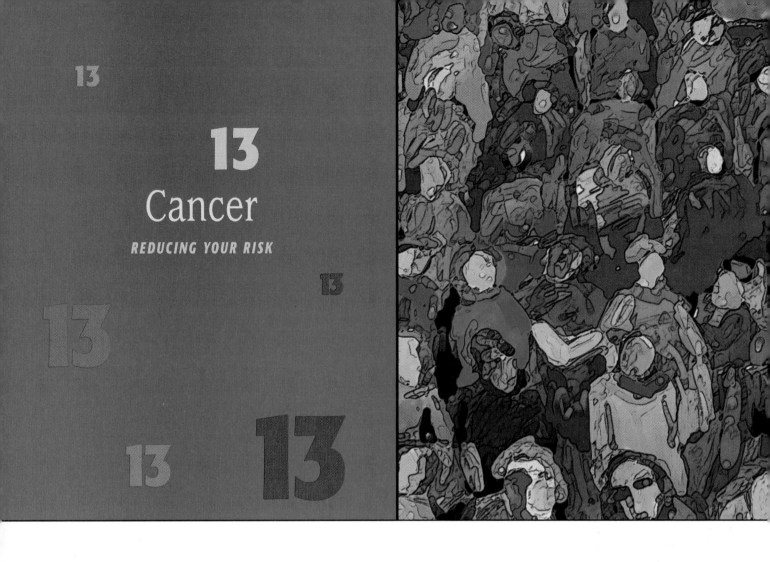

13

Cancer

REDUCING YOUR RISK

objectives

* Define cancer, and discuss how it develops.

* Discuss the causes of cancer, including biological causes, occupational and environmental hazards, lifestyle, psychological factors, chemicals in foods, viruses, medical causes, and combined causes.

* Describe the different types of cancer and the risks they pose to people at different ages and stages of life.

* Explain the importance of understanding and responding appropriately to self-exams, medical exams, and symptoms related to different types of cancer. Note how appropriate responses affect cancer survival rates.

* Discuss cancer detection and treatment, including radiation therapy, chemotherapy, immunotherapy, and other common methods of detection and treatment in use today.

As few as 50 years ago, a diagnosis of cancer was usually a death sentence. Health professionals could only guess at the cause, and treatments were often as deadly as the disease itself. Because we had no idea how a person "got" cancer, fears about possible infection led to ostracism and bigotry aimed at people who desperately needed support.

Fortunately, we've come a long way since then. Today we know that there are multiple causes of cancer and that very few are linked to any type of infectious agent. Early detection and vast improvements in technology have dramatically improved the prognosis for most cancer patients. We also know that there are many actions we can take individually and as a society to prevent cancer. Knowing the facts about cancer, recognizing your risk, and taking action to reduce your risk are important steps in the battle.

An Overview of Cancer

During 2001, approximately 553,400 Americans died of cancer, and nearly 1.3 million new cases were diagnosed. Cancer is the second leading cause of death, exceeded only by heart disease.[1] Put into perspective, these statistics mean that each day of the year, more than 1,500 people die of one of the types of cancer that affect humans. One of four deaths in the United States is from cancer; over 5 million lives have been lost since 1990.[2] However, it is important to note that although more than 2.5 million people will be diagnosed with cancer in a year, nearly four in ten will be alive five years after diagnosis. Many will be considered "cured," meaning that they have no subsequent cancer in their bodies five years after diagnosis and can expect to live a long and productive life.[3]

When adjusted for normal life expectancy (factors such as dying of heart disease, accidents, and so on), the relative five-year survival rate for all cancers is 60 percent. Some cancers that only a few decades ago presented a very poor outlook are often cured today. Acute lymphocytic leukemia in children, Hodgkin's disease, Burkitt's lymphoma, Ewing's sarcoma (a form of bone cancer), Wilms' tumor (a kidney cancer in children), testicular cancer, and osteogenic (bone) sarcoma are among the most remarkable indicators of progress.

Variations in Rates

Although cancer strikes people of all ages, races, cultures, and socioeconomic levels, some Americans are at greater risk. Overall, African Americans are more likely to develop cancer than persons of any other racial and ethnic group. In 2001, the incidence was 444.6 per 100,000 African Americans; 402.1 per 100,000 whites; 272.4 per 100,000 Hispanics; 279.3 per 100,000 Asian/Pacific Islanders; and 152.8 per 100,000 Native Americans.[4] Cancer sites for which African Americans have significantly higher incidence and mortality rates include the esophagus, uterus, cervix, stomach, liver, prostate, and larynx. African Americans are 33% more likely to die of cancer than whites and are more than twice as likely to die of cancer than Hispanics, Asian/Pacific Islanders, and American Indians. Researchers at the National Cancer Institute (NCI) believe that these differences are due more to African Americans' lower average socioeconomic status and generally more limited access to health care than to any inherent physical characteristics.[5] Some findings, however, indicate that certain cancers are simply more common in different races.

Cancer incidence and mortality rates within other minority groups, such as Hispanics, are often lower (sometimes by as much as 25 percent or more) than those of whites or African Americans. Given Hispanics' low average socioeconomic status, we might expect that they would have cancer rates similar to those of African Americans. But Hispanics seem to be "protected" from high rates. Why? No one knows for sure, but the answer may lie in differences in diet, exercise patterns, or other culturally influenced behaviors. Because cancer risk is strongly associated with lifestyle and behavior, such differences among ethnic and cultural groups can provide clues to factors involved in the development of cancer. Culturally influenced values and belief systems can also affect whether a person seeks care, participates in screenings, or follows recommended treatments. Socioeconomic factors, such as lack of health insurance or lack of transportation to treatment centers, can lead to late diagnosis and poor survival prospects.

What Is Cancer?

Cancer is the name given to a large group of diseases characterized by the uncontrolled growth and spread of abnormal cells.[6] Think of a healthy cell as a small computer programmed to operate in a particular fashion. Under normal conditions, healthy cells are protected by a powerful overseer, the immune system, as they perform their daily functions of growing, replicating, and repairing body organs. When something interrupts normal cell programming, however, uncontrolled growth and abnormal cellular development result in a new growth of tissue serving no physiologic function, which is called a **neoplasm.** This neoplasmic mass often forms a clumping of cells known as a **tumor.**

Not all tumors are **malignant** (cancerous); in fact, most are **benign** (noncancerous). Benign tumors are generally harmless unless they grow in such a fashion as to obstruct or crowd out normal tissues. A benign tumor of the brain, for instance, is life threatening when it grows in a manner that restricts blood flow and results in a stroke. The only way to determine whether a given tumor or mass is malignant is through **biopsy,** or microscopic examination of cell development.

Benign and malignant tumors differ in several key ways. Benign tumors generally consist of ordinary-looking cells enclosed in a fibrous shell or capsule that prevents their spreading to other body areas. Malignant tumors are usually not enclosed in a protective capsule and can therefore spread to other organs. This process, known as **metastasis,** makes

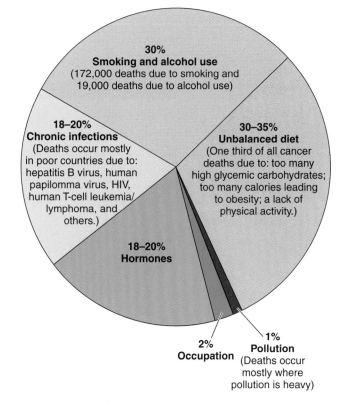

Figure 13.1

Factors Believed to Contribute to Global Causes of Cancer

Sources: Public session/panel discussion, Diet and Optimal Health International Conference, Linus Pauling Institute, May 2001 (panel participants: Steve Hecht, Bruce Ames, Jeffrey Blumberg, Barry Halliwall, Baley Irei,); American Cancer Society, *Cancer Facts & Figures 2001.*

some forms of cancer particularly aggressive in their ability to overcome the body's defenses. By the time they are diagnosed, malignant tumors have frequently metastasized throughout the body, making treatment extremely difficult. Unlike benign tumors, which merely expand to take over a given space, malignant cells invade surrounding tissue, emitting clawlike protrusions that disturb the ribonucleic acid (RNA) and deoxyribonucleic acid (DNA) within normal cells. Disrupting these substances, which control cellular metabolism and reproduction, produces **mutant cells** that differ in form, quality, and function from normal cells. Assess your own cancer risk by completing the Assess Yourself box.

What Causes Cancer?

After decades of research, most cancer epidemiologists believe that cancers are, at least in theory, preventable and that many could be avoided by suitable choices in lifestyle and environment.[7] Many specific causes of cancer are believed to be known, the most important of which are smoking, obesity, and a few organic viruses (Figure 13.1). However, a large proportion of global variation in common cancers, such as breast, prostrate, colon, and rectum, remain unexplained.[8]

Cancer A large group of diseases characterized by the uncontrolled growth and spread of abnormal cells.

Neoplasm A new growth of tissue that serves no physiological function and results from uncontrolled, abnormal cellular development.

Tumor A neoplasmic mass that grows more rapidly than surrounding tissue.

Malignant Very dangerous or harmful; refers to a cancerous tumor.

Benign Harmless; refers to a noncancerous tumor.

Biopsy Microscopic examination of tissue performed to determine whether a cancer is present.

Metastasis Process by which cancer spreads from one area to different areas of the body.

Mutant cells Cells that differ in form, quality, or function from normal cells.

Text continues on page 329

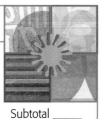

Cancer: Assessing Your Risk

You can reduce your risk of developing some types of cancer, such as lung cancer, by changing lifestyle behaviors. For other types of cancer, such as breast and colorectal cancers, your chance for cure is greatly increased if the cancer is found at an early stage through periodic screening examinations.

The following has been designed by the American Cancer Society to help you learn about (1) your risk factors for certain types of cancer and (2) the chances that cancer would be found at an early stage when a cure is possible.

Read each question concerning each site and its specific risk factors. Be honest in your responses. Circle the number in parentheses next to your response.

Individual numbers for specific questions are not to be interpreted as a precise measure of relative risk, but the totals for a given site should give a general indication of your risk.

LUNG CANCER

1. Sex:
   a. Male (2)
   b. Female (1)
2. Age:
   a. 39 or less (1)
   b. 40–49 (2)
   c. 50–59 (5)
   d. 60+ (7)
3. Exposure to any of these:
   a. Mining (3)
   b. Asbestos (7)
   c. Uranium and radioactive products (5)
   d. None (0)
4. Habits:
   a. Smoker: (10)*
   b. Nonsmoker (0)*
5. Type of smoking:
   a. Cigarettes or little cigars (10)
   b. Pipe and/or cigar, but not cigarettes (3)
   c. Nonsmoker (0)
6. Number of cigarettes smoked per day:
   a. 0 (1)
   b. less than $\frac{1}{2}$ pack per day (5)
   c. $\frac{1}{2}$–1 pack (9)
   d. 1–2 packs (15)
   e. 2+ packs (20)
7. Type of cigarette:
   a. High tar/nicotine (10)**
   b. Medium tar/nicotine (9)**
   c. Low tar/nicotine (7)**
   d. Nonsmoker (1)
8. Length of time smoking:
   a. Nonsmoker (1)
   b. Up to 15 years (5)
   c. 15–25 years (10)
   d. 25+ years (20)

Subtotal _____

REDUCING YOUR RISK

*If you stopped smoking more than 10 years ago, count yourself as a nonsmoker. If you have stopped smoking in the past 10 years, you are an ex-smoker. Ex-smokers should answer questions 4 through 8 according to how they previously smoked. Then ex-smokers may reduce their point total on questions 5 through 8 by 10% for each year they have not smoked. Current smokers also answer questions 5 through 8.

9. I am stopping smoking today.
   (If yes, subtract 2 points.)   Yes   No

Total _____

**High Tar/Nicotine: 20 mg or more tar/1.3 mg or more nicotine
Medium Tar/Nicotine: 16–19 mg tar/1.1–1.2 mg nicotine
Low Tar/Nicotine: 15 mg or less tar/1.0 mg or less nicotine

COLON AND RECTUM CANCER

RISK FACTORS

1. Age:
   a. 40 or less (2)
   b. 40–49 (7)
   c. 50 and over (12)
2. Has anyone in your family ever had:
   a. Colon cancer (18)
   b. Colon polyps (18)
   c. Neither (1)
3. Have you ever had:
   a. Colon cancer (25)
   b. Colon polyps (25)
   c. Ulcerative colitis for more than seven years (18)
   d. Cancer of the breast, ovary, uterus, or stomach (13)
   e. None of the above (1)

Total _____

SYMPTOMS

1. Do you have bleeding from the rectum?   Yes   No
2. Have you had a change in bowel habits
   (such as altered frequency, size, consistency,
   or color of stool)?   Yes   No

REDUCING YOUR RISKS AND DETECTING CANCER EARLY

1. I have altered my diet to include less fat and
   more fruits, fiber, and cruciferous vegetables
   (broccoli, cabbage, cauliflower, brussels sprouts). Yes   No
2. I have had a negative test for blood in my
   stool within the past year.   Yes   No

Continued

3. I have had a negative examination for colon cancer and polyps within the past year (proctosigmoidoscopy, colonoscopy, barium enema x-rays).   Yes   No

SKIN CANCER

1. Live in the southern part of the U.S.:   Yes   No
2. Frequent work or play in the sun: Yes   No
3. Fair complexion or freckles (natural hair color of blonde, red, or light brown, or eye color of grey, green, blue, or hazel):   Yes   No
4. Work in mines, around coal tars or radioactivity: Yes   No
5. Experienced a severe, blistering sunburn before the age of 18:   Yes   No
6. Have any family members with skin cancer or history of melanoma: Yes   No
7. Had skin cancer or melanoma in the past: Yes   No
8. Use or have used tanning beds or sun lamps: Yes   No
9. Have large, many, or changing moles: Yes   No

REDUCING YOUR RISKS AND DETECTING CANCER EARLY

10. I cover up with a wide-brimmed hat and wear long-sleeved shirts and pants.   Yes   No
11. I use sunscreens with an SPF rating of 15 or higher when going out in the sun.   Yes   No
12. I examine my skin once a month for changes in warts or moles   Yes   No

BREAST CANCER

1. Age group:
   a. under 35 (10)
   b. 35–39 (20)
   c. 40–49 (50)
   d. 50 and over (90)
2. Race:
   a. Asian (10)
   b. Hispanic (10)
   c. Black (20)
   d. White (25)
3. Family history:
   a. None (10)
   b. Mother, sister, daughter with breast cancer (30)
4. Your history:
   a. No breast disease (10)
   b. Previous lumps or cysts (15)
   c. Previous breast cancer (100)
5. Maternity:
   a. 1st pregnancy before 30 (10)
   b. 1st pregnancy at 30 or older (15)
   c. No pregnancies (20)

DETECTING CANCER EARLY

6. I practice breast self-examination monthly. (If yes, subtract 10 points.)   Yes   No
7. I have had a negative mammogram and examination by a physician in accordance with American Cancer Society Breast Health Guidelines. (If yes, subtract 25 points.)   Yes   No

Total _____

CERVICAL CANCER

(*Lower Portion of Uterus*)—These questions do not apply to a woman who has had a total hysterectomy.

1. Age group:
   a. Less than 25 (10)
   b. 25–39 (20)
   c. 40–54 (30)
   d. 55 and over (30)
2. Race:
   a. Asian or white (10)
   b. Black (20)
   c. Hispanic (20)
3. Number of pregnancies:
   a. 0 (10)
   b. 1 to 3 (20)
   c. 4 and over (30)
4. Viral infections:
   a. Viral infections of the vagina such as genital warts, herpes, or ulcer formations (10)
   b. Never (1)
5. Age at first intercourse:
   a. Before 15 (40)
   b. 15–19 (30)
   c. 20–24 (20)
   d. 25 and over (10)
   e. Never had intercourse (5)
6. Bleeding between periods or after intercourse:
   a. Yes (40)
   b. No (1)
7. Smoker:
   a. Nonsmoker (2)
   b. Smoker (3)

Subtotal _____

DETECTING CANCER EARLY

8. I have had a negative Pap smear and pelvic examination within the past year. (If yes, subtract 50 points.)   Yes   No

Total _____

ENDOMETRIAL CANCER

(*Body of Uterus*)—These questions do not apply to a woman who has had a total hysterectomy.

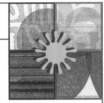

1. Age group:
   a. 39 or less (5)
   b. 40–49 (20)
   c. 50 and over (60)
2. Race:
   a. Asian (10)
   b. Black (10)
   c. Hispanic (10)
   d. White (20)
3. Births:
   a. None (15)
   b. 1 to 4 (7)
   c. 5 or more (5)
4. Weight:
   a. 50 or more pounds overweight (50)
   b. 20–49 pounds overweight (15)
   c. Normal or underweight for height (10)
5. Diabetes (elevated blood sugar):
   a. Yes (3)
   b. No (1)
6. Estrogen hormone intake*:
   a. Yes, regularly (15)
   b. Yes, occasionally (12)
   c. None (10)
7. Abnormal uterine bleeding:
   a. Yes (40)
   b. No (1)
8. Hypertension (high blood pressure):
   a. Yes (3)
   b. No (1)

Subtotal ___

DETECTING CANCER EARLY

9. I have had a negative pelvic examination and Pap smear or endometrial tissue sampling (endometrial biopsy) performed within the past year. (If yes, subtract 50 points.) Yes No

Total ___

*NOTE: This excludes birth control pills.

TEST ANALYSIS

LUNG ANSWERS

IF YOUR TOTAL IS:

24 or less . . . You have a low risk for lung cancer.

25–49 . . . You may be a light smoker and would have a good chance of kicking the habit.

50–74 . . . As a moderate smoker, your risks for lung and upper respiratory tract cancer are increased. The time to stop is now!

75 or over . . . As a heavy cigarette smoker, your chances of getting lung cancer and cancer of the upper respiratory or digestive tract are greatly increased.

REDUCING YOUR RISK

Make a decision to quit today. Join a smoking cessation program. If you are a heavy drinker of alcohol, your risks for cancer of the head and neck and esophagus are further increased. Use of "spitting" tobacco increases your risks of cancer of the mouth. Your best bet is not to use tobacco in any form. See your doctor if you have a nagging cough, hoarseness, persistent pain or sore in the mouth or throat, or lumps in the neck.

COLON AND RECTUM ANSWERS

I. RISK FACTORS*—IF YOUR TOTAL IS:

5 or less . . . You are currently at low risk for colon and rectum cancer. Eat a diet high in fiber and low in fat and follow cancer checkup guidelines.

6–15 . . . You are currently at moderate risk for colon and rectum cancer. Follow the American Cancer Society guidelines for early detection of colorectal cancer. These are (1) a digital rectal exam** every year after age 40 and (2) a fecal occult blood test every year and a sigmoido-scopic, preferably flexible, exam every 3–5 years after age 50.

16 or greater . . . You are in the high-risk group for colon and rectum cancer. This rating requires a lifetime, ongoing screening program that includes periodic evaluation of your entire colon. See your doctor for more information.

*If your answers to any of these questions change, you should reassess your risk.

**This test has an additional advantage in that it is also an early detection method for cancer of the prostate in men.

II. SYMPTOMS

The presence of rectal bleeding or a change in bowel habits may indicate colon/rectum cancer. See your physician right away if you have either of these symptoms.

III. REDUCING YOUR RISKS AND DETECTING CANCER EARLY

Regular tests for hidden blood in the stool and appropriate examinations of the colon will increase the likelihood that colon polyps are discovered and removed early and that cancers are found in an early, curable state. Modifying your diet to include more fiber, cruciferous vegetables, and foods rich in Vitamin A, and less fat and salt-cured foods, may result in a reduction of cancer risks.

Continued

SKIN ANSWERS

If you answered yes to any of the first nine questions, you need to use protective clothing and use a sunscreen with an SPF rating of 15 or greater whenever you are out in the sun and check yourself monthly for any changes in warts or moles. An answer of yes to questions 10, 11, and 12 can help reduce your risk of skin cancer or possibly detect skin cancer early.

REDUCING YOUR RISKS AND DETECTING CANCER EARLY

Numerical risks for skin cancer are difficult to state. For instance, a person with a dark complexion can work longer in the sun and be less likely to develop cancer than a person with a light complexion. Furthermore, a person wearing a long-sleeved shirt and wide-brimmed hat may work in the sun and be less at risk than a person who wears a bathing suit for only a short time. The risk for skin cancer goes up greatly with age.

Melanoma, the most serious type of skin cancer, can be cured when it is detected and treated at a very early stage. Changes in warts and moles are important and should be checked by your doctor.

BREAST ANSWERS

IF YOUR TOTAL IS:

Under 100 . . . Low-risk women (and all others). You should practice monthly breast self-examination, have your breasts examined by a doctor as part of a regular cancer-related checkup, and have mammography in accordance with ACS guidelines.

100–199 . . . Moderate-risk women. You should practice monthly BSE and have your breasts examined by a doctor as part of a cancer-related checkup, and have periodic mammography in accordance with American Cancer Society guidelines, or more frequently as your physician advises.

200 or higher . . . High risk. You should practice monthly BSE and have your breasts examined by a doctor, and have mammography more often. See your doctor for the recommended frequency of breast examinations and mammography.

DETECTING CANCER EARLY

One in 8 American women will get breast cancer in her lifetime. Being a woman is a risk factor! Most women (75 percent) who get breast cancer don't have other risk factors. BSE and mammography may diagnose a breast cancer in its earliest stage with a greatly increased chance of cure. When detected at this stage, cure is more likely and breast-saving surgery may be an option.

CERVICAL ANSWERS

IF YOUR TOTAL IS:

40–69 . . . This is a low-risk group. Ask your doctor for a Pap test and advice about frequency of subsequent testing.

70–99 . . . In this moderate-risk group, more frequent Pap tests may be required.

100 or more . . . You are in a high-risk group and should have a Pap test (and pelvic exam) as advised by your doctor.

DETECTING CANCER EARLY

Early detection of this cancer by the Pap test has markedly improved the chance of cure. When this cancer is found at an early stage, the cure rate is extremely high and uterus-saving surgery and child bearing potential may be preserved.

ENDOMETRIAL ANSWERS

IF YOUR TOTAL IS:

45–59 . . . You are at very low risk for developing endometrial cancer.

60–99 . . . Your risks are slightly higher. Report any abnormal bleeding immediately to your doctor. Tissue sampling at menopause is recommended.

100 and over . . . Your risks are much greater. See your doctor for tests as appropriate.

DETECTING CANCER EARLY

Once again, early detection improves the chance of a cure for this cancer. Regular pelvic examinations may find other female cancers such as cancer of the ovary.

Source: Reprinted by permission of the American Cancer Society, Texas Division, Inc., from *Cancer: Assessing Your Risk,* © 1981, revised 1990, 1992, 1993, 1997.

Most research supports the idea that cancer is caused by both *external* factors (chemicals, radiation, viruses, and lifestyle) and *internal* factors (hormones, immune conditions, and inherited mutations). Causal factors may act together or in sequence to promote cancer development.[9] We do not know why some people have malignant cells in their body and never develop cancer, while others may take ten years or more to develop the disease.

Anyone can develop cancer; however, most cases affect adults beginning in middle age. In fact, nearly 80 percent of cancers are diagnosed at ages 55 and over. Cancer researchers refer to one's *cancer risk* when they assess risk factors. *Lifetime risk* refers to the probability that an individual, over the course of a lifetime, will develop cancer or die from it. In the United States, men have a lifetime risk of about one in two; women have a lower risk of one in three.[10] *Relative risk* is a measure of the strength of the relationship between risk factors and a particular cancer. Basically, relative risk compares your risk if you engage in certain known risk behaviors with that of someone who does not engage in such behaviors. For example, if you are a male and smoke, you may have a 20-fold relative risk of developing lung cancer of a nonsmoker, meaning that your chances of getting lung cancer are about 20 times greater than a nonsmoker.[11]

Cellular Change/Mutation Theories

One theory of how cancer develops proposes that cancer results from spontaneous error that occurs during cell reproduction. Perhaps cells that are overworked or aged are more likely to break down, causing genetic errors that result in mutant cells.

Another theory suggests that cancer is caused by some external agent or agents that enter a normal cell and initiate the cancerous process. Numerous environmental factors, such as radiation, chemicals, hormonal drugs, immunosuppressant drugs (drugs that suppress the normal activity of the immune system), and other toxins, are considered possible **carcinogens** (cancer-causing agents); perhaps the most common carcinogen is the tar in cigarettes. The greater the dose or exposure to environmental hazards, the greater the risk of disease. People who are forced to work, live, and pass through areas that have high levels of environmental toxins may be at greater risk for several types of cancers.[12]

A third theory came out of research on certain viruses that are believed to cause tumors in animals. This research led to the discovery of **oncogenes,** suspected cancer-causing genes that are present on chromosomes. Although oncogenes are typically dormant, scientists theorize that certain conditions, such as age, stress, and exposure to carcinogens, viruses, and radiation, may activate them. Once activated, oncogenes grow and reproduce in an out-of-control manner.

Scientists are uncertain whether only people who develop cancer have oncogenes or whether we all have **protooncogenes,** genes that can become oncogenes under certain conditions. Many **oncologists** (physicians who spe-

cialize in the treatment of malignancies) believe that the oncogene theory may lead to a greater understanding of how individual cells function and bring us closer to developing effective treatments. Many factors are believed to contribute to cancer development. Combining risk factors can dramatically increase a person's risk for cancer.

Risks for Cancer—Lifestyle

Over the years, researchers have found that people who engage in certain behaviors show a higher incidence of cancer. In particular, diet, sedentary lifestyle (and resultant obesity), consumption of alcohol and cigarettes, stress, and other lifestyle factors seem to play a role. Likewise, colon and rectal cancer occur more frequently among persons with a high-fat, low-fiber diet; in those who don't eat enough fruits and vegetables; and in those who are inactive. See Chapter 9 for information about certain dietary risks related to cancer and the role of supplements in preventing cancer. More research is needed to pinpoint the mechanisms that act in the body to increase the odds of cancer. For now, there is compelling evidence that certain actions are clearly associated with a greater than average risk of developing diseases.

Smoking and Cancer Risk   Of all of the potential risk factors for cancer, smoking is among the greatest. Over the five decades since British and American epidemiologists have singled out tobacco as a cancer culprit in lung cancer and other diseases, tar levels in British cigarettes have declined dramatically, as has the prevalence of smoking in general. As a result, the lung cancer rate for British men under age 55 has fallen by two-thirds since 1955, placing it among the lowest in the developed world.[13] In the last 20 years, America's rates have shown a similar decline. Lung cancer rates among men are still increasing in most developing countries and in Eastern Europe, however, where consumption of cigarettes remains high and is still increasing in some areas.[14]

Most authorities have believed that cigarettes cause only cancers of the lung, pancreas, bladder and kidney, and (synergistically with alcohol) the larynx, mouth, pharynx, and esophagus. However, more recent evidence indicates that several other types of cancer are related to smoking. Most notably, cancer of the stomach, liver, and cervix seem to be directly related to long-term smoking.[15]

Carcinogens   Cancer-causing agents.

Oncogenes   Suspected cancer-causing genes present on chromosomes.

Protooncogenes   Genes that can become oncogenes under certain conditions.

Oncologists   Physicians who specialize in the treatment of malignancies.

Obesity and Cancer Risk   It is extremely difficult to sort through the accumulated evidence about the role of certain nutrients, obesity, sedentary lifestyle, and related variables. Nevertheless, a body of research has emerged that seems to point (albeit not with absolute certainty), to a cancer link. What is clear is that cancer is more common among people who are overweight.[16] This evidence for a link is strongest for postmenopausal breast cancer and cancers of the endometrium, gallbladder, and kidney, but obesity is also implicated in other cancers. For women, the cervix and ovaries are added to this list; for men, cancers of the colon and prostate seem to be related to obesity and/or diet.[17] The following facts seem to provide evidence of this obesity/cancer link:[18]

- The relative risk of breast cancer in postmenopausal women is 50 percent higher for obese women.
- The relative risks of colon cancer in men is 40 percent higher for obese men.
- The relative risks of gallbladder and endomentrial cancer are five times higher in obese individuals compared to individuals with "healthy" weight.
- Some studies have shown a positive association between obesity and cancers of the kidney, pancreas, rectum, esophagus, and liver.
- Obesity is believed to alter complex interactions among diet, metabolism, physical activity, hormones, and growth factors.

Biological Factors

Early theorists believed that we inherit a genetic predisposition toward certain forms of cancer.[19] Cancers of the breast, stomach, colon, prostate, uterus, ovaries, and lungs appear to run in families. For example, a woman runs a much higher risk of breast cancer if her mother or sisters (primary relatives) have had the disease, particularly if they had it at a young age. Hodgkin's disease and certain leukemias show similar familial patterns. Can we attribute these familial patterns to genetic susceptibility or to the fact that people in the same families experience similar environmental risks? To date, the research in this area is inconclusive. Recent research conducted by the University of Utah indicates that a gene for breast cancer exists. A rare form of eye cancer does appear to be passed genetically from mother to child. It is possible that we can inherit a tendency toward a cancer-prone, weak immune system or, conversely, that we can inherit a cancer-fighting potential. But the complex interaction of hereditary predisposition, lifestyle, and environment on the development of cancer makes it a challenge to determine a single cause.

Gender also affects the likelihood of developing certain forms of cancer. For example, breast cancer occurs primarily among females, although men do occasionally get breast cancer. Obviously, factors other than heredity and familial relationships affect which sex develops a particular cancer. In the 1950s, for example, women rarely contracted lung cancer. But with increases in the number of women who smoked and the length of time they had smoked, lung cancer rates soared to become the leading cause of cancer death in women. Whereas gender plays a role in certain cases of cancer, other variables, such as lifestyle, are probably more significant.

Reproductive and Hormonal Risks for Cancer   The effects of reproductive factors on breast and cervical cancer have been well documented. Pregnancy and estrogen supplementation in the form of oral contraceptives or hormone replacement therapy increase a woman's risk of breast cancer. Late menarche, early menopause, early first childbirth, and high parity (having many children) have been shown to reduce a woman's risk of breast cancer. A higher risk of endometrial cancer is also associated with hormone replacement therapy.[20]

Breast cancer incidence is much higher in most Western countries than in developing countries. This is partly—and perhaps largely—accounted for by dietary effects (consuming a diet high in calories and fat), combined with later first childbirth, lower parity (having fewer children), and shorter breastfeeding.[21]

Occupational and Environmental Factors

Overall, workplace hazards account for only a small percentage of all cancers. However, various substances are known to cause cancer when exposure levels are high or exposure is prolonged. One of the most common occupational carcinogens is asbestos, a fibrous material once widely used in the construction, insulation, and automobile industries. Nickel, chromate, and chemicals such as benzene, arsenic, and vinyl chloride have definitively been shown to be carcinogens for humans. Also, people who routinely work with certain dyes and radioactive substances may have increased risks for cancer. Working with coal tars, as in the mining profession, or working near inhalants, as in the auto painting business, is hazardous. So is working with herbicides and pesticides, although the evidence is inconclusive for low-dose exposures. Several federal and state agencies are responsible for monitoring such exposures and ensuring that businesses comply with standards designed to protect workers.

Radiation: Ionizing and Non-ionizing   Ionizing radiation (IR)—radiation from x-rays, radon, cosmic rays, and ultraviolet radiation (primarily UVB radiation)—is the only form of radiation proven to cause human cancer. (See the section on skin cancer, later in this chapter.) Incidents such as the Chernobyl accident in the 1980s focused attention on the potential risks of ionizing radiation. Evidence that high-dose IR causes cancer comes from studies of atomic bomb survivors, patients receiving radiotherapy, and certain occupational groups (for example, uranium miners). Virtually any part of the body can be affected by IR, but bone marrow and the thyroid are particularly susceptible. Radon exposures in homes can increase lung cancer risk, especially in cigarette smokers. To reduce the risk of harmful effects, diagnostic medical and dental x-rays are set at the lowest dose levels possible.[22] Although non-ionizing radiation produced by radio waves, cell phones, microwaves, computer screens, televisions, electric blankets, and other products has been a topic of great concern in recent years, research has not proven excess risk to date.

Social and Psychological Factors

Many researchers claim that social and psychological factors play a major role in determining whether a person gets cancer. Stress has been implicated in increased susceptibility to several types of cancers. By reducing stress levels in your daily life, you may, in fact, lower your risk for cancer. A number of therapists have even established preventive treatment centers where the primary focus is on "being happy" and "thinking positive thoughts." Is it possible to laugh away cancer?

Although medical personnel are skeptical of overly simplistic solutions, we cannot rule out the possibility that negative emotional states contribute to disease. People who are under chronic, severe stress or who suffer from depression or other persistent emotional problems show higher rates of cancer than their healthy counterparts. Sleep disturbances, diet, or a combination of factors may weaken the body's immune system, increasing the susceptibility to cancer.

Although psychological factors may play a part in cancer development, exposure to substances such as tobacco and alcohol are far more important. The American Cancer Society states that cigarette smoking is responsible for 30 percent of all cancer deaths—and 87 percent of all lung cancer deaths. Heavy consumption of alcohol has been related to cancers of the mouth, larynx, throat, esophagus, and liver. These cancers show up even more frequently in people whose heavy drinking is accompanied by smoking. The negative effects of smoking are not just concerns for the active smoker. Environmental (passive) tobacco smoke (ETS) causes an estimated 3,000 deaths from lung cancer, 40,000 deaths from heart disease, up to 300,000 respiratory problems, and countless deaths among nonsmokers. Cancers of the mouth and throat pose significant risks for smokers.[23]

Chemicals in Foods

Among the food additives suspected of causing cancer is *sodium nitrate,* a chemical used to preserve and give color to red meat. Research indicates that the actual carcinogen is not sodium nitrate but *nitrosamines,* substances formed when the body digests the sodium nitrates. Sodium nitrate has not been banned, primarily because it kills the bacterium *Clostridium botulinum,* which causes the highly virulent food-borne disease botulism. It should also be noted that the bacteria found in the human intestinal tract may contain more nitrates than a person could ever take in from eating cured meats or other nitrate-containing food products. Nonetheless, concern about the carcinogenic properties of nitrates has led to the introduction of meats that are nitrate-free or contain reduced levels of the substance.

Much of the concern about chemicals in foods centers on the possible harm caused by pesticide and herbicide residues. Although some of these chemicals cause cancer at high doses in experimental animals, the very low concentrations found in some foods are well within established government safety levels. Continued research regarding pesticide and herbicide use is essential, and the continuous monitoring of agricultural practices is necessary to ensure a safe food supply. Scientists and consumer groups stress the importance of a balance between chemical use and the production of quality food products. Prevention efforts should focus on policies to protect consumers, develop low-chemical pesticides and herbicides, and reduce environmental pollution. See Table 13.1 for more information on preventing cancer through diet and lifestyle.

Viral Factors

The chances of becoming infected with a "cancer virus" are very remote. However, several forms of virus-induced cancers have been observed in laboratory animals, and there is some indication that human beings display a similar tendency toward virally transmitted cancers. For example, the *herpes-related viruses* may be involved in the development of some forms of leukemia, Hodgkin's disease, cervical cancer, and Burkitt's lymphoma. The *Epstein-Barr virus,* which is associated with mononucleosis, may also contribute to cancer, and cervical cancer has been linked to *human papillomavirus,* the virus that causes genital warts.[24]

Many scientists believe that selected viruses help to provide an *opportunistic* environment for subsequent cancer development. It is likely that a combination of immunological bombardment by viral or chemical invaders and other risk factors substantially increases the risk of cancer.

Medical Factors

Some medical treatments increase a person's risk for cancer. One famous example is the prescription drug *diethylstilbestrol (DES),* widely used from 1940 to 1960 to control problems with bleeding during pregnancy and reduce the risk of miscarriage. Not until the 1970s did the dangers of this drug became apparent. Although DES caused few side effects in the millions of women who took it, their daughters were found to have an increased risk of cancers of the reproductive organs. Some scientists claim that estrogen replacement therapy in postmenopausal women is dangerous because it increases the risks for uterine cancer. Others believe that the benefits of estrogen outweigh its risks. Chemotherapy to treat one cancer may increase the risks of the patient's developing other forms of cancer.

Table 13.1
Cancer Prevention and Diet

TYPE	DECREASES RISK	INCREASES RISK	PREVENTABLE BY DIET
Lung	Vegetables, fruits	Smoking; some occupations	33–50%
Stomach	Vegetables, fruits; food refrigeration	Salt; salted foods	66–75%
Breast	Vegetables, fruits	Obesity; alcohol	33–50%
Colon/rectum	Vegetables; physical activity	Meat; alcohol; smoking	66–75%
Mouth/throat	Vegetables, fruits; physical activity	Salted fish; alcohol; smoking	33–50%
Liver	Vegetables	Alcohol; contaminated food	33–66%
Cervix	Vegetables, fruits	Smoking	10–20%
Esophagus	Vegetables, fruits	Deficient diet; smoking; alcohol	50–75%
Prostate	Vegetables	Meat or meat fat; dairy fat	10–20%
Bladder	Vegetables, fruits	Smoking; coffee	10–20%

Here are some tips issued by a panel of cancer researchers:

- Avoid being underweight or overweight, and limit weight gain during adulthood to less than 11 pounds.
- If you don't get much exercise at work, take an hour's brisk walk or similar exercise daily, and exercise vigorously for at least one hour a week.
- Eat eight or more servings a day of cereals and grains (such as rice, corn, breads, and pasta), legumes (such as peas), roots (such as beets, radishes, and carrots), tubers (such as potatoes), and plantains (including bananas).
- Eat five or more servings a day of a variety of other vegetables and fruits.
- Limit consumption of refined sugar.
- Limit alcoholic drinks to less than two a day for men and one for women.
- Limit intake of red meat to less than three ounces a day, if eaten at all.
- Limit consumption of salted foods and use of cooking and table salt. Use herbs and spices to season foods.

Sources: World Cancer Research Fund, American Institute for Cancer Research.

What do you think?

How do we determine whether a given factor is a "risk factor" for a disease? ✳ Must a clearly established "causal" link exist before consumers are warned about risk? ✳ Can you think of apparent dietary risks for cancer that seemed conclusive but have since been refuted? ✳ How does the consumer know whom or what to believe?

Types of Cancers

Classifications of Cancer

As mentioned earlier, the term *cancer* refers not to a single disease but to hundreds of different diseases. They are grouped into four broad categories based on the type of tissue from which the cancer arises.

- *Carcinomas.* Epithelial tissues (tissues covering body surfaces and lining most body cavities) are the most common sites for cancers. Carcinomas of the breast, lung, intestines, skin, and mouth are examples. These cancers affect the outer layer of the skin and mouth as well as the mucous membranes. They metastasize through the circulatory or lymphatic system initially and form solid tumors.

- *Sarcomas.* Sarcomas occur in the mesodermal, or middle, layers of tissue—for example, in bones, muscles, and general connective tissue. They metastasize primarily via the blood in the early stages of disease. These cancers are less common but generally more virulent than carcinomas. They also form solid tumors.

- *Lymphomas.* Lymphomas develop in the lymphatic system—the infection-fighting regions of the body—and metastasize through the lymphatic system. Hodgkin's disease is an example. Lymphomas also form solid tumors.

- *Leukemias.* Cancer of the blood-forming parts of the body, particularly the bone marrow and spleen, is called leukemia. A nonsolid tumor, leukemia is characterized by an abnormal increase in the number of white blood cells.

Trained oncologists determine the seriousness and general prognosis of a particular cancer. Once laboratory results and clinical observations have been made, cancers are rated by level and stage of development. Those diagnosed as "carcinoma in situ" are localized and often curable. Cancers with higher level or stage ratings have spread farther and are less likely to be cured.

Lung Cancer

Although lung cancer rates have dropped among white males during the past decade, the rate among white females and African American males and females continues to be a pervasive threat. Lung cancer killed an estimated 164,000 people in 2000. Since 1987, more women have died from lung cancer than from breast cancer, which for over 40 years had been the major cause of cancer deaths in women. Today, lung cancer continues to be the leading cancer killer for both men and women.[25] As smoking rates have declined over the past 30 years, however, we have seen significant declines in lung cancer in men. But these rates are not dropping as quickly among women. Another cause for concern is that although fewer adults are smoking, tobacco use among youth is again on the rise.

Symptoms of lung cancer include a persistent cough, blood-streaked sputum, chest pain, and recurrent attacks of pneumonia or bronchitis. Treatment depends on the type and stage of the cancer. Surgery, radiation therapy, and chemotherapy are all options. If the cancer is localized, surgery is usually the treatment of choice. If it has spread, surgery is combined with radiation and chemotherapy. Unfortunately, despite advances in medical technology, survival rates for lung cancer have improved only slightly over the past decade. Just 13 percent of lung cancer patients live five or more years after diagnosis. These rates improve to 47 percent with early detection, but only 15 percent of lung cancers are discovered in their early stages.[26]

Prevention   Smokers, especially those who have smoked for over 20 years, and people who have been exposed to industrial substances such as arsenic and asbestos or to radiation from occupational, medical, or environmental sources are at the highest risk for lung cancer. The American Cancer Society estimated that in 2000, over 430,000 cancer deaths were caused by tobacco use and an additional 20,000 cancer deaths were related to alcohol use, frequently in combination with tobacco use.[27] Exposure to sidestream cigarette smoke, known as *environmental tobacco smoke* or *ETS,* increases the risk for nonsmokers. Researchers theorize that 90 percent of all lung cancers could be avoided if people did not smoke. Substantial improvements in overall prognosis have been noted in smokers who quit at the first signs of precancerous cellular changes and allowed their bronchial linings to return to normal.

Breast Cancer

About one out of eight women will develop breast cancer at some time in her life. Although this oft-repeated ratio has frightened many women, it represents lifetime risk. Thus, not until the age of 80 does a woman's risk of breast cancer rise to one in eight.[28] Here is the risk at earlier ages:

- Birth to age 39: 1 in 227
- Ages 40–59: 1 in 25
- Ages 60–79: 1 in 15
- Birth to death: 1 in 8

In 2001, approximately 192,200 women in the United States were diagnosed with invasive breast cancer for the first time. In addition to invasive breast cancer, 46,400 new cases of in situ breast cancer, typically ductal carcinoma in situ (DCIS), a more localized cancer, will be diagnosed.[29] In the same year, about 1,500 new cases were diagnosed in men. About 40,200 women (and 400 men) would die, making breast cancer the second leading cause of cancer death for women.[30] According to the most recent data, mortality rates went down dramatically from 1990 to 1998, with the largest decrease in younger women, both white and African American.[31] The decline in rates may be due to earlier diagnosis and improved treatment, because numerous studies have shown that early detection increases survival and treatment options.

The earliest signs of breast cancer are observable on mammograms, often before lumps can be felt. Once breast cancer has grown to where it can be palpated, symptoms may include persistent breast changes, such as a lump, thickening, swelling, dimpling, skin irritation, distortion, retraction or scaliness of the nipple, nipple discharge, possible pain, or tenderness. Breast pain is commonly due to non-cancerous conditions, such as fibrocystic breasts, and is not usually a first symptom.

Risk Factors   The incidence of breast cancer increases with age. Although there are many possible risk factors, research supports the following risk factors:[32]

- Personal or family history of breast cancer (primary relatives, such as mother, daughter, sister)
- Biopsy-confirmed atypical hyperplasia (excessive increase in the number of cells)
- Long menstrual history (menstrual periods that started early and ended late in life)
- Obesity after menopause
- Recent use of oral contraceptives or postmenopausal estrogens (see the New Horizons in Health box on page 338)
- Never having children, or having a first child after age 30
- Consuming two or more drinks of alcohol per day
- Higher education and socioeconomic status

More rigorous research is needed to confirm the following possible risk factors:

- Consuming a diet high in saturated fats
- Exposure to pesticides and other chemicals
- Weight gain
- Physical inactivity
- Use of selected estrogen-receptor modulators (SERMs), such as tamoxifen and raloxifen
- Genetic predisposition through BRCA1 and BRCA2 genes

Although assessing risk factors is a useful tool, it does not always predict individual susceptibility. However, because of increased awareness, better diagnostic techniques, and

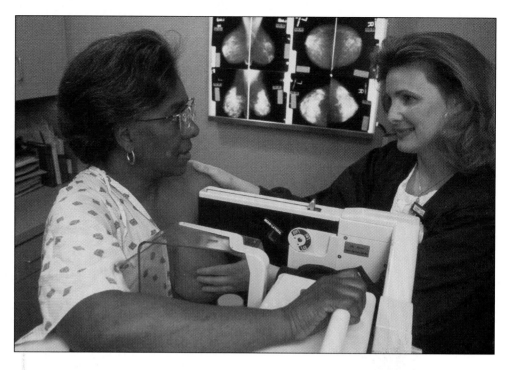

Early detection through mammography and other techniques greatly increases a woman's chance of surviving breast cancer.

improved treatments, breast cancer patients have a better chance of surviving today. The five-year survival rate for people with localized breast cancer (which includes all women living five years after diagnosis, whether the patient is in remission, disease-free, or under treatment) has risen from 72 percent in the 1940s to 96 percent today. These statistics vary dramatically, however, based on when the cancer is first detected. If the cancer has spread to surrounding tissue, the five-year survival rate is 77 percent; if it has spread to distant parts of the body, these rates fall to 21 percent; and, if the breast cancer has not spread at all, the survival rate approaches 100 percent. Survival after a diagnosis of breast cancer continues to decline beyond five years. Seventy-three percent of women diagnosed with breast cancer survive 10 years, and 59 percent survive 15 years.[33]

Prevention   A 1990 study of the role of exercise in reducing the risk of breast cancer generated much excitement in the scientific community. The study, involving 1,090 women who were 40 or younger (545 with breast cancer and 545 without) analyzed the subjects' exercise patterns since they began menstruating. The risk of those who had averaged four hours of exercise a week since menstruation was 58 percent lower than that of women who did no exercise at all. More good news: Subjects did not have to be avid joggers to have reduced risk. Their exercise included team sports, individual sports, dance, exercise classes, swimming, walking, and a variety of other activities. Researchers speculate that exercise may protect women by altering the production of the ovarian hormones estrogen and progesterone during menstrual cycles.

Other research has shown that vigorous athletics can delay the onset of menstruation and halt ovulation in some women. A woman's cumulative exposure to the sex hormones is associated with breast cancer risk.[34] Exercise can increase muscle mass and decrease body fat, which also lowers risk.[35]

Regular self-examination (Figure 13.2) and mammography are the best ways to detect breast cancer early. The American Cancer Society offers guidelines for how often women should get mammograms and other cancer checkups (see Table 13.2 on page 336). International differences in breast cancer incidence correlate with variations in diet, especially fat intake, although a causal role for these dietary factors has not been firmly established. Sudden weight gain has also been implicated. Exciting new research about the BRCA1 and BRCA2 susceptibility genes for breast cancer offers new hope for early detection.

Treatment   Today, women with breast cancer (like people with nearly any type of cancer) have many treatment options to choose from. It is important to thoroughly check out a physician's track record and his or her philosophy on the best treatment. Is the physician's recommendation consistent with that of major cancer centers in the country? Check out the doctor's credentials and the experiences of patients who have seen this doctor, as well as the surgeon who will perform your biopsy and other surgical techniques. If possible, seek a facility that has a significant number of breast cancer patients, does many surgeries, is regarded as a "teaching facility" for new oncologists, has the "latest and greatest" in terms of technology, and is highly regarded by past patients. Often, cancer support groups can provide

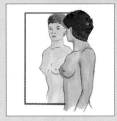
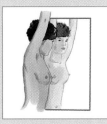
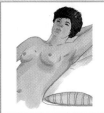
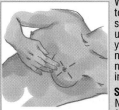
Figure 13.2
Breast Self-Examination
The illustration demonstrates breast self-examination—the ten-minute habit that could save your life.

---

invaluable information and advice. Treatments range from a lumpectomy to radical mastectomy to various combinations of radiation or chemotherapy. Figure 13.3 reviews these options. Remember that it is always a good idea to seek more than one opinion before making a decision.

Colon and Rectum Cancers

Colorectal cancers (cancers of the colon and rectum) continue to be the third most common cancers in men and women today, with over 135,400 cases diagnosed in 2001.[36] Despite an estimated 56,700 deaths from colon and rectum cancers in 2002, many people are unaware of their risk. Bleeding from the rectum, blood in the stool, and changes in bowel habits are the major warning signals. People who are over age 40, who are obese, who have a family history of colon and rectum cancer, a personal or family history of polyps (benign growths) in the colon or rectum, or inflammatory bowel problems, such as colitis, run an increased risk. Other possible risk factors include diets high in fats or low in fiber, smoking, physical inactivity, high alcohol consumption, and low intake of fruit and vegetables. Recent studies have suggested that estrogen replacement therapy and aspirin may reduce the risk of colorectal cancer.[37]

Because colorectal cancer tends to spread slowly, the prognosis is quite good if it is caught in the early stages. Colonoscopy or barium enemas are recommended screening tests for at-risk populations and for everybody over age 50. Treatment often consists of radiation or surgery. Chemotherapy, although not used extensively in the past, is today a possibility. A permanent *colostomy,* the creation of an abdominal opening to eliminate body wastes, is seldom required for people with colon cancer and even less frequently for those with rectum cancer.

Prostate Cancer

Cancer of the prostate gland is the most common type of cancer in males today, after skin cancer. In 2002, 189,000 new cases of prostate cancer will be diagnosed, and from these, about 30,200 men will die. Prostate cancer is the second leading cause of cancer death.[38]

From 1980 to 1990, prostate cancer incidence rates increased by 65 percent, largely because of earlier diagnosis in men without symptoms. This was accomplished by increased use of **prostate-specific antigen (PSA)** blood test screenings and increased public awareness.[39] Today, prostate cancer rates are declining.

Most signs of prostate cancer are nonspecific—that is, they mimic the signs of infection or enlarged prostate.

Prostate-specific antigen (PSA)   An antigen found in prostate cancer patients.

Table 13.2

Recommendations for the Early Detection of Cancer in Asymptomatic People

SITE	RECOMMENDATION
Cancer-related checkup	A cancer-related checkup is recommended every three years for people aged 20–40 and every year for people aged 40 and older. This exam should include health counseling and, depending on a person's age, might include examination for cancers of the thyroid, oral cavity, skin, lymph nodes, testes, and ovaries, as well as for some nonmalignant diseases.
Breast	Women 40 and older should have an annual mammogram and an annual clinical breast exam (CBE) performed by a health care professional and should perform monthly breast self-examination. The CBE should be conducted close to the scheduled mammogram.
	Women aged 20–39 should have a clinical breast exam performed by a health care professional every three years and should perform monthly breast self-examination.
Colon and rectum	Men and women aged 50 and older should follow *one* of the examination schedules below:
	• A fecal occult blood test every year and a flexible sigmoidoscopy every five years.*
	• A colonoscopy every ten years.*
	• A double-contrast barium enema every five to ten years.*
	*A digital rectal exam should be done at the same time as a sigmoidoscopy, colonoscopy, or double-contrast barium enema. People who are at moderate or high risk for colorectal cancer should talk with a doctor about a different testing schedule.
Prostate	The ACS recommends that both the prostate-specific antigen (PSA) blood test and the digital rectal examination be offered annually, beginning at age 50, to men who have a life expectancy of at least 10 years and to younger men who are at high risk.
	Men in high-risk groups, such as those with a strong familial predisposition (e.g., two or more affected first-degree relatives), or African Americans may begin at a younger age (e.g., 45 years).
Uterus	**Cervix:** All women who are or have been sexually active or who are 18 and older should have an annual Pap test and pelvic examination. After three or more consecutive satisfactory examinations with normal findings, the Pap test may be performed less frequently. Discuss the matter with your physician.
	Endometrium: Women at high risk for cancer of the uterus should have a sample of endometrial tissue examined when menopause begins.

Source: American Cancer Society, *Cancer Facts & Figures 2002.*

Symptoms include weak or interrupted urine flow; difficulty starting or stopping the urine flow; the need to urinate frequently; pain or difficulty in urinating; blood in the urine; and pain in the lower back, pelvis, or upper thighs. Many males mistake these symptoms for other nonspecific conditions, such as infections, and delay treatment.

Incidence of prostate cancer increases with age; over 75 percent of all cases are diagnosed in men over age 65, although increasing numbers of young men seem to be affected. African Americans have the highest prostate cancer rates in the world. The disease is most common in northwestern Europe and North America, but rare in the Near East, Africa, Central America, and South America. There seems to be a slightly increased risk if a family member has the disease, but it is unclear whether this is due to genetic or environmental factors. Recent genetic studies suggest that strong familial predisposition may be responsible for 5 to 10 percent of prostate cancers.[40] International studies suggest that dietary fat may also be a factor.

Fortunately, even with so many generalized symptoms, most prostate cancers are detected while they are still localized, and they tend to progress slowly. Because most men develop the disease in their late 60s and early 70s, it is likely that they will die of other causes first. For this reason, some health care groups question the cost-effectiveness and necessity of prostate surgeries and other costly procedures that may have little real effect on life expectancy. Prostate cancer patients have an average five-year survival rate of 80 percent. Because the incidence of prostate cancer increases with age, every man over age 40 should have an annual digital rectal prostate examination. In addition, the American Cancer Society recommends that men aged 50 and older have an annual prostate-specific antigen (PSA) test. If either result is suspicious, further evaluation in the form of transrectal ultrasound is recommended.[41]

Skin Cancer: Sun Bathers Beware

The sun seems to have betrayed its worshippers. As the primary cause of nearly 1.3 million cases of skin cancer in the United States this year, many of which will disfigure or permanently change the person's appearance, the sun may just be the skin's public enemy number one. In fact, skin cancer

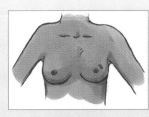

Lumpectomy
Performed when tumor is in earliest localized stages. Prognosis for recovery is better than 95 percent. Only tumor itself is removed. Some physicians may also remove normal tissue in surrounding area.

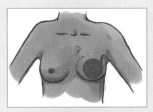

Simple mastectomy
Removal of breast and underling tissue. Prognosis for full recovery better than 80 percent.

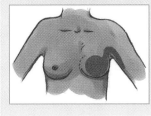

Modified radical mastectomy
Breast and lymph nodes in immediate area removed. Prognosis for full recovery dependent on level of spread.

Radical mastectomy
Removal of breast, lymph nodes, pectoral muscles, all fat and underlying tissue. Prognosis for full recovery may be as low as 60 percent dependent on level of spread.

Figure 13.3
Surgical Procedures for Diagnosed Breast Cancer
These surgeries are typically followed by radiation treatment and/or chemotherapy.

is the most common cancer in the United States today, accounting for nearly 2 percent of all cancer deaths.[42]

Although most people don't die from the highly treatable *basal* or *squamous cell* skin cancers, the highly virulent **malignant melanoma** has become the most frequent cancer in women ages 25 to 29 and runs second only to breast cancer in women ages 30 to 34. Rates of melanoma are ten times higher among whites than African Americans. In 2001, nearly 51,400 cases of melanoma were diagnosed. That year, nearly 7,800 people died of melanoma, and 2,000 died of other forms of skin cancer.[43]

In spite of these grisly statistics, over 60 percent of all Americans 25 years and under report that they are "working on a tan" at some point during the year. Fewer than one in three sunbathers bothers to wear UVB-thwarting sunscreen lotions. Are tanning booths safer than natural sunlight? No. In fact, tanning lamps emit large amounts of ultraviolet radiation that can dramatically increase the risk of skin cancer. A study in Sweden found that people under age 30 who visited a tanning booth more than ten times per year had a seven-times-greater risk of melanoma.[44]

Many people do not know what to look for when examining themselves for skin cancer. Basal and squamous cell carcinomas can be a recurrent annoyance, showing up most commonly on the face, ears, neck, arms, hands, and legs as warty bumps, colored spots, or scaly patches. Surgery may be necessary to remove them, but they are seldom life-threatening. In striking contrast is the insidious melanoma, an invasive killer that quickly spreads to regional organs and throughout the body, accounting for over 75 percent of all skin cancer deaths. Risks increase dramatically among whites after age 20.[45] Often, these moles start as normal-looking growths but quickly develop abnormal characteristics. A simple *ABCD* rule outlines the warning signs of melanoma:

- *Asymmetry*—One half of the mole does not match the other half.
- *Border irregularity*—The edges are uneven, notched, or scalloped.
- *Color*—The pigmentation is not uniform. Melanoma may vary in color from tan to deeper brown, reddish black, black, or deep bluish black.
- *Diameter*—The diameter is greater than 6 millimeters (about the size of a pea).

If you notice any of these symptoms, consult a physician promptly.

Treatment of skin cancer depends on its seriousness. Surgery is performed in 90 percent of all cases. Radiation therapy, *electrodesiccation* (tissue destruction by heat), and *cryosurgery* (tissue destruction by freezing) are also common forms of treatment. For melanoma, treatment may involve surgical removal of the regional lymph nodes, radiation, or chemotherapy.

Testicular Cancer

Testicular cancer is one of the most common types of solid tumors found in young adult males. Those between the ages of 17 and 34 are at greatest risk. There has been a steady increase in tumor frequency over the past several years in this age group.[46] Although the cause of testicular cancer is unknown, several risk factors have been identified. Males with undescended testicles appear to be at greatest risk, and some studies indicate a genetic influence.

In general, testicular tumors first appear as a painless enlargement of the testis or thickening in testicular tissue. Because this enlargement is often painless, it is extremely important that all young males practice regular testicular self-examination. This is done by placing the index and middle fingers of both hands on the underside of the testicle and the thumbs on top. Gently roll the testicle between your thumb

Malignant melanoma   A virulent cancer of the melanin (pigment-producing portion) of the skin.

What's New in Cancer Research, Prevention, and Treatment?

THE LATEST ON FIBER

Although fiber has been downplayed in the past year as a protective agent against colon and other forms of cancer, don't throw out that bran muffin just yet. A recent study of more than 68,000 women found that dietary fiber—particularly from breakfast cereals—can significantly decrease the risk of heart attacks by improving cholesterol levels, lowering blood sugar, boosting sensitivity to insulin, and lowering the risk of blood clotting. A previous study of men had similar results. Also, although some recent studies questioned fiber's benefits for cancer prevention, many experts doubt that these findings should outweigh all the previous studies that indicate it does indeed reduce risk. In short, the scientific community is unsure of the fiber–cancer link but quite sure that the benefits in other areas should more than justify a healthy high-fiber, low-fat diet.

ALCHOHOL AND CANCER

Heavy drinking is associated with an increased risk for several cancers—notably, cancer of the mouth, esophagus, pharynx, larynx, liver, and pancreas. An analysis of multiple studies found that having two alcoholic drinks per day (any type of alcohol) increased a woman's chances of developing breast cancer by nearly 25 percent. The reasons for this increased risk are unclear, but researchers speculate that alcohol influences the metabolism of estrogen and that prolonged exposure to high levels of estrogen increases breast cancer risk, particularly for women on hormone replacement therapy (HRT). The effect of one drink per day is controversial, although most experts feel that one daily drink does not increase risk. But before you toss out all of your alcohol, you

should know there is increasing evidence that a glass of red wine, with its antioxidant and HDL-boosting potential, seems to protect against heart disease.

HRT AND BREAST CANCER

The many purported benefits of hormone replacement therapy (HRT) range from relieving transitory menopausal symptoms, such as hot flashes, to lowering the long-term risk of osteoporosis and possibly heart disease. Preliminary studies also suggest that HRT may reduce the risk of Alzheimer's disease, colon cancer, and strokes. But the decision to use HRT is still clouded in controversy, particularly because its two principal components—estrogen and progestin—appear to affect breast tissue. When taken alone, estrogen significantly increases the risk of uterine cancer also, so probably the only women who should be taking estrogen alone are those who have had complete hysterectomies. Additionally, some studies have found that estrogen may cause a small increase in the risk of breast cancer, particularly in women who already are predisposed to breast cancer through family and genetic or environmental risks. Unfortunately, although many people commonly assume that HRT and increased breast cancer risk are synonymous, such is not the case. Research to date has been limited and does not provide clear associations between the two. Several long-term studies are underway through the Women's Health Initiative and other projects, but results are still at least five years away. Other researchers are concerned that progestins may also increase the risk of breast cancer, a possibility even more inconclusive than questions about estrogen. A study published in the April 2000 issue of *Obstetrics and Gynecology* suggests that women who get breast cancer while taking HRT tend to have smaller tumors and better survival rates than women with breast cancer who have never taken HRT.

What does all this mean to you? Because there is so much uncertainty about its risks and benefits, women who

are considering HRT should thoroughly check out information about dose, formulations, and length of treatment. Most experts suggest that benefits of HRT (protection from CVD and osteoporosis in particular) outweigh the small risk of breast cancer. Also, it is important to note that in studies where estrogen has appeared to slightly increase risk, women had been taking it for more than five years at relatively high doses. Today's formulations, offered under the guidance of an informed physician and combined with regular mammograms and other screenings, appear to be important elements of overall risk reduction.

NEW METHODS OF DETECTION

Several new methods of breast cancer detection are on the horizon:

- *Blood tests.* Researchers from the John Wayne Cancer Center in Santa Monica are developing biological markers that would identify microscopic tumors as they travel through the blood, before they are large enough to be picked up on conventional tests.
- *"Pap smear for the breast."* Similar to the Pap smear, which checks fluids from the cervix for abnormal cells, this newer test analyzes fluids from the breasts' milk ducts (where most tumors originate). It may be widely available soon. This test would pick up cancerous cells in their earliest, most treatable stages.
- *Better breast scans.* Researchers at the University of Chicago and elsewhere are developing better computer programs to point out questionable spots on mammograms and better, more reliable machines, such as MRIs.

Source: J. Manson, "High-Fiber Diet and Decreased Risk of Heart Disease in Women," *Journal of the American Medical Association* (1999): "The Facts About Drinking and Your Health," *Johns Hopkins Medical Health Letter—Health After 50* 12 (5) (2000): 4–6; "Latest on HRT and Breast Cancer Risks," *Johns Hopkins Medical Letter—Health After 50* 12 (3) (2000): 1–3; C. Gorman, "The Search for Smaller Tumors," *Time* (June 26, 2000): 50.

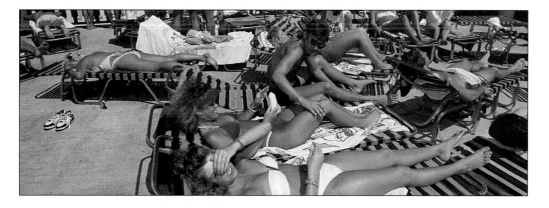

During spring break, thousands of college students try to achieve the perfect tan, often risking overexposure to sunlight and inviting potential skin cancer in later years.

and fingers. If a suspicious lump or thickening is found, consult a doctor immediately. It is best to perform an exam after a bath or shower, because the heat causes the testicles to descend and the scrotal skin to relax.

Ovarian Cancer

Ovarian cancer is the fourth leading cause of cancer death for women, killing nearly 14,000 in 2001. The most common sign is enlargement of the abdomen (or a feeling of bloating) in women over age 40. Other symptoms include vague digestive disturbances, such as gas and stomachaches that persist and cannot be explained.[47] Because its symptoms are often nonspecific, ovarian cancer frequently goes undiagnosed in its early stages.

The risk for ovarian cancer increases with age, with the highest rates found in women in their 60s. Women who have never had children are twice as likely to develop ovarian cancer as are those who have. This is because the main risk factor appears to be exposure to the reproductive hormone estrogen. Women who have multiple pregnancies or use oral contraceptives, both of which inhibit estrogen, are at lower risk. In addition, having one or more primary relatives (mother, sisters, grandmothers) who have had the disease appears to increase individual risk. With the exception of Japan, the highest incidence rates are reported in the industrialized countries of the world. Research indicates that mutations in the BRCA1 and BRCA2 genes may increase risks.[48]

Prevention An early Yale University study indicated that diet may play a role in ovarian cancer.[49] Researchers, when comparing 450 Canadian women with newly diagnosed ovarian cancer with 564 demographically similar, healthy women, found that the women without ovarian cancer had a diet lower in saturated fat. For every 10 grams of saturated fat a woman ate per day, her risk of ovarian cancer rose 20 percent. Conversely, women who lowered their saturated fat consumption by 10 grams a day experienced a 20 percent drop in risk. Every 10 grams of vegetable fiber (but not fruit or cereal fiber) added to a woman's daily menu lowered her risk by 37 percent. The study also found that each full-term pregnancy lowered risk by about 20 percent and each year of oral contraceptive use lowered it by 5 to 10 percent. So, should you go out and get pregnant or start taking birth con-

trol pills to reduce risk? Probably not. However, these results, particularly when combined with cardiovascular risks and other health information, provide yet another reason to eat plenty of vegetables and cut down on your fat intake.

To protect yourself, annual thorough pelvic examinations are important. Pap tests, although useful in detecting cervical cancer, do not reveal ovarian cancer. Women over the age of 40 should have a cancer-related checkup every year. Transvaginal ultrasound and a tumor marker, CA125, may assist in diagnosis but are not recommended for routine screening.[50] If you have any symptoms of ovarian cancer and they persist, see your doctor promptly.

Endometrium (Uterine) Cancer

In 2001, an estimated 38,300 new cases of uterine cancer were diagnosed in the United States. Most uterine cancers develop in the body of the uterus, usually in the endometrium (lining). The rest develop in the cervix, located at the base of the uterus. The overall incidence of early-stage uterine cancer—that is, cervical cancer—has increased slightly in recent years in women under the age of 50.[51] In contrast, invasive, later-stage forms of the disease appear to be decreasing. This may be due to more regular screenings of younger women using the **Pap test,** a procedure in which cells taken from the cervical region are examined for abnormal cellular activity. Although these tests are very effective for detecting early-stage cervical cancer, they are less effective for detecting cancers of the uterine lining and are not effective at all for detecting cancers of the fallopian tubes or ovaries.[52]

Risk factors for cervical cancer include early age of first intercourse, multiple sex partners, cigarette smoking, and certain sexually transmitted diseases, such as the herpesvirus and the human papillomavirus. For endometrial cancer, a history of infertility, failure to ovulate, obesity, and treatment with tamoxifen or unopposed estrogen therapy appear to be major risk factors.[53]

Pap test A procedure in which cells taken from the cervical region are examined for abnormal cellular activity.

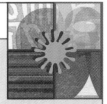

Tips for Sun Worshippers

Planning on working on your suntan? Before heading out, consider these facts.

TANNING AND THE ANATOMY OF A BURN

Ultraviolet A (UVA) and B (UVB) rays tan, burn, and age the skin. Tanning is how the skin protects itself from damage. UVA rays darken melanin grains in the epidermis, the skin's top layer. After a few days, newly pigmented skin cells, stimulated by both UVA and UVB rays, migrate to the surface. UVA rays are weaker than UVB rays, but more of them penetrate the dermis, or deepest layer of skin. Over time, exposure can break down collagen and lead to wrinkles and other signs of aging. UVB radiation is the main cause of burns and skin cancer. These shorter-wavelength rays have more energy than UVA rays, damaging cells in the epidermis.

TIME OF DAY

How long you're in the sun matters, but so does time of day. Burning is more likely between 10:00 A.M. and 3:00 P.M., when the atmosphere filters out less ultraviolet energy.

CLOUD COVER

Clouds let 80 percent of UV rays through and increase exposure by scattering the rays. It's important to protect your skin even on cloudy days.

PEAK PROTECTION

At high altitudes more UV rays get through, and snow reflects 80 percent of sunlight. Wear protective clothing and a high-SPF (sun protection factor) sunscreen.

IN THE WATER

UV rays can burn parts of your body that are under water, so use waterproof sunscreen. Wearing a shirt while swimming and wading is advisable, because UV rays reflected off water and sand intensify exposure.

SUNGLASSES

Shades not only cut glare but also reduce the risk of UV-caused cataracts.

WHAT TO WEAR

An ordinary T-shirt has an effective SPF of only 6 to 8, dropping to 4 or 5 when wet.

The more opaque the material, the fewer UV rays get through. Color, however, doesn't affect the number of UV rays that penetrate the fabric. Special sun-blocking clothing has an SPF of 30 or more.

SUNSCREEN TIPS

Apply an SPF 15 or higher sunscreen to the entire body 30 minutes before going out. Use at least a full ounce. Reapply even "waterproof" sunscreen if you're in the water longer than 80 minutes, towel off, or perspire heavily. Recent reports have highlighted the potential harmful effects of one active ingredient in some sunscreens, oxybenzone, particularly after repeated applications. The concern is based on the fact that this chemical is absorbed in the body and may have long-term negative effects.

Source: Adapted by permission from "A Sun Worshiper's Guide," *U.S. News & World Report* (June 24, 1996). Basic data from the American Academy of Dermatology, American Optometric Association, and Sun Precautions, Inc. "The Active Ingredients in Sunscreen: Is It Safe?" *Healthfacts* 23 (1998): 5.

Early warning signs of uterine cancer include bleeding outside the normal menstrual period or after menopause or persistent unusual vaginal discharge. These symptoms should be checked by a physician immediately.[54]

Cancer of the Pancreas

The incidence of cancer of the pancreas, known as a "silent" disease, has increased substantially during the last 25 years to 29,700 cases in 2002.[55] Chronic inflammation of the pancreas, diabetes, cirrhosis, and a high-fat diet may contribute to its development. Smokers have double the risk of nonsmokers.[56] Unfortunately, pancreatic cancer is one of the worst cancers to get, with only 4 percent of patients living more than five years after diagnosis, usually because the disease is well advanced by the time there are any symptoms.

Leukemia

Leukemia is a cancer of the blood-forming tissues that leads to proliferation of millions of immature white blood cells. These abnormal cells crowd out normal white blood cells (which fight infection), platelets (which control hemorrhaging), and red blood cells (which carry oxygen to the cells). As a result, symptoms such as fatigue, paleness, weight loss, easy bruising, repeated infections, nosebleeds, and other forms of hemorrhaging occur. In children, these symptoms can appear suddenly.[57]

Leukemia can be acute or chronic in nature and can strike both sexes and all age groups. Although many people think of it as a childhood disease, leukemia will strike many more adults (28,200) than children (2,500) in 2002.[58] Chronic leukemia can develop over several months and have few symptoms. The five-year survival rate for patients with leukemia had increased to 60 percent by the late 1990s.

Table 13.3
Cancer's Seven Warning Signals

1. Changes in bowel or bladder habits
2. A sore that does not heal
3. Unusual bleeding or discharge
4. Thickening or lump in breast or elsewhere
5. Indigestion or difficulty in swallowing
6. Obvious change in a wart or mole
7. Nagging cough or hoarseness

If you have a warning signal, see your doctor.

Facing Cancer

While heart disease mortality rates have declined steadily over the past 50 years, cancer mortality has increased consistently in the same period. Based on current rates, about 83 million—or one in three of us now living—will eventually develop cancer. Many factors have contributed to the rise in cancer mortality, but the increased incidence of lung cancer—a largely preventable disease—is probably the most important. Despite these gloomy predictions, recent advancements in the diagnosis and treatment of many forms of cancer have reduced much of the fear and mystery that once surrounded this disease.

Detecting Cancer

The earlier cancer is diagnosed, the better the prospect for survival. Several high-tech tools have been developed to detect cancer. They include the following:

- New high-technology diagnostic imaging techniques have replaced exploratory surgery for some cancer patients. In **magnetic resonance imaging (MRI),** a huge electromagnet detects hidden tumors by mapping the vibrations of the various atoms in the body on a computer screen. **Computerized axial tomography scanning (CAT scan)** uses x-rays to examine parts of the body. In both of these painless, noninvasive procedures, cross-section pictures can reveal a tumor's shape and location more accurately than conventional x-ray films.
- *Prostatic ultrasound* (a rectal probe using ultrasonic waves to produce an image of the prostate) is currently being investigated as a means to increase the early detection of prostate cancer. Recently, prostatic ultrasound has been combined with a blood test for prostate-specific antigen (PSA), an antigen found in prostate cancer patients.

Such medical techniques, along with regular self-examinations and checkups, play an important role in the early detection and secondary prevention of cancer. Table 13.3 shows the seven warning signals of cancer. Make sure you know which symptoms to watch for, and follow the recommendations for self-exams and medical checkups in Table 13.2.

New Hope in Cancer Treatments

Although cancer treatments have changed dramatically over the past 20 years, surgery, in which the tumor and surrounding tissue are removed, is still common. Today's surgeons tend to remove less surrounding tissue than previously and to combine surgery with either **radiotherapy** (the use of radiation) or **chemotherapy** (the use of drugs) to kill cancerous cells.

Radiation works by destroying malignant cells or stopping cell growth. It is most effective in treating localized cancer masses. Unfortunately, in the process of destroying malignant cells, radiotherapy also destroys some healthy cells. It may also increase the risks for other types of cancers. Despite these qualifications, radiation continues to be one of the most common and effective forms of treatment.

When cancer has spread throughout the body, it is necessary to use some form of chemotherapy. Currently, over 50 different anticancer drugs are in use, some of which have excellent records of success. A chemotherapeutic regimen of four anticancer drugs combined with radiotherapy has resulted in remarkable survival rates for some cancers, including Hodgkin's disease. Ongoing research will result in new drugs that are less toxic to normal cells and more potent against tumor cells. Current research indicates that some

Magnetic resonance imaging (MRI) A device that uses magnetic fields, radio waves, and computers to generate an image of internal tissues of the body for diagnostic purposes without the use of radiation.

Computerized axial tomography (CAT scan) A machine that uses radiation to view internal organs not normally visible on x-rays.

Radiotherapy The use of radiation to kill cancerous cells.

Chemotherapy The use of drugs to kill cancerous cells.

tumors may actually be resistant to certain forms of chemotherapy and that the treatment drugs do not reach the core of the tumor. Scientists are working to circumvent resistance and make tumor cells more vulnerable.

Whether used alone or in combination, radiotherapy and chemotherapy have side effects, including extreme nausea, nutritional deficiencies, hair loss, and general fatigue. Long-term damage to the cardiovascular system and other body systems can be significant. It is important to discuss these matters fully with doctors when making treatment plans.

Substances found in nature, such as taxol (originally found in Pacific Yew trees), are being synthesized in laboratories and tested on a variety of cancers. Other compounds, including those derived from sea urchins, are rich in resources for anticancer drugs.

Today, researchers are targeting cancer as a genetic disease that is brought on by some form of mutation, either inherited or acquired. Promising treatments focus on stopping the cycle of these mutant cells, targeting toxins through monoclonal antibodies, and rousing the immune system to be more effective.

Talking with Your Doctor About Cancer

Anytime the presence of cancer is suspected, people react with great anxiety, fear, and anger. Emotional distress is sometimes so intense that they are unable to make critical health care decisions. If you find it difficult to know what to ask your doctor on a routine exam, imagine how hard it would be to discuss life-or-death options for yourself or a loved one. Before you arrive at the doctor's office, prepare a list of important questions to discuss. Remember, your health care provider should be your partner and help you make the best decisions for you.

If the diagnosis is cancer, here are some suggestions for questions to ask:

- What kind of cancer do I have? What stage is it in? Based on my age and stage, what prognosis do I have?
- What are my treatment choices? Which do you recommend? Why?
- What are the benefits of each kind of treatment?
- What are the long- and short-term risks and possible side effects?
- Would a clinical trial be appropriate for me? (Clinical trials are research studies designed to answer specific questions and to find better ways to prevent or treat cancer. Often new cancer-fighting treatments are used.)

If surgery is recommended, you may want to ask these questions:

- What kind of operation will it be, and how long will it take? What form of anesthesia will be used? How many similar procedures has this surgeon done in the past month? What is his or her success rate?
- How will I feel after surgery? If I have pain, how will you help me?

- Where will the scars be? What will they look like? Will they cause disability?
- Will I have any activity limitations after surgery? What kind of physical therapy, if any, will I have? When will I get back to normal activities?

If radiation is recommended, you may want to know the following:

- Why do you think this treatment is better than my other options?
- How long will I need to have treatments, and what will the side effects be in the short and long term? What body organs or systems may be damaged?
- What can I do to take care of myself during therapy? Are there services available to help me?
- What is the long-term prognosis for people of my age with my type of cancer who are using this treatment?

Questions to ask about chemotherapy include the following:

- Why do you think this treatment is better than my other options?
- Which drug combinations pose the fewest risks and most benefits?
- What are the short- and long-term side effects on my body?
- What are my options?

Before you begin any form of cancer therapy, it is imperative to be a vigilant and vocal consumer. Read and seek information from cancer support groups. Check the skills of your surgeon, your radiation therapist, and your doctor in terms of clinical experience and interpersonal interactions.

Life After Cancer

Heightened public awareness and an improved prognosis have made the cancer experience less threatening and isolating than it once was. While you may hear stories of recovering cancer patients experiencing job discrimination and being unable to obtain health or life insurance, these cases are decreasing. Several states have even enacted legislation to prevent insurance companies from canceling policies or instituting other forms of discrimination. Health insurance can be obtained through large employers. Because large companies spread the insurance risk among many employees, insurance companies accept all new employees without underwriting.

In fact, assistance for the cancer patient is more readily available than ever before. Cancer support groups, cancer information workshops, and low-cost medical consultation are just a few of the forms of assistance now offered in many communities. The national breast cancer coalition and other groups have successfully lobbied Congress to increase cancer research dollars. As a result, government funding has increased substantially over the past decade. The battle for funds continues. Increasing efforts in cancer research, improvements in diagnostic equipment, and advances in treatment provide hope for the future.

Managing Cancer Risks

Cancer is no longer an automatic death sentence. Oncologists continually increase our chances of surviving cancer with new and improved medical care as well as better early detection tests. Nevertheless, we each hold the key to fulfilling our own hopes by doing what we can to prevent cancer. Regular checkups and monthly self-exams improve the odds of survival by providing early diagnosis. Proper diet, regular exercise, and staying clear of carcinogens also improve the odds. From the self-assessment that you completed earlier in this chapter, which factors put you at risk for cancer? What actions can you take today to reduce your risk?

Checklist for Change

Making Personal Choices

✓ *Don't smoke.* Smoking accounts for about 30 percent of all cancer deaths and 90 percent of all lung cancer deaths. People who smoke two or more packs of cigarettes a day have lung cancer mortality rates 17 to 25 times greater than those of nonsmokers.

✓ *Avoid excessive sunlight.* Almost 600,000 cases of nonmelanoma skin cancer diagnosed each year in the United States are considered to be sun related.

✓ *Avoid excessive alcohol consumption.* Oral cancer and cancers of the larynx, throat, esophagus, breast, and liver occur more frequently among heavy drinkers.

✓ *Do not use smokeless tobacco.* Use of chewing tobacco or snuff increases risk for cancer of the mouth, larynx, throat, and esophagus and is highly habit forming.

✓ *Monitor estrogen use.* Estrogen treatment to control menopausal symptoms may increase risk for endometrial cancer. Although estrogen therapy has been thought to lower women's risk for heart disease and osteoporosis, it should not be undertaken without careful discussion between a woman and her physician.

✓ *Avoid occupational carcinogens.* Exposure to any of several different industrial agents increases risk for various cancers. Risk from asbestos exposure is greatly increased when combined with cigarette smoking.

✓ *Avoid obesity.* Risk for colon, breast, ovarian, endometrial, and uterine cancers increases in obese people.

✓ *Eat your fruits and vegetables.* Eat at least five servings of fruits and vegetables every day to reduce your risk.

✓ *Cut back on fats.* Reduce fat consumption, especially saturated fats and red meats, to reduce risk for colon, breast, prostate, pancreatic, and ovarian cancers.

Making Community Choices

✓ Does your community have any major sources of carcinogens (toxic waste dumps, chemical factories, and so on)? What precautions are taken to ensure that environmental risks are reduced?

✓ Does your community have cancer support groups that you could join if you developed cancer? Where would you find out about such support groups?

Summary

✷ Cancer is a group of diseases characterized by uncontrolled growth and spread of abnormal cells. These cells may create tumors. Benign (noncancerous) tumors grow in size but do not spread; malignant (cancerous) tumors spread to other parts of the body.

✷ Several causes of cancer have been identified. Biological factors include inherited genes and gender. Occupational and environmental hazards are carcinogens present in people's home or work environments. Chemicals in foods that may act as carcinogens include preservatives and pesticides. Viruses that may be involved in the development of cancer include herpes, Epstein-Barr virus (which causes mononucleosis), and human papillomavirus (which causes genital warts). Medical factors include certain drug therapies given for other conditions that may elevate the chance of cancer. Combined risk refers to a combination of the above factors, which tends to compound the risk for cancer.

✷ There are many different types of cancer, each of which poses different risks, depending on a number of factors. Common cancers include lung, breast, colon and rectum, prostate, skin, testicular, ovarian, uterine, and pancreatic cancers, as well as leukemia.

✷ Early diagnosis improves survival rate. Self-exams for breast, testicular, and skin cancer and knowledge of the seven warning signals of cancer aid early diagnosis.

✷ New types of cancer treatments include various combinations of radiotherapy, chemotherapy, and immunotherapy.

Discussion Questions

1. What is cancer? How does it spread? What is the difference between a benign and a malignant tumor?
2. List the likely causes of cancer. Do any of them put you at greater risk? What can you do to reduce this risk? What risk factors do you share with family members? With friends?
3. What are the symptoms of lung, breast, prostate, and testicular cancer? What can you do to reduce your risk of developing these cancers or increase your chances of surviving them?
4. What are the differences between carcinomas, sarcomas, lymphomas, and leukemia? Which is the most common? Least common?
5. Why are breast and testicular self-exams important for women and men? What could be the consequences of not doing these exams regularly?
6. Discuss the seven warning signals of cancer. What could signal that you have cancer instead of a minor illness? How soon should you seek treatment for any of the warning signs?

Application Exercises

Reread the What Do You Think? scenarios at the beginning of this chapter, and answer the following questions.

1. Why do you think a tan is so important to young Americans?
2. What are the risks of tanning? What actions could be taken to reduce risks for developing skin cancer?
3. Is Nick correct when he says tanning booths are less risky than natural sunlight? Explain your answer.

Accessing Your Health on the Internet http

Visit the following Internet sites to explore further topics and issues related to personal health. To visit an organization's website, go to the Companion Website for *Health: The Basics, Fifth Edition* at www.aw.com/donatelle, click on the book image, and select "Accessing Your Health on the Internet" from the navigation menu on the left.

1. *American Cancer Society.* Home page for the leading private organization dedicated to cancer prevention. This site provides information, statistics, and resources regarding cancer.
2. *International Cancer Information Center.* Sponsored by the National Cancer Institute, this site is designed to be a comprehensive information resource on cancer for patients and health professionals.
3. *Oncolink.* Sponsored by the University of Pennsylvania Cancer Center, this site seeks to educate cancer patients and their families by offering information on support services, cancer causes, screening, prevention, and common questions.
4. *National Women's Health Information Center (NWHIC).* Provides a wealth of information about cancer in women. Cosponsored by the National Cancer Institute.

Further Reading

American Cancer Society. *Cancer Facts and Figures.* Atlanta, GA: published annually.
   A summary of major facts relating to cancer. Provides information on incidence, prevalence, symptomology, prevention, and treatment. Available through local divisions of the American Cancer Society.

American Cancer Society. *Colorectal Cancer: A Thorough and Compassionate Resource for Patients and Their Families.* New York: Random House, 2000.
   Contains up-to-date information about the disease, medical options, and emotional support.

American Cancer Institute Journal, published monthly.
   Focuses on current risk factors, prevention, and treatment research in the area of cancer.

Brownson, R., P. Remington, and J. Davis, *Epidemiology and Control of Chronic Diseases.* American Public Health Association, 1998.
   Excellent overview of major chronic diseases, risk factors for disease, and trends in prevention and control.

Nutrition and Cancer Journal, published monthly.
   Focuses on etiological aspects of various dietary factors and research on risks for cancer development. Also includes current research on dietary factors and prevention.

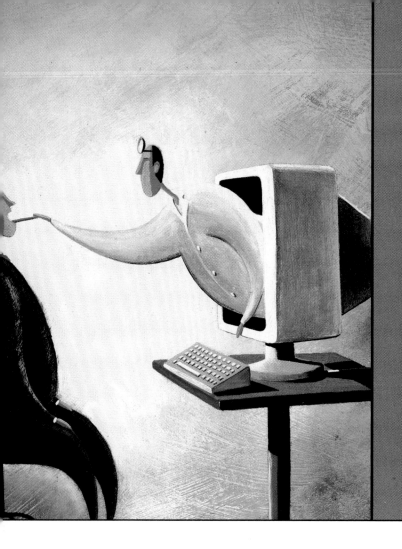

objectives

* Discuss the risk factors for infectious diseases.

* Describe the most common pathogens infecting humans today.

* Describe your immune system, how it works to protect you, and what factors may make your immune system less effective.

* Explain the major emerging and resurgent diseases affect-

ing humans; discuss why they are increasing in incidence and what actions are being taken to reduce risks.

* Discuss the various sexually transmitted infections, their means of transmission, and actions that can be taken to prevent their spread.

* Discuss human immunodeficiency virus (HIV) and acquired immune deficiency

syndrome (AIDS), trends in infection and treatment, and the impact on special populations, such as women and members of the international community.

* Discuss the chronic lung diseases, common neurological disorders, diabetes and other digestion-related disorders, and the varied musculoskeletal diseases.

Every moment of every day, you are in contact with microscopic organisms that have the ability to make you ill or even cause death. These disease-causing agents, known as **pathogens,** are found in air and food and on nearly every object or person with whom you come in contact. Although new varieties of pathogens arise all the time, scientific evidence indicates that many have existed for as long as there has been life on the planet. Fossil evidence shows that infections, cancer, heart disease, and a host of other ailments afflicted the earliest human beings. At times, infectious diseases wiped out whole groups of people through epidemics such as the Black Death, or bubonic plague, which killed more than half of the population of Europe and Asia in the 1300s. Pandemics are global epidemics of diseases such as influenza. An influenza pandemic killed more than 20 million people in 1918. Unrelenting strains of tuberculosis and cholera continue to cause premature death among populations throughout the world.

In spite of our best efforts to eradicate them, these diseases are a continuing menace to all of us. The news isn't all bad, however. Even though we are bombarded by potential pathogenic threats, our immune systems are remarkably adept at protecting us. *Endogenous microorganisms* are those that live in peaceful coexistence with their human host most of the time. For people in good health and whose immune systems are functioning properly, endogenous organisms are usually harmless. But in sick people or people with weakened immune systems, these normally harmless pathogenic organisms can cause serious health problems.

Exogenous microorganisms are organisms that do not normally inhabit the body. When they do, however, they are apt to produce an infection and/or illness. The more easily these pathogens can gain a foothold in the body and sustain themselves, the more **virulent,** or aggressive, they may be in causing disease. However, if your immune system is strong, you will often be able to fight off even the most virulent attacker. Several factors influence your susceptibility to diseases.

Assessing Your Disease Risks

Most diseases are **multifactorial diseases**—that is, they are caused by the interaction of several factors from inside and outside the person. For a disease to occur, the *host* must be *susceptible,* meaning that the immune system must be in a weakened condition; an *agent* capable of transmitting a disease must be present; and the *environment* must be hospitable to the pathogen in terms of temperature, light, moisture, and other requirements. Other risk factors also apparently increase or decrease levels of susceptibility. Figure 14.1 summarizes the body's defenses against invasion.

Risk Factors You Can't Control

Unfortunately, some risk factors are beyond our control. Some of the most common are heredity, aging, environmental conditions, and organism resistance.

Heredity Perhaps the single greatest factor influencing a person's longevity is the longevity of his or her parents. Being born into a family in which heart disease, cancer, or other illnesses are prevalent seems to increase a person's risk. Still other diseases are caused by direct chromosomal inheritance. For example, **sickle-cell anemia,** an inherited blood disease that primarily affects African Americans, is

Pathogen   A disease-causing agent.

Virulent   Strong enough to overcome host resistance and cause disease.

Multifactorial disease   Disease caused by interactions of several factors.

Sickle-cell anemia   Genetic disease commonly found among African Americans; results in organ damage and premature death.

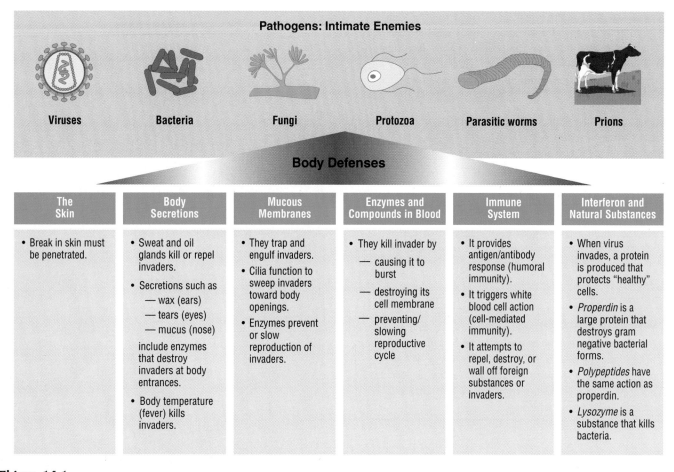

Figure 14.1
The Body's Defenses Against Disease-Causing Pathogens

often transmitted to the fetus if both parents carry the sickle-cell trait. It is often unclear whether hereditary diseases occur as a result of inherited chromosomal traits or inherited insufficiencies in the immune system.

Aging   After age 40 we become more vulnerable to most of the chronic diseases. Moreover, as we age, our immune systems respond less efficiently to invading organisms, increasing risk for infection and illness. The same flu that produces an afternoon of nausea and diarrhea in a younger person may cause days of illness or even death in an older person. The very young are also at risk for many diseases, particularly if they are not vaccinated against them.

Environmental Conditions   Unsanitary conditions and the presence of drugs, chemicals, and hazardous pollutants and wastes in food and water probably have a great effect on our immune systems. It is well documented that poor environmental conditions can weaken **immunological competence**—the body's ability to defend itself against pathogens.

Organism Resistance   Some organisms, such as the food-borne organism **botulism,** are particularly virulent, and even

tiny amounts may make the most hardy of us ill. Other organisms have mutated and are resistant to the body's defenses as well as other conventional treatments designed to protect against them. Still other, newer pathogens pose unique challenges for our immune systems—ones that our bodily defenses are ill adapted to fight.

Risk Factors You Can Control

The good news is that we all have some degree of personal control over certain risk factors for disease. Too much stress, inadequate nutrition, a low physical fitness level, lack of sleep, misuse or abuse of legal and illegal substances, poor

---

Immunological competence   Ability of the immune system to defend the body from pathogens.

Botulism   A resistant food-borne organism that is extremely virulent.

personal hygiene, high-risk behaviors, and other variables significantly increase the risk for a number of diseases. Various chapters of this text discuss these variables. Several controllable risk factors are noted with an asterisk in the following list. These factors influence a person's response to pathogens:[1]

- Dosage, virulence, and portal of entry of agent
- Age at time of infection
- Preexisting level of immunity*
- Nature and vigor of immune response*
- Genetic factors controlling immune response
- Nutritional status of host*
- Preexisting diseases*
- Personal habits: smoking, alcohol, exercise, drugs*
- Dual infection or superinfection with other agents
- Psychological factors (e.g., motivation, emotional status, and so on)

What do you think?

If you were to list your own risk factors for infectious diseases, what would they be? ✳ *What actions can you take to reduce your risks?* ✳ *Are your risks greater today than before you entered college?* ✳ *Why or why not?*

The Pathogens: Routes of Transmission

Pathogens enter the body in several ways. They may be transmitted by *direct contact* between infected persons, such as during sexual relations, kissing, or touching, or by *indirect contact,* such as by touching an object the infected person has had contact with. The hands are probably the greatest source of infectious disease transmission. You may also **autoinoculate** yourself, or transmit a pathogen from one part of your body to another. For example, you may touch a sore on your lip that is teeming with viral herpes, then transmit the virus to your eye when you scratch your itchy eyelid.

Pathogens are also transmitted by *airborne contact*—you can breathe in air that carries a particular pathogen—or by *food-borne infection* if you eat something contaminated by microorganisms. Recent episodes of food poisoning from *Salmonella* bacteria found in certain foods and *E. coli* bacteria found in undercooked beef have raised concerns about

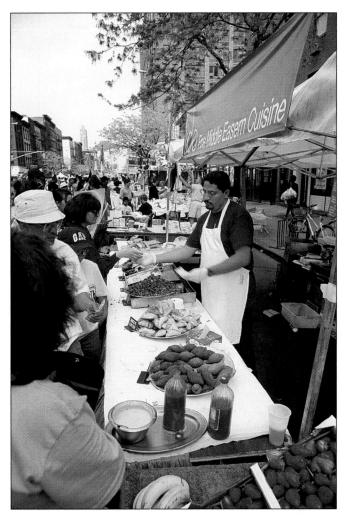

Airborne pathogens can be transmitted easily and unknowingly, thus special precautions must be taken to ensure the health and safety patrons of food markets and other public places.

the safety of the U.S. food supply. As a direct result of these concerns, food labels now caution consumers to cook meats thoroughly, wash utensils, and take other food-handling precautions.

Your best friend may be the source of *animal-borne pathogens.* Dogs, cats, livestock, and wild animals can spread numerous diseases through their bites or feces or by carrying infected insects into living areas and transmitting diseases either directly or indirectly. Although **interspecies transmission** of diseases (diseases passed from humans to animals and vice versa) is rare, it does occur. Pathogens may also be transmitted via mosquitoes, ticks, and other hosts that spread disease through sucking or biting. *Water-borne diseases* are transmitted directly from drinking water and indirectly from foods washed or sprayed with contaminated water. These pathogens can also invade your body if you wade or swim in contaminated streams, lakes, or reservoirs. Mothers may also transmit diseases *perinatally* to an infant in the womb or as the baby passes through the vagina during birth.

Autoinoculation   Transmission of a pathogen from one part of the body to another.

Interspecies transmission   Transmission of disease from humans to animals or from animals to humans.

Bacteria

Bacteria are single-celled organisms that are plantlike in nature but lack chlorophyll (the pigment that gives plants their green coloring). There are three major types of bacteria: cocci, bacilli, and spirilla. Bacteria can be viewed under a standard light microscope.

Although there are several thousand species of bacteria, only approximately 100 cause diseases in humans. In many cases, it is not the bacteria themselves that cause disease but rather the poisonous substances, called **toxins,** that they produce. The following are the most common bacterial infections.

Staphylococcal Infections   Staphylococci are normally present on our skin at all times and usually cause few problems. But when there is a cut or break in the **epidermis,** or outer layer of the skin, staphylococci may enter and cause a localized infection. If you have ever suffered from acne, boils, styes (infections of the eyelids), or infected wounds, you have probably had a staph infection.

At least one staph-caused disorder, **toxic shock syndrome,** is potentially fatal. Although most cases of toxic shock syndrome have occurred in menstruating women, the disease was first reported in 1978 in a group of children and continues to be reported in people recovering from wounds, surgery, or other injury.

To reduce the likelihood of toxic shock syndrome, take the following precautions: (1) avoid superabsorbent tampons except during the heaviest menstrual flow; (2) change tampons at least every four hours; and (3) use napkins at night instead of tampons.

Streptococcal Infections   At least five types of the **streptococcus** microorganism are known to cause bacterial infections: groups A, B, C, D, and G. Group A causes the most common diseases, such as streptococcal pharyngitis ("strep throat") and scarlet fever.[2] Group B streptococcus (GBS) can cause illness in newborn babies, pregnant women, the elderly, and adults with other illnesses such as diabetes or liver disease.[3]

Pneumonia   In the early twentieth century, **pneumonia** was one of the leading causes of death in the United States. This disease is characterized by chronic cough, chest pain, chills, high fever, fluid accumulation, and eventual respiratory failure. One of the most common forms of pneumonia is caused by bacterial infection and responds readily to antibiotic treatment in the early stages. Other forms are caused by viruses, chemicals, or other substances in the lungs and are more difficult to treat. Although medical advances have reduced the overall incidence of pneumonia, it continues to be a major threat in the United States and throughout the world. Vulnerable populations include the poor, the elderly, and those already suffering from other illnesses.[4]

Legionnaire's Disease   Legionnaire's disease is a bacterial disorder that gained widespread publicity in 1976, when several Legionnaires at the American Legion convention in Philadelphia contracted the disease and died before the invading organism was isolated and effective treatment devised. Although one of the lesser known diseases, the water-borne nature of this disease has led to several recent outbreaks in the United States.[5] The symptoms are similar to those of pneumonia, which sometimes makes identification difficult. In people whose resistance is lowered, particularly the elderly, delayed identification can have serious consequences.

Tuberculosis   One of the leading fatal diseases in the United States in the early twentieth century, **tuberculosis (TB)** was largely controlled in America by the mid-twentieth century as a result of improved sanitation, isolation of infected persons, and treatment with drugs such as *rifampin* or *isoniazid*. But though many health professionals assumed that TB had been conquered, that appears not to be the case. During the past 20 years, several factors have together led to an epidemic rise in the disease: deteriorating social conditions, including overcrowding and poor sanitation; failure to isolate active cases of TB; a weakening of public health infrastructure, which has led to less funding for screening; and migration of TB to the United States through international travel. Today, there are over 45,000 active cases of TB in the United States.[6] Newer strains of drug-resistant tuberculosis make this epidemic potentially more devastating than previous outbreaks.

Although increases in the incidence of TB in the United States are troubling, U.S. statistics pale by comparison to the staggering tuberculosis burden in the global population. Assuming no significant improvements in prevention and control between 1999 and 2020, the World Health Organization

---

Bacteria   Single-celled organisms that may cause disease.

Toxins   Poisonous substances produced by certain microorganisms that cause various diseases.

Staphylococci   Round, gram-positive bacteria, usually found in clusters.

Epidermis   The outermost layer of the skin.

Toxic shock syndrome   A potentially life-threatening bacterial infection that is most common in menstruating women who use tampons.

Streptococci   Round bacteria, usually found in chain formation.

Pneumonia   Disease of the lungs characterized by chronic cough, chest pain, chills, high fever, and fluid accumulation; may be caused by bacteria, viruses, chemicals, or other substances.

Tuberculosis (TB)   A disease caused by bacterial infiltration of the respiratory system.

(WHO) estimates that 1 billion people will acquire new tuberculosis infection, 200 million will develop active disease, and 70 million will die.[7]

Tuberculosis is caused by bacterial infiltration of the respiratory system that results in a chronic inflammatory reaction in the lungs. Airborne transmission via the respiratory tract is the primary and most efficient mode of transmitting TB. People with active cases can transmit the disease while talking, coughing, sneezing, or singing. Fortunately, tuberculosis is fairly difficult to catch, and prolonged exposure, rather than single exposure, is the typical mode of infection. Only about 20 to 30 percent of people exposed to an active case will become infected.[8] Symptoms include persistent coughing, weight loss, fever, and spitting up blood. A simple skin test will indicate infection, and treatments are effective for most nonresistant cases.

Periodontal Diseases   Diseases of the tissue around the teeth, called **periodontal diseases,** affect three out of four adults over age 35. Improper tooth care, including lack of flossing and poor brushing habits, and the failure to obtain professional dental care lead to increased bacterial growth, caries (tooth decay), and gum infections. If left untreated, permanent tooth loss may result.

> ### What do you think?
> *Why do you think we are experiencing global increases in diseases such as tuberculosis today?* ✳ *Should we be concerned about diseases in other countries?* ✳ *Do we have an obligation to help the world's population in their struggle against these diseases?* ✳ *What policies, programs, and services might help?*

Viruses

Viruses are the smallest pathogens, approximately 1/500th the size of bacteria. Because of their tiny size, they are visible only under an electron microscope and were not identified

---

Periodontal diseases   Diseases of the tissue around the teeth.

Viruses   Minute parasitic microbes that live inside another cell.

Interferon   A protein substance produced by the body that aids the immune system by protecting healthy cells.

Endemic   Describing a disease that is always present to some degree.

Influenza   A common viral disease of the respiratory tract.

---

until the twentieth century.[9] Over 150 viruses are known to cause diseases in humans. Their role in the development of various cancers and chronic diseases is still unclear.

Essentially, a virus consists of a protein structure that contains either *ribonucleic acid (RNA)* or *deoxyribonucleic acid (DNA)*. Incapable of carrying out the normal cell functions of respiration and metabolism, a virus cannot reproduce on its own and can exist only in a parasitic relationship with the cell it invades.

Viral diseases can be difficult to treat because many viruses can withstand heat, formaldehyde, and large doses of radiation with little effect on their structure. Drug treatment for viral infections is also limited. Drugs powerful enough to kill viruses generally kill the host cells too, although some medications block stages in viral reproduction without damaging the host cells.

When exposed to certain viruses, the body produces a protein substance known as **interferon.** Interferon does not destroy the invading microorganisms but sets up a protective mechanism to aid healthy cells in their struggle against the invaders. Although interferon research is promising, it should be noted that not all viruses stimulate interferon production.

The Common Cold   Colds are responsible for more days lost from work and more uncomfortable days spent at work than any other ailment.[10] Caused by any number of viruses (some experts claim there may be over 200 different viruses responsible for the common cold), colds are **endemic** (always present to some degree) among people throughout the world. In the course of a year, Americans suffer over 1 billion colds. Cold viruses are carried in the noses and throat most of the time. These viruses are held in check until the host's resistance is lowered. It is possible to "catch" a cold—from the airborne droplets of another person's sneeze or from skin-to-skin or mucous membrane contact—though recent studies indicate that the hands may be the greatest avenue of colds and transmission of other viruses.[11] Although many people believe that a cold results from exposure to cold weather or from getting chilled or overheated, experts believe that such things have little or no effect on cold development. Stress, allergy disorders that affect the nasal passages, and menstrual cycles do, however, appear to increase susceptibility.[12]

The best rule of thumb is to keep your resistance level high. Sound nutrition, adequate rest, stress reduction, and regular exercise appear to be the best bets in helping fight off infection. Avoid people with newly developed colds (colds appear to be most contagious during the first 24 hours of onset). If you contract a cold, bed rest, plenty of fluids, and aspirin to relieve pain and discomfort are the tried-and-true remedies for adults. Children should not be given aspirin for colds or the flu because of the possibility that this may lead to *Reye's syndrome,* a potentially fatal disease.

Influenza   In otherwise healthy people, **influenza,** or flu, is usually not serious. Symptoms, including aches and pains, nausea, diarrhea, fever, and coldlike ailments, generally pass very quickly. However, in combination with other disorders or among the elderly, those with respiratory or heart disease, or children under the age of five, the flu can be very serious.

To date, three major varieties of flu virus have been discovered, with many different strains existing within each variety. The "A" form of the virus is generally the most virulent, followed by the "B" and "C" varieties. If you contract one form of influenza you may develop immunity to it, but you will not necessarily be immune to other forms of the disease. Little can be done to treat flu patients once the infection has become established. Some vaccines have proved effective against certain strains of flu virus, but they are totally ineffective against others. In spite of minor risks, it is recommended that people over age 65, pregnant women, people with heart or lung disease, and those with certain other illnesses be vaccinated.

Infectious Mononucleosis   The symptoms of mononucleosis, or "mono," include sore throat, fever, headache, nausea, chills, and a pervasive weakness or tiredness in the initial stages. As the disease progresses, lymph nodes may swell, and jaundice, spleen enlargement, aching joints, and body rashes may occur.

Caused by the *Epstein-Barr virus,* mononucleosis is readily detected through a *monospot test,* a blood test that measures the percentage of specific forms of white blood cells. Because many viruses are caused by transmission of body fluids, many people once believed that young people passed the disease on by kissing (hence its nickname, "the kissing disease.") Although this is still considered a possible cause, mononucleosis is not believed to be highly contagious. It does not appear to be easily contracted through normal, everyday personal contact.

Treatment of mononucleosis is often a lengthy process that involves bed rest, balanced nutrition, and medications. Gradually, the body develops immunity to the disease, and the person returns to normal activity.

Hepatitis   One of the most highly publicized viral diseases is **hepatitis,** a virally caused inflammation of the liver. Hepatitis symptoms include fever, headache, nausea, loss of appetite, skin rashes, pain in the upper right abdomen, dark yellow (with brownish tinge) urine, and jaundice (yellowing of the whites of the eyes and the skin). In some regions of the United States and among certain segments of the population, hepatitis has reached epidemic proportions. Internationally, viral hepatitis is a major contributor to acute and chronic liver disease, accounting for high morbidity and mortality. Currently, there are seven known forms, with the following three indicating the highest rate of incidence:

- *Hepatitis A (HAV).* HAV is contracted from eating food or drinking water contaminated with human excrement. Each year, over 150,000 people in the United States are infected, typically through something in the household, sexual contact, day care attendance, or international

travel. Fortunately, people with HAV do not become chronic carriers.[13]

- *Hepatitis B (HBV).* This disease, spread primarily through body fluids, particularly during unprotected sex, can lead to chronic liver disease or a form of liver cancer. One of the fastest growing sexually transmitted infections in the United States, with over 300,000 new cases per year, HBV infection is currently more prevalent than HIV. Over 1.2 million people are chronic carriers.[14] Most people recover within 6 months, although some become chronic carriers.

- *Hepatitis C (HCV).* Hepatitis C infections are on an epidemic rise in many regions of the world, as resistant forms are emerging. Currently, it is estimated that there are 150,000 new cases of hepatitis C in the United States each year, with over 4 million people infected.[15] Over 85 percent of those infected develop chronic infections, and if the infection is left untreated, the person may develop cirrhosis of the liver, liver cancer, or liver failure. Liver failure due to chronic hepatitis C is the leading cause of liver transplants in the United States.[16] Some cases can be traced to blood transfusions or organ transplants.

In the United States, hepatitis continues to be a major threat in spite of a safe blood supply and massive efforts at education about hand washing (hepatitis A) and safer sex (primarily hepatitis B). Treatment of all forms of viral hepatitis is somewhat limited.

Measles   Measles is a viral disorder that often affects young children. Symptoms, appearing about ten days after exposure, include an itchy rash and a high fever. **German measles (rubella)** is a milder viral infection that is believed to be transmitted by inhalation, after which it multiplies in the upper respiratory tract and passes into the bloodstream. It causes a rash, especially on the upper extremities. It is not generally a serious health threat and usually runs its course in three to four days. The major exceptions to this rule are among newborns and pregnant women. Rubella can damage a fetus, particularly during the first trimester, creating a condition known as congenital rubella, in which the infant may be born blind, deaf, cognitively impaired, or with heart defects. Immunization has reduced the incidence of both measles and German measles. Infections in children not immunized against measles can lead to fever-induced

---

Hepatitis   A virally caused disease in which the liver becomes inflamed, producing symptoms such as fever, headache, and jaundice.

Measles   A viral disease that produces symptoms including an itchy rash and a high fever.

German measles (rubella)   A milder form of measles that causes a rash and mild fever in children and may cause damage to a fetus or a newborn baby.

problems such as rheumatic heart disease, kidney damage, and neurological disorders. Fortunately, progress in eradicating Rubella has been remarkable, leaving little chance for a resurgence in the United States today.

Other Pathogens

Fungi   Hundreds of species of **fungi,** multicellular or unicellular primitive plants, inhabit our environment. Many fungi are useful, providing such foodstuffs as edible mushrooms and some cheeses. But some species of fungi can produce infections. *Candidiasis* (a vaginal yeast infection), athlete's foot, ringworm, and jock itch are examples of fungal diseases. Keeping the affected area clean and dry plus treatment with appropriate medications will generally bring prompt relief.

Protozoa   Protozoa are microscopic, single-celled organisms that are generally associated with tropical diseases such as African sleeping sickness and malaria. Although these pathogens are prevalent in the developing countries of the world, they are largely controlled in the United States. The most common protozoal disease in the United States is *trichomoniasis,* which we will discuss later in this chapter's section on sexually transmitted infections. A common water-borne protozoan disease in many regions of the country is *giardiasis.* Persons who drink or are exposed to the *Giardia* pathogen may suffer intestinal pain and discomfort weeks after infection. Protection of water supplies is the key to prevention.

Parasitic Worms   Parasitic worms are the largest of the pathogens. Ranging in size from the small pinworms typically found in children to the relatively large tapeworms found in all species of warm-blooded animals, most parasitic worms are more a nuisance than a threat. Of special note today are the worm infestations associated with eating raw fish in Japanese sushi restaurants. Cooking fish and other foods to temperatures sufficient to kill the worms and their eggs can prevent infestation.

Prions   A **prion,** or unconventional virus, is a self-replicating, protein-based *agent* that can infect humans and other animals. Believed to be the underlying cause of spongiform diseases such as "mad cow disease," this agent systematically destroys brain cells. We will discuss prion-based diseases later in this chapter.

Your Body's Defenses: Keeping You Well

Although all the pathogens just described pose a threat if they take hold in your body, the chances that they will do so are actually quite small. First, they must overcome a number of effective barriers, many of which were established in your body before you were born.

Physical and Chemical Defenses

Perhaps our most critical early defense system is the skin. Layered to provide an intricate web of barriers, the skin allows few pathogens to enter. **Enzymes,** complex proteins manufactured by the body that appear in body secretions such as sweat, provide additional protection, destroying microorganisms on skin surfaces by producing inhospitable pH levels. Microorganisms that flourish at a selected pH will be weakened or destroyed as these changes occur. A third protection is our frequent slight elevations in body temperature, which create an inhospitable environment for many pathogens. Only when cracks or breaks occur in the skin can pathogens gain easy access to the body.

The linings of the body provide yet another protection. Mucous membranes in the respiratory tract and other linings of the body trap and engulf invading organisms. *Cilia,* hairlike projections in the lungs and respiratory tract, sweep invaders toward body openings, where they are expelled. Tears, nasal secretions, earwax, and other secretions found at body entrances contain enzymes designed to destroy or neutralize pathogens. Finally, any organism that manages to breach such initial lines of defense faces a formidable specialized network of defenses thrown up by the immune system.

The Immune System: Your Body Fights Back

Immunity is a condition of being able to resist a particular disease by counteracting the substance that produces the disease. Any substance capable of triggering an immune response is called an **antigen.** An antigen can be a virus, a bacterium, a fungus, a parasite, or a tissue or cell from another individual. When invaded by an antigen, the body responds by forming substances called **antibodies,** which are

---

Fungi   A group of plants that lack chlorophyll and do not produce flowers or seeds; several microscopic varieties are pathogenic.

Protozoa   Microscopic, single-celled organisms.

Parasitic worms   The largest of the pathogens, most of which are more a nuisance than a threat.

Prion   One of the newest, more frightening pathogens to infect humans and animals in recent years; a self-replicating protein-based agent that systematically destroys brain cells.

Enzymes   Organic substances that cause bodily changes and destruction of microorganisms.

Antigen   Substance capable of triggering an immune response.

Antibodies   Substances produced by the body that are individually matched to specific antigens.

matched to the specific antigen much as a key is matched to a lock. Antibodies belong to a mass of large molecules known as *immunoglobulins,* a group of nine chemically distinct protein substances, each of which plays a role in neutralizing, setting up for destruction, or actually destroying antigens. Once an antigen breaches the body's initial defenses, the body begins a process of antigen analysis. It considers the size and shape of the invader, verifies that the antigen is not part of the body itself, and then produces a specific antibody to destroy or weaken the antigen. This process, which is much more complex than described here, is part of a system called *humoral immune responses.* Humoral immunity is the body's major defense against many bacteria and bacterial toxins.

Cell-mediated immunity is characterized by the formation of a population of lymphocytes that can attack and destroy the foreign invader. These lymphocytes constitute the body's main defense against viruses, fungi, parasites, and some bacteria. Key players in this immune response are specialized groups of white blood cells known as *macrophages* (a type of phagocytic, or cell-eating, cell) and *lymphocytes,* other white blood cells in the blood, lymph nodes, bone marrow, and certain glands.

Two forms of lymphocytes in particular, the *B-lymphocytes* (B-cells) and *T-lymphocytes* (T-cells), are involved in the immune response. There are different types of B-cells, named according to the area of the body in which they develop. Most are manufactured in the soft tissue of the hollow shafts of the long bones. T-cells, in contrast, develop and multiply in the thymus, a multilobed organ that lies behind the breastbone. T-cells assist the immune system in several ways. *Regulatory T-cells* help direct the activities of the immune system and assist other cells, particularly B-cells, to produce antibodies. Dubbed "helper T's," these cells are essential for activating B-cells, other T-cells, and macrophages. Another form of T-cell, known as the "killer T" or "cytotoxic T," directly attacks infected or malignant cells. Killer T-cells enable the body to rid itself of cells that have been infected by viruses or transformed by cancer; they are also responsible for the rejection of tissue and organ grafts. The third type of T-cell, "suppressor T," turns off or suppresses the activity of B-cells, killer T-cells, and macrophages. Suppressor T-cells circulate in the bloodstream and lymphatic system, neutralizing or destroying antigens, enhancing the effects of the immune response, and helping to return the activated immune system to normal levels. After a successful attack on a pathogen, some of the attacker T- and B-cells are preserved as *memory T- and B-cells,* enabling the body to quickly recognize and respond to subsequent attacks by the same kind of organism at a later time. Thus, macrophages, T- and B-cells, and antibodies are the key factors in mounting an immune response.

Once people have survived infectious diseases, they become immune to those diseases, meaning that in all probability they will not develop them again. Upon subsequent attack by the disease-causing microorganism, their memory T- and B-cells are quickly activated to come to their defense.

Autoimmune Diseases   Although white blood cells and the antigen–antibody response generally work in our favor by neutralizing or destroying harmful antigens, the body sometimes makes a mistake and targets its own tissue as the enemy, builds up antibodies against that tissue, and attempts to destroy it. This is known as *autoimmune disease (auto* means "self"). Common autoimmune disorders are rheumatoid arthritis, lupus erythematosus, and myasthenia gravis.

In some cases, the antigen–antibody response completely fails to function. The result is a form of *immune deficiency syndrome.* Perhaps the most dramatic case of this syndrome was the "bubble boy," a youngster who died in 1984 after living his short life inside a sealed-off environment designed to protect him from all antigens. A much more common immune system disorder is *acquired immune deficiency syndrome (AIDS),* which we will discuss later in this chapter.

Fever

If an infection is localized, pus formation, redness, swelling, and irritation often occur. These symptoms indicate that the invading organisms are being fought systematically. Another indication is the development of a fever, or a rise in body temperature above the norm of 98.6°F. Fever is frequently caused by toxins secreted by pathogens that interfere with the control of body temperature. Although this elevated temperature is often harmful to the body, it is also believed to act as a form of protection. Raising body temperature by even one or two degrees provides an environment that destroys some disease-causing organisms. A fever also stimulates the body to produce more white blood cells, which destroy more invaders.

Pain

Although pain is not usually thought of as a defense mechanism, it is a response to injury, and it plays a valuable role in the body's response to invasion. Pain may be either *direct pain,* caused by the stimulation of nerve endings in an affected area, or **referred pain,** meaning that it is present in one place although the source is elsewhere. Most pain responses are accompanied by inflammation. Pain tends to be the earliest sign that an injury has occurred and often causes the person to slow down or stop the activity that was aggravating the injury, thereby protecting against further damage. Because it is often one of the first warnings of disease, persistent pain should not be overlooked or masked with short-term pain relievers.

> **Referred pain**   Pain that is present at one point, but whose source is elsewhere.

Table 14.1
Recommended Childhood Immunization Schedule

VACCINE	BIRTH	2 MOS	4 MOS	6 MOS	12 MOS	15 MOS	18 MOS	4–6 YRS	11–12 YRS	14–16 YRS
Hepatitis B (HepB)	HepB-1	HepB-2		HepB-3						
Diphtheria, tetanus, pertussis		DTP	DTP	DTP	DTP or DTaP at ≥15 months			DTP or DTaP	Td	
Haemophilus influenzae type b (Hib)		Hib	Hib	Hib	Hib					
Polio		OPV	OPV	OPV				OPV		
Measles, mumps, rubella						MMR		MMR or MMR		
Varicella zoster (VZV)					VZV	VZV	VZV			

Mothers who have tested positive for hepatitis B should consult their doctors about their infants' vaccinations.

HepB vaccine recommended at 11–12 years of age for children not previously vaccinated.

VZV recommended at 11–12 years of age for children who were not previously vaccinated and who lack a reliable history of chicken pox. Children under 13 years of age should receive a single dose; persons 13 years of age and older should receive 2 doses 4–8 weeks apart.

Source: American Academy of Pediatrics, "Recommended Childhood Immunization Schedule, United States," (Washington, DC: American Academy of Pediatrics, 1998).

Vaccines: Bolstering Your Immunity

Recall that once people have been exposed to a specific pathogen, subsequent attacks will activate their memory T- and B-cells, giving them immunity. This is the principle on which **vaccination** is based.

A vaccine consists of killed or attenuated (weakened) versions of a disease-causing microorganism, or an antigen that is similar to but less dangerous than the disease antigen. It is administered to stimulate the person's immune system to produce antibodies against future attacks—without actually causing the disease. Vaccines are given orally or by injection, and this form of artificial immunity is termed **acquired immunity,** in contrast to **natural immunity,** which a mother passes to her fetus via their shared blood supply.

Depending on the virulence of the organism, vaccines containing live, attenuated, or dead organisms are given for a variety of diseases. In some instances, if a person is already weakened by other health problems, vaccination may provoke an actual mild case of the disease. Table 14.1 shows the recommended schedule for childhood vaccinations.

Emerging and Resurgent Diseases

Although our immune systems are remarkably adept at responding to many challenges, they are threatened by an army of microbes that is so diverse, so virulent, and so insidious that the invaders appear to be gaining ground. According to the World Health Organization's *World Health Report* issued in 2000, trends such as the aging of the population (the young and old are particularly vulnerable), the urbanization of developing countries, poverty, environmental pollution, globalization of the food supply, and crumbling health care systems bode very badly for the future. As international travel increases (over 1 million people per day cross international boundaries), with germs transported from remote regions of developing countries to huge urban centers within a matter of hours, the likelihood of infection by microbes previously unknown on U.S. soil increases. Table 14.2 identifies major contributors to the emergence and resurgence of infectious diseases.

Tiny Microbes: Lethal Threats

Today's arsenal of antibiotics appears to be increasingly ineffective. Penicillin-resistant strains of diseases are on the rise

> **Vaccination** Inoculation with killed or weakened pathogens or similar, less dangerous antigens in order to prevent or lessen the effects of some disease.
>
> **Acquired immunity** Immunity developed during life in response to disease, vaccination, or exposure.
>
> **Natural immunity** Immunity passed to a fetus by its mother.

Table 14.2
Factors Contributing to Emergent/Resurgent Disease Spread and Possible Solutions

CONTRIBUTING FACTORS	POSSIBLE SOLUTIONS
Hardier bugs: tiny size, adaptability, resistant strains, misuse of antibiotics	Increased pharmaceutical efforts, new drug development, selective use of new drugs; improved vaccination rates; funding of new research
Failure to prioritize public health initiatives on national level	Increased government funding; improved efforts aimed at prevention and intervention (Less than 1 percent of the federal budget goes to prevention programs.)
Explosive population growth: resource degradation, overcrowding, land use atrocities, increased urbanization	Population control, wise use of natural resources, environmental controls, reduced deforestation and increased pollution prevention efforts
International travel	Education or risk reduction; restrictions related to unvaccinated populations; improved air quality and venting on commercial airlines
Human behaviors, particularly IV drug use and risky sexual behavior	Education about risky behaviors; incentives for improved behaviors; increased personal motivation
Vector management failures: widespread overuse/misuse of pesticides and antimicrobial agents that hasten resistance	Management of pesticide use; focus on pollution prevention; regulation; enforcement of laws
Food and water contamination; globalization of food supply and centralized processing	Control of population growth; animal controls; food controls; improved environmental legislation; food safety; pollution prevention
Complacency and apathy	Education—develop "we" mentality rather than "me" mentality
Poverty	Government support; international aid for vaccination programs early diagnosis, and treatment; care for disadvantaged
War and mass refugee migration, famine, disasters	Government intervention; international aid
Aging of population	Support for prevention/intervention against controllable age-related health problems
Irrigation, deforestation, and reforestation projects that alter habitats of disease-carrying insects and animals	Improved techniques for conservation; responsible use of resources; policies and programs that protect environment
Increased human contact with tropical rainforests and other wilderness habitats that are reservoirs for insects and animals that harbor unknown infectious agents	Increased regulation to reduce human impact; more research to improve interactions between humans and environment

Sources: Authors, plus information from U.S. Department of Health and Human Services, Centers for Disease Control and Prevention, "Preventing Emerging Infectious Diseases: A Strategy for the 21st Century" (Altanta: CDC, 1993), p. 3.

as microbes become able to outlast and outsmart even the best of our antibiotic weapons.[17] Old scourges are back, and new ones are emerging.

"Mad Cow Disease" The British beef industry is in crisis, and meat eaters from Europe to the United States are nervous about the possibility of dying from that burger they ate last year. Since 1996, evidence has been increasing that there is a relationship between ongoing outbreaks in Europe of a disease in cattle known as *bovine spongiform encephalitis* (BSE, or "mad cow disease") and a disease in humans known as *new variant Creutzfeldt-Jakob disease* (NvCJD).[18] Both disorders are invariably fatal brain diseases with unusually long incubation periods measured in years, and both are caused by unconventional transmittable agents known as prions. BSE is thought to have been transmitted when cows were fed a protein-based substance (slaughterhouse leftovers

from sheep and other cows) to help them put on weight and grow faster. Failure to treat this protein by-product sufficiently to kill the BSE organism allowed it to infect the cows. The disease is believed to be transmitted to humans through the meat of these slaughtered cows. The resultant variant of BSE in humans, known as Creutzfeldt-Jakob disease and characterized by progressively worsening neurological damage and possible death, was noted in ten people in England and linked by some studies to the BSE-diseased cows. With that, the mad-cow scare emerged. As scientists continue to look at this possible link, it should be noted that such a link has not yet been scientifically verified. In fact, the human form of BSE has not been detected in the United States despite active surveillance since 1990. It is extremely unlikely that BSE would become a food-borne hazard in the United States.[19]

Dengue and Dengue Hemorrhagic Fever   Transmitted by mosquitoes, **dengue** viruses are the most widespread arthropod viruses in the world. Today, dengue is found on most continents, and over one half of all United Nations member states are threatened.[20] Dengue symptoms include flulike nausea, aches, and chronic fatigue and weakness. As urban areas become increasingly infected with mosquitoes, nearly 1.5 billion people, including about 600 million children, are at risk. Each year, it is estimated that over 100 million people are infected, and over 8,000 die.[21] A more serious form of the disease, **dengue hemorrhagic fever,** can kill children in 6 to 12 hours, as the virus causes capillaries to leak and spill fluid and blood into surrounding tissue. Dengue is on the rise in the United States, largely because of increased international travel.

Ebola   Ebola virus, which causes fever and massive internal hemorrhaging, is fortunately not as prevalent worldwide as dengue fever. In 1995, an outbreak in Zaire killed 245 of the 316 people infected, forcing strict quarantine of the region. Subsequent infections in other regions have caused increasing concern in the global community.

Cryptosporidium   In 1993, the intestinal parasite *Cryptosporidium* infected the municipal water supply of Milwaukee, Wisconsin. The result was the largest water-borne coccidian protozoan disease outbreak ever recognized in this country, causing many deaths and sickening hundreds of thousands of people. Exactly how the water supply became infected remains in question; however, the fact that humans, birds, and animals can carry the infective agent opens the door for many possible routes.

Escherichia coli O157:H7   During the past decade, a rash of food-borne deaths and illnesses have been traced to foods contaminated with *Escherichia coli* bacteria. Once thought to be limited to uncooked meat, recent infections from apple juice were linked to cows defecating in areas where wind-fall apples are picked up for juice.

While *E. coli* organisms continue to pose threats to humans, recent findings indicate that simple changes in the way cattle are fed prior to slaughter may reduce risks. If grain is eliminated from the diet of these cattle, *E. coli* bacteria tend to die in cattle stomachs.

Cholera   Cholera, an infectious disease transmitted through fecal contamination of food or water supplies, has been rare in the United States for most of the past century. Recent epidemic outbreaks in the Western Hemisphere (over 900,000 cases), however, have started to affect the United States. Efforts to control cholera may be increasingly difficult as international travel and trade increase.

Hantavirus   Transmitted via rodent feces, this virus was responsible for many deaths in the desert areas of the southwestern United States in 1994 before experts were able to identify the culprit. Victims were believed to have come into contact with this organism through breathing the virus-laden dust created in rodent-infested homes. Within hours, victims showed serious symptoms as their lungs filled with fluid; they subsequently experienced respiratory collapse and died. Today, cases of hantavirus have been noted in over 20 states, and vaccines are being developed to counteract it.

Bioterrorism: The New Global Threat   The idea of using infectious microorganisms as weapons is not new. In fact, in the English wars with Native Americans, blankets impregnated with scabs from patients with smallpox were traded to Native Americans in hopes of causing disease.[22] In the 1980s, a large community outbreak of salmonellosis in Oregon was believed to originate in intentional contamination of salad bars in multiple restaurants, carried out by followers of an extremist religious group.[23]

The threat of delivering a lethal load of anthrax or other deadly microorganisms in the warheads of missiles is a topic of much discussion among today's world leaders, particularly after the cases of anthrax delivered via the mail following the September 11, 2001, terrorist attacks. For a complete listing of those biological threats considered to pose the greatest risk, see the Bioterrorism box in Chapter 7.

Sexually Transmitted Infections

Sexually transmitted infections (STIs) have been with human beings since earliest recorded history. Today, there are more than 20 known types of STIs. Once referred to as "venereal diseases" and then "sexually transmitted diseases," the most current terminology is more reflective of the number and types of these communicable diseases. More virulent strains and more antibiotic-resistant forms spell trouble for at-risk populations in the days ahead.

A report issued by the Centers for Disease Control and Prevention (CDC) in 2000 indicates that there were 16.2 million new occurrences of STIs in 1999, an increase of over 3.5 million since 1988.[24] According to Felicia Stewart of the Kaiser Family Health Foundation, "[T]here is no indication that STIs are coming rapidly under control. . . . In fact, people vastly underestimate risks and fail to take precautions. A . . . Kaiser survey found that just 14% of men and 8% of women felt at risk for STIs, even though at least one third will get one."[25]

Dengue   A disease transmitted by mosquitoes, which causes flulike symptoms.

Dengue hemorrhagic fever   A more serious form of dengue.

Sexually transmitted infections (STIs)   Infectious diseases transmitted via some form of intimate, usually sexual, contact.

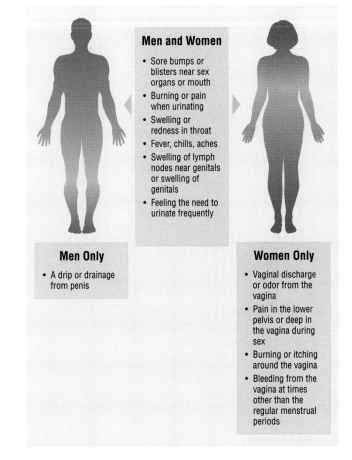

Men and Women
- Sore bumps or blisters near sex organs or mouth
- Burning or pain when urinating
- Swelling or redness in throat
- Fever, chills, aches
- Swelling of lymph nodes near genitals or swelling of genitals
- Feeling the need to urinate frequently

Men Only
- A drip or drainage from penis

Women Only
- Vaginal discharge or odor from the vagina
- Pain in the lower pelvis or deep in the vagina during sex
- Burning or itching around the vagina
- Bleeding from the vagina at times other than the regular menstrual periods

Figure 14.2
Signs or Symptoms of an STI

Early symptoms of an STI are often mild (Figure 14.2). Left untreated, some of these infections can have grave consequences, such as sterility, blindness, central nervous system destruction, disfigurement, and even death. Infants born to mothers carrying the organisms for these infections are at risk for a variety of health problems. As with many communicable diseases, much of the pain, suffering, and anguish associated with STIs can be eliminated through education, responsible action, simple preventive strategies, and prompt treatment.

Possible Causes: Why Me?

Several reasons have been proposed to explain the present high rates of STIs. The first relates to the moral and social stigma associated with these infections. Shame and embarrassment often keep infected people from seeking treatment. Unfortunately, these people usually continue to be sexually active, thereby infecting unsuspecting partners. People who are uncomfortable discussing sexual issues may also be less likely to use and ask their partners to use condoms to protect against STIs and pregnancy.

Another reason proposed for the STI epidemic is our culture's casual attitude about sex. Bombarded by media hype that glamorizes easy sex, many people take sexual partners without considering the consequences. Others are pressured into sexual relationships they don't really want. Generally, the more sexual partners a person has, the greater the risk for contracting an STI. Evaluate your own attitude about STIs by completing the accompanying Assess Yourself box.

Ignorance—about the infections, their symptoms, and the fact that someone can be asymptomatic but still be infected—is also a factor. A person who is infected but asymptomatic can unknowingly spread an STI to an unsuspecting partner, who may in turn ignore or misinterpret any symptoms. By the time either partner seeks medical help, he or she may have infected several others.

Modes of Transmission

Sexually transmitted infections are generally spread through some form of intimate sexual contact. Sexual intercourse, oral–genital contact, hand–genital contact, and anal intercourse are the most common modes of transmission. More rarely, pathogens for STIs are transmitted from mouth to mouth or through contact with fluids from body sores. Although each STI is a different infection caused by a different pathogen, all STI pathogens prefer dark, moist places, especially the mucous membranes lining the reproductive organs. Most of them are susceptible to light, excess heat, cold, and dryness, and many die quickly on exposure to air. (The toilet seat is not a likely breeding ground for most bacterial or viral STIs!) Although most STIs are passed on by sexual contact, other kinds of close contact, such as sleeping on sheets used by someone who has pubic lice, may also infect you. Like other communicable infections, STIs have both pathogen-specific incubation periods and periods of time during which transmission is most likely, called periods of communicability.

Chlamydia

Chlamydia, a disease that often presents no symptoms, tops the list of the most commonly reported infections in the United States. Chlamydia infects about 4 million people annually in the United States, the majority of cases being women.[26] Public health officials believe that the actual number of cases is probably higher because these figures represent only those cases reported. College students account for over 10 percent of infections, and these numbers seem to be increasing yearly.

The name of the disease is derived from the Greek verb *chlamys,* meaning "to cloak," because, unlike most bacteria, *Chlamydia* bacteria can live and grow only inside other cells. Although many people classify chlamydia as either *nonspecific* or *nongonococcal urethritis (NGU),* a person may

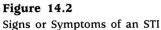

Chlamydia   Bacterially caused STI of the urogenital tract.

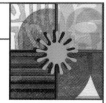

Sexually Transmitted Infections Attitude and Belief Scale

The following quiz will help you evaluate whether your beliefs and attitudes about STIs lead you to take risks that increase your risk of infection.

DIRECTIONS

Indicate that you believe the following items are true or false by circling the T or the F. Then consult the answer key that follows.

1. You can usually tell whether someone is infected with an STI, especially HIV infection.   T   F
2. Chances are that if you haven't caught an STI by now, you probably have a natural immunity and won't get infected in the future.   T   F
3. A person who is successfully treated for an STI needn't worry about getting it again.   T   F
4. So long as you keep yourself fit and healthy, you needn't worry about STIs.   T   F
5. The best way for sexually active people to protect themselves from STIs is to practice safer sex.   T   F
6. The only way to catch an STI is to have sex with someone who has one.   T   F
7. Talking about STIs with a partner is so embarrassing that it's better not to raise the subject and instead hope the other person will.   T   F
8. STIs are mostly a problem for people who have numerous sex partners.   T   F
9. You don't need to worry about contracting an STI so long as you wash yourself thoroughly with soap and hot water immediately after sex.   T   F
10. You don't need to worry about AIDS if no one you know has ever come down with it.   T   F
11. When it comes to STIs, it's all in the cards. Either you're lucky or you're not.   T   F
12. The time to worry about STIs is when you come down with one.   T   F
13. As long as you avoid risky sexual practices, such as anal intercourse, you're pretty safe from STIs.   T   F
14. The time to talk about safer sex is before any sexual contact occurs.   T   F
15. A person needn't be concerned about an STI if the symptoms clear up on their own in a few weeks.   T   F

SCORING KEY

1. **False.** While some STIs have telltale signs, such as the appearance of sores or blisters on the genitals or disagreeable genital odors, others do not. Several STIs, such as chlamydia, gonorrhea (especially in women), internal genital warts, and even HIV infection in its early stages cause few if any obvious signs or symptoms. You often cannot tell whether your partner is infected with an STI. Many of the nicest-looking and well-groomed people carry STIs, often unknowingly. The only way to know whether a person is infected with HIV is by means of an HIV-antibody test.
2. **False.** If you practice unprotected sex and have not contracted an STI to this point, count your blessings. The thing about good luck is that it eventually runs out.
3. **False.** Sorry. Successful treatment does not render immunity against reinfection. You still need to take precautions to avoid reinfection, even if you have had an STI in the past and were successfully treated. If you answered true to this item, you're not alone. About one in five college students polled in a recent survey of more than 5,500 college students across Canada believed that a person who gets an STI cannot get it again.
4. **False.** Even people in prime physical condition can be felled by the tiniest of microbes that cause STIs. Physical fitness is no protection against these microscopic invaders.
5. **True.** If you are sexually active, practicing safer sex is the best protection against contracting an STI.
6. **False.** STIs can also be transmitted through nonsexual means, such as by sharing contaminated needles or, in some cases, through contact with disease-causing organisms on towels and bed sheets or even toilet seats.

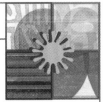

7. False. Because of the social stigma attached to STIs, it's understandable that you may feel embarrassed about raising the subject with your partner. But don't let embarrassment prevent you from taking steps to protect your own and your partner's welfare.

8. False. While it stands to reason that people who are sexually active with numerous partners stand a greater chance that one of their sexual partners will carry an STI, all it takes is one infected partner to pass along an STI to you, even if he or she is the only partner you've had or even if the two of you had sex only once. STIs are a potential problem for anyone who is sexually active.

9. False. While washing your genitals immediately after sex may have some limited protective value, it is no substitute for practicing safer sex.

10. False. You can never know whether you may be the first among your friends and acquaintances to become infected. Moreover, symptoms of HIV infection may not appear for years after initial infection with the virus, so you may have sexual contacts with people who are infected but don't know it and who are capable of passing along the virus to you. You in turn may then pass it along to others, whether or not you are aware of any symptoms.

11. False. Nonsense. While luck may play a part in determining whether you have a sexual contact with an infected partner, you can significantly reduce your risk of contracting an STI.

12. False. The time to start thinking about STIs (thinking helps, but worrying only makes you more anxious than you need be) is now, not after you have contracted an infection. Some STIs, like herpes and AIDS, cannot be cured. The only real protection you have against them is prevention.

13. False. Any sexual contact between the genitals, or between the genitals and the anus, or between the mouth and genitals, is risky if one of the partners is infected with an STI.

14. True. Unfortunately, too many couples wait until they have commenced sexual relations to have "a talk." By then it may already be too late to prevent the transmission of an STI. The time to talk is before any intimate sexual contact occurs.

15. False. Several STIs, notably syphilis, HIV infection, and herpes, may produce initial symptoms that clear up in a few weeks. But while the early symptoms may subside, the infection is still at work within the body and requires medical attention. Also, as noted previously, the infected person is capable of passing along the infection to others, regardless of whether noticeable symptoms were ever present.

INTERPRETING YOUR SCORE

First, add up the number of items you got right. The higher your score, the lower your risk. The lower your score, the greater your risk. A score of 13 correct or better may indicate that your attitudes toward STIs would probably decrease your risk of contracting them. Yet even one wrong response on this test may increase your risk of contracting an STI. You should also recognize that attitudes have little effect on behavior unless they are carried into action. Knowledge alone isn't sufficient to protect yourself from STIs. You need to ask yourself how you are going to put knowledge into action by changing your behavior to reduce your chances of contracting an STI.

Source: From Jeffrey S. Nevid with Fern Gotfried, *Choices: Sex in the Age of STDs* (Boston: Allyn and Bacon, 1995), p. 10–13.
© Copyright 1995 by Allyn and Bacon. Reprinted by permission.

have NGU without having the organism for chlamydia. In males, early symptoms may include painful and difficult urination, frequent urination, and a watery, puslike discharge from the penis. Symptoms in females may include a yellowish discharge, spotting between periods, and occasional spotting after intercourse. Unfortunately, many chlamydia victims display no symptoms and therefore do not seek help until the disease has done secondary damage. Females are especially likely to be asymptomatic; over 70 percent do not realize they have the disease until secondary damage occurs.

The secondary damage resulting from chlamydia is serious in both sexes. Men can suffer damage to the prostate gland, seminal vesicles, and bulbourethral glands as well as arthritislike symptoms and damage to the blood vessels and heart. In women, chlamydia-related infection can injure the cervix or fallopian tubes, causing sterility, and can damage the inner pelvic structure, leading to pelvic inflammatory disease (PID). If an infected woman becomes pregnant, she has a high risk for miscarriage and stillbirth. *Chlamydia* bacteria may also be responsible for one type of **conjunctivitis,** an eye infection that affects not only adults but also infants, who can contract the disease from an infected mother during delivery. Untreated conjunctivitis can cause blindness. If detected early, chlamydia is easily treatable with antibiotics such as tetracycline, doxycycline, or erythromycin.

What do you think?

Even though many college students have heard about the risks of STIs and HIV infection, why do so many fail to use condoms and take other precautions? ✳ *What actions could you, other individuals, or your college community take to make more of your friends heed the warnings about STIs?*

Pelvic Inflammatory Disease (PID)

Pelvic inflammatory disease (PID) is a term used to describe a number of infections of the uterus, fallopian tubes, and ovaries. Although PID often results from an untreated sexually transmitted infection, especially chlamydia or gonorrhea, it is not actually an STI. Nonsexual causes of PID are also common, including excessive vaginal douching, cigarette smoking, and substance abuse.

In the United States, an estimated 500,000 to 1,000,000 cases of PID occur annually.[27] Symptoms vary but generally include acute inflammation of the pelvic cavity, severe pain in the lower abdomen, menstrual irregularities, fever, nausea, painful intercourse, tubal pregnancies, and severe depression.[28] Major consequences of untreated PID are infertility, ectopic pregnancy, chronic pelvic pain, and recurrent upper genital infections. Risk factors include young age at first sexual intercourse, multiple sex partners, high frequency of sexual intercourse, and change of sexual partners within the past 30 days. Regular gynecological examinations and early treatment for STI symptoms reduce risk.

Conjunctivitis   Serious inflammation of the eye caused by any number of pathogens or irritants; can be caused by STIs such as chlamydia.

Pelvic inflammatory disease (PID)   Term used to describe various infections of the female reproductive tract.

Gonorrhea   Second most common STI in the United States; if untreated, may cause sterility.

Syphilis   One of the most widespread STIs; characterized by distinct phases and potentially serious results.

Gonorrhea

Gonorrhea is one of the most common STIs in the United States, surpassed only by chlamydia in number of cases. The Institute of Medicine estimates that there are over 800,000 cases per year and that large numbers go unreported.[29] Health economists estimate that the annual cost of gonorrhea and its complications is over $1.1 billion.[30] Caused by the bacterial pathogen *Neisseria gonorrhoeae,* this infection primarily infects the linings of the urethra, genital tract, pharynx, and rectum. It may spread to the eyes or other body regions via the hands or body fluids, typically during vaginal, oral, or anal sex. Most victims are males between the ages of 20 and 24. Sexually active females between the ages of 15 and 19 are also at high risk.[31]

In males, a typical symptom is a white milky discharge from the penis accompanied by painful, burning urination two to nine days after contact. This is usually enough to send most men to the physician for treatment. However, about 20 percent of all males with gonorrhea are asymptomatic.

In females, the situation is just the opposite: only 20 percent experience any discharge, and few develop a burning sensation upon urinating until much later in the course of the infection (if ever). The organism can remain in the woman's vagina, cervix, uterus, or fallopian tubes for long periods with no apparent symptoms other than an occasional slight fever. Thus a woman can be unaware that she has been infected and that she is infecting her sexual partners.

If the infection is detected early, antibiotic treatment is generally effective within a short period of time. If the infection goes undetected in a woman, it can spread throughout the genital–urinary tract to the fallopian tubes and ovaries, causing sterility or, at the very least, severe inflammation and PID. The bacteria can also spread up the reproductive tract or, more rarely, can spread through the blood and infect the joints, heart valves, or brain. If an infected woman becomes pregnant, the infection can cause conjunctivitis in her infant. To prevent this, physicians routinely administer silver nitrate or penicillin preparations to the eyes of newborn babies.

Untreated gonorrhea in the male may spread to the prostate, testicles, urinary tract, kidney, and bladder. Blockage of the vasa deferentia due to scar tissue formation may cause sterility. In some cases, the penis develops a painful curvature during erection.

Syphilis

Syphilis is also caused by a bacterial organism, the *spirochete* known as *Treponema pallidum.* Because it is extremely delicate and dies readily upon exposure to air, dryness, or cold, the organism is generally transferred only through direct sexual contact. Typically, this means contact between sexual organs during intercourse, but in rare instances, the organism enters the body through a break in the skin, through deep kissing in which body fluids are exchanged, or through some other transmission of body fluids.

Syphilis is called the "great imitator" because its symptoms resemble those of several other infections. Left untreated, syphilis generally progresses through distinct stages. It should be noted, however, that some people experience no symptoms at all.

Primary Syphilis   The first stage of syphilis, particularly for males, is often characterized by the development of a **chancre** (pronounced "shank-er"), a sore at the site of the initial infection. This dime-sized chancre is painless, but it oozes with bacteria, ready to infect an unsuspecting partner. Usually the chancre appears three to four weeks after contact.

In males, the site of the chancre tends to be the penis or scrotum because this is the site where the organism first enters the body. But if the infection was contracted through oral sex, the sore can appear in the mouth, throat, or other "first contact" area. In females, the site of infection is often internal, on the vaginal wall or high on the cervix. Because the chancre is not readily apparent, the likelihood of detection is not great. In both males and females, the chancre will completely disappear in three to six weeks.

Secondary Syphilis   From a month to a year after the chancre disappears, secondary symptoms may appear, including a rash or white patches on the skin or on the mucous membranes of the mouth, throat, or genitals. Hair loss may occur, lymph nodes enlarge, and the victim may develop a slight fever or a headache. In rare cases, sores develop around the mouth or genitals. As during the active chancre phase, these sores contain infectious bacteria, and contact with them can spread the infection. In a few cases, there may be arthritic pain in the joints. Because symptoms vary so much and appear so much later than the sexual contact that caused them, the victim seldom connects the two. The infection thus often goes undetected even at this second stage. Symptoms may persist for a few weeks or months and then disappear, leaving the victim thinking that all is well.

Latent Syphilis   After the secondary stage, the syphilis spirochetes begin to invade body organs. Symptoms, including infectious lesions, may reappear periodically for two to four years after the secondary period. After this period, the infection is rarely transmitted to others, except during pregnancy, when it can be passed on to the fetus. The child will then be born with *congenital syphilis,* which can cause death or severe birth defects such as blindness, deafness, or disfigurement. Because in most cases the fetus does not become infected until after the first trimester, treatment of the mother during this period will usually prevent infection of the fetus.

In some instances, a child born to an infected mother will show no apparent signs of the infection at birth but within several weeks will develop body rashes, a runny nose, and symptoms of paralysis. Congenital syphilis is usually detected before it progresses much further. But sometimes the child's immune system will ward off the invading organism, and further symptoms may not surface until the teenage

years. Fortunately, most states protect against congenital syphilis by requiring prospective marriage partners to be tested for syphilis prior to obtaining a marriage license.

If untreated, latent syphilis will progress and infect more and more organs.

Late Syphilis   Years after syphilis has entered the body, its effects become all too evident. Late-stage syphilis indications include heart damage, central nervous system damage, blindness, deafness, paralysis, premature senility, and, ultimately, insanity.

Treatment for Syphilis   Because the organism is bacterial, it is treated with antibiotics, usually penicillin, benzathine penicillin G, or doxycycline. The major obstacle to treatment is misdiagnosis of this "imitator" infection.

Pubic Lice

Pubic lice, often called "crabs," are small parasites that are usually transmitted during sexual contact. More annoying than dangerous, they move easily from partner to partner during sex. They have an affinity for pubic hair, attaching themselves to the base of these hairs, where they deposit their eggs (nits). One to two weeks later, these nits develop into adults that lay eggs and migrate to other body parts, thus perpetuating the cycle.

Treatment includes washing clothing, furniture, and linens that may harbor the eggs. It usually takes two to three weeks to kill all larval forms. Although sexual contact is the most common mode of transmission, you can "catch" pubic lice from lying on sheets that an infected person has slept on. Sleeping in hotel and dormitory rooms in which sheets are not washed regularly or sitting on toilet seats where the nits or larvae have been dropped and lie in wait for a new carrier will put you at risk.

Genital HPV

Genital warts (also known as venereal warts or condylomas) are caused by a small group of viruses known as **human papillomaviruses (HPVs).** A person becomes infected when an

---

Chancre   Sore often found at the site of syphilis infection.

Pubic lice   Parasites that can inhabit various body areas, especially the genitals; also called "crabs."

Genital warts   Warts that appear in the genital area or the anus; caused by the human papillomaviruses (HPVs).

Human papillomaviruses (HPV)   A small group of viruses that cause genital warts.

HPV penetrates the skin and mucous membranes of the genitals or anus through sexual contact. HPV is among the most common forms of STI. The virus appears to be relatively easy to catch. The typical incubation period is from six to eight weeks after contact. Many people have no symptoms, particularly if the warts are located inside the reproductive tract. Others may develop a series of itchy bumps on the genitals, ranging in size from small pinheads to large cauliflowerlike growths. On dry skin (such as the shaft of the penis), the warts are commonly small, hard, and yellowish-gray, resembling warts that appear on other parts of the body.

Genital warts are of two different types: (1) *full-blown genital warts* that are noticeable as tiny bumps or growths, and (2) the much more prevalent *flat warts* that are not usually visible to the naked eye.

Risks and Treatments of Genital Warts Many genital warts eventually disappear on their own. Others grow and generate unsightly flaps of irregular flesh on the external genitalia. If they grow large enough to obstruct urinary flow or become irritated by clothing or sexual intercourse, they can cause significant problems.

The greatest threat from genital warts lies in the apparent relationship between them and a tendency for *dysplasia,* or changes in cells that may lead to a precancerous condition. It is known that within five years after infection, 30 percent of all HPV cases progress to the precancerous stage. If precancerous cases are left untreated, 70 percent of them will result in actual cancer. In addition, venereal warts pose a threat to a pregnant woman's fetus if the fetus is exposed to the virus during birth. Cesarean deliveries may be considered in serious cases.

Genital warts can be treated with topical medications or removed by being frozen with liquid nitrogen. Large warts may require surgical removal.

Candidiasis (Moniliasis)

Unlike many STIs, which are caused by pathogens that come from outside the body, the yeastlike fungus caused by the *Candida albicans* organism normally inhabits the vaginal tract in most women. Only under certain conditions, in which the normal chemical balance of the vagina is disturbed, will these organisms multiply and begin to cause problems.

The likelihood of **candidiasis** (also known as moniliasis or a *yeast infection*) increases if a woman has diabetes, if her immune system is overtaxed or malfunctioning, if she is taking birth control pills or other hormones, or if she is taking broad-spectrum antibiotics. All of these factors decrease the acidity of the vagina and create favorable conditions for a yeastlike infection.

Symptoms of candidiasis include severe itching and burning of the vagina and vulva, swelling of the vulva, and a white, cheesy vaginal discharge. These symptoms are collectively called **vaginitis,** or inflammation of the vagina. When this microbe infects the mouth, whitish patches form, and the condition is referred to as *thrush.* This monilial infection also occurs in males and is easily transmitted between sexual partners.

Candidiasis strikes at least half a million American women a year. Antifungal drugs applied on the surface or by suppository usually cure it in just a few days. For approximately one out of ten women, however, nothing seems to work, and the infection returns again and again. Symptoms can be aggravated by contact of the vagina with soaps, douches, perfumed toilet paper, chlorinated water, and spermicides. Tight-fitting jeans and pantyhose can provide the combination of moisture and irritant that the organism thrives on.

Trichomoniasis

Unlike many STIs, **trichomoniasis** is caused by a protozoan. Although as many as half of the men and women in the United States may carry this organism, most remain free of symptoms until their bodily defenses are weakened. Both men and women may transmit the infection, but women are the more likely candidates for infection. Symptoms include a foamy, yellowish, unpleasant-smelling discharge accompanied by a burning sensation, itching, and painful urination. These symptoms are most likely to occur during or shortly after menstruation, but they can appear at any time or be absent altogether. Although usually transmitted by sexual contact, the "trich" organism can also be spread by toilet seats, wet towels, or other items that have discharged fluids on them. You can also contract trichomoniasis by sitting naked on the locker room bench at your local gym. Treatment includes oral metronidazole, usually given to both sexual partners to avoid the possible "ping-pong" effect of repeated cross-infection so typical of STIs.

General Urinary Tract Infections

Although *general urinary tract infections (UTIs)* can be caused by various factors, some forms are sexually transmitted. Anytime invading organisms enter the genital area, they can travel up the urethra and enter the bladder. Similarly, organisms normally living in the rectum, urethra, or bladder may travel to the sexual organs and eventually be transmitted to another person.

Candidiasis Yeastlike fungal disease often transmitted sexually.

Vaginitis Set of symptoms characterized by vaginal itching, swelling, and burning.

Trichomoniasis Protozoan infection characterized by foamy, yellowish discharge and unpleasant odor.

You can also get a UTI through autoinoculation, often during the simple task of wiping yourself after defecating. Wiping from the anus forward can transmit organisms found in feces to the vaginal opening or the urethra. Contact between the hands and the urethra and between the urethra and other objects are also common means of autoinoculation. Women, with their shorter urethras, are more likely to contract UTIs. Hand washing with soap and water prior to sexual intimacy, foreplay, and so on, is recommended. Treatment depends on the nature and type of pathogen.

Herpes

Herpes is a general term for a family of infections characterized by sores or eruptions on the skin. Herpes infections range from mildly uncomfortable to extremely serious. **Genital herpes** is an infection caused by the herpes simplex virus (HSV).

There are two types of herpes simplex virus (HSV). Historically, the herpes simplex type 2 virus was considered the primary culprit in genital herpes, and herpes simplex virus type 1 was thought to affect the area of the lips and other body areas.[32] We now know that both type 1 and type 2 can infect any area of the body, producing lesions (sores) in and around the vaginal area, on the penis, around the anal opening, and on the buttocks or thighs. Occasionally, sores appear on other parts of the body. HSV remains in certain nerve cells for life and can flare up, or cause symptoms, when the body's ability to maintain itself is weakened.

The prodromal (precursor) phase of the infection is characterized by a burning sensation and redness at the site of infection. During this time, prescription medicines will often keep the disease from spreading. However, this phase of the disease is quickly followed by the second phase, in which a blister filled with a clear fluid containing the virus forms. If you pick at this blister or otherwise touch the site and spread this fluid with fingers, lipstick, lip balm, or other products, you can autoinoculate other body parts. Particularly dangerous is the possibility of spreading the infection to your eyes, because a herpes lesion on the eye can cause blindness.

Over a period of days, the unsightly blister will crust over, dry up, and disappear, and the virus will travel to the base of an affected nerve supplying the area and become dormant. Only when the victim becomes overly stressed, when diet and sleep are inadequate, when the immune system is overworked, or when excessive exposure to sunlight or other stressors occurs will the virus become reactivated (at the same site every time) and begin the blistering cycle all over again. These sores cast off (shed) viruses that can be highly infectious. However, it is important to note that a herpes site can shed the virus even when no overt sore is present, particularly during the prodromal stages (the interval between the earliest symptoms and blistering). People may get genital herpes by having sexual contact with others who don't know they are infected or who are having outbreaks of herpes without any sores. A person with genital herpes can

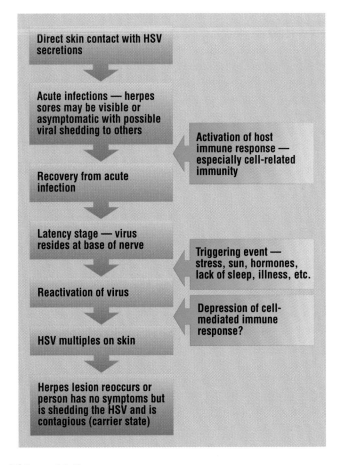

Figure 14.3
The Herpes Cycle
Source: Adapted by permission of Lippincott-Raven Publishers from "Sexually Transmitted Diseases in the 1990s," *STD Bulletin* 11 (1992): 4.

also infect a sexual partner during oral sex. The virus is spread only rarely, if at all, by touching objects such as a toilet seat or hot tub seat.[33] In fact, if you are seated on a toilet seat properly, your genitals should make contact only with air, and thus the likelihood of contact exposure would be exceedingly rare. Figure 14.3 summarizes the herpes cycle.

Genital herpes is especially serious in pregnant women because the baby could be infected as it passes through the vagina during birth. Many physicians recommend cesarean deliveries for infected women. Additionally, women who have a history of genital herpes appear to have a greater risk of developing cervical cancer.

Although there is no cure for herpes at present, certain drugs can reduce symptoms. Unfortunately, they seem to work only if the infection is confirmed during the first few hours after contact. As you may guess, this is rather rare. The effectiveness of other treatments, such as L-lysine, is largely

Genital herpes STI caused by the herpes simplex virus.

unsubstantiated. Newer over-the-counter medications seem to be moderately effective in reducing the severity of symptoms. Although lip balms and cold-sore medications may provide temporary anesthetic relief, remember that rubbing anything on a herpes blister can spread herpes-laden fluids to other body parts.

Preventing Herpes You can take precautions to reduce your risk of herpes:

- Avoid any form of kissing if you notice a sore or blister on your partner's mouth. Kiss no one, not even a peck on the cheek, if you know that you have a herpes lesion. Allow time after the sores go away before you start kissing again.
- Be extremely cautious if you have casual sexual affairs. Not every partner will feel obligated to tell you that he or she has a problem. It's up to you to protect yourself.
- Wash your hands immediately with soap and water after any form of sexual contact.
- If you have questionable sores or lesions, seek medical help at once. Do not be afraid to name your contacts.
- If you have herpes, be responsible in your sexual contacts with others. If you have any suspicious lesions that might put your partner at risk, say so. Find an appropriate time and place, and hold a candid discussion.
- Reduce your risk of herpes outbreaks by avoiding excessive stress, sunlight, or whatever else appears to trigger an episode.

HIV/AIDS

Acquired immune deficiency syndrome (AIDS) is a significant global health threat. Since 1981, when AIDS was first recognized, over 60 million people in the world have become infected with **human immunodeficiency virus (HIV),** the virus that causes AIDS. Over 18 million of these people have died, and another 14 million struggle with the disease.[34] In the United States, as of December 2000, over 775,000 men, women, and children with AIDS have been reported to the Centers for Disease Control and Prevention (CDC), and at least 449,000 have died.[35] The CDC estimates that at least 40,000 new infections occur each year in the United States.

A Shifting Epidemic

Under old definitions, people with HIV were diagnosed as having AIDS only when they developed blood infections, the

Acquired immune deficiency syndrome (AIDS) Extremely virulent sexually transmitted disease that renders the immune system inoperative.

Human immunodeficiency virus (HIV) The slow-acting virus that causes AIDS.

cancer known as Kaposi's sarcoma, or any of 21 other indicator diseases, most of which were common in males. The CDC has expanded the indicator list to include pulmonary tuberculosis, recurrent pneumonia, and invasive cervical cancer. Perhaps the most significant new indicator is a drop in the level of the body's master immune cells, called CD4s, to 200 per cubic millimeter (one-fifth the level in a healthy person).

AIDS cases have been reported state by state throughout the United States since the early 1980s as a means of tracking the disease. While the numbers of actual reported cases have always been suspect, improved reporting and surveillance methods have helped increase accuracy. Today, the CDC recommends that all states report HIV infections as well as AIDS. Because of medical advances in treatment and increasing numbers of HIV-infected persons who do not progress to AIDS, it is believed that AIDS incidence statistics may not provide a true picture of the epidemic, the long-term costs of treating HIV-infected individuals, and other key information. HIV incidence data also provide a better picture of infection trends. Currently, most states mandate that those who test positive for the HIV antibody be reported.

Women and AIDS

HIV is an equal-opportunity pathogen that can attack anyone who engages in high-risk behaviors. This is true regardless of race, gender, sexual orientation, or social economic status. Consider the following facts:[36]

- Women are four to ten times more likely than men to contract HIV through unprotected sexual intercourse with an infected partner.[37]
- By 2000, women accounted for over 43 percent of all AIDS cases in the United States.
- HIV/AIDS due to heterosexual sexual transmission is increasing faster in rural America than in any other part of the country. Women most at risk are ethnic minorities and the economically disadvantaged. Among sexually active heterosexual teenagers, college students, and health care workers, nearly 60 percent of HIV cases are women.
- Females aged 13 to 24 accounted for 44 percent of new HIV cases in 1997.
- Most women with AIDS were infected through heterosexual exposure to HIV, followed by injection drug use (sharing needles).
- Women of color are disproportionately affected by HIV; African American and Hispanic women together account for 76 percent of AIDS cases among women in the United States, though comprising less than 25 percent of all U.S. women.
- Of all AIDS cases among women, 61 percent were reported from five states: New York (26 percent), Florida (13 percent), New Jersey (10 percent), California (7 percent), and Texas (5 percent).

Staggering Toll of HIV/AIDS in the Global Community

In spite of noteworthy progress in stemming the tide of infectious diseases such as HIV/AIDS in the United States, epidemics of these diseases have had an increasingly devastating impact on other regions of the world. By the year 2000, over 35 million people from all regions of the world were infected with HIV, translating to nearly 1 out of every 100 men, women, and children. Through 1997, women, children, and teenagers seemed to be on the periphery of the HIV/AIDS pandemic. However, by 2000, they were at the center of the epidemic. Consider the following.

AFRICA

- In South Africa, one in every three people is now infected.
- In seven other African countries, at least one-fifth of the population is infected.
- According to the National Institute of Allergy and Infectious Diseases (NIAID), more than 10 percent of the population in over 16 African countries are

infected. More than 6,500 new cases occur every day among people 15 to 24 years old worldwide—5.4 million in 1999 alone.

- The AIDS epidemic is expected to wipe out about half the current population of teenagers in the worst-hit African nations, devastating economies and shattering societies. A child born in Botswana in 2010 can expect to live 29 years—the lowest life expectancy seen in a century. Men in several sub-Saharan countries will soon greatly outnumber women.
- Almost two-thirds of the 35 million people worldwide who are infected with HIV live in sub-Saharan Africa. By 2000, 55 percent of all HIV infections were in women, primarily due to heterosexual contact with their infected male partners.
- Since the start of the HIV/AIDS pandemic, approximately 8.2 million children younger than age 15 have been orphaned worldwide due to the premature death of parents infected with HIV.

NORTH AMERICA

- An estimated 900,000 people were living with AIDS at the end of 1999.

The United States has an infection rate of 0.61 percent of the adult population, and Canada has an infection rate of 0.30 percent.

- Public health workers were alarmed to note that there appears to be an increase in high-risk behavior among young homosexuals and a rise in gonorrhea, indicating that our numbers may increase after a long downward trend.

LATIN AMERICA AND THE CARIBBEAN

- An estimated 1.67 million people were living with AIDS virus at the end of 1999. The epidemic was mainly spread through heterosexual intercourse.
- Haiti was worst hit, with 5.1 percent of adults infected, followed by Barbados with 4.1 percent.

EUROPE

- An estimated 940,000 people were living with AIDS virus at end of 1999.
- Rates of infection are increasing among drug users sharing needles in eastern Europe and the former Soviet Union.

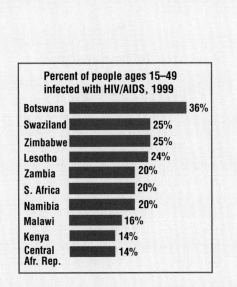

Percent of people ages 15–49 infected with HIV/AIDS, 1999

Botswana	36%
Swaziland	25%
Zimbabwe	25%
Lesotho	24%
Zambia	20%
S. Africa	20%
Namibia	20%
Malawi	16%
Kenya	14%
Central Afr. Rep.	14%

Adults and children estimated to be living with HIV/AIDS as of 1999

Sub-Saharan Africa	24.5 million
South and Southeast Asia	5.6 million
Latin America	1.3 million
North America	900,000
East Asia and Pacific	530,000
Western Europe	520,000
Eastern Europe and Central Asia	420,000
Caribbean	360,000
North Africa and Middle East	220,000
Australia and New Zealand	15,000

Continued

ASIA

- An estimated 6.13 million people were living with AIDS virus at the end of 1999.
- Cambodia has the highest rate, with 4.4 percent infected, largely through heterosexual intercourse.

- Thailand has an infection rate of 2.15 percent, and good prevention campaigns have slowed the spread of disease through heterosexual intercourse.
- An estimated 3.7 million people in India live with the virus, the second highest

national total behind South Africa, with an infection rate of 0.7 percent.

Source: National Institute of Allergy and Infectious Diseases, "HIV/AIDS Statistics," 2000 (http://www.nih.gov).

- AIDS is the leading cause of death among African American women aged 25 to 44, and the fourth leading cause of death among all American women in this age group.

Compounding the problems are serious deficiencies in our health and social service systems, including inadequate treatment for women addicts and lack of access to child care, health care, and social services for families headed by single women. Women with HIV/AIDS are of special interest because they are the major source of infection in infants. Virtually all new HIV infections among children in the United States are attributable to perinatal transmission of HIV.[38]

Although contracting HIV is a serious problem for both males and females, women often have an even more difficult time protecting themselves from infection and taking care of themselves once they become ill. Irrefutable evidence indicates that HIV/AIDS disproportionately affects women. This discrepancy can be traced to two sets of factors: biological factors and social and economic factors.

Biological factors include the following:

- HIV can enter through mucous membrane surfaces of the genital tract; the vagina has a greater exposed mucous membrane than does the urethra of the penis.
- The vaginal area is more likely to incur micro-tears during sexual intercourse, which facilitate entry of HIV.
- During intercourse, a woman is exposed to more semen than is the male to vaginal fluids.
- Semen is more likely to enter the vagina with force, whereas vaginal fluids do not enter the penis with force.
- Women who have STIs are more likely to be asymptomatic and therefore unaware they have an STI; STIs increase the risk of HIV transmission.

Social and economic factors include the following:

- Currently there are more HIV-infected men than HIV-infected women in the United States; thus, it is more likely for a woman to have an HIV-infected male partner.
- Women have been underrepresented in clinical trials for HIV treatment and prevention.
- Many cultural norms place women in subordination to men, especially in developing nations. This reduces

women's decision-making power and ability to negotiate safer sex.
- Women are more vulnerable to sexual abuse from their male partners.
- Women are more likely to be economically dependent on men.
- Women may be less likely to seek medical treatment because of lack of money, caregiving burden, and transportation problems.
- In the United States, HIV-positive women are more likely than are HIV-positive men to be younger and less educated.

What do you think?

Why do you think HIV/AIDS is increasing so rapidly in America? * Why are some women particularly vulnerable to diseases such as AIDS? * What actions can we take as a nation to reduce the spread of HIV/AIDS among women and minority groups? * Should Americans be concerned about the global HIV/AIDS epidemic? Why or why not?

How HIV Is Transmitted

HIV typically enters one person's body when another person's infected body fluids (in particular, semen, vaginal secretions, or blood) gain entry through a breach in body defenses. Mucous membranes of the genital organs and the anus provide the easiest route of entry. If there is a break in the mucous membranes (as can occur during sexual intercourse, particularly anal intercourse), the virus enters and begins to multiply. After initial infection, the HIV multiplies rapidly, invading the bloodstream and cerebrospinal fluid. It progressively destroys helper T-lymphocytes, weakening the body's resistance to disease. The virus also changes the genetic structure of the cells it attacks. In response to this invasion, the body quickly begins to produce antibodies.

Despite some myths, HIV is not a highly contagious virus. Studies of people living in households with a person with HIV/AIDS have turned up no documented cases of HIV infection due to casual contact. Other investigations provide overwhelming evidence that insect bites do not transmit HIV.

Engaging in High-Risk Behaviors   AIDS is not a disease of gay people or minority groups. If you engage in high-risk behaviors, you increase your risk for the disease. If you do not practice these behaviors, your risk is minimal. Anyone who engages in unprotected sex is at risk, especially sex with a partner who has engaged in other high-risk behaviors. Sex with multiple partners is the greatest threat.

Exchange of Body Fluids   The exchange of HIV-infected body fluids during vaginal and anal intercourse is the greatest risk factor. Substantial research evidence indicates that blood, semen, and vaginal secretions are the major fluids of concern. Most health officials state that saliva is not a high-risk body fluid unless blood is present. But the fact that the virus has been found in isolated samples of saliva does provide a good rationale for using caution when engaging in deep, wet kissing.[39]

Initially, public health officials also included breast milk in the list of high-risk fluids because a few infants apparently contracted HIV while breast-feeding. Subsequent research has indicated that HIV transmission could have been caused by bleeding nipples as well as by actual consumption of breast milk and other fluids. Infection through contact with feces and urine is believed to be highly unlikely though technically possible.

Receiving a Blood Transfusion Prior to 1985   A small group of people became infected with HIV after receiving blood transfusions. In 1985, the Red Cross and other blood donation programs implemented a stringent testing program for all donated blood. Today, because of these massive screening efforts, the risk of receiving HIV-infected blood is almost nonexistent.

Injecting Drugs   A significant percentage of AIDS cases in the United States are believed to result from sharing or using HIV-contaminated needles and syringes. Though users of illegal drugs are commonly considered the only members of this category, others may also share needles—for example, people with diabetes who inject insulin or athletes who inject steroids. People who share needles and also engage in sexual activities with members of high-risk groups, such as those who exchange sex for drugs, increase their risks dramatically.

Mother-to-Infant Transmission (Perinatal)   Approximately one in three of the children who has contracted AIDS received the virus from an infected mother while in the womb or while passing through the vaginal tract during delivery.

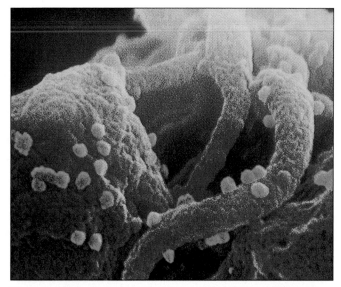

Viruses attach themselves to host cells and inject their own DNA or RNA in order to reproduce new cells. Some viruses run their course and expire. Others, such as HIV, shown here, are destructive over the long term.

Symptoms of HIV Disease

A person may go for months or years after infection by HIV before any significant symptoms appear. The incubation time varies greatly from person to person. Children have shorter incubation periods than adults. Newborns and infants are particularly vulnerable to AIDS because human beings do not become fully immunocompetent (that is, their immune system is not fully developed) until they are 6 to 15 months old. New information suggests that some very young children show the "adult" progression of AIDS.[40] For adults who receive no medical treatment, it takes an average of eight to ten years for the virus to cause the slow, degenerative changes in the immune system that are characteristic of AIDS. During this time, the person may experience a large number of opportunistic infections (infections that gain a foothold when the immune system is not functioning effectively). Colds, sore throats, fever, tiredness, nausea, night sweats, and other generally non–life-threatening conditions commonly appear. People who show these combinations of symptoms have been described as having pre-AIDS symptoms.

Testing for HIV Antibodies

Once antibodies have formed in reaction to HIV, a blood test known as the **ELISA** test may detect their presence. If sufficient antibodies are present, the ELISA test will be positive.

ELISA   Blood test that detects presence of antibodies to HIV virus.

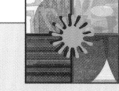

Staying Safe in an Unsafe Sexual World

HIV transmission depends on specific behaviors; this is true of other STIs as well. You can do several things to protect yourself and reduce your risk.

- Avoid casual sexual partners. Ideally, have sex only if you are in a long-term mutually monogamous relationship with someone who is equally committed to the relationship and whose HIV status is negative.
- Avoid unprotected sexual activity involving the exchange of blood, semen, or vaginal secretions with people whose present or past behaviors put them at risk for infection. Do not be afraid to ask intimate questions about your partner's sexual past. You expose yourself to your partner's history whenever you choose to have sexual relations. Postpone sexual involvement until you are assured that he or she is not infected.
- If you are sexually active and not in a lifelong monogamous relationship, practice safer sex by using latex condoms. Remember, however, that condoms still do not provide 100 percent safety.
- Never share injecting needles with anyone for any reason.
- Never share any devices through which the exchange of blood could occur, including needles, razors, tattoo instruments, and other body-piercing instruments.
- Avoid injury to body tissue during sexual activity. HIV can enter the bloodstream through microscopic tears in anal or vaginal tissues.
- Avoid unprotected oral sex or any sexual activity in which semen, blood, or vaginal secretions could penetrate mucous membranes through breaks in the membrane. Always use a condom or a dental dam during oral sex.
- Avoid using drugs that may dull your senses and affect your ability to make decisions about responsible precautions with potential sex partners.
- Wash your hands before and after sexual encounters. Urinate after sexual relations and, if possible, wash your genitals.
- Although total abstinence is the only absolute means of preventing the sexual transmission of HIV, abstinence can be a difficult choice to make. If you have any doubt about the potential risks of having sex, consider other means of intimacy, at least until you can assure your safety. Enjoyable and safer alternatives include massage, dry kissing, hugging, holding and touching, and masturbation (alone or with a partner).
- When receiving care from medical professionals such as dentists or doctors, make sure they take appropriate precautions to prevent potential transmission, including washing their hands and wearing gloves and masks. Be sure that all equipment used for treatment is properly sterilized.
- If you are worried about your own HIV status, have yourself tested rather than risk infecting others inadvertently.
- If you are a woman and HIV positive, take the steps necessary to ensure that you do not become pregnant.
- If you suspect that you may be infected or if you test positive for HIV antibodies, do not donate blood, semen, or body organs.

At no time in your life is it more important to communicate openly than when you are considering an intimate relationship. Do not be afraid to ask questions so that you can then make an informed decision about whether to get involved. Remember that you can't tell whether someone has a sexually transmitted infection. Anyone who has ever had sex with anyone else or has injected drugs is at risk, and he or she may not even know it.

The following tips can help you communicate about potential risks:

- *Remember that you have a responsibility to your partner to disclose your status.* You also have a responsibility to yourself to stay healthy. Do not be afraid to ask about your partner's HIV status. If either person's status is unknown, suggest going through the testing together as a means of sharing something important.
- *Be direct, honest, and determined in talking about sex before you become involved.* Do not act silly or evasive. Get to the point, ask clear questions, and do not be put off in receiving a response. Remember, a person who does not care enough to talk about sex probably does not care enough to take responsibility for his or her actions.
- *Discuss the issues without sounding defensive or accusatory.* Develop a personal comfort level with the subject prior to raising the issue with your partner. Be prepared with complete information and articulate your feelings clearly. Reassure your partner that your reasons for desiring abstinence or safer sex arise from respect and not distrust. Sharing feelings is easier in a calm, suspicion-free environment in which both people feel comfortable.
- *Encourage your partner to be honest and to share feelings.* This will not happen overnight. If you never had a serious conversation with this person before getting into an intimate situation, you cannot expect honesty and openness when the lights go out.
- *Analyze your own beliefs and values ahead of time.* The worst thing you can do is to get into an awkward situation before you have had time to think about what is important to you. Know where you will draw the line on

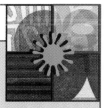

certain actions, and be very clear with your partner about what you expect. If you believe that using a condom is necessary, make sure you communicate this.

- *Decide what you will do if your partner does not agree with you.* Anticipate potential objections or excuses, and prepare your responses accordingly.
- *Ask questions about your partner's history.* Although it may seem as though you are prying into another per-

son's business, your own future depends upon knowing basic information about your partner's past. An idea of your partner's past sexual practices and use of drug injections is very valuable. Again, it is important to let your partner know why you are concerned and that you are not inquiring because of jealousy or other ulterior motives.

- *Ask about the significance of monogamy in your partner's relationships.* A basic question to ask before

becoming involved in a regular sexual relationship is: "How important is a committed relationship to you?" You will need to decide early how important this relationship is to you and how much you are willing to work at arriving at an acceptable compromise on lifestyle.

When a person who previously tested *negative* (no HIV antibodies present) has a subsequent test that is *positive,* seroconversion is said to have occurred. In such a situation, the person would typically take another ELISA test, followed by a more expensive, more precise test known as the **Western blot,** to confirm the presence of HIV antibodies.

It should be noted that these tests are not AIDS tests per se. Rather, they detect antibodies for the disease, indicating the presence of HIV in the person's system. Whether the person will develop AIDS depends to some extent on the strength of the immune system. However, the vast majority of all infected people develop some form of the disease.

As testing for HIV antibodies has been perfected, scientists have explored various ways of making it easier for individuals to be tested. Health officials distinguish between *reported* and *actual* cases of HIV infection because it is believed that many HIV-positive people avoid being tested. One reason may be fear of knowing the truth. Another is the fear of recrimination from employers, insurance companies, and medical staff if a positive test becomes known to others. However, early detection and reporting are important, because immediate treatment for someone in the early stages of HIV disease is critical.

New Hope and Treatments

New drugs have slowed the progression from HIV to AIDS and have prolonged life expectancies for many AIDS patients. While these new therapies offered the promise of life for many, they may have inadvertently led to increases in risky behaviors and a noteworthy rise in cases in 2000. Although AIDS fell to 14th place among the leading causes of death in 1997 and has held steady at that ranking, many fear that we are taking steps backward. Advocates for AIDS patients believe the medications still cost too much money and cause too many side effects. Multidrug treatment for AIDS for

one person now exceeds $20,000 per year. Medical costs for people with AIDS, from the time of diagnosis until death, exceed $102,000.[41]

Current treatments combine selected drugs, especially protease inhibitors and reverse transcriptase inhibitors. Protease inhibitors (for example, Amprenavir, Ritonavir, and Saquinavir) resemble pieces of the protein chain that the HIV protease normally cuts. They block the HIV protease enzyme from cutting the protein chains needed to produce new viruses. Older AIDS drugs work by preventing the virus from infecting new cells.

Although protease inhibitors show promise, they have proved difficult to manufacture, and some have failed while others have been successful. Side effects vary, and getting the right dose is critical for effectiveness. All of the protease drugs seem to work best in combination with other therapies. These combination treatments are still quite experimental, and no combination has proved to be absolute for all people as yet. Also, as with other antiviral treatments, resistance to the drugs can develop. Individuals who already show resistance to AZT may not be able to use a protease-AZT combination. This can pose a problem for many people who have been taking the common drugs and then find their options for combination therapy limited.

Although these drugs provide new hope and longer survival rates for people living with HIV, we are still a long way from a cure. In addition, the number of people becoming HIV-infected each year has not declined, meaning that we are still a long way from beating this disease.

Western blot   A test more accurate than the ELISA to confirm presence of HIV antibodies.

Preventing HIV Infection

Although scientists have been searching for an HIV vaccine since 1983, they have had no success so far. The only way to prevent HIV infection is to avoid risky behaviors. HIV infection and AIDS are not uncontrollable conditions. You can reduce your risk by the choices you make in sexual behaviors and taking responsibility for your health and the health of your loved ones. The Skills for Behavior Change box on page 368 presents ways to reduce your risk for contracting HIV.

Noninfectious Diseases

Typically, when we think of major noninfectious ailments, we think of "killer" diseases such as cancer and heart disease. Clearly, these diseases make up the major portion of life-threatening diseases—accounting for nearly two-thirds of all deaths. Yet although these diseases capture much media attention, other chronic conditions can cause substantial pain, suffering, and disability. Fortunately, most of them can be prevented or their symptoms relieved.

Generally, noninfectious diseases are not transmitted by a pathogen or by any form of personal contact. Lifestyle and personal health habits are often implicated as underlying causes. Healthy changes in lifestyle and public health efforts aimed at research, prevention, and control can minimize the effects of these diseases.

Chronic Lung Disease

Chronic lung diseases pose a serious and significant threat to Americans today. Collectively, they have become the fourth leading cause of death, with most sufferers living with a condition known as chronic **dyspnea,** or chronic breathlessness. Depending on the situation, dyspnea may result in the inability to climb stairs, walk unassisted, or sleep without fear of stopping breathing. Chronic lung disease can result in major disability and lack of function as the lungs fill with mucus, be-

---

Dyspnea   Chronic breathlessness.

Chronic obstructive pulmonary diseases (COPDs) A collection of chronic lung diseases including asthma, emphysema, and chronic bronchitis.

Allergy   Hypersensitive reaction to a specific antigen or allergen in the environment in which the body produces excessive antibodies to that antigen or allergen.

Histamines   Chemical substances that dilate blood vessels, increase mucous secretions, and produce other symptoms of allergies.

Hay fever   A chronic respiratory disorder that is most prevalent when ragweed and flowers bloom.

---

come susceptible to bacterial or viral infections, or cause acute stress on the heart as they struggle to get valuable oxygen. Chronic cough, excessive phlegm, wheezing, or coughing up blood also may occur. Over time, many of these underlying conditions lead to hospitalization and possible death.

Among the more deadly chronic lung diseases are the **chronic obstructive pulmonary diseases (COPDs):** asthma, emphysema, and chronic bronchitis. Other chronic lung diseases also cause significant health risks, the most common of which are allergy-induced problems and hay fever. Each of these may exacerbate or contribute to the development of COPD.

Allergy-Induced Respiratory Problems

An **allergy** occurs as a part of the body's attempt to defend itself against a specific *antigen* or *allergen* by producing specific *antibodies.* When foreign pathogens such as bacteria or viruses invade the body, the body responds by producing antibodies to destroy these invading antigens. Under normal conditions, the production of antibodies is a positive element in the body's defense system. However, for unknown reasons, in some people the body overreacts by developing an overly elaborate protective mechanism against relatively harmless allergens or antigens. The resultant *hypersensitivity reaction* to specific allergens or antigens in the environment is fairly common, as anyone who has awakened with a runny nose or itchy eyes will testify. Most commonly, these hypersensitivity, or allergic, responses occur as a reaction to environmental antigens such as molds, animal dander (hair and dead skin), pollen, ragweed, or dust. Once excessive antibodies to these antigens are produced, they trigger the release of **histamines,** chemical substances that dilate blood vessels, increase mucous secretions, cause tissues to swell, and produce other allergylike symptoms, particularly in the respiratory system (Figure 14.4).

Although many people think of allergies as childhood diseases, in reality allergies tend to become progressively worse with time and with increased exposure to allergens. In these circumstances, allergic responses become chronic in nature, and treatment becomes difficult. Many people take allergy shots to reduce the severity of their symptoms, with some success. In most cases, once the offending antigen has disappeared, allergy-prone people suffer few symptoms. Although allergies can cause numerous problems, one of the most significant effects is on the immune system.

Hay Fever

Perhaps the best example of a chronic respiratory disease is **hay fever.** Usually considered a seasonally related disease (most prevalent when ragweed and flowers are blooming), hay fever is common throughout the world. Hay fever attacks, which are characterized by sneezing and itchy, watery eyes and nose, cause a great deal of misery for countless

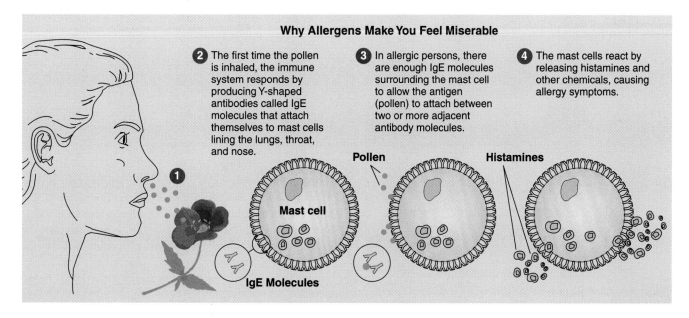

Why Allergens Make You Feel Miserable

2 The first time the pollen is inhaled, the immune system responds by producing Y-shaped antibodies called IgE molecules that attach themselves to mast cells lining the lungs, throat, and nose.

3 In allergic persons, there are enough IgE molecules surrounding the mast cell to allow the antigen (pollen) to attach between two or more adjacent antibody molecules.

4 The mast cells react by releasing histamines and other chemicals, causing allergy symptoms.

1

Mast cell

Pollen

Histamines

IgE Molecules

Figure 14.4
Steps of an Allergy Response

people. Hay fever appears to run in families, and research indicates that lifestyle is not as great a factor in developing hay fever as it is in other chronic diseases. Instead, an overzealous immune system and exposure to environmental allergens including pet dander, dust, pollen from various plants, and other substances appear to be the critical factors that determine vulnerability. For those people who are unable to get away from the cause of their hay fever response, medical assistance in the form of injections or antihistamines may provide the only possibility of relief.

Asthma

Unfortunately, for many persons who suffer from allergies such as hay fever, their condition often becomes complicated by the development of one of the major COPDs: asthma, emphysema, or bronchitis. **Asthma** is a long-term, chronic inflammatory disorder that blocks air flow in and out of the lungs. Asthma causes tiny airways in the lung to overreact with spasms in response to certain triggers. Symptoms include wheezing, difficulty in breathing, shortness of breath, and coughing spasms. Although most asthma attacks are mild and non–life-threatening, they can trigger bronchospasms (contractions of the bronchial tubes in the lungs) that are so severe that without rapid treatment, death may occur. Between attacks, most people have few symptoms.

A number of things can trigger an attack, including air pollutants; particulate matter, such as wood dust; indoor air pollutants, such as sidestream smoke from tobacco; and allergens, such as dust mites, cockroach saliva, and pet dander. Stress is also believed to trigger an asthmatic attack in some individuals.[42]

Asthma can occur at any age, but it is most likely to occur in children between infancy and age 5 and in adults before the age of 40. In childhood, asthma strikes more boys than girls; in adulthood, it strikes more women than men. Also, the asthma rate is 50 percent higher among African Americans than whites, and four times as many African Americans die of asthma than do whites. Midwesterners appear to be more prone to asthma than are people from other areas of the country. In recent years, concern over the rise in incidence of asthma has grown considerably. How serious is the problem? Consider these points:[43]

- Asthma has become the most common chronic disease of childhood, accounting for one-fourth of all school absences.
- Asthma is the number one cause of hospitalization and absenteeism.
- Asthma affects over 15 million Americans, including 5 million children.
- Overall, 13 percent of all students aged 5 to 19 have asthma.
- The number of asthma sufferers has increased by more than 65 percent since the 1980s; one in ten new asthma cases is diagnosed in people over age 65.
- The death toll from asthma has nearly doubled since 1980, to more than 5,000 persons per year.

Asthma   A chronic respiratory disease characterized by attacks of wheezing, shortness of breath, and coughing spasms.

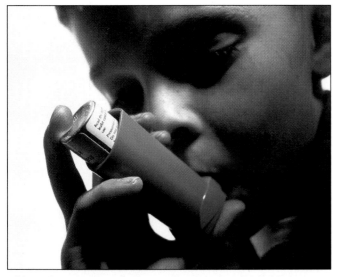

Although a number of new medications are available to relieve the symptoms of asthma, the marked increase of this respiratory problem among young children worries health officials.

People with asthma fall into one of two distinctly different types of asthma development. The most common type, known as *extrinsic* (or *slow onset*) *asthma,* is most commonly associated with allergic triggers. This type tends to run in families and begins to develop in childhood. Often, by adulthood, a person has few episodes, or the disorder completely goes away. *Intrinsic asthma* also may have allergic triggers, but the main difference is that any unpleasant event or stimulant may trigger an attack. A common form of extrinsic asthma is *exercise-induced asthma (EIA),* which may or may not have an allergic connection. Some athletes have no allergies yet live with asthma. Cold, dry air is believed to exacerbate EIA; thus, keeping the lungs moist and warming up prior to working out may reduce risk. The warm, moist air around a swimming pool is one of the best environments for people with asthma.

Relaxation techniques appear to help some asthma sufferers. Drugs may be necessary for serious cases. Determining whether a specific allergen provokes asthma attacks, taking steps to reduce exposure to it, avoiding triggers such

as certain types of exercise or stress, and finding the most effective medications are big steps in asthma prevention and control. Numerous new drugs are available that cause fewer side effects than older medications. Finding a doctor who specializes in asthma treatment and stays up-to-date on possible options is critical.

Emphysema

Emphysema involves the gradual destruction of the **alveoli** (tiny air sacs) of the lungs. As the alveoli are destroyed, the affected person finds it more and more difficult to exhale. The victim typically struggles to take in a fresh supply of air before the air held in the lungs has been expended. The chest cavity gradually begins to expand, producing the barrel-shaped chest characteristic of the chronic emphysema victim.

The exact cause of emphysema is uncertain. There is, however, a strong relationship between emphysema and long-term cigarette smoking and exposure to air pollution. Victims of emphysema often suffer discomfort over a period of many years. In fact, studies have shown that lung function decline may begin well before the age of 50 and an early morning "smoker's cough" may signal that the damage has already begun.[44] What most of us take for granted—the easy, rhythmic flow of air in and out of the lungs—becomes a continuous struggle for people with emphysema. Inadequate oxygen supply, combined with the stress of overexertion on the heart, eventually takes its toll on the cardiovascular system and leads to premature death.

Bronchitis

Bronchitis refers to an inflammation of the lining of the bronchial tubes. These tubes, the bronchi, connect the windpipe with the lungs. When the bronchi become inflamed or infected, less air is able to flow from the lungs, and heavy mucus begins to form. *Acute bronchitis* is the most common of the bronchial diseases, resulting in millions of visits to the doctor every year at a cost of over $300 million per year.[45] Over 95 percent of these acute cases are caused by viruses; however, they are often misdiagnosed and treated with antibiotics, even though little evidence supports this treatment. Typically, misdiagnosis occurs when a cluster of symptoms is labeled as bronchitis, despite the fact that there is no true laboratory diagnosis. *Chronic bronchitis,* in contrast, is defined by the presence of a productive (mucus-laden) cough most days of the month, over 3 months of a year for two successive years without underlying disease to explain the cough. Typically, cigarette smoking is the cause of chronic bronchitis, and once bronchitis begins, secondary bacterial or viral infections often make the condition worse. Air pollution and industrial dusts and fumes are also risk factors.

Emphysema   A respiratory disease in which the alveoli become distended or ruptured and are no longer functional.

Alveoli   Tiny air sacs of the lungs.

Bronchitis   An inflammation of the lining of the bronchial tubes.

Neurological Disorders

Headaches

Almost all of us have experienced at least one major headache. In fact, over 80 percent of women and 65 percent of men experience headaches on a regular basis.[46] Common types of headaches and their treatments are described below.

Tension Headache Tension headaches, also referred to as muscular contraction headaches, are generally caused by muscle contractions or tension in the neck or head. This tension may be caused by actual strain placed on neck or head muscles due to overuse, static positions held for long periods of time, or tension triggered by stress. Recent research indicates that tension headaches may be a product of a more "generic mechanism" in which chemicals deep inside the brain may cause the muscular tension, pain, and suffering often associated with an attack. Triggers for this chemical assault may be red wine, lack of sleep, fasting, menstruation, or other factors. The same symptoms (sensitivity to light and sound, nausea, and/or throbbing pain) may be characteristic of different types of headaches and may vary in intensity and duration. Relaxation, hot water treatment, and massage have surfaced as the new holistic treatments, while aspirin, Tylenol, Aleve, and Advil remain the old standby forms of pain relief. Although such painkillers may bring temporary relief of symptoms, it is believed that, over time, the drugs may dull the brain's own pain-killing weapons and result in more headaches rather than fewer.

Migraine Headache Migraine is not just a name for an unusually bad headache; it is a specific diagnosis, involving pain that begins on one side of the head, often accompanied by nausea and sensitivity to light and sounds. Many migraine sufferers experience the sensation of an "aura" in their visual field, typically some form of disturbance such as flashing lights or blind spots, along with numbness or weakness on one side of the body or slurred speech,[47] all signals of an ensuing bad headache. Most people report pain behind or around one eye and always on the same side of the head—a pain that can last for hours or days and then disappear. A migraine can strike at any time, although the hormonal changes around menstrua-

tion and ovulation often seem to set off migraines in women, who are three times more likely to get migraines than men.[48]

Patients report that migraines can be triggered by emotional stress, the weather, certain foods, lack of sleep, and a litany of other causes. When tested under laboratory settings, however, much of this evidence is inconclusive. What is known is that migraines occur when blood vessels dilate in the membrane that surrounds the brain. Historically, treatments have centered on reversing or preventing this dilation, with the most common treatment derived from the rye fungus *ergot*. Today, many fast-acting ergot compounds are available by nasal spray, vastly increasing the speed of relief to patients. However, ergot drugs have many side effects, the least of which may be that they are habit forming, causing users to wake up with "rebound" headaches each morning after use.[49]

Critics of the blood vessel dilation theory question why only blood vessels of the head are dilated in these situations. They also wonder why, if the dilation causes vessels to press against nerves and inflict pain, aren't joggers and people who take a lot of hot baths more prone to migraine attacks? Opponents of blood vessel dilation theory suggest that the key to understanding the origin of migraines lies in the cortex of the brain, where certain pain sensors are stimulated.

When true migraines occur, relaxation is only minimally effective as a treatment. Often, strong pain-relieving drugs prescribed by a physician are necessary. Imitrex, a drug tailor-made for migraines, works for about 80 percent of those who try it. Recently, treatment with lidocaine has also shown promising results, and newer drugs called triptans, such as Zomig, Amerge, and Maxalt, are now available.[50]

Secondary Headaches Secondary headaches arise as a result of some other underlying condition. Hypertension, blocked sinuses, allergies, low blood sugar, diseases of the spine, the common cold, poorly fitted dentures, problems with eyesight, and other types of pain or injury can trigger this condition. Relaxation and pain relievers such as aspirin are of little help in treating secondary headaches. Rather, medications or other therapies designed to relieve the underlying organic cause of the headache must be included in the treatment regimen.

Seizure Disorders

The word **epilepsy** is derived from the Greek *epilepsia,* meaning "seizure." Approximately 1 percent of all Americans

Migraine A condition characterized by localized headaches that possibly result from alternating dilation and constriction of blood vessels.

Epilepsy A neurological disorder caused by abnormal electrical brain activity; can be accompanied by altered consciousness or convulsions.

suffer from some form of seizure-related disorder. These disorders are generally caused by abnormal electrical activity in the brain and are characterized by loss of control of muscular activity and unconsciousness. Symptoms vary widely from person to person. Common forms of epilepsy include the following:

- *Grand mal, or major motor seizure.* These seizures are often preceded by a shrill cry or a seizure aura (body sensations such as ringing in the ears or a specific smell or taste that occurs prior to a seizure). Convulsions and loss of consciousness generally occur and may last from 30 seconds to several minutes or more. Keeping track of the length of time elapsed is one aspect of first aid.
- *Petit mal, or minor seizure.* These seizures involve no convulsions. Rather, a minor loss of consciousness that may go unnoticed occurs. Minor twitching of muscles may take place, usually for a shorter time than the duration of grand mal convulsions.
- *Psychomotor seizure.* These seizures involve both mental processes and muscular activity. Symptoms may include mental confusion and a listless state characterized by activities such as lip smacking, chewing, and repetitive movements.
- *Jacksonian seizure.* This is a progressive seizure that often begins in one part of the body, such as the fingers, and moves to other parts, such as the hand or arm. Usually only one side of the body is affected.

In most cases, people afflicted with seizure disorders can lead normal, seizure-free lives when under medical supervision. Public ignorance about these disorders is one of the most serious obstacles confronting people with seizure disorders. Improvements in medication and surgical interventions to reduce some causes of seizures are among the most promising treatments today.

Gender-Related Disorders

Premenstrual Syndrome (PMS)

Premenstrual syndrome (PMS) is a syndrome describing a series of characteristic symptoms that occur prior to menstruation in some women. PMS has generated a great deal of controversy in recent years. It is characterized by as many as 150 possible physical and emotional symptoms that vary from

person to person and from month to month. These symptoms usually appear a week to 10 days preceding the menstrual period and affect between 20 and 40 percent of U.S. women of menstruating age to some degree. They include depression, tension, irritability, headaches, tender breasts, bloated abdomen, backache, abdominal cramps, acne, fluid retention, diarrhea, and fatigue. It is believed that women who have PMS develop a predictable pattern of symptoms during the menstrual cycle and that the severity of their symptoms may be influenced by external factors, such as stress. For many women, the first day of their period brings immediate relief. For others, the depressive symptoms persist all month and are only heightened prior to the menstrual period.

Most authorities believe that the most plausible cause of PMS is a hormonal imbalance related to the rise in estrogen levels preceding the menstrual period. This theory is substantiated by the fact that progesterone often relieves the symptoms. Critics of this theory argue that controlled research has not yet been conducted on the effects of progesterone on PMS.

Common treatments for PMS include hormonal therapy in addition to drugs and behaviors designed to relieve the symptoms. These include aspirin for pain, diuretics for fluid buildup, decreases in caffeine and salt intake, increases in intake of complex carbohydrates, stress reduction techniques, and exercise.

Endometriosis

Whether the incidence of **endometriosis** is on the rise in the United States or whether the disorder is simply attracting more attention is difficult to determine. Victims of endometriosis tend to be women between the ages of 20 and 40. Symptoms include severe cramping during and between menstrual cycles, irregular periods, unusually heavy or light menstrual flow, abdominal bloating, fatigue, painful bowel movements with periods, painful intercourse, constipation, diarrhea, menstrual pain, infertility, and low back pain.

Although much remains unknown about the causes of endometriosis, we do know that the disease is characterized by the abnormal growth and development of endometrial tissue (the tissue lining the uterus) in regions of the body other than the uterus. There are several widely accepted theories concerning the causes of endometriosis: the transmission of endometrial tissue to other regions of the body during surgery or through the birthing process; the movement of menstrual fluid backward through the fallopian tubes during menstruation; and abnormal cell migration through the movement of body fluids. Women with cycles shorter than 27 days and those with flows lasting over a week are at increased risk. The more aerobic exercise a woman engages in and the earlier she starts it, the less likely she is to develop endometriosis.

Treatment of endometriosis ranges from bed rest and stress reduction to **hysterectomy** (the removal of the uterus) and/or the removal of one or both ovaries and fallopian tubes. Recently, physicians have been criticized by

Premenstrual syndrome (PMS)   A series of physical and emotional symptoms that may occur in women prior to their menstrual periods.

Endometriosis   Abnormal development of endometrial tissue outside the uterus, resulting in serious side effects.

Hysterectomy   Surgical removal of the uterus.

some segments of the public for being too quick to select hysterectomy as the treatment of choice. More conservative treatments that involve dilation and curettage, surgically scraping endometrial tissue off the fallopian tubes and other reproductive organs, and combinations of hormone therapy have become more acceptable. Hormonal treatments include gonadotropin-releasing hormone (GnRH) analogs, various synthetic progesterone-like drugs (Provera), and oral contraceptives.

Digestion-Related Disorders

Diabetes

In healthy people, the *pancreas,* a powerful enzyme-producing organ, produces the hormone **insulin** in sufficient quantities to allow the body to use or store glucose (blood sugar). When this organ fails to produce enough insulin to regulate sugar metabolism or when the body fails to use insulin effectively, a disease known as **diabetes mellitus** occurs. Diabetics exhibit **hyperglycemia,** or elevated blood sugar levels, and high glucose levels in their urine. Other symptoms include excessive thirst, frequent urination, hunger, tendency to tire easily, wounds that heal slowly, numbness or tingling in the extremities, changes in vision, skin eruptions, and, in women, a tendency toward vaginal yeast infections. Each year an average of 650,000 new cases are identified, with rapidly rising incidence rates in recent decades. Diabetes mellitus is among the leading causes of death in America and is a major contributor to cardiovascular disease, blindness, and renal (kidney) failure. A recent CDC study indicated an alarming increase in diabetes cases; the prevalence in diagnosed cases increased from 4.9 percent in 1990 to 6.5 percent in 1998. Of grave concern was the fact that for people in their 40s, diabetes cases increased by 40 percent during the eight-year study, and by over 70 percent for those in their 30s.[51] Of the estimated 16 million people with diabetes in the United States today, nearly 6 million are unaware that they have a problem.

The most serious form, known as type I (insulin-dependent) diabetes, is an autoimmune disease in which the immune system destroys the insulin-making beta cells.[52] Type I diabetics typically must depend on insulin injections or oral medications for the rest of their lives because insulin is not present in their bodies. Type II (non–insulin-dependent) diabetes, in which insulin production is deficient or the body *resists* or is unable to utilize available insulin, tends to develop in later life. People with this form of diabetes can often control the symptoms of their disease with minimal medical intervention by maintaining a regimen of proper diet, weight control, and exercise. They may be able to avoid oral medications or insulin indefinitely. A third type of diabetes, *gestational diabetes,* can develop in a woman during pregnancy. The condition usually disappears after childbirth, but it does leave the woman at greater risk of developing type II diabetes at some point.

Risk Factors Diabetes tends to run in families, and a tendency toward being overweight, coupled with inactivity, dramatically increases a person's risk. Older persons and mothers of babies weighing over 9 pounds also run an increased risk. Approximately 80 percent of all patients are overweight at the time of diagnosis. Weight loss and exercise are important factors in lowering blood sugar and improving the efficiency of cellular use of insulin. Both can help to prevent overwork of the pancreas and the development of diabetes. African Americans, Hispanics, and Native Americans have the highest rates of type II diabetes in the world—much higher than that of Caucasians. The reasons for this increased risk are not clear.[53]

Controlling Diabetes Most physicians attempt to control diabetes with a variety of insulin-related drugs. Most of these drugs are taken orally, although self-administered hypodermic injections are prescribed when other treatments are inadequate. Recent breakthroughs in individual monitoring and the implanting of insulin monitors and insulin infusion pumps that regulate insulin intake "on demand" have provided many people with diabetes the opportunity to lead normal lives. Newer forms of insulin that last longer in the body and have fewer side effects are now available. An insulin inhaler is being tested and may soon be available. In addition, many people have found that they can help control their diabetes by eating foods that are rich in complex carbohydrates, low in sodium, and high in fiber; by losing weight; and by getting regular exercise.

Lactose Intolerance

As many as 50 million Americans are unable to eat dairy products such as milk, cheese, ice cream, and other foods that the rest of us take for granted. These people suffer from **lactose intolerance,** meaning that they have lost the ability to produce the digestive enzyme lactase, which is necessary for the body to convert milk sugar (lactose) into glucose. That cold glass of milk becomes a source of stomach cramping, diarrhea, nausea, gas, and related symptoms. Once diagnosed, however, lactose intolerance can be treated by introducing low-lactose or lactose-free foods into the diet.

Insulin   A hormone produced by the pancreas; required by the body for the metabolism of carbohydrates.

Diabetes mellitus   A disease in which the pancreas fails to produce enough insulin or the body fails to use insulin effectively.

Hyperglycemia   Elevated blood sugar levels.

Lactose intolerance   The inability to produce lactase, an enzyme needed to convert milk sugar into glucose.

Through trial and error, individuals usually find that they can tolerate one type of low-lactose food better than others. As an alternative to eating foods without lactose, some people find that they can purchase special products that contain the missing lactase and thus eat dairy foods without serious side effects. Most large grocery chains, food cooperatives, and drug stores have these products available in liquid or tablet form. It should be noted, however, that these products do not work for everyone. Someone who is lactose intolerant may need to experiment before settling into a diet that works.

Colitis and Irritable Bowel Syndrome (IBS)

Ulcerative colitis is a disease of the large intestine in which the mucous membranes of the intestinal walls become inflamed. Victims with severe cases may have as many as 20 bouts of bloody diarrhea a day. Colitis can also produce severe stomach cramps, weight loss, nausea, sweating, and fever. Although some experts believe that colitis occurs more frequently in people with high stress levels, this theory is controversial. Hypersensitivity reactions, particularly to milk and certain foods, have also been considered as a possible cause. It is difficult to determine the cause of colitis because the disease goes into unexplained remission and then recurs without apparent reason. This pattern often continues over periods of years and may be related to the later development of colorectal cancer. Because the cause of colitis remains unknown, treatment focuses exclusively on relieving the symptoms. Increasing fiber intake and taking anti-inflammatory drugs, steroids, and other medications designed to reduce inflammation and soothe irritated intestinal walls have been effective in relieving symptoms.

Many people develop a related condition known as **irritable bowel syndrome (IBS),** characterized by nausea, pain, gas, diarrhea attacks, or cramps that occur after eating certain foods or when a person is under unusual stress. IBS symptoms commonly begin in early adulthood. Symptoms may vary from week to week and can fade for long periods of time, only to return. The cause is unknown, but researchers suspect that people with IBS have digestive systems that are overly sensitive to what they eat and drink, to stress, and to certain hormonal changes. They may also be more sensitive to pain signals from the stomach. Stress management, relaxation techniques, regular activity, and diet can bring IBS under control in the vast majority of cases. Problems with diarrhea can be reduced by cutting down on fat and avoiding caffeine and excessive amounts of sorbitol, a sweetener found in dietetic foods and chewing gum.

Peptic Ulcers

An ulcer is a lesion or wound that forms in body tissue as a result of some form of irritant. A **peptic ulcer** is a chronic ulcer that occurs in the lining of the stomach or the section of the small intestine known as the *duodenum*. It has been thought to be caused by the erosive effect of digestive juices on these tissues. The lining of these organs becomes irritated, the protective covering of mucus is reduced, and the gastric acid begins to digest the dying tissue, just as it would a piece of food. Typically, this irritation causes pain that disappears when the person eats but returns about an hour later.

In 1994, the National Institutes of Health (NIH) announced that a common bacterium, *Helicobacter pylori,* may be the cause of most ulcers. The NIH called for the use of powerful antibiotics to treat the disorder, which affects over 4 million Americans every year. This was a dramatic departure from the typical treatment of using acid-reducing drugs. The new treatment recommends a two-week course of antibiotics and antacids in ulcer cases in which excess stomach acid or overuse of drugs such as aspirin and ibuprofen have caused an irritation. The good news is that by treating ulcers with germ-killing drugs, the ulcers appear less likely to recur. People with ulcers should avoid high-fat foods, alcohol, and substances such as aspirin that may irritate organ linings or cause increased secretion of stomach acids.

Musculoskeletal Diseases

Arthritis

Called the "nation's primary crippler," **arthritis** strikes one in seven Americans, or over 38 million people. Symptoms range from the occasional tendinitis of the weekend athlete to the horrific pain of rheumatoid arthritis. Arthritis accounts for over 30 million lost workdays annually and costs the U.S. economy over $12 billion per year, including $5.5 billion in hospital and nursing home services. In addition, arthritis sufferers spend more than $1 billion a year on dubious cures.

Osteoarthritis, also known as degenerative joint disease, is a progressive deterioration of bones and joints that has been associated with the wear-and-tear theory of aging.

Ulcerative colitis   An inflammatory disorder that affects the mucous membranes of the large intestine, producing bloody diarrhea.

Irritable bowel syndrome (IBS)   Condition characterized by nausea, pain, gas, or diarrhea caused by certain foods or stress.

Peptic ulcer   Damage to the stomach or intestinal lining, usually caused by digestive juices.

Arthritis   Painful inflammatory disease of the joints.

Osteoarthritis   A progressive deterioration of bones and joints that has been associated with the wear-and-tear theory of aging.

More recent research indicates that as joints are used, they release enzymes that digest cartilage while other cells in the cartilage try to repair the damage. When the enzymatic breakdown overpowers cellular repair, the pain and swelling characteristic of arthritis may occur. Weather extremes, excessive strain, and injury often lead to osteoarthritis flare-ups. But a specific precipitating event does not seem to be necessary. Obesity, joint trauma, and repetitive joint usage all contribute to increased risk, and thus are important targets for prevention.

Although age and injury are undoubtedly factors in the development of osteoarthritis, heredity, abnormal use of the joint, diet, abnormalities in joint structure, and impaired blood supply to the joint may also contribute. Joint replacement and bone fusion are common surgical repair techniques. For most people, anti-inflammatory drugs and pain relievers such as aspirin and cortisone-related agents ease discomfort. In some sufferers, applications of heat, mild exercise, and massage may also relieve the pain.

Rheumatoid arthritis is an autoimmune disease involving chronic inflammation. It can occur at any age, but it most commonly appears between the ages of 20 and 45. Rheumatoid arthritis is three times more common among women than among men during early adulthood but equally common among men and women in the over-70 age group. Symptoms include stiffness, pain, and swelling of multiple joints, often including the joints of the hands and wrists, and can be gradually progressive or sporadic, with occasional unexplained remissions.

Treatment for rheumatoid arthritis is similar to that for osteoarthritis. Emphasis is placed on pain relief and attempts to improve the functional mobility of the patient. In some instances, immunosuppressant drugs are given to reduce the inflammatory response.

Fibromyalgia

Fibromyalgia is a chronic, painful, rheumatoidlike disorder that affects as many as 5 to 6 percent of the general population. Persons with fibromyalgia experience an array of symptoms including headaches, dizziness, numbness and tingling, itching, fluid retention, chronic joint pain, abdominal or pelvic pain, and even occasional diarrhea. Suspected causes have ranged from sleep disturbances, stress, emotional distress, viruses, and autoimmune disorders; however, none has been proved in clinical trials. Because of fibromyalgia's multiple symptoms, it is usually diagnosed only after myriad tests have ruled out other disorders. The American College of Rheumatology identifies the major diagnostic criteria as the following:[54]

- History of widespread pain of at least three months' duration in the axial skeleton as well as in all four quadrants of the body
- Pain in at least 11 of 18 paired tender points on digital palpation of about 4 kilograms of pressure

Fibromyalgia primarily affects women in their 30s and 40s. It can be extremely debilitating, causing unrelieved pain, feelings of bloating or swelling, and fatigue in its victims. Many people with fibromyalgia also become depressed and report chronic fatiguelike symptoms. Treatment varies based on the severity of symptoms. Typically, adequate rest, stress management, relaxation techniques, dietary supplements and selected herbal remedies, and pain medications are prescribed.

Systemic Lupus Erythematosus (SLE)

Systemic lupus erythematosus (SLE), or, more simply, **lupus,** is a disease in which the immune system attacks the body, producing antibodies that destroy or injure organs such as the kidneys, brain, and heart. The symptoms vary from mild to severe and may disappear for periods of time. A butterfly-shaped rash covering the bridge of the nose and both cheeks is common. Nearly all SLE sufferers have aching joints and muscles, and 60 percent of them develop redness and swelling that move from joint to joint. The disease affects 1 in 700 Caucasians but 1 in 250 African Americans; 90 percent of all victims are females. Extensive research has not yet found a cure for this sometimes fatal disease.

Low Back Pain

Approximately 80 percent of all Americans will experience low back pain at some point. Some of these low back pain (LBP) episodes result from muscular damage and may be short-lived and acute. Other episodes may involve dislocations, fractures, or other problems with spinal vertebrae or discs, resulting in chronic pain or requiring surgery. Low back pain is epidemic throughout the world. It is the major cause of disability for people aged 20 to 45 in the United States, who suffer more frequently and severely from this problem than older people do.[55] LBP causes more lost work time in the United States than any other illness except upper respiratory infections. In fact, costs associated with back injury exceeded those associated with all other industrial injuries combined.[56]

Almost 90 percent of all back problems occur in the lumbar spine region (lower back). You can avoid many

---

Rheumatoid arthritis A serious inflammatory joint disease.

Fibromyalgia A chronic, painful rheumatoidlike disorder that can be highly painful and difficult to diagnose.

Lupus A disease in which the immune system attacks the body, producing antibodies that destroy or injure organs such as the kidneys, brain, and heart.

Table 14.3
Other Modern Afflictions

DISEASE	DESCRIPTION	TREATMENT
Cystic fibrosis	Inherited disease occurring in 1 out of every 1,600 births. Characterized by pooling of large amounts of mucus in lungs, digestive disturbances, and excessive sodium excretion. Results in premature death.	Most treatments are geared toward relief of symptoms. Antibiotics are administered for infection. Recent strides in genetic research suggest better treatments and potential cure in the near future.
Sickle-cell anemia	Inherited disease affecting 8–10 percent of all African Americans. Disease affects hemoglobin, forming sickle-shaped red blood cells that interfere with oxygenation. Results in severe pain, anemia, and premature death.	Reduce stress, and attend to minor infections immediately. Seek genetic counseling.
Cerebral palsy	Disorder characterized by the loss of voluntary control over motor functioning. Believed to be caused by a lack of oxygen to the brain at birth, brain disorders or an accident before or after birth, poisoning, or brain infections.	Follow preventive actions to reduce accident risks; improved neonatal and birthing techniques show promise.
Graves' disease	A thyroid disorder characterized by swelling of the eyes, staring gaze, and retraction of the eyelid. Can result in loss of sight. The cause is unknown, and the disease can occur at any age.	Medication may help control symptoms. Radioactive iodine supplements also may be administered.

problems by consciously maintaining good posture. Other preventive hints include the following:

- Purchase a firm mattress, and avoid sleeping on your stomach.
- Avoid high-heeled shoes, which often tilt the pelvis forward.
- Control your weight.
- Lift objects with your legs, not your back.
- Buy a good chair for doing your work, preferably one with lumbar support.
- Move your car seat forward so your knees are elevated slightly.
- Warm up before exercising.
- Engage in regular exercise, particularly exercises that strengthen the abdominal muscles and stretch the back muscles.

Other Maladies

During the past decade, numerous afflictions have surfaced that seem to be products of our times. Some of these health problems relate to specific groups of people; some are due to technological advances; and others have not been explained (see Table 14.3).

Chronic Fatigue Syndrome (CFS)

Fatigue is a subjective condition in which people feel tired before they begin activities, lack the energy to accomplish tasks that require sustained effort and attention, or become abnormally exhausted after normal activities. In the late 1980s, several U.S. clinics noted a characteristic set of symptoms including chronic fatigue, headaches, fever, sore throat, enlarged lymph nodes, depression, poor memory, general weakness, nausea, and symptoms remarkably similar to mononucleosis.

Despite extensive testing, no viral cause has been found.[57] In the absence of a known pathogen, many researchers believe that the illness, commonly referred to as *chronic fatigue syndrome (CFS)*, may have strong psychosocial roots. Our heightened awareness of health makes some of us scrutinize our bodies so carefully that the slightest deviation becomes amplified. In addition, the growing number of people who suffer from depression seem to be good candidates for chronic fatigue syndrome. Experts worry, however, that too many people approach CFS as something that is "in the person's head" and that such an attitude may prevent scientists from doing the serious research needed to find a cure.

The diagnosis of chronic fatigue syndrome depends on two major criteria and eight or more minor criteria. The major criteria are debilitating fatigue that persists for at least six months and the absence of diagnoses of other illnesses that could cause the symptoms. Minor criteria include headaches, fever, sore throat, painful lymph nodes, weakness, fatigue after exercise, sleep problems, and rapid onset of these symptoms. Treatment focuses on improved nutrition, rest, counseling for depression, judicious exercise, and development of a strong support network.

Repetitive Stress Injuries (RSIs)

The Bureau of Labor Statistics estimates that 25 percent of all injuries in the labor force that result in lost work time are due to **repetitive stress injuries (RSIs).** RSIs are injuries to nerves, soft tissue, or joints that result from the physical stress of repeated motions. They are estimated to cost employers over $22 billion a year in workers' compensation and an additional $85 billion in related costs, such as absenteeism.

One of the most common RSIs is **carpal tunnel syndrome.** Hours spent typing at the computer, flipping groceries through computerized scanners, or other jobs "made simpler" by technology can irritate the median nerve in the wrist, causing numbness, tingling, and pain in the fingers and hands. Although carpal tunnel syndrome risk can be reduced by proper placement of the keyboard, mouse, wrist pads, and other techniques, RSIs are often overlooked until significant damage has been done. Better education and ergonomic workplace designs can eliminate many injuries of this nature.

> **Repetitive stress injury (RSI)**   An injury to nerves, soft tissue, or joints due to the physical stress of repeated motions.
>
> **Carpal tunnel syndrome**   A common occupational injury in which the median nerve in the wrist becomes irritated, causing numbness, tingling, and pain in the fingers and hands.

Taking Charge

14   14   14

Managing Your Disease Risks

Infectious and noninfectious diseases pose serious challenges in the U.S. and throughout the world. In particular, sexually transmitted infections, including HIV infection, present an increasing health risk to our nation's youth. Nearly all infectious diseases can be prevented by practicing safe and responsible behaviors. The following are sensible steps you can take to avoid infectious diseases.

Checklist for Change

Making Personal Choices

✓ Be aware of factors that can threaten your health status.

✓ Know your disease and immunization history.

✓ Take the proper precautions to protect yourself from exposure to infectious pathogens.

✓ Know the health status of your intimate partners.

✓ Communicate openly and honestly with your partners about your feelings regarding sexual intimacy.

✓ If you have an infectious disease that can be spread through casual contact, remember to wash your hands frequently.

✓ Avoid traveling to places where outbreaks of infectious diseases have not been controlled.

✓ Follow a healthy routine of sleep, nutrition, and exercise.

✓ Follow safe measures when involved with someone with an infectious disease.

✓ Cook and store foods at their appropriate temperatures.

✓ Respect the symptoms that indicate a possible infection, and seek treatment immediately.

✓ Recognize your responsibility for the health of others.

✓ Behave in sexually responsible ways.

✓ Limit your sexual partners.

✓ Avoid using alcohol or other drugs during intimate sexual encounters.

✓ Assess your level of risk for acquiring an STI, including HIV infection.

✓ Respect the rights and needs of individuals affected by an infectious disease.

✓ Follow your physician's instructions completely when seeking help.

Making Community Choices

✓ What services does your student health service offer for testing for STIs? For HIV?

✓ Name any local free clinics where you could be tested for STIs or HIV.

✓ What have you done to support government spending for HIV research and health promotion (education)? What else could you do?

✓ Have you written to your congressional representatives regarding your support of funding?

✓ Does your local school system offer a sex education curriculum including discussion about how

to stop the spread of the HIV virus?

Summary

* The major uncontrollable risk factors for contracting infectious diseases are heredity, age, environmental conditions, and organism resistance. The major controllable risk factors are stress, nutrition, fitness level, sleep, hygiene, avoidance of high-risk behaviors, and drug use.

* The major pathogens are bacteria, viruses, fungi, protozoa, prions, and parasitic worms. Bacterial infections include staphylococcal infections, streptococcal infections, pneumonia, Legionnaire's disease, tuberculosis, and periodontal diseases. Major viruses include the common cold, influenza, mononucleosis, hepatitis, and measles.

* Your body uses a number of defense systems to keep pathogens from invading. The skin is the body's major protection, helped by enzymes. The immune system creates antibodies to destroy antigens. In addition, fever and pain play a role in defending the body. Vaccines bolster the body's immune system against specific diseases.

* Emerging and resurgent diseases pose significant threats for future generations. Many factors contribute to these risks. Possible solutions focus on a public health approach to prevention.

* Sexually transmitted infections are spread through intercourse, oral sex, anal sex, hand–genital contact, and sometimes through mouth-to-mouth contact. Major STIs include chlamydia, pelvic inflammatory disease, gonorrhea, syphilis, pubic lice, venereal warts, candidiasis, trichomoniasis, and herpes. Sexual transmission may also be involved in some general urinary tract infections.

* Acquired immune deficiency syndrome (AIDS) is caused by the human immunodeficiency virus (HIV). HIV is not confined to certain high-risk groups. Globally, HIV/AIDS has become a major threat to the world's population. Anyone can get HIV by engaging in high-risk sexual activities that include exchange of body fluids, by having received a

blood transfusion before 1985, and by injecting drugs (or having sex with someone who does). Women appear to be particularly susceptible to infection. You can cut your risk for AIDS by deciding not to engage in risky sexual activities.

* Chronic lung diseases include allergies, hay fever, asthma, emphysema, and chronic bronchitis. Allergies are part of the body's natural defense system. Chronic obstructive pulmonary diseases are the fifth leading cause of death in the United States.

* Neurological conditions include headaches and seizure disorders. Headaches may be caused by a variety of factors, the most common of which are tension, dilation and/or rapid contraction of blood vessels in the brain, chemical influences on muscles and vessels that cause inflammation and pain, and underlying physiological and psychological disorders.

* Premenstrual syndrome (PMS) is the name given to a wide variety of symptoms that appear to be related to the menstrual cycle. Endometriosis is the buildup of endometrial tissue in regions of the body other than the uterus.

* Diabetes occurs when the pancreas fails to produce enough insulin to regulate sugar metabolism. Other conditions, such as colitis, irritable bowel syndrome, and peptic ulcers, are the direct result of functional problems in various digestion-related organs or systems.

* Musculoskeletal diseases such as arthritis, lower back pain, repetitive stress injuries, and other problems cause significant pain and disability in millions of people. Chronic fatigue syndrome (CFS) and repetitive stress injuries (such as carpal tunnel syndrome) have emerged in the past decade as major chronic maladies. CFS is associated with depression. Repetitive stress injuries are preventable by proper equipment placement and usage.

Discussion Questions

1. What are the major controllable risk factors for contracting infectious diseases? Using this knowledge, how would you change your current lifestyle to prevent such infection?

2. What is a pathogen? What are the similarities and differences between pathogens and antigens? Discuss uncon-

trollable and controllable risk factors that can threaten your health.

3. What are the six types of pathogens? What are the various means by which they can be transmitted? How have social conditions among the poor and homeless increased the risks for certain diseases, such as tuberculosis,

influenza, and hepatitis? Why are these conditions a challenge to the efforts of public health officials?

4. Identify possible reasons for the spread of emerging and resurgent diseases. Indicate public policies and programs that might reduce this trend.

5. Identify five sexually transmitted infections. What are their symptoms? How do they develop? What are their potential long-term effects?

6. Should Americans be concerned about soaring HIV/AIDS rates elsewhere in the world? Explain your answer.

7. What are some of the major noninfectious chronic diseases affecting Americans today? Do you think there is a pattern in the types of diseases that we get? What are the common risk factors?

8. List common respiratory diseases affecting Americans. Which of these diseases has a genetic basis? An environmental basis? An individual basis? What, if anything, is being done to prevent, treat, and control each of these conditions?

9. Describe the symptoms and treatment of diabetes. What is the difference between type I diabetes and type II diabetes?

10. What are the major disorders of the musculoskeletal system? Why do you think there aren't any cures? Describe the difference between osteoarthritis and rheumatoid arthritis.

Application Exercises

Reread the What Do You Think? scenario at the beginning of this chapter, and answer the following questions:

1. Historically, public health practice has required reporting and contact tracing of people with certain contagious diseases. Do you believe that the right to protect confidentiality supersedes the duty to warn others of possible infection? Under what circumstances? What might Debbie discover from such a tracing of contacts?

2. What obligations do health care workers have to tell patients and co-workers about their own health problems such as herpes or HIV? Do patients have the right to know whether the doctor who is doing surgery is HIV infected? Do health care workers have the right to know whether a patient is infected?

Accessing Your Health on the Internet

Visit the following Internet sites to explore further topics and issues related to personal health. To visit an organization's website, go to the Companion Website for *Health: The Basics, Fifth Edition* at www.aw.com/donatelle, click on the book image, and select "Accessing Your Health on the Internet" from the navigation menu on the left.

1. ***Centers for Disease Control and Prevention (CDC).*** Home page for the government agency dedicated to disease intervention and prevention, with links to all the latest data and publications put out by the CDC, including the *MMWR, HIV/AIDS Surveillance Report,* and the *Journal of Emerging Infectious Diseases,* and access to the CDC research database, Wonder.

2. ***The New England Journal of Medicine Online.*** Online version of a weekly journal reporting the results of important medical research worldwide; includes articles from current and past publications.

3. ***World Health Organization.*** Access to the latest information on world health issues as put out by WHO. Provides direct access to publications and fact sheets, with keywords to help users find topics of interest.

Further Reading

Benenson, A. *Control of Communicable Diseases in Man,* 16th ed. Washington, DC: American Public Health Association, 1998.
Outstanding pocket reference for information on infectious diseases. Published every three to five years in new edition.

Stine, G. *Acquired Immune Deficiency Syndrome.* Englewood Cliffs, NJ: Prentice Hall, 2002.
Excellent text describing the biological, medical, social, and legal issues relating to HIV infection and the AIDS epidemic.

National Center for Health Statistics. *Monthly Vital Statistics Report* and *Advance Data from Vital and Health Statistics.* Hyattsville, MD: Public Health Service.
Detailed government reports, usually published monthly, concerning mortality and morbidity data for the United States, including changes occurring in the rates of particular diseases and in health practices so patterns and trends can be analyzed.

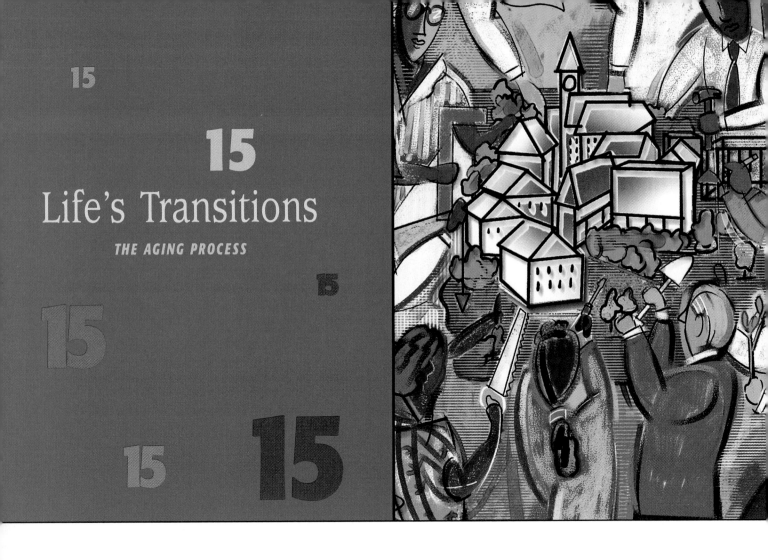

15

15
Life's Transitions
THE AGING PROCESS

objectives

* Review the definition of aging, and explain the related concepts of biological, psychological, social, legal, and functional age.

* Explain the impact on society of the growing population of the elderly.

* Discuss the unique health challenges faced by the elderly, such as alcohol abuse, use of prescription and over-the-counter drugs, osteoporosis, urinary incontinence, depression, senility, and Alzheimer's disease.

* Discuss strategies for healthy aging that can begin during young adulthood.

* Define *death,* and analyze why people deny death in Western culture.

* Discuss the stages of the grieving process, and describe strategies for coping more effectively with death.

* Describe the ethical concerns that arise from the concepts of the right to die and rational suicide.

* Review the decisions that need to be made when someone is dying or has died, including hospice care, funeral arrangements, wills, and organ donations.

Ruth, aged 55, has been smoking for nearly 25 years and has regular flare-ups of bronchitis and other respiratory problems. Fiercely independent, she has a large circle of friends. She also enjoys several hobbies, such as gardening and traveling. Since her divorce seven years ago, Ruth has not found time for a serious romantic relationship and is not worried about finding another person to make her "happy."

Harry, aged 65, is a musician and an avid weightlifter. He spends hours every day working out to stay in shape. He has had two affairs with younger women, and although his wife has warned him that another affair will end their marriage, he is constantly looking for something to make him feel younger. He is dissatisfied with the choices he has made in life and wishes he could do things over.

Which of these people do you think is aging successfully? ✳ *What lifestyle choices have Ruth and Harry made that will help them cope effectively with aging?* ✳ *Which choices may cause significant risks and difficulties?*

Grow old along with me!
The best is yet to be,
The last of life, for which the first was made. . . .
—Robert Browning, *Rabbi Ben Ezra*

In a society that seems to worship youth, researchers have begun to offer good—even revolutionary—news about the aging process. Growing old doesn't have to mean a slow slide to disability, loneliness, and declining physical and mental health. Health promotion, disease prevention, and wellness-oriented activities can prolong vigor and productivity, even among those who haven't always led model lifestyles or made healthful habits a priority. In fact, getting older can mean getting better in many ways—particularly socially, psychologically, and intellectually.

The manner in which you view aging (either as a natural part of living or an inevitable decline toward disease and death) is a crucial factor in how successfully you will adapt to life's transitions. If you view these transitions as periods of growth in your development as a human being, your journey through even the most difficult times will be easier. Explore your own notions about aging in the Assess Yourself box on page 384.

Aging has traditionally been described as the patterns of life changes that occur in members of all species as they grow older. Some people believe that aging begins at the moment of conception. Others contend that it starts at birth. Still others believe that true aging does not begin until we reach our 40s. Typically, experts and laypersons alike have used chronological age to assign a person to a particular life-cycle stage.

Redefining Aging

Discrimination against people based on age is known as **ageism.** When directed against the elderly, this type of discrimination carries with it social ostracism and negative portrayals of older people.

The study of individual and collective aging processes, known as **gerontology,** explores the reasons for aging and the ways in which people cope with and adapt to this process. Gerontologists have identified several age-related characteristics that define where a person is in terms of biological, psychological, social, legal, and functional life-stage development:[1]

- *Biological age* refers to the relative age or condition of the person's organs and body systems. There are 70-year-old runners who have the cardiovascular system of a 40-year-old, and 40-year-olds who have less energy than their elders. Arthritis and other chronic conditions can accelerate the aging process.
- *Psychological age* refers to a person's adaptive capacities, such as coping abilities and intelligence, and to the person's awareness of his or her individual capabilities, self-efficacy, and general ability to adapt to situations. Although chronic illness may render people physically handicapped, they may possess tremendous psychological reserves and remain alert and fully capable of making decisions.

Aging The patterns of life changes that occur in members of all species as they grow older.

Ageism Discrimination based on age.

Gerontology The study of individual and collective aging processes.

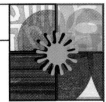

Where Do You Want to Be?

During the peak of youth, aging most likely is the furthest thing from our minds. However, thinking about aging and what we expect from life are important elements of a satisfying adult development process. Take a few minutes to answer the following questions. Your answers may tell you a great deal about yourself.

1. At this point in your life, what do you value most?
2. What do you think will be most important to you when you reach your 40s? 50s? 60s? What similarities and differences do you notice, and what causes these similarities and differences?
3. Do you think your parents are happy and content with the way their lives have turned out? If they could change anything, what do you think they might do differently?
4. What about your own direction so far in life is similar to that of your parents? What have you done differently? Are the similarities and differences good? Why or why not?
5. What do you think are the keys to a happy and satisfying life?
6. What do you want to accomplish by the time you are 40? 50? 60?
7. Have you ever thought of retirement? Describe your retirement.
8. Describe the "you" that you would like to be at the age of 70. How is that "you" similar to or different from the "you" of today? What actions will you need to take to be that "you" in the future?

- *Social age* refers to a person's habits and roles relative to society's expectations. People in a particular life stage usually share similar tastes in music, television shows, and politics.
- *Legal age* is probably the most common definition of age in the United States. Based on chronological years, legal age is used as a factor in determining voting rights, driving privileges, drinking age, eligibility for Social Security payments, and a host of other rights and obligations.
- *Functional age* refers to the ways in which people compare to others of a similar age. It is difficult to separate functional aging from many of the other types of aging, particularly chronological and biological aging.

What Is Successful Aging?

Many of today's "elderly" individuals lead active, productive lives. Typically, people who have aged successfully have the following characteristics:

- In general, they have managed to avoid serious, debilitating diseases and disability.

- They maintain a high level of physical functioning, live independently, and engage in most normal activities of daily living.
- They have maintained cognitive functioning and are actively engaged in mentally challenging and stimulating activities.
- They are actively engaged in social and productive activities.
- They are resilient and able to cope reasonably well with physical, social, and emotional changes.

The process of aging has often been viewed with dread because of changes that result from ordinary biological or disease processes. Only in the past decade have we begun to fully appreciate the gains and positive aspects of normal adult development throughout the life span. According to gerontologist Dr. Karen Hooker, the elderly as a population display much more differentiation in personalities, coping styles, and "possible selves" than any other age group. She states that "successful aging and development as individuals can be viewed as dynamic processes of adaptation between the self and the environment. Throughout our lives we make choices and respond to changes in vastly different ways. Each person is born with certain traits that stay reasonably stable throughout life, but character is deeply affected by personal action constructs that change with time and life history."[2]

Aging is not a static process, but one in which we change and become someone uniquely fashioned by our life's story. Gerontologists have devised several categories for specific age-related characteristics. People aged 65 to 74 are viewed as the **young-old**; those aged 75 to 84 are the **middle-old** group; those 85 and over are classified as the **old-old.**

Young-old   People aged 65 to 74.

Middle-old   People aged 75 to 84.

Old-old   People aged 85 and over.

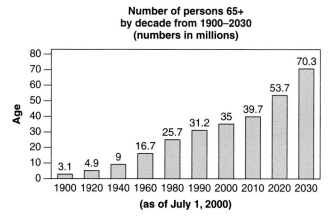

Figure 15.1

Number of Older Americans (in Millions)

Sources: U.S. Bureau of the Census, "Projections of the Total Resident Population by 5 Year Age Groups, Race, and Hispanic Origin with Special Age Categories: Middle Series, 1999 to 2000," U.S. Census Internet release date: January 13, 2000; "Population Projections of the United States by Age, Sex, Race, and Hispanic Origin: 1995–2050," *Current Population Reports,* P. 25–1130. Data for 2000 are from the 2000 Census.

What do you think?

What factors influence the aging process? ✳ *Which of these factors do you have the power to change through your behavior right now?*

The Elderly: A Growing Population

In 2000, there were an estimated 35 million people aged 65 or older in the United States, nearly 13 percent of the total population. The number of older Americans has increased more than tenfold since 1900, when there were only about 3 million people age 65 or older, comprising 4 percent of the total population.[3] (See Figure 15.1). Despite the growth of the older population, the United States is a relatively young country compared to many developed nations, where older persons account for 15 percent or more of the population.[4] According to researchers at the National Institute on Aging, "[T]he aging of the 75 million–strong baby boomer generation could have an impact on our society of equal magnitude to that of immigration at the turn of the century."[5]

Health Issues for an Aging Society

Life expectancy for a person born in 2000 is 76.9 years, about 29 years longer than a child born in 1900.[6] Whereas people aged 65 and older comprise 13 percent of the U.S. population today, they are projected to make up over 21 percent of the population by 2030. Where will these elderly people live, and how will they support themselves?

Health Care Costs

Today, the elderly account for approximately 38 percent of total national health care costs, with estimated costs in excess of $6,800 per person. Out-of-pocket health expenses for the elderly have risen by 33 percent since 1990.[7] As people live longer, the chances of developing a costly chronic disease increase. In 2000, 26.3 percent of older persons assessed their health as fair or poor, compared to 9.2 percent of all age groups taken together. Nearly 29 percent of older people also reported activity limitations.[8] As our technology improves, chronic illnesses that once were quickly fatal may now be treated successfully for years. Projected future costs from these two trends are staggering.

Will working Americans be willing to pay an increased share of the health care costs for people on fixed incomes who cannot pay for themselves? If not, what will become of older Americans? Perhaps most important, who will ultimately pay?

Housing and Living Arrangements Contrary to popular opinion, most elderly people (over 95 percent) never live in a nursing home. Community living, assisted living, skilled nursing care, and other options are new possibilities for those who have financial means or who have purchased some form of long-term care insurance.[9] However, the low-income elderly continue to face housing problems. Who will provide the necessary social services, and who will pay the bill? Will the family of the future be forced to coexist with several generations under one roof? Will there be an increase in support for caretakers of the elderly?

Ethical and Moral Considerations Difficult ethical questions arise when we consider the implications for an already overburdened health care system. Given the shortage of donor organs, will we be forced to decide whether a 75-year-old should receive a heart transplant instead of a 50-year-old? Questions have already surfaced regarding the efficacy of hooking up a terminally ill older person to costly machines that prolong life for a few weeks or months but overtax health care resources. Is the prolongation of life at all costs a moral imperative, or will future generations be forced to devise a set of criteria for deciding who will be helped and who will not? Understanding the process of aging and knowing what actions we all can take to prolong our own healthy years are a part of our collective responsibility.

What do you think?

Do you currently have health insurance? If not, why not? ✳ *What do you think people over 65 would do if they suddenly didn't have Medicare?* ✳ *Should elderly Americans be left out of the health insurance industry because they are at high risk for illness and disability?* ✳ *Why are the aging of the population and the impending difficulties with health care costs and access important to everyone?*

Aging: The World's Oldest Countries

The numerical and proportional growth of older populations around the world is a result of major achievements—reliable birth control that has decreased fertility rates, improvements in medical care and sanitation that have reduced infant and maternal mortality and infectious and parasitic diseases, and improvements in nutrition and education. Every month, the net increase in the world's population aged 60 and over is more than 1 million; 70 percent of this increase occurs in developing countries and 30 percent in developed countries. Based on projected estimates, the percentage increase in world population over the age of 60 will be 59 percent for the developed countries of the world and 159 percent for the less developed countries between 1991 and 2020.

The world's elderly population—defined here as persons aged 60 and over—numbers 495 million today and is expected to exceed 1 billion by the year 2020. Almost half of today's elderly population lives in just four nations: the People's Republic of China, India, the Commonwealth of Soviet States, and the United States. There is intense debate over issues—social security costs, health care, educational investments, and so on—that are directly linked to this changing age structure of societies.

Sources: U.S. Department of Commerce, Bureau of the Census, Economics and Statistics Administration, *Global Aging: Comparative Indicators and Future Trends* (Washington, D.C.: Government Printing Office, 1991); U.S. Bureau of the Census, International Programs Center, International Data Base, 1998; United Nations, *International Plan of Action on Aging: Demographic Background,* March 2002. http://www.un.org/esa/socdev/ageing/ageipaa.htm.

Theories on Aging

Biological Theories

Explanations for the biological causes of aging include the following:

- The *wear-and-tear theory* states that, like everything else in the universe, the human body wears out. Inherent in this theory is the idea that the more you abuse your body, the faster it will wear out. Fortunately, today's elderly can achieve high levels of fitness without having to be marathon runners. Strength training, walking, gardening, vigorous shopping, and other activities allow even the most out of shape to improve.
- The *cellular theory* states that at birth we have only a certain number of usable cells, which are genetically programmed to divide or reproduce a limited number of times. Once these cells reach the end of their reproductive cycle, they die, and the organs they make up begin to deteriorate. The rate of deterioration varies from person to person, and its impact depends on the system involved.
- The *autoimmune theory* attributes aging to the decline of the body's immunological system. Studies indicate that as we age, our immune systems become less effective in fighting disease. Eventually, bodies that are subjected to too much stress, lack of sleep, and so on—especially if these stressors are coupled with poor nutrition—show signs of disease and infirmity. In some instances, the immune system appears to lose control and turn its protective mechanisms inward, actually attacking the person's own body. Although this type of disorder may occur in all age groups, some gerontologists believe that the condition increases in frequency and severity with age.
- The *genetic mutation theory* proposes that the number of cells exhibiting unusual or different characteristics increases with age. Proponents of this theory believe that aging is related to the amount of mutational damage within the genes. The greater the mutation, the greater the chance that cells will not function properly, leading to eventual dysfunction of body organs and systems.

Psychosocial Impacts on Aging

Numerous psychological and sociological factors also influence the manner in which people age. Psychologists Erik Erikson and Robert Peck have formulated theories of personality development that emphasize adaptation and adjustment. In his developmental model, Erikson states that people must progress through eight critical stages during a lifetime. If a person does not receive the proper stimulus or develop effective methods of coping with life's turmoil from infancy onward, problems are likely to develop later in life. According to this theory, maladjustments in old age are often a result of problems encountered in earlier stages of a person's life.

Peck argues that during middle and old age, people face a series of increasingly stressful tasks. Those who are poorly adjusted psychologically or who have not developed appropriate coping skills are likely to undergo a painful aging process. Both Erikson and Peck suggest that a combination of psychosocial and biological factors and environmental "trigger mechanisms" causes each of us to age in a unique manner. But what is normal and what is unique in aging? How much change is inevitable, and how much can we avoid?

Changes in the Body and Mind

Typical Physical Changes

Although the physiological consequences of aging can differ in severity and timing, certain standard changes occur as a result of the aging process.

The Skin   As a normal consequence of aging, the skin becomes thinner and loses elasticity, particularly in the outer surfaces. Fat deposits, which add to the soft lines and shape of the skin, diminish. Starting at about age 30, lines develop on the forehead as a result of smiling, squinting, and other facial expressions. These lines become more pronounced, with added "crow's feet" around the eyes, during the 40s. During a person's 50s and 60s, the skin begins to sag and lose color, leading to pallor in the 70s. Body fat in underlying layers of skin continues to be redistributed away from the limbs and extremities into the trunk region of the body. Age spots become more numerous because of excessive pigment accumulation under the skin, particularly in people who have experienced heavy sun exposure.

Bones and Joints   Throughout the life span, bones are continually changing because of the accumulation and loss of minerals. By the third or fourth decade of life, mineral loss from bones becomes more prevalent than mineral accumulation, resulting in a weakening and porosity (diminishing density) of bony tissue. This loss of minerals (particularly calcium) occurs in both sexes, although it is much more common in females. Loss of calcium can contribute to **osteoporosis,** a disease characterized by low bone density and structural deterioration of bone tissue. These porous, fragile bones are susceptible to fracture. Osteoporosis can, however, occur at any age.[10] (See the accompanying Reality Check box on page 388.)

The Head   With age, features of the head enlarge and become more noticeable. Increased cartilage and fatty tissue cause the nose to grow a half inch wider and another half inch longer. Earlobes get fatter and grow longer, while overall head circumference increases one quarter of an inch per decade, even though the brain itself shrinks. The skull becomes thicker with age.

The Urinary Tract   At age 70, the kidneys can filter waste from the blood only half as fast as they could at age 30. The need to urinate more frequently occurs because the bladder's capacity declines from 2 cups of urine at age 30 to 1 cup at age 70.

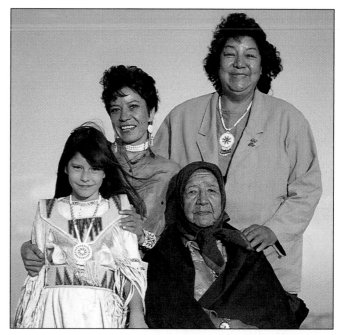

In most cases, you need look no further than your family tree to get an idea of the effects that aging will have on you.

One problem often associated with aging is **urinary incontinence,** which ranges from passing a few drops of urine while laughing or sneezing to having no control over urination. As many as 19 percent of older men and 38 percent of older women have some degree of urinary incontinence.[11]

Incontinence can pose major social, physical, and emotional problems. Embarrassment and fear of wetting oneself may cause an older person to become isolated and avoid social functions. Caregivers may become frustrated with incontinent elderly patients. Prolonged wetness and the inability to properly care for oneself can lead to irritation, infections, and other problems.

However, incontinence is not an inevitable part of aging. Most cases are caused by highly treatable neurological problems that affect the central nervous system, by medications, by infections of the pelvic muscles, by weakness in the pelvic walls, or by other problems. When the problem is treated, the incontinence usually vanishes.[12]

The Heart and Lungs   Resting heart rate stays about the same over the course of a person's life, but the stroke volume (the amount of blood the muscle pushes out per beat) diminishes as heart muscles deteriorate. Vital capacity, or the amount of air that moves when you inhale and exhale at

---

Osteoporosis   A degenerative bone disorder characterized by increasingly porous bones.

Urinary incontinence   The inability to control urination.

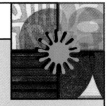

Osteoporosis: Preventing an Age-Old Problem

Although many people consider osteoporosis to be a disease of elderly women, osteoporosis can occur at any age, and increasingly it poses a problem for men, too. When people hear that someone has osteoporosis, the image that comes to mind is a slumped-over individual with a characteristic "dowager's hump" in the upper back; however, this is a relatively rare, extreme version of the disease. Osteoporosis is progressive and occurs over many years. Without proper prevention in the form of diet, weight-bearing exercise, and overall fitness improvements, each of us risks developing this condition. As awareness increases, millions of Americans are demanding "bone density" tests to determine just how far gone their bones and joints really may be. Health care providers, responding to the estimated $14 billion in direct and indirect costs that osteoporosis patients incur, are also motivated to focus on controlling risks.

EPIDEMIOLOGY OF THE DISEASE

Prevalence data about osteoporosis indicate the following:

- Recent results from the National Osteoporosis Risk Assessment (NORA), the largest osteoporosis study in the United States to date, indicates that as many as 40 percent of postmenopausal women have osteopenia (an early precursor to bone loss/weakening), and another 7 percent have significant bone loss characteristic of the more severe form, osteoporosis.
- The hips, wrists, and spine are most vulnerable to the ravages of osteoporosis.

- In the United States, osteoporosis affects over 28 million Americans, 80 percent of whom are women.
- Each year osteoporosis causes 1.5 million fractures: 300,000 at the hip; 700,000 in the vertebrae; 250,000 in the wrists; and more than 300,000 at other sites.
- One out of every two women and one in eight men over age 50 will have an osteoporosis fracture sometime in life.
- More than 2 million American men have osteoporosis, and millions more are at risk. Each year, 80,000 men suffer a hip fracture, and one-third of them die within a year.

RISK FACTORS

A number of factors may predispose a person to developing osteoporosis. Risk factors that we cannot control include the following:

- *Gender.* Your chances of developing osteoporosis are greater if you are a woman. Women have less bone tissue and lose bone more rapidly than men because of the hormonal changes resulting from menopause.
- *Age.* The older you are, the greater your risk of osteoporosis. Your bones become less dense and weaker as you age.
- *Body size.* Small, thin-boned women are at greater risk.
- *Ethnicity.* Caucasian and Asian women are at highest risk; African American and Latina women have a lower but still significant risk.
- *Family history.* Susceptibility to fracture may be, in part, hereditary. People

whose parents have a history of fractures also seem to have reduced bone mass.

However, we can modify several other risk factors by our choices in lifestyle behaviors, medication, and diet:

- Levels of sex hormones—abnormal absence of menstrual periods (amenorrhea), low estrogen level (menopause), and low testosterone level in men may signal potential problems
- Anorexia
- A lifetime diet low in calcium and vitamin D
- Use of certain medications, such as glucocorticoids or some anticonvulsants
- An inactive lifestyle or extended bed rest
- Cigarette smoking
- Excessive use of alcohol

The following preventive measures can help everyone reduce the risk of osteoporosis.

INCREASE CALCIUM AND VITAMIN D INTAKE

Many studies support the notion that if you don't consume enough calcium, you will be at increased risk for osteoporosis. Calcium needs change over the course of a lifetime. The need is greater during childhood and adolescence, when the skeleton is growing, and during pregnancy and breast-feeding. Postmenopausal women and older men also need more calcium. Medications also may deplete calcium reserves. Because Vitamin D helps with calcium absorption, taking in adequate amounts of vitamin D will ensure that the body uses the calcium that it ingests.

EXERCISE

Like muscle, bone is living tissue that responds to exercise by becoming stronger. The best exercise for the bones is weight-bearing exercise that forces you to work against gravity. Examples include walking, jogging, weight training, tennis, and dancing.

Research conducted by Dr. Christine M. Snow, director of Oregon State University's bone research lab and internationally known exercise scientist, has shed interesting light on the importance of exercise for residents of nursing homes in Oregon. Residents were given modest exercises to do while wearing weighted vests. Subjects not only improved bone density but also balance and strength, which together can reduce risk of falling and fracturing bones. In addition, residents developed a faster gait, which makes them less likely to fall to the side if they lose balance. In studies of young gymnasts, Snow has found that bone density can be increased through various types of exercise. She emphasizes that it is vitally important that exercise begin early in life to ensure bone health in later years.

Sources: National Institutes of Health, Osteoporosis and Related Bone Diseases National Resource Center, December 2000 (http://www.osteo.org/osteo.html); B. Demyan, "The Graying of America: Can Exercise Stem the Aging Process?" 2 (2) (2000): 4. E. Siris, P. Miller, et al., "Identification and Fracture Outcomes of Undiagnosed Low Bone Mineral Density in Postmenopausal Women: Results of the National Osteoporosis Risk Assessment," *Journal of the American Medical Association* 286 (2001): 2815; C. Chestnut, "Osteoporosis: An Underdiagnosed Disease," *Journal of the American Medical Association* 286 (2001): 2825.

---

maximum effort, also declines with age. Exercise can do a great deal to preserve heart and lung function.

Eyesight By age 30, the lens of the eye begins to harden, causing problems by the early 40s. The lens begins to yellow and loses transparency, while the pupil of the eye shrinks, allowing less light to penetrate. Activities such as reading become more difficult, particularly in dim light. By age 60, depth perception declines, and farsightedness often develops. A need for glasses usually develops in the 40s, and this evolves into a need for bifocals in the 50s and trifocals in the 60s. **Cataracts** (clouding of the lens) and **glaucoma** (elevated pressure within the eyeball) become more likely. Eventually, a tendency toward color blindness may develop, especially for shades of blue and green.

Hearing The ability to hear high-frequency consonants (for example, *s, t,* and *z*) diminishes with age. Much of the actual hearing loss lies in the ability to distinguish extreme ranges of sound rather than normal conversational tones.

Sexual Changes As men age, they experience notable changes in sexual functioning. Whereas the degree and rate of change vary greatly from person to person, the following changes generally occur:

1. The ability to obtain an erection is slowed.
2. The ability to maintain an erection is diminished.
3. The length of the refractory period between orgasms increases.
4. The angle of the erection declines with age.
5. The orgasm itself grows shorter in duration.

Women also experience several changes:

1. Menopause usually occurs between the ages of 45 and 55. Women may experience symptoms such as hot flashes, mood swings, weight gain, development of facial hair, and other hormone-related problems.
2. The walls of the vagina become less elastic, and the epithelium thins, possibly making intercourse painful.
3. Vaginal secretions, particularly during sexual activity, diminish.
4. The breasts become less firm. Loss of fat in various areas leads to fewer curves, with a decrease in the soft lines of the body contours.

While these physiological changes may seem somewhat discouraging, a recent study by the National Council on Aging indicates that older Americans continue to be sexually active. This study refutes long-held beliefs that sexual desire decreases as we age. Results indicate that nearly half of Americans over age 60 engage in sexual activity at least once a

---

Cataracts Clouding of the lens that interrupts the focusing of light on the retina, resulting in blurred vision or eventual blindness. This condition is correctable with surgery.

Glaucoma Elevation of pressure within the eyeball, leading to hardening of the eyeball, impaired vision, and possible blindness.

month and that four out of ten would like to have sex more frequently than they currently do.[13] With the advent of drugs designed to treat sexual dysfunction, such as Viagra, many older adults may get their wish.

Body Comfort   Because of the loss of body fat, thinning of the epithelium, and diminished glandular activity, elderly people experience greater difficulty in regulating body temperature. This limits their ability to withstand extreme cold or heat, increasing the risks of hypothermia, heatstroke, and heat exhaustion.

> ### What do you think?
> *Of the health conditions discussed in this section, which ones can you prevent?* ✳ *Which ones can you delay?* ✳ *What actions can you take now to protect yourself from these problems?*

Mental Changes

Intelligence   Today it is commonly recognized that much of our previous knowledge about the intelligence of older people was based on inappropriate testing procedures. Given an appropriate length of time, elderly people may learn and develop skills in a similar manner to younger people. It is also widely believed that what many elderly people lack in speed of learning they make up for in practical knowledge—that is, the "wisdom of age."

Memory   Have you ever wondered why your grandfather seems unable to remember what he did last weekend even though he can graphically describe an event that occurred 40 years ago? This phenomenon is not unusual among the elderly. Research indicates that although short-term memory may fluctuate on a daily basis, the ability to remember events from past decades seems to remain largely unchanged.

Flexibility Versus Rigidity   Although it is widely believed that people become more like one another as they age, noth-

Senility   A term associated with loss of memory and judgment and orientation problems occurring in a small percentage of the elderly.

Dementias   Progressive brain impairments that interfere with memory and normal intellectual functioning.

Alzheimer's disease (AD)   A chronic condition involving changes in nerve fibers of the brain that results in mental deterioration.

ing could be further from the truth. Having lived through a multitude of experiences and faced diverse joys, sorrows, and obstacles, the typical elderly person has developed unique methods of coping with life. These unique adaptive variations make for interesting differences in how they confront the many changes brought on by the aging process. As a group, the elderly are extremely heterogeneous.

Depression   Most adults continue to lead healthy, fulfilling lives as they grow older. However, some elderly people do suffer from mental and emotional disturbances. Some research indicates that depression may be the most common psychological problem facing older adults.[14] Depression typically occurs in conjunction with other medical illnesses, such as cardiovascular disease, stroke, diabetes, and cancer. Older people who face significant personal losses, economic problems, and social isolation are at greatest risk. Support systems, community resources, and proper medication are critical factors in prevention. However, the rate of major depression is actually lower among older people than among younger adults.

Senility: Getting Rid of Ageist Attitudes   Over the years, the elderly have often been victims of ageist attitudes. People who were chronologically old were often labeled "senile" whenever they displayed memory failure, errors in judgment, disorientation, or erratic behaviors. Today scientists recognize that these same symptoms can occur at any age and for various reasons, including disease or the use of over-the-counter and prescription drugs. When the underlying problems are corrected, the memory loss and disorientation also improve. Currently, the term **senility** is seldom used except to describe a very small group of organic disorders.

Alzheimer's Disease   **Dementias** are progressive brain impairments that interfere with memory and normal intellectual functioning. Although there are many types of dementia, one of the most common forms is **Alzheimer's disease (AD)**. Attacking over 4 million Americans, and killing over 100,000 of them every year, this disease is one of the most painful and devastating conditions that families can endure. It kills its victims twice: first through a slow loss of personhood (memory loss, disorientation, personality changes, and eventual loss of the ability to function independently), and then through the deterioration of bodily systems as they gradually succumb to the powerful impact of neurological problems. On average, patients with AD live for eight to ten years after diagnosis, though the disease can last for up to 20 years.[15]

Currently, Alzheimer's afflicts an estimated one in ten people over age 65 and one in five people over age 85; over 360,000 new cases occur per year.[16] These numbers are certain to increase. Alzheimer's disease is estimated to cost society over $100 billion a year currently.[17] With the U.S. population gradually aging, the economic burden of the future seems even more dismal. Although the disease is associated in most people's minds strictly with the elderly,

Alzheimer's has been diagnosed in people in their late 40s. In fact, over 5 percent of all cases occur before age 65.[18]

Contrary to what many people think, Alzheimer's is not a new disease. Named after Alois Alzheimer, a German neuropathologist who recorded it as early as 1906, Alzheimer's disease refers to a degenerative disease of the brain in which nerve cells stop communicating with one another. This lack of communication occurs when nerves collect a form of *amyloid protein plaque,* and *neurofibrillary tangles* (abnormal collections of twisted cells) disrupt nerve transmission.[19] Ordinarily, brain cells communicate by releasing chemicals that allow the cells to receive and transmit messages for various types of behavior. In Alzheimer's patients, the brain doesn't produce enough of these chemicals; cells can't communicate; and eventually the cells die. This degeneration happens in the sections of the brain that affect memory, speech, and personality, leaving the parts that control other bodily functions, such as heartbeat and breathing, working just fine. Thus, the mind begins to go as the body lives on. It all happens in a slow, progressive manner, and it may be as long as 20 years before symptoms are noticed. Alzheimer's is generally detected first by families, who note changes, particularly memory lapses and personality changes, in their loved ones. Medical tests rule out underlying causes, and certain neurological tests help confirm the diagnosis.

Alzheimer's disease characteristically progresses in three stages. During the *first stage,* symptoms include forgetfulness, memory loss, impaired judgment, increasing inability to handle routine tasks, disorientation, lack of interest in one's surroundings, and depression. These symptoms accelerate in the *second stage,* which also includes agitation and restlessness (especially at night), loss of sensory perceptions, muscle twitching, and repetitive actions. Many patients become depressed, combative, and aggressive. In the *final stage,* disorientation is often complete. The person becomes completely dependent on others for eating, dressing, and other activities. Identity loss and speech problems are common symptoms. Eventually, control of bodily functions may be lost.

Once Alzheimer's disease strikes, the victim's life expectancy is cut in half. Tragically, little can be done at present to treat the disorder. Researchers are investigating a number of possible causes, including genetic predisposition, malfunction of the immune system, a slow-acting virus, chromosomal or genetic defects, oxidative stress, chronic inflammation, and neurotransmitter imbalance.[20]

Health Challenges of the Elderly

Some health problems common in the elderly are brought on by failing health, others by society. Some problems result when people do not develop the ability to cope properly with life's hurdles. Still other problems come from the elderly person's perceived loss of control over life's events—watching loved ones die, facing health problems, and confronting an uncertain economy on a fixed income. Developing life skills and a network of social support during earlier years can significantly reduce problems in old age.

Alcohol Use and Abuse

Although alcohol abuse continues to be a major health concern in the United States today, the problem is highest among young adults and lowest among adults ages 65 and older. The younger you start drinking, the greater your risks of late-life problem drinking.[21] Early studies reported that 2 to 10 percent of the elderly were alcoholics, but the exact percentages are controversial today. However, a person who is prone to alcoholism during the younger and middle years is more likely to continue during later years. The old alcoholic is probably no more common in American society than the young alcoholic, despite the stereotype of the old, lost soul, hiding his or her sorrows in a bottle.

Men tend to have higher risks for alcoholism at all ages. Alcohol abuse is five times more common among elderly men than among elderly women. Yet as many as half of all elderly men and an even higher proportion of elderly women don't drink at all.[22] Those who do drink do so less than younger persons, consuming only five to six drinks weekly. It is important to note that most of the elderly who consume alcohol are neither alcoholics nor people who drink to cope with their losses. Most drinking among the elderly is social and may, in fact, be much less of a problem than previously thought.[23]

Prescription Drug Use

It is extremely rare for elderly people to use illicit drugs, but some do overuse and grow dependent upon prescription drugs. Anyone who combines different drugs runs the risk of dangerous drug interactions. The risks of adverse effects are even greater for people with impaired circulation and declining kidney and liver function. Elderly people displaying symptoms of these drug-induced effects, which may include bizarre behavior patterns or disorientation, are all too often dismissed as senile rather than examined for underlying causes and treated. Doctors often have difficulty medicating elderly individuals, particularly when the patient is taking several different drugs at the same time.

Over-the-Counter Remedies

A substantial segment of the over-60 population avoids orthodox medical treatment, viewing it as a last resort. This is becoming increasingly true as Medicare coverage becomes less adequate and the elderly are forced to pay larger medical bills out of their own resources. The poor are particularly prone to turn to folk medicine and over-the-counter preparations as cheaper, less intimidating alternatives.

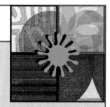

Aging and Exercise

Whether you're 20, 50, or 80 years old, you can exercise and improve your health. Staying physically active is key to good health well into later years. Yet only about one in four older adults exercises regularly. Many older people think they are too old or too frail to exercise. Nothing could be further from the truth. Physical activity of any kind—from heavy-duty exercises such as jogging or bicycling to easier efforts like walking—is good for you. Vigorous exercise can help strengthen your heart and lungs. Talk to your doctor before you begin, especially if you are over 60 or have a medical problem. Thirty minutes of moderate activity each day is a good goal.

Include a mix of stretching, strength training, and aerobic or endurance exercises in your exercise plan. People who are weak or frail should start slowly. Start with stretching and strength training; add aerobics later. Aerobics are safer and easier once you feel balanced and your muscles are stronger.

Stretching improves flexibility, eases movement, and lowers the risk of injury and muscle strain. Stretching increases blood flow and gets your body ready for exercise. Warm up and cool down for 5 to 15 minutes, slowly and carefully, before and after all types of exercise. Stretching can help loosen muscles in the arms, shoulders, back, chest, stomach, buttocks, thighs, and calves. It's also very relaxing.

Strength training (also called resistance training or weight lifting) builds muscle and bone, both of which decline with age. Strengthening exercises for the upper and lower body can be done by lifting weights or working out with machines or an elastic band. It is very important to have an expert teach you how to work with weights. Without help, you can get hurt. With help, older adults can work their way up to many of the same weight-lifting routines as younger adults. Once you know what to do, simple strength training exercises can be done at home. Strength training activities do not have to take a lot of time; 30 to 40 minutes at least two or three times each week is all that's needed. Try not to exercise the same muscles two days in a row.

Aerobic exercises (also called endurance exercises) strengthen the heart and improve overall fitness by increasing the body's ability to use oxygen. Swimming, walking, and dancing are "low-impact" aerobic activities. They avoid the muscle and joint pounding of more "high-impact" exercises, such as jogging and jumping rope. Aerobic exercises raise the number of heartbeats each minute (heart rate). It's best to get your heart rate to a certain point and keep it there for 20 minutes or more. If you have not exercised in a while, start slowly. As you get stronger, you can try to increase your heart rate. Aerobics should be done for 20 to 40 minutes at least three times each week. Before starting any aerobics program, check with your doctor, and ask about your own target heart rate. Some blood pressure medicines, for example, can affect how you calculate your target heart rate.

Local gyms, universities, or hospitals can help you find a teacher or program that works for you. You can also check with local churches or synagogues, senior and civic centers, parks, recreation associations, YMCAs, YWCAs, and even local shopping malls for exercise and wellness programs. Many community centers also offer programs for older people who may be worried about special health problems such as heart disease or falling. Look for books and tapes at your local library.

Source: Adapted from U.S. Department of Health and Human Services, National Institute on Aging, "Don't Take It Easy—Exercise!" (Gaithersburg, MD: National Institute on Aging, n.d.). Available at MedAccess Age Page, http://www.medaccess.com/seniors/agepg/ap41.htm.

Preventive Actions for Healthy Aging

As you know from reading this book, you can do many things to prolong your life and improve the quality of your life. Some factors, however, are especially important. To provide for healthy older years, each of the following should be part of your younger years.

Develop and Maintain Healthy Relationships

Social bonds lend vigor and energy to life. Be willing to give to others, and seek variety in your relationships rather than befriending only people who agree with you. By experiencing diverse people and interacting with different points of view, we gain a new perspective on life.

Enrich the Spiritual Side of Life

Although we often take this for granted, cultivating a relationship with nature, the environment, a higher being, and yourself is a key factor in personal growth and development. Take time for thought and quiet contemplation, and enjoy the sunsets, sounds, and energy of life. These moments spent in time prioritized for "you" will leave you invigorated and fresh—better able to cope with the ups and downs of life. If you don't take time for yourself now, it just may be that you won't have time in the later years.

Improve Fitness

If you're basically sedentary, just about any moderate-intensity exercise that gets your heart beating faster and increases strength and/or flexibility will maximize your

For many, the secret to aging well is to stay active and enjoy the company of good friends.

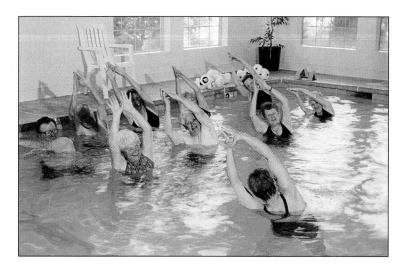

physical health and functional years. One of the inevitable physical changes that the body undergoes is **sarcopenia,** age-associated loss of muscle mass. The less muscle you have, the less energy you will burn even while resting. The lower your metabolic rate, the more likely the weight gain. With regular strength training, you can increase your muscle mass, boost your metabolism, strengthen your bones, prevent osteoporosis, and, in general, feel better and function more efficiently. The Skills for Behavior Change box provides tips for exercise.

Eat for Health

Although other chapters in this text provide detailed information about nutrition and weight control, certain nutrients are especially essential to healthy aging.

- *Calcium.* Bone loss tends to increase in women, particularly in the hip region, shortly before menopause. During perimenopause and menopause, this bone loss accelerates rapidly, with an average of about 3 percent of skeletal mass lost per year over a five-year period. The result is an increased risk for fracture and disability. Few women actually consume the 1,000 milligrams of calcium recommended during the younger years, or the 1,500 milligrams recommended during and after menopause.
- *Vitamin D.* Vitamin D is necessary for adequate calcium absorption, yet as people age, particularly in their 50s and 60s, they do not absorb vitamin D from foods as readily as they did in their younger years. If vitamin D is unavailable, calcium levels are also likely to be lower.
- *Protein.* As the elderly become more concerned about cholesterol and fatty foods, as their budgets shrink, one nutrient that often takes the "hit" is protein. Many elderly cut back on protein to a point that is below the recommended daily amount. Because protein is necessary for muscle mass, protein insufficiencies can spell trouble.

Other nutrients, including vitamin E, folic acid (folate), iron, potassium, and vitamin B_{12}, are important to the aging process, and most of these are readily available in any diet that follows food pyramid recommendations.

Caring for the Elderly

Elderly women far outnumber elderly men in American society, and the discrepancy increases with age. Because women live seven years longer than men on average, elderly women are more likely to be living alone. Further, they are more likely to experience poverty and multiple chronic health problems, a situation referred to as **comorbidity.** Consequently, more elderly women than men are likely to need assistance from children, other relatives, friends, and neighbors.

Women have usually been the primary caregivers for elderly Americans, often for their ailing husbands. Research also indicates that women spend more hours than men (38 hours versus 27 hours per week) in caregiving activities and perform a wider range of activities. Regardless of the time spent, caregiving is a difficult and stressful experience for both women and men. **Respite care,** or care that is given by someone who relieves the primary caregiver, should be available to ease the burden.

Sarcopenia Age-related loss of muscle mass.

Comorbidity The presence of a number of diseases at the same time.

Respite care The care provided by substitute caregivers to relieve the principal caregiver from his or her continuous responsibility.

Understanding Death

Death eventually comes to everyone, but if you live life to the fullest and learn as much about end-of-life issues as you can, you will be better able to accept the inevitable. To cope effectively with dying, we must address the individual needs of those who are facing life's final transition. Let's begin by investigating what death means, at least in medical terms.

Defining Death

Dying is the process of decline in body functions resulting in the death of an organism. **Death** can be defined as the "final cessation of the vital functions" and also refers to a state in which these functions are "incapable of being restored."[24] This definition has become more significant as medical advances make it increasingly possible to postpone death.

In response to legal and ethical questions related to death and dying, a presidential commission developed the Uniform Determination of Death Act in 1981, which was endorsed by the American Medical Association, the American Bar Association, and the National Conference for Commissioners on Uniform State Laws. This act, which has been adopted by several states, reads as follows: "An individual who has sustained either (1) irreversible cessation of circulatory and respiratory functions, or (2) irreversible cessation of all functions of the entire brain, including the brain stem, is dead. A determination of death must be made in accordance with accepted medical standards."[25]

The concept of **brain death,** defined as the irreversible cessation of all functions of the entire brain stem, has gained increasing credence. As defined by the Ad Hoc Committee of the Harvard Medical School, brain death occurs when the following criteria are met:

- Unreceptivity and unresponsiveness—that is, no response even to painful stimuli
- No movement for a continuous hour after observation by a physician and no breathing after three minutes off a respirator
- No reflexes, including brain stem reflexes; fixed and dilated pupils
- A "flat" electroencephalogram (EEG) for at least 10 minutes

---

Dying The process of decline in body functions, resulting in the death of an organism.

Death The permanent ending of all vital functions.

Brain death The irreversible cessation of all functions of the entire brain stem.

- All of these tests repeated at least 24 hours later with no change
- Certainty that hypothermia (extreme loss of body heat) and depression of the central nervous system caused by use of drugs such as barbiturates are not responsible for these conditions[26]

The Harvard report provides useful guidelines; however, the definition of *death* and all its ramifications continue to concern us.

> ### What do you think?
> *Why is there so much concern over the definition of* death? ✳ *How does modern technology complicate the understanding of when death occurs?*

Denying Death

Attitudes toward death tend to fall on a continuum. At one end of the continuum, death is viewed as the mortal enemy of humankind. Both medical science and certain religions have promoted this idea. At the other end of the continuum, death is accepted and even welcomed[27] by some religious groups and segments of the population. For people whose attitudes fall at this end, death is a passage to a better state of being. But most of us perceive ourselves to be in the middle of this continuum. From this perspective, death is a bewildering mystery that elicits fear and apprehension while profoundly influencing beliefs and actions throughout life.

In the United States, a high level of discomfort is associated with death and dying. We may avoid speaking about death to limit our own discomfort. Those who deny death tend to exhibit the following behaviors:

- Avoiding people who are grieving after the death of a loved one so that they won't have to talk about it
- Failing to validate a dying person's frightening situation by talking to the person as though nothing were wrong
- Substituting euphemisms for the word *death* (a few examples are "passing away," "kicking the bucket," "no longer with us," "going to heaven," or "going to a better place")
- Giving false reassurance to people who are dying by saying such things as, "Everything is going to be okay"
- Shutting off conversations about death
- Avoiding touching people who are dying

Death denial has always been a predominant characteristic of our society. However, recent years have shown a greater effort on the part of the American public to mourn openly, as indicated by roadside memorials placed at the sites of violent or unexpected deaths. Although these are fairly new additions to the American landscape, these memorials have long been popular in other parts of the world, particularly in predominantly Catholic countries.[28]

The Process of Dying

Dying is a complex process that includes physical, intellectual, social, spiritual, and emotional dimensions. Now that we have examined the physical indicators of death, we must consider the emotional aspects of dying and "social death."

Coping Emotionally with Death

Although emotional reactions to dying vary, many people share similar experiences during this process. Much of our knowledge about reactions to dying stems from the work of Elisabeth Kübler-Ross, a major figure in modern **thanatology,** the study of death and dying. In 1969, Kübler-Ross published *On Death and Dying,* a sensitive analysis of the reactions of terminally ill patients. This pioneering work encouraged the development of death education as a discipline and prompted efforts to improve the care of dying patients. Kübler-Ross identified five psychological stages that terminally ill patients often experience as they approach death:

1. *Denial.* ("Not me, there must be a mistake.") This is usually the first stage, experienced as a sensation of shock and disbelief. A person intellectually accepts the impending death but rejects it emotionally. The patient is too confused and stunned to comprehend "not being" and thus rejects the idea. Within a relatively short time, the anxiety level may diminish, enabling the patient to sort through the powerful web of emotions.
2. *Anger.* ("Why me?") Anger is another common reaction. The person becomes angry at having to face death when others, including loved ones, are healthy and not threatened. The dying person perceives the situation as "unfair" or "senseless" and may be hostile to friends, family, physicians, or the world in general.
3. *Bargaining.* ("If I'm allowed to live, I promise . . . ") This stage generally occurs at about the middle of the progression. The dying person may resolve to be a better person in return for an extension of life or may secretly pray for a short reprieve from death in order to experience a special event, such as a family wedding or birth.
4. *Depression.* ("It's really going to happen to me, and I can't do anything about it.") Depression eventually sets in as vitality diminishes and the person begins to experience distressing symptoms with increasing frequency. The person's deteriorating condition becomes impossible for him or her to deny, and feelings of doom and tremendous loss may become unbearable. Feelings of worthlessness and guilt are also common because the dying person may feel responsible for the emotional suffering of loved ones and the arduous but seemingly futile efforts of caregivers.
5. *Acceptance.* ("I'm ready.") This is often the final stage. The patient stops battling with emotions and becomes tired and weak. The need to sleep increases, and wakeful periods become shorter and less frequent. With acceptance, the person does not "give up" and become sullen or resentfully resigned to death, but rather becomes passive. According to one dying person, the acceptance stage is "almost void of feelings . . . as if the pain had gone, the struggle is over, and there comes a time for the final rest before the long journey."[29] As he or she lets go, the dying person may no longer welcome visitors and may not wish to engage in conversation. Death usually occurs quietly and painlessly while the victim is unconscious.

Some of Kübler-Ross's contemporaries consider her stage theory too neat and orderly. The experiences of dying people do not always fit easily into specific stages, and patterns vary from person to person. Even if it is not accurate in all its particulars, however, Kübler-Ross's theory offers valuable insights for those seeking to understand or deal with the process of dying.

> ### What do you think?
> *Do you agree with Elisabeth Kübler-Ross's stages of dying?* ✳ *Do you think it is important to help a person get through all the stages that Kübler-Ross has identified? Why or why not?*

Social Death

The need for recognition and appreciation within a social group is nearly universal. Although the size and nature of the social group may vary widely, the need to belong exists in all of us. Loss of being valued or appreciated by others can lead to **social death,** an irreversible situation in which a person is not treated like an active member of society. Dramatic examples of social death include the exile of nonconformists from their native countries or the excommunication of dissident members of religious groups. More often, however, social death is inflicted by denying a person normal social interaction. Numerous studies indicate that people are treated differently when they are dying. The following common behaviors contribute to the social death that often isolates people who are terminally ill:

- The dying person is referred to as if he or she were already dead.
- The dying person may be inadvertently excluded from conversations.
- Dying patients are often moved to terminal wards and given minimal care.

Thanatology   The study of death and dying.

Social death   An irreversible situation in which a person is not treated like an active member of society.

Death-Related Customs Around the World

Each culture recognizes death as a significant rite of passage. Yet the traditions associated with death vary a great deal in different places, often reflecting religious views and ancient customs. Here is a sampling of practices related to death.

- The Maori of New Zealand place the dying in special huts. After a person dies, the body is dressed in nice clothes and placed in a seated position to be viewed by the public. The mourners wear wreaths of green leaves. They cry out, cut themselves with knives, chant praises, and give gifts to the relatives of the deceased. Later, the hut, together with the body, is burned.
- Muslims in the Middle East place the body of the deceased on its side and wash it with warm soap and water an

odd number of times. Generally, members of the same sex of the deceased must perform the washings. The body is then dried off, perfumed, and wrapped in white cloth. Mourners face Mecca and recite prayers, and then a silent procession takes the body to its burial place. All of the mourners participate in filling the grave with soil.

- In Judaism, seven immediate family members are expected to observe the mourning period: mother, father, son, daughter, brother, sister, and husband or wife. *Shiva*, or the mourning period, lasts for seven days, beginning with the funeral, which should take place as soon as possible after death occurs. During *shiva*, family members do not shave, bathe, wear makeup, use perfume, wear leather shoes, get haircuts, or engage in sexual relations. During this period, family members and friends come to comfort the bereaved and usually bring food.
- In China, when a death occurs in the family all statues of deities in the house are covered with red paper (so

that they will not be exposed to the body or to the coffin), and mirrors are removed from sight. This custom comes from the belief that if someone sees the reflection of the coffin in a mirror, that person will soon have a death in her or his family. A white cloth is hung across the doorway of the house, and a gong is placed at the entrance.

- The New Orleans jazz funeral began in the days of slavery. Mourners, singing spirituals and somber hymns, followed the funeral procession. After the burial, the tone shifted to more joyous songs and dances as mourners returned home. The farewell celebrated the belief that the deceased had passed over into a better existence, free of slavery. The procession ceremony is still celebrated today, although it tends to be more celebratory and less solemn, and the old hymns and spirituals, though still used, have been adapted as they have passed from generation to generation of New Orleans musicians.

- Bereaved family members are avoided, often for extended periods, because friends and neighbors are uncomfortable in the presence of grief.
- Medical personnel may make degrading comments about patients in their presence.[30]

This decrease in meaningful social interaction often strips dying and bereaved people of their identity as valued members of society at a time when belonging is critical. Some dying people choose not to speak of their inevitable fate in an attempt to make others feel more comfortable and thus preserve vital relationships.

Coping with Loss

The losses resulting from the death of a loved one are extremely difficult to cope with. The dying person, as well as

close family and friends, frequently suffers emotionally and physically from the impending loss of critical relationships and roles. Words used to describe feelings and behavior related to losses resulting from death include *bereavement, grief, grief work,* and *mourning.* These terms are related but not identical in meaning. Understanding them may help in comprehending the emotional processes associated with loss and the cultural constraints that often inhibit normal coping behavior. Figure 15.2 depicts the stages of grief that many people commonly experience.

Bereavement is generally defined as the loss or deprivation experienced by a survivor when a loved one dies. Because relationships vary in type and intensity, reactions to losses also vary. In the lives of the bereaved or of close survivors, "holes" will be left by the loss of loved ones. We can think of bereavement as the awareness of these holes. Time and courage are necessary to fill these spaces.

A special case of bereavement occurs in old age. Loss is an intrinsic part of growing old. The longer we live, the more losses we are likely to experience. They include physical, social, and emotional losses as our bodies deteriorate and more and more of our loved ones die. The theory of *bereavement overload* has been proposed to explain the effects of

Bereavement The loss or deprivation experienced by a survivor when a loved one dies.

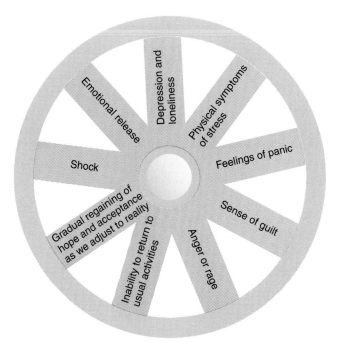

Figure 15.2
The Stages of Grief
People react differently to losses, but most eventually adjust. Generally, the stronger the social support system, the smoother the progression through the stages of grief.

multiple losses and the accumulation of sorrow in the lives of some elderly people. This theory suggests that the gloomy outlook, disturbing behavior patterns, and apparent apathy that characterize these people may be related more to bereavement overload than to intrinsic physiological degeneration in old age.[31]

Grief is a state of mental distress that occurs in reaction to significant loss, including one's own impending death, the death of a loved one, or a quasi-death experience (a loss, such as the end of a relationship or job, that resembles death in that it involves separation, grief, or change in personal identity). Grief reactions include any adjustments needed for one to "make it through the day" and may include changes in patterns of eating, sleeping, working, and even thinking.

When a person experiences a loss that cannot be openly acknowledged, publicly mourned, or socially supported, coping may be much more difficult. This type of grief is referred to as **disenfranchised grief**.[32] It may occur among those who miscarry, are developmentally disabled, or are close friends rather than relatives of the deceased. It may also include those relationships that are not socially approved, such as those between extramarital lovers or homosexual couples. When society does not assign significance to a high-grief death, grieving is made more difficult for the bereaved.

The term **mourning** is often incorrectly equated with the term *grief*. As we have noted, *grief* refers to a wide variety of feelings and actions that occur in response to bereavement. *Mourning,* in contrast, refers to culturally prescribed and accepted time periods and behavior patterns for the

expression of grief. In Judaism, for example, "sitting *shivah*" is a designated mourning period of seven days that involves prescribed rituals and prayers. Depending on a person's relationship with the deceased, various other rituals may continue for up to a year.

Symptoms of grief vary in severity and duration, depending on the situation and the individual. However, the bereaved person can benefit from emotional and social support from family, friends, clergy, employers, and the traditional support organizations, including the medical community and the funeral industry. The larger and stronger the support system, the easier readjustment is likely to be.

What Is "Normal" Grief?

Grief responses vary widely from person to person, but frequently include the following symptoms:

- Periodic waves of physical distress lasting from 20 minutes to an hour
- A feeling of tightness in the throat
- Choking and shortness of breath
- A frequent need to sigh
- A feeling of emptiness in the abdomen
- A feeling of muscular weakness
- An intense feeling of anxiety that is described as actually painful

Other common symptoms of grief include insomnia, memory lapse, loss of appetite, difficulty in concentrating, a tendency to engage in repetitive or purposeless behavior, an "observer" sensation or feeling of unreality, difficulty in making decisions, lack of organization, excessive speech, social withdrawal or hostility, guilt feelings, and preoccupation with the image of the deceased. Susceptibility to disease increases with grief and may even be life threatening in severe and enduring cases.

A bereaved person may suffer emotional pain and exhibit a variety of grief responses for many months after the death. The rate of the healing process depends on the amount and quality of grief work that a person does. **Grief work** is the process of integrating the reality of the loss into everyday life

---

Grief   The state of mental distress that occurs in reaction to significant loss, including one's own impending death, the death of a loved one, or a quasi-death experience.

Disenfranchised grief   Grief concerning a loss that cannot be openly acknowledged, publicly mourned, or socially supported.

Mourning   The culturally prescribed behavior patterns for the expression of grief.

Grief work   The process of accepting the reality of a person's death and coping with memories of the deceased.

and learning to feel better. Often, the bereaved person must deliberately and systematically work at reducing denial and coping with the pain that results from memories of the deceased. This process takes time and requires emotional effort.

Life-and-Death Decision Making

Many complex, and often expensive, life-and-death decisions must be made during a highly distressing -period in people's lives. We will not attempt to present definitive answers to moral and philosophical questions about death; instead, we offer these topics for your consideration. We hope that this discussion of the needs of the dying person and the bereaved will help you negotiate these difficult decisions in the future.

The Right to Die

Few people would object to a proposal for the right to a dignified death. Going beyond that concept, however, many people today believe that they should be allowed to die if their condition is terminal and their existence depends on mechanical life support devices or artificial feeding or hydration systems. Artificial life support techniques that may be legally refused by competent patients in some states include the following:

- Electrical or mechanical heart resuscitation
- Mechanical respiration by machine
- Nasogastric tube feedings
- Intravenous nutrition
- Gastrostomy (tube feeding directly into the stomach)
- Medications to treat life-threatening infections

As long as a person is conscious and competent, he or she has the legal right to refuse treatment, even if this decision will hasten death. However, when a person is in a coma or is otherwise incapable of speaking on his or her own behalf, medical personnel and administrative policy will dictate treatment. This issue has evolved into a battle involving personal freedom, legal rulings, health care administration policy, and physician responsibility. The living will was developed to assist in solving conflicts among these people and agencies.

Rational suicide   The decision to kill oneself rather than endure constant pain and slow decay.

Dyathanasia   The passive form of "mercy killing," in which life-prolonging treatments or interventions are not offered or are withheld, thereby allowing a terminally ill person to die naturally.

Active euthanasia   "Mercy killing" in which a person or organization knowingly acts to hasten the death of a terminally ill person.

Cases have been reported in which the wishes of people who have signed a living will (also called an advanced directive) indicating their desire not to receive artificial life support were not honored by their physician or medical institution. This problem can be avoided by choosing both a physician and a hospital that will carry out the directives of the living will. Taking this precaution and discussing your wishes with your family should eliminate anxiety about how you will be treated at the end of your life. Many legal experts suggest that you take the following steps to ensure that your wishes are carried out:

1. *Get specific.* Rather than signing an advanced directive (which speaks only in generalities), fill out a directive that permits you to make specific choices about a variety of procedures under different circumstances. Attach this document to a completed copy of the standard advance directive for your state.
2. *Get an agent.* Even the most detailed directive cannot anticipate every situation that may arise. You may want to also appoint a family member or friend to act as your agent, or *proxy,* by making out a form known as either a *durable power of attorney for health care* or a *health care proxy.*
3. *Discuss your wishes.* Discuss your wishes in detail with your proxy and your doctor. Going over the situations described in the form will give them a clear idea of just how much you are willing to endure to preserve your life.
4. *Deliver the directive.* Distribute several copies, not only to your doctor and your agent but also to your lawyer and to immediate family members or a close friend. Make sure *someone* knows to bring a copy to the hospital in the event you are hospitalized.[33]

Rational Suicide

We have discussed suicide in earlier chapters. The concept of **rational suicide** as an alternative to an extended dying process, however, deserves mention here. Although exact numbers are not known, medical ethicists and specialists in forensic medicine (the study of legal issues in medicine) estimate that thousands of terminally ill people every year decide to kill themselves rather than endure constant pain and slow decay. To these people, the prospect of an undignified death is unacceptable. This issue has been complicated by advances in death prevention techniques that allow terminally ill patients to exist in an irreversible disease state for extended periods of time. Medical personnel, clergy, lawyers, and patients all must struggle with this ethical dilemma.

Dyathanasia is a form of "mercy killing" in which someone plays a passive role in the death of a terminally ill person. This passive role may include withholding life-prolonging treatments or withdrawing life-sustaining medical support, thereby allowing the person to die. Euthanasia is often referred to as "mercy killing." The term **active euthanasia** has been given to end the life of a person (or animal) that is suffering greatly and has no chance of recovery. An example might be a physician-prescribed lethal injection. **Passive euthanasia** refers to the intentional withholding of treatment that would prolong life. Deciding not to place a person with massive brain trauma on life support is an example of passive euthanasia.

Dr. Jack Kevorkian, a physician in Michigan, has started a one-person campaign to force the medical profession to change its position regarding physician-assisted death. Kevorkian has assisted many terminally ill patients in dying and, until recently, had escaped conviction despite being taken into court several times for his actions. Kevorkian has argued that the Hippocratic oath is not binding. He believes that the present situations in our society demand a shift in the thinking and practices that medicine has carried out throughout most of human history. He believes that acceptance of euthanasia, specifically physician-assisted death, is one of those changes. In 1998, Kevorkian took his argument to prime time, as the CBS News program *60 Minutes* broadcast his latest case of assisting a terminally ill patient with ending his life. This time, however, the courts determined that Kevorkian's methods had gone too far, and in 1999 he was convicted of murder and sentenced to prison.

Kevorkian's actions have focused a great deal of attention on the issue, causing many to speculate on the merits of physician-assisted suicide. A study in Michigan revealed that a greater number of physicians were in favor of legalizing assisted suicide than were against it.[34] A similar study in Oregon found that physicians have a more favorable attitude toward legalized physician-assisted suicide, are more willing to participate, and are currently participating in greater numbers than other surveyed groups in the United States.[35] In both studies, however, a sizable minority of physicians had a number of reservations about the practical applications of the proposed law.

> **What do you think?**
>
> *Are there any end-of-life situations in which you would ask a physician to help you die? Explain your answer.* ✳ *Do you believe people should have the right to ask a physician to help them die? Why or why not?*

Taking Care of Business

Caring for dying people and dealing with the practical and legal questions surrounding death can be difficult and painful. The problems of the dying person and the bereaved loved ones involve a wide variety of psychological, legal, social, spiritual, economic, and interpersonal issues.

Hospice Care: Positive Alternatives

Since the mid-1970s, **hospice** programs have grown from a mere handful to more than 2,500, and are available in nearly every community. To a greater extent than even only ten years ago, families facing terminal illness are often expected to make difficult medical decisions, including where their loved ones will die. Improving the quality of care at the end of life is a top priority of the American Medical Association.

The primary goals of hospice programs are to relieve the dying person's pain, offer emotional support to the dying person and loved ones, and restore a sense of control to the dying person, family, and friends. Although home care with maximum involvement by loved ones is emphasized, hospice programs are directed by cooperating physicians, coordinated by specially trained nurses, and fortified with the services of counselors, clergy, and trained volunteers. Hospital inpatient beds are available if necessary. Hospice programs usually include the following characteristics:

1. The patient and family constitute the unit of care, because the physical, psychological, social, and spiritual problems of dying confront the family as well as the patient.
2. Emphasis is placed on symptom control, primarily the alleviation of pain. Curative treatments are curtailed as requested by the patient, but sound judgment must be applied to avoid a feeling of abandonment.
3. There is overall medical direction of the program, with all health care being provided under the direction of a qualified physician.
4. Services are provided by an interdisciplinary team because no one person can provide all the needed care.
5. Coverage is provided 24 hours a day, seven days a week, with emphasis on the availability of medical and nursing skills.
6. Carefully selected and extensively trained volunteers are an integral part of the health care team, augmenting staff service but not replacing it.
7. Care of the family extends through the bereavement period.
8. Patients are accepted on the basis of their health needs, not their ability to pay.

Despite the growing number of people considering the hospice option, many people prefer to go to a hospital to die. Others choose to die at home, without the intervention of medical staff or life-prolonging equipment. Each dying person and his or her family should decide as early as possible what type of terminal care is most desirable and feasible. This will allow time for necessary emotional, physical, and financial preparations. Hospice care may also help the survivors cope better with the death experience.

Passive euthanasia   The intentional withholding of treatment that would prolong life.

Hospice   A concept of care for terminally ill patients designed to maximize quality of life.

Making Funeral Arrangements

Anthropological evidence indicates that all cultures throughout history have developed some sort of funeral ritual. For this reason, social scientists agree that funerals assist survivors of the deceased in coping with their loss.

In the United States, with its diversity of religious, regional, and ethnic customs, funeral patterns vary. In some faiths, the deceased may be displayed to formalize last respects and increase social support of the bereaved. This part of the funeral ritual is referred to as a *wake* or *viewing*. The funeral service may be held in a church, in a funeral chapel, or at the burial site. Some people choose to replace the funeral service with a simple memorial service held within a few days of the burial. Social interaction associated with funeral and memorial services is valuable in helping survivors cope with their losses.

Common methods of body disposal include burial in the ground, entombment above ground in a mausoleum, cremation, and anatomical donation. Expenses vary according to the method chosen and the available options. It should be noted that if burial is selected, an additional charge may be assessed for a burial vault. Burial vaults—concrete or metal containers that hold the casket—are required by most cemeteries to limit settling of the gravesite as the casket disintegrates and collapses. The actual container for the remains is only one of many things that must be dealt with when a person dies. There are many other decisions concerning the funeral ritual that can be burdensome for survivors.

Pressures on Survivors

Funeral practices in the United States today are extremely varied. A great number of decisions have to be made, usually within 24 hours. These decisions relate to the method and details of body disposal, the type of memorial service, display of the body, the site of burial or body disposition, the cost of funeral options, organ donation decisions, ordering floral displays, contacting friends and relatives, planning for guests, choosing markers, gathering and submitting obituary information to newspapers, printing memorial folders, and many other details. In our society, people who make their own funeral arrangements can save their loved ones from having to deal with unnecessary problems. Even making the decision regarding the method of body disposal can greatly reduce the stress on survivors.

Wills

The issue of inheritance is controversial in some families and should be resolved before the person dies in order to reduce conflict and needless expense. Unfortunately, many people are so intimidated by the thought of making a will that they never do so and die **intestate** (without a will). This is tragic, especially because the procedure for establishing a legal will is relatively simple and inexpensive. In addition, if you don't make up a will before you die, the courts (as directed by state laws) will make up a will for you. Legal issues, rather than your wishes, will preside.

In some cases, other types of wills may substitute for the traditional legal will. One of these alternatives is the **holographic will,** which is written in the handwriting of the **testator** (person who leaves a will) and unwitnessed. Caution should be taken concerning holographic wills and other alternatives to legally written and witnessed wills because they are not honored in all states. For example, holographic wills are contestable in court. Think of the parents who never approved of the fact that their child lived with someone outside marriage; they could successfully challenge the holographic will in court.

> ### What do you think?
> *What can you do to ensure that your wishes will be carried out at the time of your death?*

Organ Donation

Another decision concerns organ donation. Organ transplant techniques have become so refined, and the demand for transplant tissues and organs has become so great, that many people are being encouraged to donate these "gifts of life" upon death. Uniform donor cards are available through the National Kidney Foundation; donor information is printed on the backs of drivers' licenses; and many hospitals include the opportunity for organ donor registration as a part of their admission procedures. Although some people are opposed to organ transplants and tissue donation, others experience a feeling of personal fulfillment from knowing that their organs may extend and improve someone else's life after their own deaths.

Intestate   Not having made a will.

Holographic will   A will written in the testator's own handwriting and unwitnessed.

Testator   A person who leaves a will or testament at death.

Taking Charge

Reducing Age-Related Risks

There is no one right way to age. Most people who do age successfully, however, pay attention to their physical, spiritual, emotional, mental, and social well-being.

Checklist for Change

Making Personal Choices

✓ Keep active mentally. For some people, mentally active equals socially active. Take time for quiet reflection, concentrated thought, and idle musing.

✓ Schedule regular medical checkups. One of the best ways to pre-vent major health problems is to take care of minor problems early.

✓ Develop a sense of self. Maintaining a sense of yourself as a worthwhile, productive member of society can be a challenge in the face of changes that appear to diminish individual prestige.

✓ Learn to accept help when you need it.

✓ Make optimal use of your time and energy. Take steps now to plan for a secure retirement. Living for the moment can result in financial problems that will seriously limit your options later in life.

✓ Become familiar with services that are available to assist the elderly. Do not allow yourself to stagnate. The willingness to encounter change and undertake new activities can add pleasure at any age.

Making Community Choices

✓ What community services are available to promote health at each of the different levels and stages of life?

✓ What services do you think are needed to help people achieve optimal health through the years?

✓ Do you keep up with the federal government's plans for Social Security and Medicare? Have you taken the time to learn how these programs will affect you in the future?

Summary

* Aging can be defined in terms of biological age, referring to a person's physical condition; psychological age, referring to a person's coping abilities and intelligence; social age, referring to a person's habits and roles relative to society's expectations; legal age, based on chronological years; or functional age, relative to how other people function at varied ages.

* The growing numbers of elderly (people aged 65 and older) will have a growing impact on society in terms of economy, health care, housing, and ethical considerations.

* Two broad groups of theories—biological and psychosocial—purport to explain the physiological and psychological changes that occur with aging. Biological explanations include the wear-and-tear theory, the cellular theory, the autoimmune theory, and the genetic mutation theory. Psychosocial theories center on adaptation and adjustments related to self-development.

* Aging changes the body and mind in many ways. Physical changes occur in the skin, bones and joints, head, urinary tract, heart and lungs, senses, sexual functioning, and temperature regulation. Major physical concerns are osteoporosis and urinary incontinence. The elderly maintain a high level of intelligence and memory. Potential mental problems include depression and Alzheimer's disease.

* Special challenges for the elderly include alcohol abuse, prescription and over-the-counter drug interactions, questions about vitamin and mineral supplementation, and issues regarding caregiving.

* Lifestyle choices we make today will affect health status later in life. Choosing to exercise, eat a healthy diet, and foster lasting relationships will contribute to healthy aging. Decisions about caring for the elderly and stresses related to caregiving are ongoing concerns as the elderly population increases in the United States.

* *Death* can be defined biologically in terms of brain death and/or the final cessation of vital functions. Denial of death results in limited communication about death, which can lead to further denial.

* Death is a multifaceted process, and individuals may experience emotional stages of dying, which include denial, anger, bargaining, depression, and acceptance. Social death results when a person is no longer treated as living. Grief is the state of distress felt after loss.

* The right to die by rational suicide involves ethical, moral, and legal issues. Dyathanasia involves passive help in suicide for a terminally ill patient; euthanasia involves direct help.

* Practical and legal issues surround dying and death. Choices of care for the terminally ill include hospice care. After death, funeral arrangements must be made almost immediately, adding to pressures on survivors. Decisions should be made in advance of death through wills and organ donation cards.

Discussion Questions

1. Discuss the various definitions of aging. At what age would you place your parents for each category?
2. As the elderly population grows, how will it affect your life? Would you be willing to pay higher taxes to support government social programs for the elderly? For example, do you believe that Social Security should continue its yearly increases in payments, which are pegged to inflation? Why or why not?
3. Which of the biological theories of aging do you think is most correct? Why?
4. List the major physiological changes that occur with aging. Which of these, if any, can you change?
5. Explain the major health challenges that the elderly may face. What advice would you give to your grandparents before they took a prescription or over-the-counter drug?
6. Discuss actions you can start taking now to ensure a healthier aging process.
7. Discuss why so many of us deny death. How could death become a more acceptable topic to discuss?
8. Debate whether or not rational suicide should be legalized for the terminally ill. What restrictions would you include in a law?
9. Compare and contrast the hospital experience with hospice care. What must one consider before arranging for hospice care?
10. Discuss the legal matters surrounding death, including wills, physician directives, organ donations, and funeral arrangements.

Application Exercise

Reread the What Do You Think? scenarios at the beginning of the chapter, and answer the following questions.

1. If you could change aspects of Ruth and/or Harry to make them into someone you might like to be, what would you change?
2. Which of their behaviors and attitudes make them likely to age successfully? Which do not?
3. What things would you need to change about yourself to help you achieve your vision of successful and happy aging?

Accessing Your Health on the Internet http

Visit the following Internet sites to explore further topics and issues related to personal health. To visit an organization's website, go to the Companion Website for *Health: The Basics, Fifth Edition* at www.aw.com/donatelle, click on the book image, and select "Accessing Your Health on the Internet" from the navigation menu on the left.

1. *Administration on Aging.* A link to the Health and Human Services agency dedicated to addressing the health needs of the elderly.
2. *Alzheimer's Association.* Media releases, position statements, fact sheets, and research on Alzheimer's disease.
3. *SeniorCom.* Home page to a link to numerous resources for senior citizens, including chatrooms, databases, and services dedicated to assisting the aging.
4. *Social Security Online.* Provides information about Social Security benefits and entitlements. Also offers links to related sites.
5. *Funerals: A Consumer Guide.* This site guides the consumer through the thinking process of planning for a funeral, including preplanning, types of funerals, costs, choosing a casket, burial, and many other aspects of funeral preparation.
6. *Loss, Grief, and Bereavement.* This site from the National Cancer Institute covers a variety of topics related to loss, grief, and bereavement. Among the contents is a summary written by cancer experts.
7. *Terminal Illness and Hospice.* This site addresses all aspects of dealing with terminal illness, including loss, ALS (Lou Gehrig's disease), Alzheimer's disease, legal issues, and funeral planning.
8. *Hospice Web.* Information and links about hospice, including frequently asked questions.

Further Reading

The Johns Hopkins Medical Letter—Health After 50.
Comprehensive, accurate overview of health topics relevant for this population.

Jacobs Altman, L. *Death: An Introduction to Medical–Ethical Dilemmas.* Berkeley Heights, NJ: Enslow, 2000.
A multifaceted exploration of death that gives the reader much to consider.

Muth, A. S. (ed.). *Death and Dying Sourcebook: Basic Consumer Health Information for the Layperson About End-of-Life Care and Related Ethical and Legal Issues.* Omnigraphics, 2000.
Provides up-to-date information on the issues of nursing care, living wills, pain management, and counseling.

16

Environmental Health

THINKING GLOBALLY, ACTING LOCALLY

16   16   16   16   16   16

objectives

* Identify the problems and ethical issues associated with current levels of global population growth.

* Discuss major causes of air pollution, including photo-chemical smog and acid rain, and the global consequences of the accumulation of greenhouse gases and of ozone depletion.

* Identify sources of water pollution and the chemical contaminants often found in water.

* Describe the physiological consequences of noise pollution.

* Distinguish between municipal solid waste and hazardous waste.

* Discuss the health concerns associated with ionizing and non-ionizing radiation.

Human health, well-being, and the survival of all living things depend on the health and integrity of the planet on which we live. Today the natural world is under siege from the pressures of a burgeoning population that requires massive use of natural resources to survive. In response to public and political concerns, there has been a surge in federal and state regulations, along with a multibillion-dollar national infrastructure—but doubt remains as to the effectiveness of that infrastructure in reducing environmental health risks.[1] An informed citizenry with a strong commitment to be responsible for the planet and maintain it for future generations is essential to the survival of the earth and all living things.

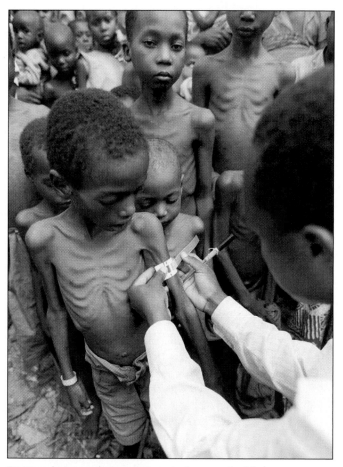

Burgeoning population puts a strain on valuable resources and leaves many parts of the world unable to meet the needs of their citizens.

Overpopulation

Anthropologist Margaret Mead wrote, "Every human society is faced with not one population problem but two: how to beget and rear enough children and how not to beget and rear too many."[2] The United Nations projects that the world population will grow from 6.1 billion in the year 2000 to 9.4 billion in 2050.[3] Though the population is expanding, the earth's resources are not. Population experts believe that many areas of the world are already struggling with "demographic fatigue" and that the most critical environmental challenge today is to slow the population growth of the world.[4]

The population explosion is not distributed equally. The United States and western Europe have the lowest birth rates. At the same time, these two regions produce more grain and other foodstuffs than their populations consume. Countries that can least afford a high birth rate in economic, social, health, and nutritional terms are the ones with the most rapidly expanding populations.

The bulk of population growth in developing countries is occurring in urban areas. Populations in the cities with developing countries are doubling every 10 to 15 years, overwhelming their governments' attempts to provide clean water, sewage facilities, adequate transportation, and other basic services. Every week, the population of the world's urban centers grows by more than 1 million.[5] In 1800, London was the only city in the world with 1 million people; today, 14 cities each have populations of over 10 million.[6]

As the global population expands, so does competition for the earth's resources. Environmental degradation caused by loss of topsoil, pesticides, toxic residues, deforestation, global warming, air pollution, acid rain, a rapidly expanding population, and increasing poverty is exerting heavy pressure on natural resources and the capacity of natural resources to support human life and world health.[7]

Overpopulation threats are more evident in Latin America, Africa, and Asia. The country projected to have the largest increase in population is India, which could add another 600 million people by the year 2050 and surpass China as the most populous country in the world.[8] These projections could change, however, if governments are not able to cope with the increased resource and economic demands. For example, the AIDS epidemic has stabilized in industrial countries to an adult infection rate of under 1 percent, but countries such as Zimbabwe, Botswana, and Zambia may lose one-fifth or more of their adult population within the next decade to AIDS.[9] The loss of a significant part of the workforce would have devastating economic as well as health consequences. Diseases such as AIDS are not the only threats to countries with unstable population growth. As governments

Population Control

In 1999, the world's population surpassed 6 billion. Ninety-seven percent of each year's population growth occurs in the poorest parts of the world. The following statistics are based on the current population:

- 300 million women desire family planning but lack the information or the means to obtain it.
- 1 billion people have no access to health care.
- 1.3 billion people live in poverty.
- 840 million people are malnourished.
- 85 countries lack the ability to grow or purchase enough food to feed their citizens.
- 1.5 billion people lack access to safe drinking water.
- 2.3 billion live without adequate sanitation.

The Population Reference Bureau projects that world population will increase to over 9 billion by 2050. The statistics listed above are sure to rise as the population increases. According to many scientists, overpopulation has led to environmental degradation, resulting in the loss of immense tracts of forest and tons of arable topsoil. Additionally, some scientists suggest that increased industrialization and consumption threaten the atmosphere and world climate. Many people fear that unrestricted population growth will lead to worldwide shortages of food and energy.

Already women, particularly in the developing world, suffer the ill health effects of having too many children too close together. Often these children live in poverty and are malnourished. Particularly in areas of the world where HIV and poverty are rampant, many women neglect their own health in order to care for sick partners and children.

For the past half century, those concerned about overpopulation have called for population control. A number of organizations, such as the International Planned Parenthood Federation, have been advocating women's access to family planning information and contraception. Unfortunately, even if many of these women had access to family planning services, cultural mores or religious beliefs could prevent their use of these resources.

Another solution some have offered is government regulation of population growth. In the 1970s, China instituted a strictly enforced one child–one family policy that allowed each family to have only a single child. Although the policy has been effective in cities, where people tend to be more educated and where space is already extremely limited, it has not been successful in rural areas, where families whose survival depends on having enough labor continue to have multiple children. One unintended consequence of this policy has been female infanticide by families who want to make sure that their one child will be a boy.

Other recommendations are under consideration. One of these gives each woman born the right to have two babies. If the woman chooses not to exercise this right, she can sell her rights on the open market. If people want a large family, they must have enough resources to buy the baby rights and therefore, in all likelihood, would also have the ability to pay to support these children. Paying women not to have children has also been suggested. Each year of her childbearing years that a woman does not have a child, she is rewarded financially.

Finally, some people suggest that the problem is not overpopulation but the unequal consumption of resources by a small majority of the world's population. These people believe that poverty is not a consequence of overpopulation but of the inequitable distribution of wealth.

Students Speak Up

Do you think overpopulation is a problem? ✳ Do you think population control is the answer? ✳ How do you think population control should be effected? ✳ Do you think inequality is a greater problem than overpopulation? If so, what do you think should be done to bring about greater equality worldwide?

strain to support growing numbers of people, they are at increased risk of developing significant problems should any new or increased demands be placed on resources.

What can we do to alleviate these conditions? We can do our part by recognizing that the United States consumes far more energy and raw materials per person than any other nation on earth. Many of these resources come from other countries, and our consumption is depleting the resource balances of those countries.

Perhaps the simplest course of action is to control our own reproductivity. The concept of zero population growth (ZPG) was born in the 1960s. Proponents of this idea believed that each couple should produce only two offspring. When the parents die, the two offspring are their replacements, and the population stabilizes.

The continued preference for large families in many developing nations is related to several factors: high infant mortality rates; the traditional view of children as "social security" (they work from a young age to assist families in daily survival, and they support parents when the parents grow too old to work); the low educational and economic status of women; and the traditional desire for sons, which keeps parents of daughters reproducing until they get male offspring.

Air Pollution

The daily impact of a growing population makes clean air more difficult to find. Concern about air quality prompted Congress to pass the Clean Air Act in 1970 and to amend it in 1977 and again in 1990. The object was to develop standards for six of the most widespread air pollutants that seriously affect health: sulfur dioxide, particulates, carbon monoxide, nitrogen dioxide, ozone, and lead.

Sources of Air Pollution

Sulfur Dioxide **Sulfur dioxide** is a yellowish brown gas that is a by-product of burning fossil fuels. Electricity generating stations, smelters, refineries, and industrial boilers are the main source points. In humans, sulfur dioxide aggravates symptoms of heart and lung disease, obstructs breathing passages, and increases the incidence of respiratory diseases such as colds, asthma, bronchitis, and emphysema. Sulfur dioxide is toxic to plants, destroys some paint pigments, corrodes metals, impairs visibility, and is a precursor to acid rain, which we discuss later in this chapter.

Particulates **Particulates** are tiny solid particles or liquid droplets that are suspended in the air. Cigarette smoke releases particulates. Industrial processes and the internal combustion engine also release particulates as by-products. Particulates irritate the lungs and can carry heavy metals and carcinogenic agents deep into the lungs. When combined with sulfur dioxide, they exacerbate respiratory diseases. Particulates can also corrode metals and obscure visibility.

Numerous scientific studies have found significant links between exposure to air particulate concentrations at or below current standards and adverse health effects, including premature death.[10]

Carbon Monoxide **Carbon monoxide** is an odorless, colorless gas that originates primarily from motor vehicle emissions. Carbon monoxide interferes with the blood's ability to absorb and carry oxygen and can impair thinking, slow reflexes, and cause drowsiness, unconsciousness, and death. Many people have purchased home monitors to test for carbon monoxide.

Ozone Ground-level **ozone** is a form of oxygen that is produced when nitrogen dioxide reacts with hydrogen chloride. These gases release oxygen, which is altered by sunlight to produce ozone. In the lower atmosphere, ozone irritates the mucous membranes of the respiratory system, causing coughing and choking. It can impair lung functioning, reduce resistance to colds and pneumonia, and aggravate heart disease, asthma, bronchitis, and pneumonia. One of the irritants found in smog, this ozone corrodes rubber and paint and can injure or kill vegetation. The natural ozone found in the upper atmosphere (sometimes called "good" ozone), however, serves as a protective membrane against heat and radiation from the sun. We will discuss this atmospheric ozone layer later in the chapter.

Nitrogen Dioxide **Nitrogen dioxide** is an amber-colored gas emitted by coal-powered electrical utility boilers and motor vehicles. High concentrations of nitrogen dioxide can be fatal. Lower concentrations increase susceptibility to colds and flu, bronchitis, and pneumonia. Nitrogen dioxide is also toxic to plant life and causes a brown discoloration of the atmosphere. It is a precursor of ozone and, along with sulfur dioxide, of acid rain.

Lead **Lead** is a metal pollutant found in paint, batteries, drinking water, pipes, and dishes with lead-glazed bases. The elimination of lead from gasoline and auto exhaust in the

---

Sulfur dioxide A yellowish brown gaseous by-product of the burning of fossil fuels.

Particulates Nongaseous air pollutants.

Carbon monoxide An odorless, colorless gas that originates primarily from motor vehicle emissions.

Ozone A gas formed when nitrogen dioxide interacts with hydrogen chloride.

Nitrogen dioxide An amber-colored gas found in smog; can cause eye and respiratory irritations.

Lead A metal found in the exhaust of motor vehicles powered by fuel containing lead and in emissions from lead smelters and processing plants.

1970s was one of the great public health accomplishments of all time. Although stricter standards for all of the above prevail, almost 1 million children in the United States had elevated blood lead levels in 1997.[11] Lead affects the circulatory, reproductive, and nervous systems. It can also affect the blood and kidneys and can accumulate in bone and other tissues. Lead is particularly detrimental to children and fetuses. It can cause birth defects, behavioral abnormalities, and decreased learning abilities.

Hydrocarbons   Sometimes known as *volatile organic compounds* (VOCs), **hydrocarbons** are chemical compounds containing different combinations of carbon and hydrogen. Although not listed as one of the six major air pollutants in the Clean Air Act, hydrocarbons encompass a wide variety of chemical pollutants in the air. The principal source is the internal combustion engine. Most automobile engines emit hundreds of different hydrocarbon compounds. By themselves, hydrocarbons seem to cause few problems, but when they combine with sunlight and other pollutants, they form such poisons as formaldehyde, ketones, and peroxyacetylnitrate (PAN), all of which are respiratory irritants. Hydrocarbon combinations such as benzene and benzo(a)pyrene are carcinogenic. In addition, hydrocarbons play a major part in the formation of smog.

> **What do you think?**
>
> *Should auto makers be responsible for developing cars with low emissions?* ✳ *As a motorist, how can you help eliminate carbon monoxide emissions?*

Photochemical Smog

Photochemical smog is a brown, hazy mix of particulates and gases that forms when oxygen-containing compounds of nitrogen and hydrocarbons react in the presence of sunlight. It is sometimes called *ozone pollution* because ozone is created when vehicle exhaust reacts with sunlight. In most cases, smog forms in areas that experience a **temperature**

Hydrocarbons   Chemical compounds that contain carbon and hydrogen.

Photochemical smog   The brownish yellow haze resulting from the combination of hydrocarbons and nitrogen oxides.

Temperature inversion   A weather condition occurring when a layer of cool air is trapped under a layer of warmer air.

Acid rain   Precipitation contaminated with acidic pollutants.

---

inversion, a weather condition in which a cool layer of air is trapped under a layer of warmer air, preventing the air from circulating. When gases such as the hydrocarbons and nitrogen oxides are released into the cool air layer, they remain suspended until wind conditions move away the warmer air layer. Sunlight filtering through the air causes chemical changes in the hydrocarbons and nitrogen oxides, which results in smog. Smog is more likely to be produced in valley regions blocked by hills or mountains—for example, the Los Angeles basin, Denver, and Tokyo.

The most noticeable adverse effects of exposure to smog are difficulty in breathing, burning eyes, headaches, and nausea. Long-term exposure poses serious health risks, particularly for children, the elderly, pregnant women, and people with chronic respiratory disorders such as asthma and emphysema.

Acid Rain

Acid rain is precipitation that has fallen through acidic air pollutants, particularly those containing sulfur dioxides and nitrogen dioxides. This precipitation, in the form of rain, snow, or fog, is more acidic than unpolluted precipitation. When introduced into lakes and ponds, acid rain gradually acidifies the water. When the acid content of the water reaches a certain level, plant and animal life cannot survive. Ironically, acidified lakes and ponds become a crystal-clear deep blue, giving the illusion of beauty and health.

Sources of Acid Rain   More than 95 percent of acid rain originates in human actions, chiefly the burning of fossil fuels. The greatest sources of acid rain in the United States are coal-fired power plants, ore smelters, and steel mills.

When these and other industries burn fuels, the sulfur and nitrogen in the emissions combine with the oxygen and sunlight in the air to become sulfur dioxide and nitrogen oxides (precursors of sulfuric acid and nitric acids, respectively). Small acid particles are then carried by the wind and combine with moisture to produce acidic rain or snow. Rain is more acidic in the summertime because of higher concentrations of sunlight. The ability of a lake to cleanse itself and neutralize its acidity depends on several factors, the most critical of which is bedrock geology.

Effects of Acid Rain   In addition to damaging lakes and ponds, every year acid rain destroys millions of trees in Europe and North America. Scientists have concluded that 75 percent of Europe's forests are now experiencing damaging levels of sulfur deposition by acid rain. Forests in every country on the continent are affected.[12]

Doctors believe that acid rain aggravates and may even cause bronchitis, asthma, and other respiratory problems. People with emphysema and those with a history of heart disease may also suffer from exposure to acid rain. In addition, it may be hazardous to a pregnant woman's unborn child.

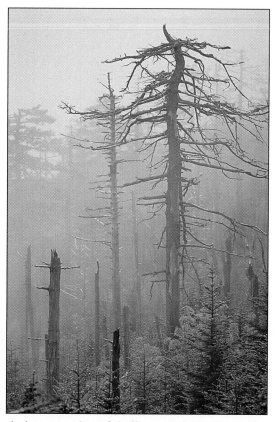
Acid rain has many harmful effects on the environment. Because its toxins seep into groundwater and enter the food chain, it also poses health hazards to humans.

Acidic precipitation can cause metals such as aluminum, cadmium, lead, and mercury to **leach** (dissolve and filter) out of the soil. If these metals make their way into water or food supplies (particularly fish), they can cause cancer in humans who consume them. Acid rain also damages crops; laboratory experiments show that it can reduce seed yield by up to 23 percent. Actual crop losses are being reported with increasing frequency. A final consequence of acid rain is the destruction of public monuments and structures, with billions of dollars in projected building damage each year.

Indoor Air Pollution

In the last several years, a growing body of scientific evidence has indicated that the air within homes and other buildings can be more seriously polluted than the outdoor air in even the most industrialized cities. Other research indicates that some of the most vulnerable people, particularly the young, elderly and those who are already sick, often spend over 90 percent of their time indoors.[13]

The greatest culprits in indoor air pollution are sources that release gases or particles into the air. Woodstoves, furnaces, asbestos, formaldehyde, and radon cause the majority of indoor air problems. Inadequate ventilation, particularly in heavily insulated buildings with airtight windows may increase pollution by not allowing the entry of outdoor air, as their drafty older counterparts once did. Some of the major sources of indoor air pollution and possible health effects from these pollutants are described in Table 16.1 on page 410.

Preventing indoor air pollution generally focuses on three major areas: (1) source control, including eliminating or reducing individual contaminants; (2) ventilation improvements, which often focus on increasing the amount of outdoor air coming indoors, and (3) the use of air cleaners for removal of particulates.[14]

Woodstove Smoke   Woodstoves emit significant levels of particulates and carbon monoxide in addition to other pollutants, such as sulfur dioxide. If you rely on wood for heating, make sure that your stove is properly installed, vented, and maintained. Burning properly seasoned wood reduces particulates.

Furnace Emissions   People who rely on oil- or gas-fired furnaces also need to make sure that these appliances are properly installed, ventilated, and maintained. Inadequate cleaning and maintenance can lead to a buildup of carbon monoxide in the home, which can be deadly.

Asbestos   Asbestos is a mineral that was commonly used in insulation materials in buildings constructed before 1970. When bonded to other materials, asbestos is relatively harmless, but if its tiny fibers become loosened and airborne, they can embed themselves in the lungs. Their presence leads to cancer of the lungs, stomach, and chest lining and is the cause of a fatal lung disease called mesothelioma.

Formaldehyde   Formaldehyde is a colorless, strong-smelling gas present in some carpets, draperies, furniture, particle board, plywood, wood paneling, countertops, and many adhesives. It is released into the air in a process called *outgassing*. Outgassing is highest in new products, but the process can continue for many years.

Exposure to formaldehyde can cause respiratory problems, dizziness, fatigue, nausea, and rashes. Long-term exposure can lead to central nervous system disorders and cancer. Ask about the formaldehyde content of products you

Leach   To dissolve and filter through soil.

Asbestos   A substance that separates into stringy fibers and lodges in the lungs, where it can cause various diseases.

Formaldehyde   A colorless, strong-smelling gas released through outgassing; causes respiratory and other health problems.

Table 16.1
Indoor Air Pollution: Health Effects

TYPE OF POLLUTANT	SOURCES	HEALTH EFFECTS
Radon	Uranium in the soil or rock on which homes are built; well water can also be a source	Lung cancer from air, other health risks from swallowing radon in water
Environmental Tobacco Smoke (ETS)	Smoke that comes from burning end of cigarette, pipe, or cigar	Complex mixture of over 4,000 compounds, over 40 of which cause cancer
Biological Contaminants (molds, mildew, viruses, animal dander and cat saliva, dust mites, cockroaches, and pollen	Improper ventilation and moisture buildup, lack of cleanliness/sanitation, contaminated heating systems, household pets, rodents, insects, damp carpets	Allergic reactions, including hypersensitivity rhinitis, asthma, infectious illnesses, sneezing, watering eyes, coughing, shortness of breath, dizziness, lethargy, fever, digestive problems
Stoves, heaters, fireplaces, chimneys	Unvented kerosene heaters, woodstoves, fireplaces, gas stoves	Carbon monoxide: headaches, dizziness, weakness, nausea, confusion and disorientation, chest pain, death; nitrogen dioxide: irritation of nose, eyes, respiratory distress; particles: damage and/or irritation to lungs
Household chemicals (see partial list below)	Paints, varnishes, cleaning products, solvents, degreasers, and hobby products	Variable symptoms, depending on exposure level: eye and respiratory tract problems, headaches, dizziness, visual disorders and memory impairment
Benzene	Paint, new carpet, new drapes, upholstery, fast-drying glues, caulks	Headaches, eye/skin irritation, fatigue, cancer
Formaldehyde	Tobacco smoke, plywood, cabinets, furniture, particle board, new carpet and drapes, wallpaper, ceiling tile, paneling	Headaches, eye/skin irritation, drowsiness, fatigue, respiratory problems, memory loss, depression, gynecological problems, cancer
Chloroform	Paint, new drapes, new carpet, upholstery	Headaches, asthma attacks, dizziness, eye/skin irritations
Toluene	All paper products, most finished wood products	Headaches, eye/skin irritation, sinus problems, dizziness, cancer
Hydrocarbons	Tobacco smoke, gas burners and furnaces	Headaches, fatigue, nausea, dizziness, breathing difficulty
Ammonia	Tobacco smoke, cleaning supplies, animal urine	Eye/skin irritation, headaches, nosebleeds, sinus problems
Trichloroethylene	Paints, glues, caulking, vinyl coatings, wallpaper	Headaches, eye/skin irritation, upper respiratory irritation

purchase, and avoid those that contain this gas. Some houseplants, such as philodendrons and spider plants, help clean formaldehyde from the air. If you experience symptoms of formaldehyde exposure, have your home tested by a city, county, or state health agency.

Radon Radon, an odorless, colorless gas, is the natural by-product of the decay of uranium and radium in the soil. Radon penetrates homes through cracks, pipes, sump pits,

and other openings in the foundation. An estimated 30,000 cancer deaths per year have been attributed to radon, making it second only to smoking as the leading cause of lung cancer.[15]

The EPA estimates that 1 in 15 American homes has an elevated radon level.[16] A home-testing kit from a hardware store will enable you to test your home yourself. "Alpha track" detectors are commonly used for this type of short-term testing. They must remain in your home for 2 to 90 days, depending on the device.

> **Radon**   A naturally occurring radioactive gas resulting from the decay of certain radioactive elements.

Household Chemicals Use cleansers and other cleaning products in a well-ventilated room, and be conservative in their use. All those caustic chemicals that zap mildew and grease cause a major risk to water and the environment.

Avoid buildup. Regular cleanings will reduce the need to use potentially harmful substances. Cut down on dry cleaning; the chemicals used by many cleaners can cause cancer. If your newly cleaned clothes smell of dry-cleaning chemicals, return them to the cleaner or hang them in the open air until the smell is gone. Avoid household air freshener products containing the carcinogenic agent *dichlorobenzene*.

Indoor air pollution is also a concern in the classroom and workplace. Studies show that one in five U.S. schools has problems with indoor air quality, which affect an estimated 8.4 million students.[17] Poor air quality in classrooms may lead to drowsiness, headaches, and lack of concentration. It may also affect physical growth and development. Children with asthma are particularly at risk. Many people who work indoors complain of maladies that tend to lessen or vanish when they leave the building. **Sick building syndrome (SBS)** is said to exist when 80 percent of a building's occupants

report problems. One of the primary causes of sick building syndrome is poor ventilation. Symptoms include eye irritation, sore throat, queasiness, and worsened asthma.[18]

Ozone Layer Depletion

The ozone layer in the stratosphere protects our planet and its inhabitants from ultraviolet B (UVB) radiation, a primary cause of skin cancer. Ultraviolet B radiation may also damage DNA and weaken immune systems in both humans and animals. Thus, the ozone layer is crucial to life on the planet's surface.

In the early 1970s, scientists began to warn of a depletion of the earth's ozone layer. Instruments developed to test atmospheric contents indicated that chemicals used on earth, **chlorofluorocarbons (CFCs),** were contributing to its rapid depletion.

Chlorofluorocarbons were used as refrigerants (Freon), as aerosol propellants in products such as hairsprays and deodorants, as cleaning solvents, and in medical sterilizers, rigid foam insulation, and Styrofoam. Along with halons (found in many fire extinguishers), methyl chloroform, and carbon tetrachloride (found in cleaning solvents), CFCs were eventually found to be a major cause of ozone depletion. When released into the air through spraying or outgassing, CFCs migrate upward toward the ozone layer, where they decompose and release chlorine atoms. These atoms cause ozone molecules to break apart (Figure 16.1).

In the early 1970s, the U.S. government banned the use of aerosol sprays containing CFCs. The discovery of an "ozone hole" over Antarctica led to the 1987 Montreal Protocol treaty, whereby the United States and other nations agreed to reduce the use of CFCs and other ozone-depleting chemicals. The treaty was amended in 1995 to ban CFC production in developed countries. Today, over 160 countries have signed the treaty, as the international community strives to preserve the ozone layer.[19]

Global Warming

More than 100 years ago, scientists theorized that carbon dioxide emissions from burning of fossil fuels would create a buildup of *greenhouse gases* in the earth's atmosphere that could have a warming effect on the earth's surface. The century-old predictions are now coming true, with alarming results. Average global temperatures are higher today than at any time since global temperatures were first recorded, and the change in atmospheric temperature may be taking a

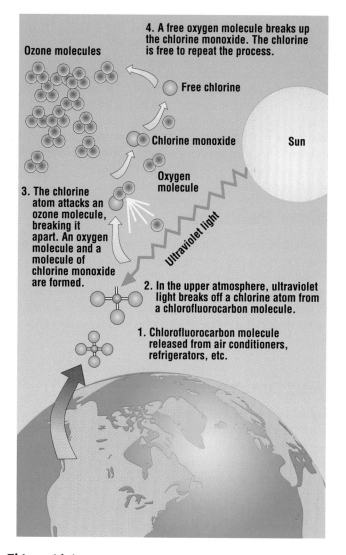

Figure 16.1
How the Ozone Layer Is Being Depleted

Sick building syndrome (SBS) Problem that exists when 80 percent of a building's occupants report maladies that tend to lessen or vanish when they leave the building.

Chlorofluorocarbons (CFCs) Chemicals that contribute to the depletion of the ozone layer.

heavy toll on human beings and crops. Climate researchers predicted in 1975 that the buildup of greenhouse gases would produce life-threatening natural phenomena, including drought in the midwestern United States, more frequent and severe forest fires, flooding in India and Bangladesh, extended heat waves over large areas of the earth, and killer hurricanes. Recently, the planet has experienced all five of these phenomena, although whether they were connected to global warming remains a matter of debate.

Greenhouse gases include carbon dioxide, CFCs, ground-level ozone, nitrous oxide, and methane. They become part of a gaseous layer that encircles the earth, allowing solar heat to pass through and then trapping it close to the earth's surface. The most predominant of these gases is carbon dioxide, which accounts for 49 percent of all greenhouse gases. Eastern Europe and North America are responsible for approximately half of all carbon dioxide emissions. Since the late nineteenth century, carbon dioxide concentrations in the atmosphere have increased by 25 percent, with half of this increase occurring since the 1950s. Carbon emissions from the burning of oil, coal, and gas continue to climb. By 1997, carbon dioxide concentrations in the atmosphere reached their highest levels in 160,000 years.[20] Not surprisingly, these greater concentrations coincide with world industrial growth.

Rapid deforestation of the tropical rain forests of Central and South America, Africa, and Southeast Asia is also contributing to the rapid increase of greenhouse gases. Trees take in carbon dioxide, transform it, store the carbon for food, and then release oxygen into the air. As we lose forests, at the rate of hundreds of acres per hour, we lose the capacity to dissipate carbon dioxide.[21]

Reducing Air Pollution

Our national air pollution problems are rooted in our energy, transportation, and industrial practices. We must develop comprehensive national strategies to address the problem of air pollution in order to clean the air for the future. We must support policies that encourage the use of renewable resources such as solar, wind, and water power as the providers of most of the world's energy. Table 16.2 indicates global trends in sources of energy consumption.

Most experts agree that shifting away from automobiles as the primary source of transportation is the only way to reduce air pollution significantly. Many cities have taken steps in this direction by setting high parking fees, imposing bans on

> **Greenhouse gases** Gases that contribute to global warming by trapping heat near the earth's surface.
>
> **Point source pollutants** Pollutants that enter waterways at a specific point.
>
> **Nonpoint source pollutants** Pollutants that run off or seep into waterways from broad areas of land.

Table 16.2
Global Trends in Energy Use, by Source, 1990–1997

ENERGY SOURCE	ANNUAL RATE OF GROWTH (%)
Wind power	25.7
Solar power	16.8
Geothermal power	3.0
Natural gas	2.1
Hydroelectric power	1.6
Oil	1.4
Nuclear power	0.6

Source: C. Flavin and S. Dunn, *Vital Signs Brief 98–6: Merger Signals Beginning of Geriatric Era for Oil Industry* (Washington, DC: Worldwatch Institute, 1998).

city driving, and establishing high road usage tolls. Community governments should be encouraged to provide convenient, inexpensive, and easily accessible public transportation.

Auto makers must be encouraged to manufacture automobiles that provide good fuel economy and low rates of toxic emissions. Incentives given to manufacturers to produce such cars, tax breaks for purchasers who buy them, and gas-guzzler taxes on inefficient vehicles are three promising measures in this area. Another promising initiative is "bicycle power." Bicycles are gaining popularity. Currently, China leads the world in bicycle use, followed by India. In Germany, bicycle use has increased by 50 percent, and England has a plan to quadruple bicycle use by the year 2012.[22]

Water Pollution

Seventy-five percent of the earth is covered with water in the form of oceans, seas, lakes, rivers, streams, and wetlands. Beneath the landmass are reservoirs of groundwater. We draw our drinking water from either this underground source or from surface freshwater sources. The status of our water supply reflects the pollution level of our communities and, ultimately, of the whole earth.

Water Contamination

Any substance that gets into the soil can potentially enter the water supply. Industrial pollutants, acid rain, and pesticides eventually work their way into the soil, then into the groundwater. Spills of oil and other hazardous wastes flow into local rivers. Underground storage tanks for gasoline may leak. The list continues.

Congress has coined two terms, *point source* and *nonpoint source,* to refer to the two general sources of water pollution. **Point source pollutants** enter a waterway at a specific point through a pipe, ditch, culvert, or other conduit. The two major sources of this type of pollution are sewage treatment plants and industrial facilities. **Nonpoint source pollutants—**

What is the AQI?

Local air quality affects how we live and breathe. Like the weather, it can change from day to day or even hour to hour. The U.S. Environmental Protection Agency (EPA) and others are working to make information about outdoor air quality as available to the public as information about the weather. A key tool in this effort is the Air Quality Index, or AQI. EPA and local officials use the AQI to provide the public with timely and easy-to-understand information on local air quality and whether air pollution levels pose a health concern.

The AQI is an index for reporting daily air quality. It tells you how clean or polluted your air is, and what associated health concerns you should be aware of. The AQI focuses on health effects that can happen within a few hours or days after breathing polluted air. EPA uses the AQI for five major air pollutants regulated by the Clean Air Act: ground-level ozone, particulate matter, carbon monoxide, sulfur dioxide, and nitrogen dioxide. For each of these pollutants, EPA has established national air quality standards to protect against harmful health effects.

HOW DOES THE AQI WORK?

You can think of the AQI as a yardstick that runs from 0 to 500. The higher the AQI value, the greater the level of air pollution and the greater the health danger. For example, an AQI value of 50 represents good air quality and little potential to affect public health, while an AQI value over 300 represents hazardous air quality.

An AQI value of 100 generally corresponds to the national air quality standard for the pollutant, which is the level EPA has set to protect public health. So, AQI values below 100 are generally thought of as satisfactory. When AQI values are above 100, air quality is considered to be unhealthy—at first for certain sensitive groups of people, then for everyone as AQI values get higher.

UNDERSTANDING THE AQI

The purpose of the AQI is to help you understand what local air quality means to your health. To make the AQI as easy to understand as possible, EPA has divided the AQI scale into six categories, shown below:

AIR QUALITY INDEX (AQI) VALUES	LEVELS OF HEALTH CONCERN	COLORS
WHEN THE AQI IS IN THIS RANGE:	AIR QUALITY CONDITIONS ARE:	AS SYMBOLIZED BY THIS COLOR:
0 to 50	Good	Green
51 to 100	Moderate	Yellow
101 to 150	Unhealthy for Sensitive Groups	Orange
151 to 200	Unhealthy	Red
201 to 300	Very Unhealthy	Purple
301 to 500	Hazardous	Maroon

Each category corresponds to a different level of health concern. For example, when the AQI for a pollutant is between 51 and 100, the health concern is "Moderate." Here are the six levels of health concern and what they mean:

- *"Good"* The AQI value for your community is between 0 and 50. Air quality is considered satisfactory and air pollution poses little or no risk.

- *"Moderate"* The AQI for your community is between 51 and 100. Air quality is acceptable; however, for some pollutants there may be a moderate health concern for a very small number of individuals. For example, people who are unusually sensitive to ozone may experience respiratory symptoms.

- *"Unhealthy for Sensitive Groups"* Certain groups of people are particularly sensitive to the harmful effects of certain air pollutants. This means they are likely to be affected at lower levels than the general public. For example, children and adults who are active outdoors and people with respiratory disease are at greater risk from exposure to ozone, while people with heart disease are at greater risk from carbon monoxide. Some people may be sensitive to more than one pollutant. When AQI values are between 101 and 150, members of sensitive groups may experience health effects. The general public is not likely to be affected when the AQI is in this range.

- *"Unhealthy"* AQI values are between 151 and 200. Everyone may begin to experience health effects. Members of sensitive groups may experience more serious health effects.

- *"Very Unhealthy"* AQI values between 201 and 300 trigger a health alert, meaning everyone may experience more serious health effects.

- *"Hazardous"* AQI values over 300 trigger health warnings of emergency conditions. The entire population is more likely to be affected.

Source: Excerpt from Air Quality Index: A Guide to Air Quality and Your Health, 2-3. United States Environmental Protection Agency, June 2000.

commonly known as *runoff* and *sedimentation*—run off or seep into waterways from broad areas of land rather than through a discrete conduit. It is estimated that 99 percent of the sediment in our waterways, 98 percent of the bacterial contaminants, 84 percent of the phosphorus, and 82 percent of the nitrogen come from nonpoint sources.[23]

Nonpoint pollution results from a variety of human land use practices. It includes soil erosion and sedimentation, construction wastes, pesticide and fertilizer runoff, urban street runoff, wastes from engineering projects, acid mine drainage, leakage from septic tanks, and sewage sludge.[24] (See Figure 16.2.)

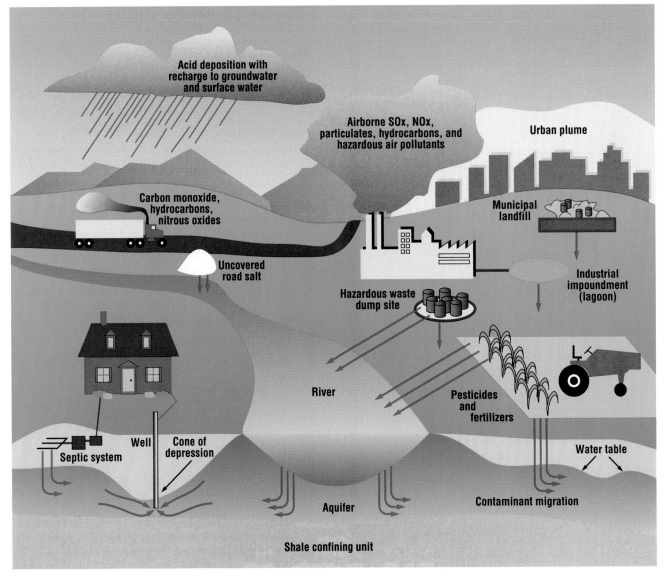

Figure 16.2
Sources of Groundwater Contamination

Septic Systems   Bacteria from human waste can leach into the water supply from improperly installed septic systems. Toxic chemicals that are dumped into septic systems can also enter groundwater.

Landfills   Landfills and dumps generate a liquid called **leachate,** a mixture of soluble chemicals from household garbage, office waste, biological waste, and industrial

waste. If a landfill has not been properly lined, leachate trickles through its layers of garbage and eventually into the water supply as acid and into the atmosphere as methane gas.

Gasoline and Petroleum Products   In the United States, there are more than 2 million underground storage tanks for gasoline and petroleum products, most of which are located at gasoline filling stations. One quarter of these underground tanks are thought to be leaking.[25]

Most of these tanks were installed 25 to 30 years ago. They were made of fabricated steel that was unprotected from corrosion. Over time, pinpoint holes develop in the steel, and the petroleum products leak into the groundwater. The most common way to detect the presence of petroleum

Leachate   A liquid consisting of soluble chemicals that come from garbage and industrial waste that seeps into the water supply from landfills and dumps.

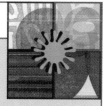

Speaking Out on the Environment

Here are eight ways to get involved in the crusade against environmental pollution:

- Monitor legislation. All of the key environmental organizations keep tabs on state and national laws being considered in order to offer testimony and to generate letter-writing campaigns on behalf of (or against) proposed laws. [You can ask them for information.] . . .

- Write letters. It may not seem like a potent weapon, but letters to state and federal legislators on pending bills do influence their opinions. When writing to any public official, keep your letter simple. Focus on one subject and identify a particular piece of legislation. . . . Request a specific action . . . and state your reasons for taking your position. If you live or work in the legislator's district, make sure to say so. . . . Keep the letter to one or two paragraphs, and never write more than one page. [You can send your letters to:]
[To U.S. Representatives]
Hon. _____
House Office Building
Washington, D.C. 20515
[To U.S. Senators] Senator _____
Senate Office Building
Washington, D.C. 20515

- Fill out customer comment cards and/or phone toll-free numbers on packages [to let companies know your concerns].
- Educate others. You can do this in a variety of ways, from talking to your friends, coworkers, and neighbors to organizing an educational activity. . . .
- Campaign for environmental candidates. Don't just be concerned about someone claiming to be an "environmental president." Look at the environmental positions of candidates at all levels of government. . . .
- Launch a campaign at school or work. At Rutgers University, for example, members of the law association decided to target the use of plastic foam in the cafeterias. The students spoke with the director of food services, who readily agreed to stop using foam cups and foam food containers. Sometimes all you have to do is ask.
- Invite speakers to your organization. Most environmental organizations offer speakers on a wide range of topics who will speak at no charge to your civic, school, religious, or social organization. For maximum impact, consider scheduling a debate or panel discus-

sion among representatives of environmental groups, government agencies, and industry.
- Get involved with government. Most communities offer a variety of boards, commissions, and committees that deal with environmental issues: planning commissions, zoning and land-use commissions, parks commissions, transit boards, and so on. Each can play a role in setting policies that affect the quality of the environment in your area.

products in the water supply is to test for benzene, a component of oil and gasoline. Benzene is highly toxic and is associated with the development of cancer.

Chemical Contaminants

Chemicals designed to dissolve grease and oil are called *organic solvents*. These extremely toxic substances, such as carbon tetrachloride, tetrachloroethylene, and trichloroethylene (TCE), are used to clean clothing, painting equipment, plastics, and metal parts. Many household products, such as stain and spot removers, degreasers, drain cleaners, septic system cleaners, and paint removers, also contain these toxic chemicals.

Organic solvents work their way into the water supply in different ways. Consumers often dump leftover products

into the toilet or into street drains. Industries pour leftovers into large barrels, which are then buried. After a while, the chemicals eat their way out of the barrels and leach into the groundwater system.

One related group of toxic substances contains chlorinated hydrocarbons. The most notorious of these substances are the **polychlorinated biphenyls (PCBs),** their cousins the *polybromated biphenyls (PBBs),* and the *dioxins*. Pesticides and lead are also sources of chemical contamination.

Polychlorinated biphenyls (PCBs)   Toxic chemicals that were once used as insulating materials in high-voltage electrical equipment.

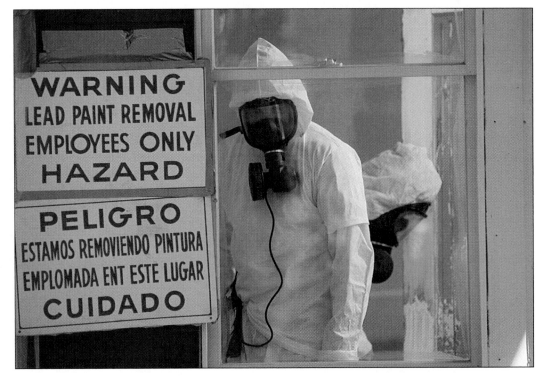

Although an expensive and cumbersome project, de-leading a house is now one the most important considerations of prospective homeowners, especially those with children.

PCBs Fire resistant and stable at high temperatures, PCBs were used for many years as insulating materials in high-voltage electrical equipment such as transformers. PCBs bioaccumulate, meaning that the body does not excrete them but rather stores them in fatty tissues and the liver. PCBs are associated with birth defects, and exposure to them is known to cause cancer. The manufacture of PCBs was discontinued in the United States in 1977, but approximately 500 million pounds of them have been dumped into landfills and waterways, where they continue to pose an environmental threat.[26]

Dioxins Dioxins are chlorinated hydrocarbons found in herbicides (chemicals that are used to kill vegetation) and produced during certain industrial processes. Dioxins have the ability to bioaccumulate and are much more toxic than PCBs.

The long-term effects of bioaccumulation of these toxic substances include possible damage to the immune system and increased risk of infections and cancer. Exposure to high concentrations of PCBs or dioxins for a short period of time can also have severe consequences, including nausea, vomiting, diarrhea, painful rashes and sores, and chloracne, an ailment in which the skin develops hard, black, painful pimples that may never go away.

Pesticides Pesticides are chemicals that are designed to kill insects, rodents, plants, and fungi. Americans use more than 1.2 billion pounds of pesticides each year, but only 10 percent actually reach the targeted organisms. The remaining 1.1 billion pounds of pesticides settle on the land and in our water supplies. Pesticide residues also cling to many fresh fruits and vegetables and are ingested when people eat these items.

Most pesticides remain in the environment and accumulate in the body. A recent study found a correlation between breast cancer and Dieldrin, a popular pesticide used until the 1970s.[27] Women who had the highest traces of Dieldrin in their blood were twice as likely as women with the lowest levels to develop breast cancer. Other potential hazards associated with exposure to pesticides include birth defects, cancer, liver and kidney damage, and nervous system disorders.

Lead The Environmental Protection Agency has issued new standards to reduce dramatically the levels of lead in U.S. drinking water. These standards are already in place in many municipalities and will eventually reduce lead exposure for approximately 130 million people. The new rules stipulate that tap water lead values must not exceed 15 parts per billion (the previous standard allowed an average lead level of

Dioxins Highly toxic chlorinated hydrocarbons contained in herbicides and produced during certain industrial processes.
Pesticides Chemicals that kill pests.

50 parts per billion). When water suppliers identify problem areas, they will have to lower the water's acidity with chemical treatment (because acidity increases water's ability to leach lead from the pipes through which it passes), or they will have to replace old lead plumbing in the service lines.

If lead does exist in your home's water, you can reduce your risk by running tap water for several minutes before taking a drink or cooking with it. This flushes out water that has been standing overnight in lead-contaminated lines. Although leaded paints and ceramic glazes used to pose health risks, particularly for small children who put painted toys in their mouths, the use of lead in such products has been effectively reduced in recent years.

> **What do you think?**
> *Who should bear the financial responsibility for cleaning up hazardous waste leaks?* ✳ *What can you do to avoid contributing to water contamination?*

Noise Pollution

Our bodies have definite physiological responses to noise, and noise can become a source of physical or mental distress. Short-term exposure to loud noise reduces productivity, concentration levels, and attention spans and may affect mental and emotional health. Symptoms of noise-related distress include disturbed sleep patterns, headaches, and tension. Physically, our bodies respond to noises in a variety of ways. Blood pressure increases, blood vessels in the brain dilate, and vessels in other parts of the body constrict. The pupils of the eye dilate. Cholesterol levels in the blood rise, and some endocrine glands secrete additional stimulating hormones, such as adrenaline, into the bloodstream.

Sounds are measured in decibels. A jet takeoff from 200 feet has a noise level of approximately 140 decibels, while voice in normal conversation has a level of about 60 decibels. Hearing can be damaged by varying lengths of exposure to sound. If the duration of allowable daily exposure to different decibel levels is exceeded, hearing loss will result.

Unfortunately, despite increasing awareness that noise pollution is more than just a nuisance, noise control programs at federal, state, and local levels have been given a low budgetary priority. To protect your hearing, you must take it upon yourself to avoid voluntary and involuntary exposure to excessive noise.

> **What do you think?**
> *What do you currently do that places your hearing at risk?* ✳ *What changes can you make in your lifestyle to lower your risk?*

Land Pollution

Solid Waste

Each day, every person in the United States generates about four pounds of **municipal solid waste**—containers and packaging, discarded food, yard debris, and refuse from residential, commercial, institutional, and industrial sources. By the year 2000, solid waste generation was projected to reach 216 million tons daily, or 4.2 pounds per person.[28] Approximately 73 percent of this waste is buried in landfills. Cities and smaller communities throughout the country are in danger of exhausting their landfill space.

As communities run out of landfill space, it is becoming more common to haul garbage out to sea to dump it or ship it to landfills in developing countries. Although experts believe that up to 90 percent of our trash is recyclable, only 26 percent of it is currently recycled. In today's throwaway society, we need to become aware of the amount of waste we generate every day and to look for ways to recycle, reuse, and—most desirable of all—reduce the products we use.

Hazardous Waste

The community of Love Canal, New York, has come to symbolize **hazardous waste** dump sites. The Hooker Chemical Company used Love Canal as a chemical dump site for nearly 30 years, starting in the 1920s. Then the area was filled in by land developers and built up with homes and schools.

In 1976, homeowners began noticing strange seepage in their basements and strong, chemical odors. Babies were born with abnormal hearts and kidneys, two sets of teeth, mental handicaps, epilepsy, liver disease, and abnormal rectal bleeding. The rate of cancer and miscarriages was far above normal.

The New York State Department of Health investigated the Love Canal area and found high concentrations of PCBs in the storm sewers near the old canal, but it took the department another two years to order the evacuation of Love Canal homes. Over 900 families were evacuated, and the state purchased their homes. Finally, in 1978, the expensive process of cleaning up the waste dump began. Many lawsuits for damages are still being litigated.

Municipal solid waste   Solid wastes such as durable goods, nondurable goods, containers and packaging, food wastes, yard wastes, and miscellaneous wastes from residential, commercial, institutional, and industrial sources.

Hazardous waste   Solid waste that, because of its toxic properties, poses a hazard to humans or to the environment.

Environmental Racism

Environmental racism has meant, among other things, that toxic waste dumps, landfills, and industrial plants are much more likely to be placed in communities of color and in the developing world than in predominantly white communities. The interconnectedness of race and poverty has contributed to the disparities in risks faced by ethnic minority communities. In the United States, minorities bear a disproportionate risk of living in an unhealthy environment because race of the local population has been a significant determining factor in the location of hazardous waste facilities nationwide.

The adverse health effects of environmental racism have been devastating for people of color in the United States and throughout the world. A clear example comes from the Amazon rain forest of Ecuador. Over a 21-year period, an American oil company systematically dumped more than 16 million gallons of oil and toxic wastewater into the Ecuadorian Amazon. Three indigenous groups lived in the area where the oil company operated—the Cofan, the Secoya, and the Siona. The Cofan, who numbered approximately 15,000 when the oil company built its first well in 1971, now number only a few hundred. The Secoya and Siona have likewise experienced reductions in their populations. Each of these three groups was a fishing culture when the oil company first came to the Amazon. Now, because of oil contamination, they can no longer fish in the rivers and so face malnourishment.

Often young people migrate to the cities and take low-wage jobs. The result of the contamination of the environment has been the practical decimation of these three indigenous cultures.

In the mid-1990s, the remaining indigenous people filed suit against the oil company, claiming that they had violated the people's right to a healthy environment. They said that the company's decision to dump millions of gallons of toxins in the rain forest led to the cultural genocide of the three tribes; this, they claimed, amounts to racial and ethnic discrimination. One of the tribes' attorneys commented, "The fact is when [the oil company] drills for oil where white people live, they do it safely and according to industry standards. When they drilled in the headwaters of the Amazon river, however, they blatantly ignored these standards while knowingly wreaking havoc on the local people, almost all of whom are people of color." As late as September 1999, the oil company was continuing to fight the lawsuit and refusing to clean up the Amazon. Indigenous leaders launched a national media campaign in the United States, charging the oil company with racism. The company denied that race played any role in its actions.

Scientific literature clearly demonstrates that crude oil and toxic wastewater produced by oil drilling are highly carcinogenic. A September 1999 public health study of San Carlos, an Ecuadorian town containing more than 30 oil wells, found cancer rates 30 times greater than normal, despite the fact that local inhabitants do not smoke, have a healthy diet, and are not exposed to urban contamination.

Additionally, no other industries in the area release cancer-causing toxins. The water in San Carlos had nearly 150 times the amount of hydrocarbons considered safe by internationally recognized limits.

Examples of environmental racism can also be found throughout the United States. Consider these examples.

- In Los Angeles, recycling plants were located in low-income, primarily Latino neighborhoods. Residents consistently complained of dustlike glass particles in the air throughout the community.
- In Augusta, Georgia, a wood preservant factory leaked creosote into the ground, and a scrap metal company leaked arsenic. This ethnic minority community now evidences high rates of cancer and skin disease. The plants are also located near an elementary school, and students there experience high rates of learning disabilities, allergies, and asthma.
- In the predominantly African American area of Chester, Pennsylvania, four hazardous and municipal waste facilities are located. That area has the highest percentage of low-weight births in the state as well as mortality and lung cancer rates 60 percent higher than in the rest of the county.

Many health, civil rights, and environmental activists have become proponents of environmental justice. Proponents of environmental justice argue that people of color have the right to be protected from hazardous substances and that public policy be developed based on mutual respect and justice for all people.

In 1980, the Comprehensive Environmental Response Compensation and Liability Act (Superfund) was enacted to provide funds for cleaning up chemical dump sites that endanger public health and land. This fund is financed through taxes on the chemical and petroleum industries (87 percent) and through general federal tax revenues (13 percent). Cleanup cost estimates from the year 1990 through 2020 range from $106 billion to as high as $500 billion.[29]

To date, 32,500 potentially hazardous waste sites have been identified across the nation. After investigation, 17,800 of these sites were determined to require no further action. But about 1,300 sites are listed on the National Priorities List (NPL), and 46 percent of the sites assessed from 1992

Superfund Fund established under the Comprehensive Environmental Response Compensation and Liability Act to be used for cleaning up toxic waste dumps.

through 1996 are a hazard to human health.[30] The large number of hazardous waste dump sites in the United States indicates the severity of our toxic chemical problem. American manufacturers generate more than 1 ton of chemical waste per person per year (approximately 275 million tons). The *Agency for Toxic Substances and Disease Registry (ATSDR)* and the EPA evaluate and rank the chemicals that are considered hazardous substances. The EPA and the states have undertaken a "cradle-to-grave" program to manage hazardous wastes by monitoring their generation, transportation, storage, treatment, and final disposal.[31]

> **What do you think?**
>
> *What items do you currently recycle? ✳ What are some of the reasons you do not recycle? ✳ What might encourage you to recycle more than you do? ✳ What concerns would you have about living near a landfill or hazardous waste production or disposal site?*

Radiation

A substance is said to be radioactive when it emits high-energy particles from the nuclei of its atoms. There are three types of radiation: alpha particles, beta particles, and gamma rays. *Alpha* particles are relatively massive and are not capable of penetrating human skin. They pose health hazards only when inhaled or ingested. *Beta* particles can penetrate the skin slightly and are harmful if ingested or inhaled. *Gamma* rays are the most dangerous because they can pass straight through the skin, causing serious damage to organs and other vital structures.

Ionizing Radiation

Exposure to ionizing radiation is an inescapable part of life on this planet. **Ionizing radiation** is caused by the release of particles and electromagnetic rays from atomic nuclei during the normal process of disintegration. Some naturally occurring elements, such as uranium, emit radiation. Radiation can wreak havoc on human cells, leading to mutations, cancer, miscarriages, and other problems.

Reactions to radiation differ from person to person. Exposure is measured in **radiation absorbed doses,** or **rads** (also called roentgens). Recommended maximum "safe" dosages range from 0.5 rad to 5 rads per year. Approximately 50 percent of the radiation to which we are exposed comes from natural sources, such as building materials. Another 45 percent comes from medical and dental x-rays. The remaining 5 percent comes from computer display screens, microwave ovens, television sets, luminous watch dials, and radar screens and waves. Most of us are exposed to far less radiation than the "safe" maximum dosage per year.

Radiation can cause damage at dosages as low as 100 to 200 rads. At this level, signs of radiation sickness include nausea, diarrhea, fatigue, anemia, sore throat, and hair loss, but death is unlikely. At 350 to 500 rads, these symptoms become more severe, and death may result because the radiation hinders bone marrow production of the white blood cells we need to protect us from disease. Dosages above 600 to 700 rads are invariably fatal. The effects of long-term exposure to relatively low levels of radiation are unknown. Some scientists believe that such exposure can cause lung cancer, leukemia, skin cancer, bone cancer, and skeletal deformities.

EMFs: Emerging Risks?

If you believe what you hear on TV or read in the papers, electric and magnetic fields (EMFs) generated by electric power delivery systems are responsible for risks for cancer (particularly among children), reproductive dysfunction, birth defects, neurological disorders, Alzheimer's disease, and other ailments. But does research support these claims about EMFs? A six-year study by the National Institute of Environmental Health Sciences (NIEHS) found that the evidence for a link between cancer and EMFs is "weak," although the director of NIEHS warned that efforts to reduce exposure should continue. The study did find a slight increase in risk for childhood leukemia, as well as chronic lymphocytic leukemia in occupationally exposed adults such as utility workers, machinists, and welders. However, NIEHS suggests that the lack of consistent, positive findings weakens the contention that this association is actually due to EMFs.[32]

Nuclear Power Plants

Nuclear power plants account for less than 1 percent of the total radiation to which we are exposed. Other producers of radioactive waste include medical facilities that use radioactive materials as treatment and diagnostic tools and nuclear weapons production facilities.

Proponents of nuclear energy believe that it is a safe and efficient way to generate electricity. Initial costs of building nuclear power plants are high, but actual power generation is relatively inexpensive. A 1,000-megawatt reactor produces enough energy for 650,000 homes and saves 420 million gallons of fossil fuels each year. In some areas where nuclear power plants were decommissioned, electricity bills

---

Ionizing radiation Radiation produced by photons having energy high enough to ionize atoms.

Radiation absorbed doses (rads) Units that measure exposure to radioactivity.

tripled when power companies turned to hydroelectric or fossil fuel sources to generate electricity.

Nuclear reactors also discharge fewer carbon oxides into the air than fossil-fuel-powered generators. Advocates believe that conversion to nuclear power could help slow the global warming trend. Over the past 15 years, carbon emissions were reduced by 298 million tons, or 5 percent.

All these advantages of nuclear energy must be weighed against the disadvantages. First, disposal of nuclear wastes is extremely problematic for the entire world. Additionally, a reactor core meltdown could pose serious threats to a plant's immediate environment and to the world in general.

A **meltdown** occurs when the temperature in the core of a nuclear reactor increases enough to melt both the nuclear fuel and the containment vessel that holds it. Most modern facilities seal their reactors and containment vessels in concrete buildings having pools of cold water on the bottom. If a meltdown occurs, the building and the pool are supposed to prevent the escape of radioactivity.

Two serious nuclear accidents within seven years of each other caused a steep decline in public support for nuclear energy. The first occurred in 1979 at Three Mile Island near Harrisburg, Pennsylvania, when a mechanical failure caused a partial meltdown of one reactor core and small amounts of radioactive steam were released into the atmosphere. No loss of human life was reported, although residents in the area were evacuated. Miscarriages, birth defects, and cancer rates in the area are reported to have increased, but no public health statistics have been released.

Human error and mechanical failure were the reported causes of the 1986 reactor core fire and explosion at the Chernobyl nuclear power plant in the Soviet Union. In just 4.5 seconds, the temperature in the reactor rose to 120 times normal, causing the explosion. Eighteen people were killed immediately, 30 workers died later from radiation sickness, and 200 other workers were hospitalized for severe radiation sickness. Soviet officials evacuated towns and villages near the plant. Some medical workers estimate that the eventual death toll from radiation-induced cancers related to the Chernobyl incident could top 100,000.

Radioactive fallout from the Chernobyl disaster spread over most of the northern hemisphere. Milk, meat, and vegetables in Scandinavian countries were contaminated with radioactive iodine and cesium and were declared unfit for human consumption. Thousands of reindeer in Lapland were contaminated and had to be destroyed. In Great Britain, thousands of sheep had to be destroyed, and three years later sheep in the northern regions of the country were still found to be contaminated. Direct costs of the disaster totaled more than $13 billion, including lost agricultural output and the cost of replacing the power plant. Nuclear accidents continue to pose risks to human health, even in well-controlled settings.

Meltdown   An accident that results when the temperature in the core of a nuclear reactor increases enough to melt the nuclear fuel and the containment vessel housing it.

What do you think?
How much exposure do you have to ionizing and non-ionizing radiation a year? ✷ *What measures could you take to reduce this exposure?* ✷ *Do you feel the advantages outweigh the disadvantages of nuclear power?* ✷ *Explain why or why not.*

Taking Charge

16   16   16

Managing Environmental Pollution

Checklist for Change

Assessing Personal Choices

✓ Do you recycle newspaper, tin cans, glass, paper, plastic, and cardboard?

✓ Do you take short showers?

✓ Do you heat only rooms that are being used?

✓ Do you turn off lights when you leave a room?

✓ Do you use cold water and run your washing machine fully loaded?

✓ Do you dry clothes on a line when possible?

✓ Do you carpool or take public transportation whenever possible?

✓ Do you drive a car that gets good gas mileage?

✓ Do you purchase only the things you need?

✓ Do you recycle used oil?

✓ Do you use low-phosphorus fertilizers?

Taking Charge

✓ Do you compost leaves, clippings, and kitchen scraps?

✓ Do you dispose of household chemicals safely?

✓ Do you buy products in recyclable packaging?

✓ Do you reuse containers rather than buy new ones?

✓ Do you refuse to use products that contribute to deforestation, wetland extinction, and water or air pollution?

Assessing Community Choices

✓ Do you write or call politicians to advocate for environmental legislation?

✓ Do you protest the location of hazardous waste sites and toxic chemical use in communities of color?

✓ Do you support candidates who have strong environmental records?

✓ Do you contact manufacturers to discourage overpackaging, non-recyclable packaging, and environmentally harmful products?

✓ Do you encourage your school to recycle?

Summary

☀ Population growth is the single largest factor affecting the demands made on the environment. Demand for more food, products, and energy—as well as places to dispose of waste, particularly in the industrialized world—places great strains on the earth's resources.

☀ The primary constituents of air pollution are sulfur dioxide, particulate matter, carbon monoxide, nitrogen dioxide, ozone, lead, and hydrocarbons. Air pollution takes the forms of photochemical smog and acid rain, among others. Indoor air pollution is caused primarily by woodstove smoke, furnace emissions, asbestos, passive smoke, formaldehyde, and radon. Pollution is depleting the earth's protective ozone layer, causing global warming.

☀ Water pollution can be caused by either point sources (direct entry through a pipeline, ditch, etc.) or nonpoint sources (runoff or seepage from a broad area of land).

Chemicals that are major contributors to water pollution include dioxins, pesticides, and lead.

☀ Noise pollution affects our hearing and produces other symptoms such as reduced productivity, reduced concentration, headaches, and tension.

☀ Solid waste pollution includes household trash, plastics, glass, metal products, and paper. Limited landfill space creates problems. Hazardous waste is toxic; its improper disposal creates health hazards for those in surrounding communities.

☀ Ionizing radiation results from the natural erosion of atomic nuclei. Non-ionizing radiation is caused by the electric and magnetic fields around power lines and household appliances, among other sources. The disposal and storage of radioactive wastes from nuclear power plants and weapons production pose serious potential problems for public health.

Discussion Questions

1. How are the rapidly increasing global population and consumption of resources related? Is population control the best solution? Why or why not?

2. What are the primary sources of air pollution? What can be done to reduce air pollution?

3. What causes poor indoor air quality? How does indoor air pollution affect schoolchildren?

4. What are the causes and consequences of global warming?

5. What are point and nonpoint sources of water pollution? What can be done to reduce or prevent water pollution?

6. What are the physiological consequences of noise pollution? What can you do to lessen your exposure to noise pollution?

7. Why do you think so little recycling occurs in the United States?

8. Would you feel comfortable living near a nuclear power plant? Do you think nuclear power is an important source of energy in the future? Why or why not?

Application Exercise

Reread the What Do You Think? scenario at the beginning of the chapter, and answer the following questions.

1. What are the arguments in favor of and against population growth?
2. Which signs show that renewable resources are being depleted?

3. A larger population creates greater demand for resources and in turn generates greater amounts of waste. What steps could be taken worldwide to prevent population growth from depleting resources and polluting the environment? Describe components of a U.S. program to decrease consumption and pollution.

Accessing Your Health on the Internet

Visit the following Internet sites to explore further topics and issues related to personal health. To visit an organization's website, go to the Companion Website for *Health: The Basics, Fifth Edition* at www.aw.com/donatelle, click on the book image, and select "Accessing Your Health on the Internet" from the navigation menu on the left.

1. ***National Center for Environmental Health.*** A section of the Centers for Disease Control and Prevention, with information on a wide variety of environmental health issues, including a series of helpful fact sheets.

2. ***National Environmental Health Association.*** This organization provides educational resources and opportunities for environmental health professionals. The NEHA website lists conferences, trainings, and publications and offers informational position papers.

3. ***Environmental Protection Agency.*** Government agency responsible for overseeing environmental regulation and protection issues in the United States.

Further Reading

Godish, T. *Indoor Environmental Quality.* Boca Raton, FL: Lewis Publishers, 2000.
    Explores the scope of the indoor environment, both in the home and workplace, and major indoor contaminants.

Hofrichter, R., ed. *Reclaiming the Environmental Debate: The Politics of Health in a Toxic Culture.* Boston: MIT Press, 2000.
    Examines the links between the threat of hazardous substances to public health and the social arrangements that encourage and excuse the deterioration of human health and the environment.

Nadakavukaren, N. *Our Global Environment: A Health Perspective.* Prospect Heights, IL: Waveland, 2000.
    A survey of major global environmental issues and their ecological impact on personal and community health.

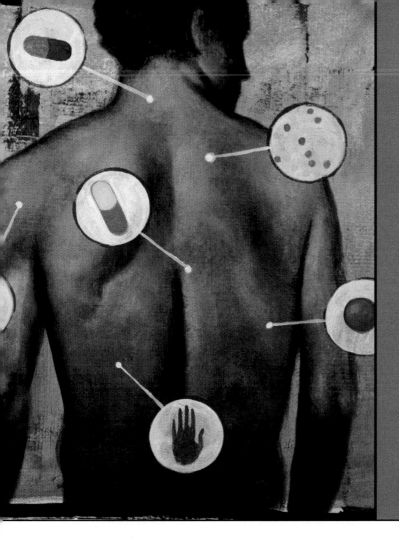

17

Consumerism

SELECTING HEALTH CARE PRODUCTS AND SERVICES

objectives

* Explain why responsible consumerism is important to Americans and how to encourage consumers to take action.

* Explain why self-diagnosis, self-help, and self-care are becoming increasingly important in the individual's quest for health and well-being.

* Discuss the choices available to Americans who seek health care through allopathic avenues, as well as factors that should be considered in making decisions about health care.

* Describe the U.S. health care system in terms of types of medical practice, provider groups, and the changing structures of managed care and other options.

* Discuss key issues in American health care services in terms of cost, quality, and access to services.

* Discuss the different types of health insurance available in the United States and the role that they play in providing health care to American citizens.

There are many reasons for you to be an informed health care consumer. Most important, you have only one body, and if you don't treat it with care, you will pay a major price in terms of financial costs and health consequences. Doing everything you can to prevent illness, stay healthy, and recover rapidly when you do get sick will enhance every other part of your life.

To obtain high-quality health care at an affordable cost, you need to be both informed and assertive. But, as you know, medical services are much harder to evaluate for need, availability, cost, and quality than are, say, clothing or vegetables. In addition, you may seek health care services in circumstances of physical or emotional distress, when your decision-making powers are compromised and you may find yourself very vulnerable.

This chapter will help you make better decisions that affect your health and health care. Our health care system is a maze of health care providers, payers (insurance, government, and individuals), and products. Many of us find it hard to thread our way through the maze. Health care is the fifth largest industry in our country, accounting for over 10 percent of our workforce, and many different companies aggressively market health products and services to the public. Increasingly, health care organizations are "for-profit" businesses, sold and traded on the stock market, and making a profit is their goal. Medical professionals and consumers report that they feel overwhelmed, confused, and frustrated by the multitude of choices, seemingly divergent interests, and lack of coordination in our system.

Responsible Consumerism: Choices and Challenges

Perhaps the single greatest difficulty that we face as health consumers is the sheer magnitude of choices available to us. If you try to select a general practitioner from the telephone book, you may have to thumb through dozens of pages of specialists. When you want to purchase cough syrup, you are confronted with hundreds of options, each claiming to do more for you than the brand next to it. Even trained pharmacists sometimes find it impossible to keep up with the explosion of new drugs and health-related products. Because there are so many profit-seekers competing for a share of the lucrative health market and because misinformation is so common, wise health consumers use every means at their disposal to ensure that they are acting responsibly and economically.

Attracting Consumers' Dollars

Health care products and services are often marketed using the same techniques that are used to market other consumer products. Today's marketing specialists can identify a target audience for a given product and carefully go after it with a whole arsenal of gimmicks, subtle persuaders, and sophisticated strategies. Different techniques are used to attract new customers, maintain existing customers, and encourage former consumers of the product to come back. Advertisements may present a product as a status symbol or play on inner fears and insecurities, causing you to wonder whether your deodorant is working, your breath is bad, or your skin is greasy.

Putting Cure into Better Perspective

People often fall victim to false health claims because they mistakenly believe that a product or provider has helped them. Frequently this belief arises from two conditions: spontaneous remission and the placebo effect.

Spontaneous Remission It is commonly said that if you treat a cold, it will disappear in a week, but if you leave it alone, it will last seven days. A **spontaneous remission** from an ailment refers to the disappearance of symptoms without any apparent cause or treatment. Many illnesses, like the common cold and even back strain, are self-limiting and will improve in time, with or without treatment. Other illnesses, such as multiple sclerosis and some cancers, are characterized by alternating periods of severe symptoms and sudden remissions. People experiencing spontaneous remissions can easily attribute their "cure" to a treatment that in fact had no real effect.

Placebo Effect The **placebo effect** is an apparent cure or improved state of health brought about by a substance, product, or procedure that has no generally recognized therapeutic value. It is not uncommon for patients to report improvements based on what they expect, desire, or were told would happen after taking simple sugar pills that they believed were powerful drugs. About 10 percent of the population is believed to be exceptionally susceptible to the power of suggestion and may be easy targets for such aggressive marketing. Although the placebo effect is generally harmless, it does account for the expenditure of millions of dollars on health products and services every year. Megadoses of vitamin C have never been proven to treat cancer. Mud baths do not smooth wrinkled skin, nor do electric shocks reduce muscle pain. People who mistakenly use placebos when medical treatment is urgently needed increase their risk for health problems.

Taking Responsibility for Your Health Care

As the health care industry has become more sophisticated about seeking your business, so must you become more sophisticated about purchasing its products and services. Learn how, when, and where to enter the massive technological maze that is our health care system without incurring unnecessary risk and expense. Acting responsibly in times of illness can be difficult, but the person best able to act on your behalf is you.

If you are not feeling well, you must first decide whether you really need to seek medical advice. Not that long ago, as many as 70 percent of all trips to the doctor and nearly half of all hospital stays were believed to be unnecessary and potentially harmful.[1] These figures have been reduced considerably, however, with the advent of managed care, which carries with it a degree of out-of-pocket shared costs. Theoretically, patients who have to pay for a portion of their care will not seek care that is not needed. Managed care involves a number of measures designed to keep people out of the hospitals and emergency rooms.[2] Although there are no exact figures, respected sources indicate that the number of emergency room visits has decreased dramatically and that the cost of emergency room care for nonemergencies has declined as well.[3]

Yet critics of managed care point to cost savings as a part of the problem with quality and access. Not seeking treatment, whether because of high costs or limited coverage, or trying to medicate oneself when more rigorous methods of treatment are needed, is dangerous. Being knowledgeable about the benefits of and limits to self-care is critical for responsible consumerism.

Self-Help or Self-Care

A recent concept in health consumerism proposes that the patient is the primary health care provider or first line of defense. We can practice behaviors that promote health, prevent disease, and minimize reliance on the formal medical system. We can also interpret basic changes in our own physical and emotional health and treat minor afflictions without seeking professional help. Self-care consists of knowing your body, paying attention to its signals, and taking appropriate action to stop the progression of illness or injury. Common forms of self-care include the following:

- Diagnosing symptoms or conditions that occur frequently but may not need physician visits (e.g., the common cold, minor abrasions)
- Performing breast and testicular self-examinations (monthly)
- Learning first-aid for common, uncomplicated injuries and conditions
- Checking blood pressure, pulse, and temperature
- Using home pregnancy and ovulation kits and HIV test kits
- Doing periodic checks for blood cholesterol
- Using home stool test kits for blood and early colon cancer detection
- Using self-help books, tapes, software, websites, and videos
- Benefiting from relaxation techniques, including meditation, nutrition, rest, and exercise

When to Seek Help

Effective self-care also means understanding when to seek medical attention rather than treating a condition yourself. Deciding which conditions warrant professional advice is not always easy. Generally, you should consult a physician if you experience any of the following:

Spontaneous remission The disappearance of symptoms without any apparent cause or treatment.

Placebo effect An apparent cure or improved state of health brought about by a substance or product that has no medicinal value.

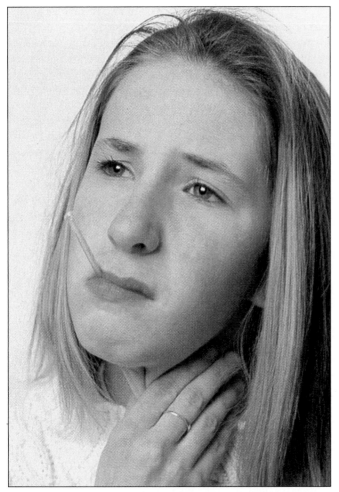

Deciding when to contact a physician can be difficult. Most people first try to diagnose and treat their condition themselves.

- A serious accident or injury
- Sudden or severe chest pains causing breathing difficulties
- Trauma to the head or spine accompanied by persistent headache, blurred vision, loss of consciousness, vomiting, convulsions, or paralysis
- Sudden high fever or recurring high temperature (over 102°F for adults and 103°F for children) and/or sweats
- Tingling sensation in the arm accompanied by slurred speech or impaired thought processes
- Adverse reactions to a drug or insect bite (shortness of breath, severe swelling, dizziness)
- Unexplained bleeding or loss of bodily fluid from any body opening
- Unexplained sudden weight loss
- Persistent or recurrent diarrhea or vomiting
- Blue-colored lips, eyelids, or nail beds
- Any lump, swelling, thickness, or sore that does not subside or that grows for over a month
- Any marked change or pain in bowel or bladder habits
- Yellowing of the skin or the whites of the eyes

- Any symptom that is unusual and recurs over time
- Pregnancy

With the vast array of home diagnostic devices currently available, it appears to be relatively easy for most people to take care of themselves. But some caution is in order here: Although many of these devices are valuable for making an initial diagnosis, home health tests cannot substitute for regular, complete examinations by a trained practitioner. The accompanying Skills for Behavior Change box offers valuable information about taking an active role in your own health care.

Assessing Health Professionals

Suppose you decide that you do need medical help. You must then identify what type of help you need and where to obtain it. Initially, selecting a professional may seem a simple matter, yet many people have no idea how to assess the qualifications of a health care provider.

Knowledge of both traditional medical specialties and alternative, or complementary, medical treatment is critical to making an intelligent selection. You also need to be aware of your own criteria for evaluating a health professional. Several studies have pointed to bedside manner and positive interactions with doctors as key to patient satisfaction. In a survey of HMO members, it was shown that even in a setting of limited physician choice, the opportunity to select one's personal physician had a positive influence on patient satisfaction with that physician.[4] When selecting from a network of providers, make sure you fully understand your coverage options. Carefully consider the following factors about all prospective health care providers:

- What professional educational training have they had? What license or board certification do they hold? Note that there is a difference between "board eligible" and "board certified." *Board certified* indicates that the practitioner has passed the national board examination for his or her specialty (e.g., pediatrics) and has been certified as competent in that specialty. In contrast, *board eligible* merely means that the practitioner is eligible to take the specialty board's exam or that he or she may have failed the exam.
- Are they affiliated with an accredited medical facility or institution? The Joint Commission on the Accreditation of Healthcare Organizations (JCAHO) requires these institutions to verify all education, licensing, and training claims of their affiliated practitioners. What other doctors are in their group, and who will assist in your treatment?
- Are they open to complementary or alternative strategies? Would they refer you for different treatment modalities, when appropriate?
- Do they indicate clearly how long a given treatment may last, what side effects you might expect, and what things you should be on the alert for?
- Do their diagnoses, treatments, and general statements appear to be consistent with established scientific theory and practice?

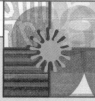

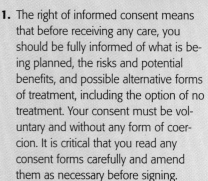

Being Proactive in Your Health Care

Throughout this book, we have emphasized the importance of healthy preventive behaviors. Sometimes, however, regardless of the steps you take to care for yourself, you still get sick. At such a time, it is important that you continue to be actively involved in your care. The more you know about your body and the factors that can affect your health, the better you will be at communicating with your doctor. Being proactive also helps you make informed decisions and recognize when a certain treatment may not be right for you. The following points can help:

- Know your own and your family's medical history.
- Be knowledgeable about your condition—causes, physiological effects, possible treatments, prognosis. Don't rely on the doctor for this information. Do some research.
- Bring a friend or relative along for medical visits to help you review what the doctor says. Or take notes if you go alone.
- Ask the practitioner to explain the problem and possible treatments, tests, and drugs in a clear and understandable way. If you don't understand something, ask for clarification.
- If the doctor prescribes any medications, ask whether you can take generic equivalents that cost less.
- Ask for a written summary of the results of your visit and any lab tests.
- If you have any doubt about the doctor's recommended treatment, seek a second opinion.

- If you will need to take a prescription medication for an extended time, ask for the maximum number of doses allowed by your plan if you have a small pharmacy copayment.

After seeing a health care professional, consider these ideas:

- Write down an accurate account of what happened and what was said. Be sure to include the names of the doctor and all other people involved in your care, the date, and the place.
- Shop around drugstores for the best prices in the same way that you would when shopping for clothes.
- When filling prescriptions, ask to see the pharmacist's package inserts that list medical considerations concerning the medicines. Request detailed information about any potential drug interactions.
- Write clear instructions on the label to avoid risk to others who may take the drug in error.

Just like you, doctors are human. Their decisions are based on the best information they have available to them and may be influenced by a number of factors—for example, workload, limited information, and personal views. Therefore, in addition to following the practical steps listed above, being proactively involved in your health care also means that you should be aware of your rights as a patient. Your rights include the following:

1. The right of informed consent means that before receiving any care, you should be fully informed of what is being planned, the risks and potential benefits, and possible alternative forms of treatment, including the option of no treatment. Your consent must be voluntary and without any form of coercion. It is critical that you read any consent forms carefully and amend them as necessary before signing.
2. You are entitled to know whether the treatment you are receiving is standard or experimental. In experimental conditions, you have the legal and ethical right to know whether the study is one in which some people receive treatment while others do not in order to compare the results and whether any drug is being used in the research project for a purpose not approved by the Food and Drug Administration (FDA).
3. You have the right to privacy, which includes the source of payment for treatment and care. It also includes protecting your right to make personal decisions concerning all reproductive matters.
4. You have the right to receive care. You also have the legal right to refuse treatment at any time and to cease treatment at any time.
5. You are entitled to access all your medical records and to have those records remain confidential.
6. You have the right to seek the opinions of other health care professionals regarding your condition.

- Who will be responsible for your care when the doctor is on vacation or off call?
- Do they listen to you, respect you as an individual, and give you time to ask questions? Do they return your calls, and are they available to answer questions?
- How often has the doctor performed this test, surgery, or procedure, and with what proportion of successful outcome?

When a doctor orders a test, treatment, or medication, you might ask questions like these:

- What are the side effects, and can these side effects be treated or reduced?
- Does this procedure require an overnight stay at a hospital, or can it be performed in a doctor's office?
- Why has this test been ordered? What is the doctor trying to find or exclude?

Table 17.1
Allopathic/Traditional Medical Professionals

Allergist	A specialist who diagnoses and treats allergies
Anesthesiologist	A specialist who administers drugs during surgical procedures to reduce pain or induce unconsciousness
Cardiologist	A specialist in the diagnosis and treatment of heart and blood vessel disorders
Dermatologist	A specialist in the diagnosis and treatment of skin disorders
Dietitian	A specialist in the field of diet and human nutrition
Endocrinologist	A specialist in the diagnosis and treatment of glandular disorders
Family practitioner	A physician who offers routine medical service for a variety of ailments
Gastroenterologist	A specialist who diagnoses and treats disorders of the stomach and intestinal tract
Geneticist	A specialist who diagnoses and treats genetic diseases
Health educator	A specialist in the field of health education and health promotion who holds a degree in a health-related area (look for Comprehensive Health Education Specialist [CHES] certification)
Hematologist	A specialist who diagnoses and treats blood-related disorders
Neurologist	A specialist who diagnoses and treats diseases of the brain, nervous system, and spinal cord
Nurse practitioner	Nurse specialist with additional training in a specified area, such as OB/GYN
Obstetrician/gynecologist (OB/GYN)	A specialist who diagnoses and treats problems of the female reproductive system
Oncologist	A specialist who diagnoses and treats cancerous growths and tumors
Ophthalmologist	A specialist who diagnoses, treats, and provides general care of eye disorders
Orthopedist/orthopedic surgeon	A specialist who diagnoses, treats, or provides surgical care for bone and joint injuries and problems
Otolaryngologist	A specialist who specializes in ear, nose, and throat disorders
Pediatrician	A physician who treats childhood diseases
Physical therapist	A specialist who rehabilitates people after impairment due to injury or disease
Physician assistant	Health care professional trained to assist physicians
Plastic surgeon	A specialist who provides corrective surgery for irregularities of body or facial contours
Podiatrist	A specialist who diagnoses and treats disorders of the feet
Psychiatrist	A physician who diagnoses and treats mental and emotional disorders
Pulmonary specialist	A specialist who diagnoses and treats disorders of the respiratory system
Radiologist	A specialist in diagnosing disease by using x-rays and other imaging techniques
Rheumatologist	A specialist who diagnoses and treats medical conditions of joints and surrounding tissues
Urologist	A specialist who diagnoses and treats disorders of the urinary tract

Asking the right questions at the right time may save you personal suffering and expense. Many patients find that writing their questions down before an appointment helps them get answers to all their questions. You should not accept a defensive or hostile response; asking questions is your right as a patient.

Allopathic medicine Traditional, Western medical practice; in theory, based on scientifically validated methods and procedures.

Choices in Medical Care

How can you choose the right provider for your needs? Familiarize yourself with the various health professions and subspecialties (see the list in Table 17.1). These professionals all subscribe to allopathic medical procedures. Most people believe that **allopathic medicine,** or traditional Western medical practice, is based on scientifically validated methods, but you should consider the fact that not all allopathic treatments have had the benefit of the extensive clinical trials and long-term studies of outcomes that would be necessary to conclusively prove effectiveness in different populations. In fact, a treatment provided in one facility may differ

Doc.com Surfer Beware

Mary, an avid fitness proponent with no formal academic training in health, took her first webpage-building class in August. Today, because of her interest in and enthusiasm for health topics, she has a website offering comprehensive medical advice, on which she talks with great authority about a variety of interesting topics. The site includes self-assessment exercises and numerous links to other health sites. But does her glitzy, interactive page provide accurate, well-researched advice? Or is she just picking up bits and pieces of information from the same, often questionable sites to which we all have access? Mary is just as vulnerable to bad information as the rest of us. She may not even know that her information may be based on weak science. So, while her intentions are good, Mary's advice has the potential to harm others seriously.

Although Mary is a fictional character invented to make a point, such a scenario is more than possible. A great many "Marys" abound on the Internet today, because anyone capable of creating a webpage has the tools to put up anything he or she wants. Sometimes what is put online for the world lacks the backing of reputable scientists, medical and health care groups, or educational counsel. It can be misleading and may even be harmful. This is certainly the case with the surge of sites devoted to health and medical information. The World Wide Web is filled with self-appointed health experts, with legitimate professional health agencies, and, more recently, with what has come to be known as Doc.coms—websites that provide everything from online diagnoses, chatroom support groups, and detailed information on conditions and procedures, to opportunities to watch surgical procedures. Today, millions of people throughout the world have information at their fingertips and often turn to that source for help with the self-diagnosis of symptoms. Although this availability of information could encourage people to be more proactive in their own care, the potential for harm should make us proceed with caution.

Browsers in the e-marketplace of medical information will find that the quality is very diverse. Some sites offer depth of data, with credentials to back them up. Others display nice site design or easy access but have thin content. Just because a site is glitzy and professional looking does *not* mean that it is reputable or scientifically valid. Look for sites affiliated with recognized universities, professional groups, or associations. Cross-check references whenever possible, and look for credentials for the person administering the site.

How can you make sure you get the best information possible? Follow these tips:

- Don't forget the wealth of information at your school's library. Ask the reference librarian at your school about health-related information data banks that the school subscribes to. Institutions of higher education generally subscribe to peer-reviewed journals, which are written by professionals and reviewed by the writers' colleagues. In addition, universities often subscribe to services that compile journal articles from the social and health sciences and meet the criteria for peer review. Many of these publications are online. Those that are not will probably be on your library's shelves.
- Seek information from several different types of sources. Check author credentials, and cross-check information from different sources to find areas of consensus. Taking information from only one source, assuming it to be true, is a bad idea.
- Reputable information in the health area often includes complete references. Find out whether the site is professionally managed, peer-reviewed, and updated regularly.
- Professional and nationally recognized organizations, including government agencies, are good places to start. Although still possessing inaccuracies, many of these sites include the latest data-based statistics from randomized, clinical trials.
- Remember that just because a site is "linked" to a government source doesn't mean that the government source is aware of the site or endorses it.
- Look at the credentials of the authors of any papers posted online. With what organizations, if any, are they affiliated?
- Avoid online health professionals who will diagnose or make blanket statements about your health without requiring a formal examination or referring you to others.
- Look at the advertisements on the page. If they are part of the text or if they appear to promise quick cures or easy solutions, beware.
- Note the date of the article and all references. Citations that are more than a couple of years old are too old.
- If the site is from a reputable institution of higher education, determine whether it is managed by faculty, students, or laboratories on campus.
- Look to see whether the site provides both sides of controversial issues, including references. Reputable sites don't try to force you into buying their product or endorsing their view; they want you to be aware of and consider your options.
- Use caution when purchasing health products and services over the Internet. Check out your options, consider the costs and the benefits, and proceed with caution.
- For personal health issues, weigh all the information you gather from the Internet with what you learn from your health care provider. Your health care providers are still some of the best resources at your disposal.

markedly from that provided in another. What is true is that allopathic practitioners receive similar training and are bound by a consistent professional code of ethics.

Traditional Western (Allopathic) Medicine

Selecting a **primary care practitioner**—a medical practitioner whom you can go to for routine ailments, preventive care, general medical advice, and appropriate referrals—is not an easy task. The primary care practitioner for most people is a family practitioner, an internist, a pediatrician, or an obstetrician/gynecologist. Many people routinely see nurse practitioners or physician assistants who work for an individual doctor or a medical group, and others use nontraditional providers as their primary source of care.

Active participation in your own treatment is the only sensible course in a health care environment that encourages "defensive medicine." That is, physicians will frequently order tests to rule out rare or unlikely diagnoses simply because they are worried about possible malpractice suits. Researchers have documented that this practice often leads to unnecessary tests and overtreatment. It has been well documented that most medical treatments carry risks and that there is no 100 percent guarantee of improved health outcomes. You may find that your condition worsens or that the treatment may create an iatrogenic disease (an illness caused by the medical treatment itself). *Informed consent* refers to

your right to have explained to you—in nontechnical language you can understand—all possible side effects, benefits, and consequences of a procedure as well as available alternatives to it. It also means that you have the right to refuse a treatment and to seek a second or even third opinion from unbiased, noninvolved providers.[5]

What do you think?

Have you ever opted for a treatment other than what was recommended by your allopathic medical provider? ✳ *How did you go about checking on the safety of the treatment? What was the result?* ✳ *Did your health insurer cooperate fully and pay the bill?*

Other Forms of Allopathic Specialties

Although Table 17.1 provides an overview of common sources of health care, it is by no means all-inclusive. Other specialists include **osteopaths,** general practitioners who receive training similar to a medical doctor's but who put special emphasis on the skeletal and muscular systems. Their treatments may involve manipulation of the muscles and joints. Osteopaths receive the degree of doctor of osteopathy (D.O.) rather than doctor of medicine (M.D.).

Much confusion exists about the roles of optometrists and ophthalmologists. An **ophthalmologist** holds a medical degree and can perform surgery and prescribe medications. An **optometrist** typically evaluates visual problems and fits glasses but is not a trained physician. If you have an eye infection, glaucoma, or other eye condition needing diagnosis and treatment, you need to see an ophthalmologist.

Dentists are specialists who diagnose and treat diseases of the teeth, gums, and oral cavity. They attend dental school for four years and receive the title of doctor of dental surgery (D.D.S.) or doctor of medical dentistry (D.M.D.). They must also pass both state and national board examinations before receiving their licenses to practice. The field of dentistry includes many specialties. For example, **orthodontists** are specialists in the alignment of teeth. **Oral surgeons** perform surgical procedures to correct problems of the mouth, face, and jaw.

Nurses are highly trained and strictly regulated health practitioners who provide a wide range of services for patients and their families, including patient education, counseling, community health and disease prevention information, and administration of medications. Nurses may today choose from several training options.

There are over 2.4 million licensed registered nurses (R.N.) in the United States who have completed either a four-year program leading to a bachelor of science in nursing (B.S.N.) degree or a two-year associate degree program. More than 0.5 million lower-level licensed practical or vocational nurses (L.P.N. or L.V.N.) have completed a one- to two-year

Primary care practitioner   A medical practitioner who treats routine ailments, advises on preventive care, gives general medical advice, and makes appropriate referrals when necessary.

Osteopath   General practitioner who receives training similar to a medical doctor's but with an emphasis on the skeletal and muscular systems; often uses spinal manipulation as part of treatment.

Ophthalmologist   Physician who specializes in the medical and surgical care of the eyes, including prescriptions for glasses.

Optometrist   Eye specialist whose practice is limited to prescribing and fitting lenses.

Dentist   Specialist who diagnoses and treats diseases of the teeth, gums, and oral cavity.

Orthodontist   Dentist who specializes in the alignment of teeth.

Oral surgeon   Dentist who performs surgical procedures to correct problems of the mouth, jaw, and face.

Nurse   Health practitioner who provides many services for patients and who may work in a variety of settings.

training program, which may be community college–based or hospital-based.

Nurse practitioners (N.P.) are professional nurses having advanced training obtained through either a master's degree program or a specialized nurse practitioner program. Nurse practitioners have the training and authority to conduct diagnostic tests and prescribe medications (in some states). They work in a variety of settings, particularly in HMOs, clinics, and student health centers. Nurses may also earn the clinical doctor of nursing degree (N.D.) or a doctorate of nursing science (D.N.S. or D.N.Sc.), or a research-based Ph.D. in nursing.

More than 30,000 **physician assistants** (P.A.) currently practice in the United States. Most of these are in office-based practices, including school health centers, but approximately 40 percent practice in areas where physicians are in short supply. Studies have shown that this relatively new class of midlevel practitioners may competently care for the majority of patients seeking primary care. All physician assistants must work under the supervision of a licensed physician, but most states do allow physician assistants to prescribe drugs.[6]

Health Care Organizations, Programs, and Facilities

Today, managed care is the dominant health payer system in the United States, even though its position has weakened in recent years. Patient dissatisfaction over lack of provider choice and consumer complaints about care have eroded many of the rapid increases and growth that HMOs experienced in the 1990s. Selective contracting between insurers or employers and health providers has limited the freedom of choice that some Americans previously enjoyed under a fee-for-service system. Two critical decisions to make are (1) choosing an insurance carrier or type of plan, and then (2) choosing from among the health care providers who participate in that plan. This section lists the most common choices.

Types of Medical Practices

In the highly competitive market for patients, many health care providers have found it essential to combine resources into a **group practice,** which can be single-specialty or multi-speciality. Physicians share offices, equipment, utility bills, and staff costs. Besides sharing costs, they may also share profits. Proponents of group practice maintain that it provides better coordination of care, reduces unnecessary duplication of equipment, and improves the quality of health care through peer review. Critics argue that group practice may limit competition and patients' access to services.

Solo practitioners are medical providers who practice independently of other practitioners. It is hard for solo practitioners to survive in today's high-cost, high-technology health

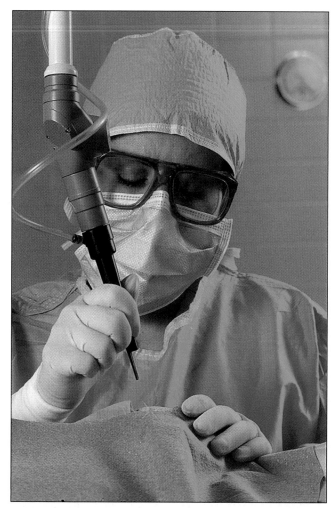

Modern technology has vastly improved treatment for many illnesses, but it has also played a major role in the escalating costs of medical care.

care market. Additionally, solo practitioners often have little time away from their offices and have to trade on-call hours with other doctors. For these reasons, there are far fewer solo practices today than in the past. Most solo practitioners are doctors who established their practices years ago, have a specialty that's in high demand, or work in a rural or underserved area.

Physician assistant   A midlevel practitioner trained to handle most standard cases of care.

Group practice   A group of physicians who combine resources, sharing offices, equipment, and staff costs to render care to patients.

Solo practitioner   Physician who renders care to patients independently of other practitioners.

Integrated Health Care Organizations

Both hospitals and clinics provide a range of health care services, including emergency treatment, diagnostic tests, and inpatient and outpatient (ambulatory) care. Your selection of a hospital or clinic will depend on your needs, income, and insurance coverage, plus the availability of services in your community. The number of hospitals has decreased in recent years because of an oversupply of hospital beds, a decreasing need for inpatient care, and an increase in competition. As a result, the number of hospital-based outpatient clinics has grown. These integrated health care organizations range from groups of loosely affiliated health service organizations and hospitals to HMOs that control their own very tightly joined hospitals, clinics, pharmacies, and even home health agencies.

There are several ways to classify hospitals: by profit status (nonprofit or for-profit), by ownership (private, city, county, state, federal), by specialty (children's, maternity, chronic care, psychiatric, general acute), by teaching status (teaching-affiliated or not), by size, and by whether they are part of a chain of hospitals. **Nonprofit (voluntary) hospitals** have traditionally been run by religious or other humanitarian groups. Earnings have generally been reinvested in the hospital to improve health care. These hospitals have often provided care regardless of a patient's ability to pay.

The number of **for-profit (proprietary) hospitals** has multiplied over the past two decades. Today they constitute over 20 percent of nongovernmental acute-care hospitals. For-profit hospitals, which do not receive tax breaks, are not compelled to operate as a charity and typically provide fewer free services to the community than do nonprofit hospitals. Historically, some for-profit hospitals have quickly transferred indigent (poor) or uninsured patients to public hospitals or to nonprofit hospitals.[7] This practice, known as *patient dumping,* was prohibited by federal law in 1986. Today, all hospital emergency rooms are required to perform a screening medical exam on all patients, regardless of their ability to pay. Patients must be determined to be "medically stable" before they can be transferred to another facility or discharged from the emergency room.

More treatments or services, including surgery, are delivered on an **outpatient (ambulatory) care** basis (care that does not involve an overnight stay) by hospitals, traditional clinics, student health clinics, and nontraditional clinical centers. One type of ambulatory facility that is becoming common is the *surgicenter*—a place where minor, low-risk procedures such as vasectomies, tubal ligations, tissue biopsies, cosmetic surgery, abortions, and minor eye operations are performed. In 1982, nearly 85 percent of all surgeries in the United States involved an overnight hospital stay; in 2000, fewer than 30 percent of surgeries did so.

To reduce the distance patients have to travel, many hospitals locate satellite clinics in cities' outlying areas, sometimes in large shopping centers. A few hospitals have designated their satellites as freestanding emergency centers, or surgicenters, that function like hospital emergency rooms for uncomplicated immediate-care cases but have lower operating costs. Some consumers refer to these as "doc-in-the-box" centers.

Many hospitals and group practices have freestanding imaging and diagnostic laboratory centers affiliated with them through either direct ownership or other profit-sharing arrangements. Significant debate surrounds this practice. Critics argue that when doctors own the diagnostic and laboratory services to which they refer patients, they may order an excessive number of tests. Today, such practices amount to "conflict of interest situations" and are largely prohibited by anti-kickback legislation.

Most health clinics were once located within hospitals. Today they are more likely to be independent facilities run by medical practitioners. Other health clinics are run by county health departments; these offer low-cost diagnosis and treatment for financially needy patients. Additionally, some 1,500 college campuses have student health centers that, along with county, city, or community clinics, supply low-cost family planning, tests and services related to sexually transmitted infection, gynecological services, and vaccination services.

Consumers who consider using a hospital or clinic should scrutinize the facility's accreditation. Accredited hospitals have met rigorous standards set by the Joint Commission on the Accreditation of Healthcare Organizations (JCAHO). If you choose an institution having this form of accreditation, you have a high likelihood of obtaining quality care.

With the growth of managed care organizations, concerns have arisen about the quality of care offered under this type of payment system. These concerns compelled consumer groups and public health organizations to require managed care insurers to compile quality care "report cards," known as HEDIS Reports (Health Employer Data Information Set), so that health outcomes could be compared across different plans. The quality measures include preventive services (childhood immunizations, Pap smears, mammograms), disease indicators (eye exams and glucose control tests for diabetics), and screening exams (routine physical exams, including gynecological exams).

Consumers can obtain additional information regarding the provider's malpractice insurance or sanctions from state licensure boards and the National Practitioner Data Bank, on request. Report concerns about billing-related fraud or abuse directly to the Health Care Finance Administration (HCFA).

Nonprofit (voluntary) hospitals   Hospitals run by religious or other humanitarian groups that reinvest their earnings in the hospital to improve health care.

For-profit (proprietary) hospitals   Hospitals that provide a return on earnings to the investors who own them.

Outpatient (ambulatory) care   Treatment that does not involve an overnight stay in a hospital.

Issues Facing Today's Health Care System

Many Americans believe that our health care system needs fundamental reform. What are the problems that have brought us to this point? Cost, access, malpractice, restriction in choice of provider and treatment modality, unnecessary procedures, complicated and cumbersome insurance rules, and dramatic ranges in quality are among the issues of concern. One of the most frequently voiced criticisms concerns lack of access to adequate health insurance, as many Americans have had increasing difficulty obtaining comprehensive coverage from their employers. Until recently, insurance benefits were often lost when employees changed jobs, causing many to remain in undesirable positions in order to avoid losing health benefits. This phenomenon, known as *job lock,* led the federal government to pass legislation mandating the "portability" of health insurance benefits from one job to the next, thereby guaranteeing coverage during the transition.

Over 80 million people in the United States suffer from chronic health conditions that should be at least monitored by medical practitioners. Their access to care is largely determined by whether they have health insurance. Catastrophic or chronic illness among only 10 percent of the population accounts for 70 percent of all health expenditures.[8] Because we cannot perfectly predict who will fall into that 10 percent, every American is potentially vulnerable to the high cost and devastating effects of such illnesses.

Cost

Both per capita and as a percentage of gross domestic product (GDP), we spend more on health care than does any other nation. Yet, unlike the rest of the industrialized world, we do not provide access for our entire population. In 1998, we spent over $1.1 trillion on health care, up nearly 6 percent since 1997.[9] This translates into nearly 15 percent of our GDP, up from 5 percent of the GDP in 1960. Why do health care costs continue to spiral upward? There are many factors involved: excess administrative costs; duplication of services; an aging population; demand for new diagnostic and treatment technologies; an emphasis on crisis-oriented care instead of preventive care; inappropriate utilization of services by consumers; and related factors.

Our system has more than 2,000 health insurance companies, each with different coverage structures and administrative requirements. This lack of uniformity prevents our system from achieving *economies of scale* (bulk purchasing at a reduced cost) and administrative efficiency realized in countries where there is a single-payer delivery system. According to the Health Insurance Association of America (HIAA), commercial insurance companies commonly experience administrative costs greater than 10 percent of the total health care insurance premium, whereas the administrative cost of the government's Medicare program is less than 4 percent. Administrative expenses in the private sector contribute to the high cost of health care and force companies to require employees to share more of the costs, cut back on benefits, and drop some benefits altogether. These costs are largely passed on to consumers in the form of higher prices.

The declining availability of health insurance coverage means more Americans are uninsured or underinsured. These people are unable to access preventive care and seek care only in the event of an emergency or crisis. Because emergency care is extraordinarily expensive, they often are unable to pay, and the cost is absorbed by those who *can* pay—the insured or taxpayers. This process is known as *cost shifting.*

Access

Access to health care is determined by numerous factors, including the supply of providers and facilities, proximity to care, ability to maneuver in the system, health status, and insurance coverage. Although there are approximately 700,000 physicians in the United States, many Americans do not have adequate access to care or other health services because of insurance barriers or maldistribution of providers. There is an oversupply of higher-paid specialists and a shortage of lower-paid primary care physicians (family practitioners, pediatricians, internists, OB/GYNs, geriatricians, and gerontologists). Inner cities and some rural areas face constant shortages of physicians and supporting health professionals.

Managed-care health plans determine access on the basis of participating providers, health plan benefits, and administrative rules. Often this means that consumers do not have the freedom to choose specialists, facilities, or treatment options beyond those contracted with the health plan and recommended by their primary care provider (also known as *gatekeeper*). In the United States, consumer demand has led to an expansion of benefits to include nonallopathic therapies, such as chiropractic and acupuncture (see Chapter 18). However, many nonallopathic treatments remain unavailable, even to a limited degree, through available health plans.

Quality and Malpractice

Patient injuries that result from preventable medical errors have received increasing attention in recent years. A recent Institute of Medicine report indicated that more than one in

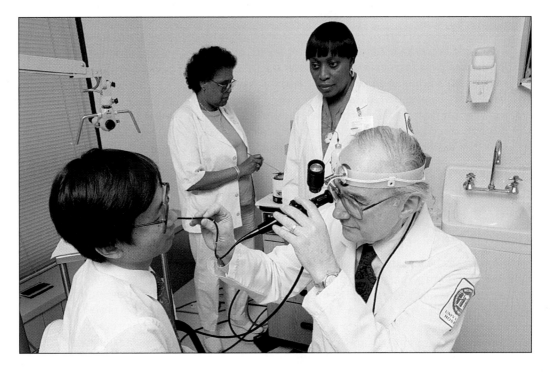

People who rely largely on student health centers, clinics, and hospital emergency rooms for treatment miss out on the benefits of continuity of care offered by a primary care physician.

six hospitalized patients suffered medical injuries that prolonged their hospital stays. Large numbers of deaths were also directly attributable to mistakes in medical practice.[10] The total annual costs associated with injuries resulting from medical error are estimated to be in excess of $200 billion, the equivalent of nearly one out of every five dollars spend on health care in America. However, this estimate does not account for the costs of death and permanent disability.[11] The elderly are at greatest risk when it comes to malpractice; in fact, they experience medical injury at a rate that is believed to be two to four times greater than other age groups.[12] How great is our concern over this issue?

A 1997 national survey indicated that Americans believe our health care system is only moderately safe—safer than nuclear power and food handling, but less safe than airplane travel and the workplace. Forty-two percent of those surveyed said that they had been involved, either personally or through a friend or relative, in a situation where a medical mistake was made.[13] Since the 2001 Institute of Medicine Report brought injury and death rates into the national limelight, Americans have become even more concerned about a health care system that is costly, mistake-prone, and inaccessible to many Americans.

The U.S. health care system employs several mechanisms for ensuring quality services: education, licensure, certification/registration, accreditation, peer review, and, as a last resort, the legal system of malpractice litigation. Some of these mechanisms are mandatory before a professional or organization may provide care, whereas others are purely voluntary. (Be aware that licensure, although mandated for some practitioners and facilities by the state in which they reside, is only a minimum guarantee of quality.) Insurance

companies and government payers may require a higher level of quality by linking payment to whether a practitioner is board certified or a facility is accredited by the appropriate agency. In addition, most insurance plans now require prior authorization and/or second opinions not only to reduce costs but also to improve quality of care.

Many people believe that malpractice is a leading cause of our health care crisis. Although the U.S. Department of Health and Human Services estimates that the total cost of malpractice is less than 1 percent of total health outlays, these figures do not account for the previously described practice of *defensive medicine*. In addition, they do not account for the costs of inappropriately prescribed medications (which, research indicates, are given to up to one in five elderly persons)[14] or for the costs of medical mistakes that result in increasing numbers of deaths each year. A recent Institution of Medicine report indicates that as many as 44,000 to 98,000 people die in U.S. hospitals each year as a result of medical errors—more than the number who die from motor vehicle accidents, breast cancer, or AIDS![15] Defensive medicine not only costs money and places patients at additional risk, but also has changed the standards of care, in that people expect these extra, but unnecessary, tests and procedures.

What do you think?

*Do you believe prospective patients should have access to information about practitioners' and facilities' malpractice records? * How about their success and failure rates or outcomes of various procedures?*

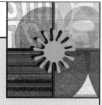

"Actionable" Medical Malpractice: What Is It, and When Should You Consider It?

Actionable medical malpractice or medical negligence occurs when a physician fails to properly treat a medical condition and the negligent act or omission causes a new or aggravated injury to the patient. Obviously, the physician cannot be responsible for the original underlying medical condition. The negligence in medical malpractice cases can occur in a variety of situations including, but not limited to, the following:

✓ A delay or failure in diagnosing a disease

✓ A surgical or anesthesia-related mishap during an operative procedure

✓ Failure to gain the informed consent of the patient for an operation or surgical procedure

✓ Failing to properly treat the disease process after making the correct diagnosis

✓ Misuse of prescription drugs or a medical device or implant

Typically, patients must secure an attorney who is well versed in medical law and who can quickly determine whether there is an actionable case. Usually a medical expert who is well qualified to give medical opinion and is board certified in the relevant field of medicine is also necessary. The attorney agrees up front to advance costs, to be repaid in the event the case is won, with a percentage of the gross recovery as the established fee for service. Medical malpractice lawsuits are costly, are complex, and may take years to win. Careful record-keeping of procedures and actions is an important part of the entire case. Having a health advocate who has witnessed the events is also another key element in determining future litigation success.

Source: "Actionable Medical Malpractice: Civil Rights and the Law," January 2002. *Http://www.civilrights.com/medical.html*

Third-Party Payers

The fundamental principle of insurance underwriting is that the cost of health care can be predicted for large populations. This is how health care premiums (payments) are determined. Policyholders pay premiums into a pool, which fills as reserves until needed. When you are sick or injured, the insurance company pays out of the pool, regardless of your total amount of contribution. Depending on circumstances, you may never pay for what your medical care costs, or you may pay much more for insurance than your medical bills ever total. The idea is that you pay in affordable premiums so that you never have to face catastrophic bills. In today's profit-oriented system, insurers prefer to have healthy people in their plans who pour money into risk pools without taking money out.

Unfortunately, not everyone has health insurance. Almost 40 million Americans are uninsured at any given point in time—that is, they have no private health insurance and are not eligible for Medicare, Medicaid, or other health programs. The number of the uninsured has been growing since the late 1970s. Lack of health insurance has been associated with delayed health care and increased mortality. *Underinsurance* (i.e., the inability to pay out-of-pocket expenses despite having insurance) also may result in adverse health consequences. Findings from the CDC's latest Behavior Risk Factor Surveillance System (BRFSS) indicate that a large proportion of all adults are either uninsured or underinsured. People lacking any type of health insurance make up nearly 17 percent of the nonelderly population, or 16.8 percent of the total population.[16] Another 20 to 40 million Americans are estimated to be underinsured (at risk for spending more than 10 percent of their income on medical care because their insurance is inadequate).[17]

Contrary to the common belief that the uninsured are unemployed, 75 percent of them are either workers or the dependents of workers. Twenty-five percent are children under age 16. College students are one of the largest groups of the uninsured who are not in the labor force. Large numbers of college students, either uninsured or underinsured and in a crisis, must come up with major out-of-pocket funds for treatment. This presents a difficult dilemma for both universities and students when they must seek care because most university insurance plans are designed as short-term, noncatastrophic plans having low upper limits of benefits. As a full-time student, you should consider purchasing a higher level catastrophic plan to protect yourself in the event of a rare, but very costly, illness or accident.

Early Private Health Insurance

Our current health system began in the past century, and its growth accelerated in the post–World War II era to its current massive, complex web. Hospitals became the engines of medicine during the middle of the twentieth century. Doctors became the drivers or conductors of this rapidly moving system. The system was fueled by a variety of funding sources but, chiefly, first by the growth of tax-exempt nonprofit private insurance companies established in the 1940s and later by the growth of for-profit insurance companies.

Health insurance originally consisted solely of coverage for hospital costs (it was called *major medical*), but gradually coverage was extended to routine physicians' treatment and to other areas such as dental services and pharmaceuticals. Payment mechanisms used until recently laid the groundwork for today's steadily rising health care costs. Hospitals were reimbursed on a cost-plus basis after services were rendered; that is, they billed for the costs of providing care plus an amount for profit. This system provided no incentive to contain costs, limit the number of procedures, or curtail capital investment in redundant equipment and facilities. Physicians were reimbursed on a fee-for-service (indemnity) basis determined by "usual, customary, and reasonable" fees. This system encouraged physicians to charge high fees, raise them often, and perform as many procedures as possible. At the same time, because most insurance did not cover routine or preventive services, consumers were encouraged to use hospitals whenever possible (the coverage was better) and to wait until illness developed to seek care instead of seeking preventive care. Consumers were also free to choose any provider or service they wished, including even inappropriate—and often very expensive—levels of care.

Private insurance companies have increasingly employed several mechanisms to control costs. These mechanisms include deductibles, copayments, coinsurance, exclusions, "preexisting condition" clauses, waiting periods, and upper limits on payments. *Deductibles* are front-end payments (commonly $250 to $1,000) that you must make to your provider before your insurance company will start paying for any services you use. *Copayments* are set amounts that you pay per service received, regardless of the cost of the services (e.g., $5 per doctor visit or $10 per prescription). *Coinsurance* is the percentage of the bill that you must pay throughout the course of treatment (e.g., 20 percent of whatever the total is). *Preexisting condition clauses* limit the insurance company's liability for medical conditions that a consumer had before obtaining coverage (i.e., if a woman takes out coverage while she is pregnant, the insurance company may cover pregnancy complications and infant care but

not charges related to "normal pregnancy"). Because many insurance companies use a combination of these mechanisms, keeping track of the costs you are responsible for can become very difficult.

Group plans of large employers (government agencies, school districts, and corporations, for example) generally do not have preexisting condition clauses in their plans. But smaller group plans (a group may be as small as two) often do. Some plans never cover services for preexisting conditions, whereas others specify a *waiting period* (such as six months) before they will provide coverage. All insurers set some limits on the types of services they will cover (e.g., most exclude cosmetic surgery, private rooms, and experimental procedures). Some insurance plans may also include an *upper* or *lifetime limit,* after which coverage will end. Although $250,000 may seem like an enormous sum, medical bills for a sick child or chronic disease can easily run this high within a few years.

Medicare and Medicaid (Social Insurance versus Welfare)

After years of debate about whether we should have a national health program like those of most industrialized countries, the U.S. government directed the system toward a mixed private and public approach in the 1960s. Most Americans obtained their health insurance through their employers. But this left out two groups—the nonworking poor and the aged. In 1965, amendments to the 1935 Social Security Act established Medicare and Medicaid. Although enacted simultaneously, these programs were vastly different.

Medicare is basically a federal social insurance covering 99 percent of the elderly over 65 years of age, all totally and permanently disabled people (after a waiting period), and all people with end-stage renal failure. Medicare is a universal program that covers a broad range of services except long-term care and pharmaceuticals. It currently covers 36 million people. Medicare is widely accepted by physicians and hospitals and has relatively low administrative costs.

In contrast, **Medicaid,** which covers approximately 35 million people, is a federal–state matching funds welfare program for people who are defined as poor. Because each state determines income eligibility levels and payments to providers, there are vast differences in the way Medicaid operates from state to state.

To control hospital costs, in 1983 the federal government set up a prospective payment system based on **diagnosis related groups (DRGs)** for Medicare. Using a complicated formula, nearly 500 groupings of diagnoses were created to establish how much a hospital would be reimbursed for a particular patient. If a hospital can treat the patient for less than that amount, it can keep the difference. However, if a patient's care costs more than the set amount, the hospital must absorb the difference (with a few exceptions that must be reviewed by a panel). This system gives hospitals the incentive to discharge patients quickly after doing as little as

---

Medicare   Federal health insurance program for the elderly and the permanently disabled.

Medicaid   Federal–state health insurance program for the poor.

Diagnosis related groups (DRGs)   Diagnostic categories established by the federal government to determine in advance how much hospitals will be reimbursed for the care of a particular Medicare patient.

---

possible for them, provide more ambulatory care, and admit only patients with favorable (profitable) DRGs.

In its continued efforts to control rising costs, HCFA has encouraged the growth of prepaid health maintenance organization (HMO) senior plans for Medicare-eligible persons. Under this system, commercial managed care insurance plans receive a fixed per-capita premium from HCFA and then offer more preventive services with lower out-of-pocket copayments. These managed care plans encourage providers and patients to utilize health care resources under administrative rules similar to commercial HMO plans. Similarly, states have encouraged the growth of managed Medicaid programs.

Managed Care

Managed care describes a health care delivery system consisting of the following elements:

1. A budget based on an estimate of the annual cost of delivering health care for a given population
2. A network of physicians, hospitals, and other providers and facilities linked contractually to deliver comprehensive health benefits within that predetermined budget, sharing economic risk for any budget deficit or surplus
3. An established set of administrative rules requiring patients to follow the advice of participating health care providers in order to have their health care paid for under the terms of the health plan

Many such plans pay their contracted health care providers through **capitation,** that is, prepayment of a fixed monthly amount for each patient without regard of the type or number of health services provided. Some plans pay health care providers' salaries, and some are still fee-for-service plans. As with other insurance plans, enrollees are members of a risk pool, and it is expected that some persons will use no services, some will use a modest amount of services, and others will have high-cost utilization over a given year. Doctors have the incentive to keep their patient pool healthy and avoid catastrophic ailments that are preventable; usually such incentives come back in terms of increased salaries, bonuses, and other benefits. As such, prevention and health education to reduce risk and intervene early to avoid major problems should be capstone components of such plans.

Today, managed care plans are sweeping the nation, with over 60 million Americans enrolled in one type of plan, the health maintenance organization, and another 90 million in other forms of managed care. Four million beneficiaries are in Medicare HMOs, with enrollment growing by about 80,000 people a month.[18] Types of managed care plans include HMO plans, point of service (POS) plans, and preferred provider organization (PPO) plans.

Health Maintenance Organizations (HMOs)   HMOs provide a wide range of covered health benefits, such as check-

ups, surgery, doctor visits, and lab tests, for a fixed amount prepaid by you, the employer, Medicaid, or Medicare.[19] Usually, HMO premiums are the least expensive (saving between 10 and 40 percent more than other plans), but HMOs are the most restrictive type of managed care. There are low or no deductibles or coinsurance payments, and copayments are $5 to $10 per office visit. HMOs contract with providers to supply health services for enrollees through various systems,[20] such as following:

- *The staff model.* You receive care from salaried staff doctors at the HMO's facility.
- *The group network model.* The HMO contracts with one or several groups of doctors who provide care for a fixed amount per plan member. Groups often practice in one facility.
- *The independent practice association (IPA).* Doctors in private practice form an association that contracts with HMOs. The physicians generally work in their own offices.

The downside of these plans is that patients are typically required to use the plan's doctors and hospitals and to get approval from a "gatekeeper" or primary care physician for treatment and referrals. Although more and more people are opting for HMOs, some people continue to be skeptical about them, leveling questions such as these:

- Do highly paid administrators and stockholders ration care, allocating more care to those who are better able to pay and have better health ?
- Does the huge administrative structure imposed by the HMO make it virtually impossible for patients to sue in the event of clear violations?
- Are patients denied costly diagnostic tests because such tests cut into bottom-line profits? Are some tests given too late because of concerns over costs?
- Are HMOs really focused on prevention or intervention? Evidence exists that the fee structure of many HMOs actually discourages basic preventive services, such as immunizations.
- Are doctors allowed to treat patients using their best judgment and skills, or do policies and profit-motivated concerns interfere with the doctors' roles as advocates for their patients?
- Are the obstacles imposed by HMOs too daunting for patients in need of urgent care?
- Do HMO cost-saving policies force patients out of hospitals and treatment centers too early?

Managed care   Cost-control procedures used by health insurers to coordinate treatment.

Capitation   Prepayment of a fixed monthly amount without regard to the type or number of services provided.

Point of Service (POS)   Point of Service (POS) plans often provide a more acceptable form of managed care for those used to the traditional indemnity plan of insurance. This is probably why POS is among the fastest growing of the managed care plans. Under POS, patients can go to providers outside of their HMO for care but must pay for the extra cost. Usually this is a reasonable alternative for middle-class or wealthy Americans who are willing to pay the extra cost for choices in care.[21]

Preferred Provider Organizations (PPOs)   PPOs are networks of independent doctors and hospitals that contract to provide care at discounted rates. Although they offer greater choices in doctors than HMOs do, they are less likely to coordinate a patient's care. In addition, although members have a choice of seeing doctors who are not on the preferred list, this choice may come at considerable cost (such as having to pay 30 percent of the charges out of pocket, rather than 10 to 20 percent for PPO doctors and services).[22]

What do you think?

Why is it important that private insurance cover preventive or lower-level care as well as hospitalization and high-technology interventions? ✷ What kinds of incentives would cause you to seek early care rather than to delay care?

Taking Charge   17   17   17

Managing Your Health Care Needs

Throughout this text, we have emphasized behaviors important to staying healthy. How can you promote your health when seeking medical attention? Many people wait until a problem arises to seek medical care, and they either take the first available physician or go to the nearest medical facility. This is not always the best choice. When you have a medical problem (even a minor one), you need to decide how best to treat it. Do your research. Be aware of your options. Then you will be able to make informed decisions that will lead to better health care.

Some health care decisions are dictated by physicians, insurance companies, and government agencies, but many decisions still rest with you. Are you a good health consumer? Start by learning about your own insurance protection. What coverage do you currently have? If you don't have coverage, how would you pay for a medical emergency? What coverage is available to you as a student? Learn how your insurance plan works and what it does and does not cover. Can you choose your physicians and hospitals? Remember that you have rights as a patient and a consumer. Don't be afraid to ask questions. Consider the following issues.

Checklist for Change

Assessing Personal Choices

✓ Do you feel comfortable discussing your problems with your health care provider?

✓ Are you confident that your doctor knows what he or she is talking about?

✓ Is the doctor willing to talk about issues such as credentials, hospital affiliations, qualifications of referrals for special problems, and fees?

✓ Are you able to understand answers to your questions? Does the doctor seem interested in whether you understand? Is he or she willing to answer questions?

✓ Does the physician tell you why one test is being given rather than another? About risks of the test? About preparation for the tests? About what to expect concerning certain results?

✓ Is the physician willing to refer you to a nongroup specialist in a location of your choice?

✓ Does the doctor support your obtaining a second opinion, or does he or she seem irritated by the request?

Assessing Community Choices

✓ How long has your doctor been in your community?

✓ How many hospitals are within a 30-minute drive from your home? Are any of them teaching hospitals?

✓ What percentage of people in your community don't have health insurance?

Taking Charge

17   **17**   **17**

✓ What services are available in your community to help people who are underinsured or uninsured?

✓ What are the policies of local hospitals concerning the treatment of uninsured individuals who need care?

✓ Have you written to your congressional leaders concerning your views about health care legislation?

Summary

* Advertisers of health care products and services use sophisticated tactics to attract attention and get business. Advertising claims sometimes appear to be supported by spontaneous remission (symptoms disappearing without any apparent cause) or the placebo effect (symptoms disappearing because you think they should), rather than the efficacy of the product or service.

* Self-care and individual responsibility are key factors in reducing rising health care costs and improving health status. Advance planning can help a person navigate health care treatment in unfamiliar situations or emergencies. Assess health professionals by considering their qualifications, their record of treating problems like yours, and their ability to work with you.

* In theory, allopathic ("traditional") medicine is based on scientifically validated methods and procedures. Medical doctors, specialists of various kinds, nurses, physician as-

sistants, and other health professionals practice allopathic medicine.

* Health care providers may provide services as solo practitioners or in group practices (which share overhead cost). Hospitals and clinics are classified by profit status, ownership, specialty, and teaching status.

* Concerns about the U.S. health care system include cost, access, choice of treatment modality, quality and malpractice, and fraud and abuse.

* Health insurance is based on the concept of spreading risk. Insurance is provided by private insurance companies (who charge premiums) and the government Medicare and Medicaid programs (funded by taxes). Managed care (in the form of HMOs and PPOs) attempts to keep costs lower by streamlining administrative procedures and stressing preventive care (among other initiatives).

Discussion Questions

1. What claims do marketers use to get people to try their health-related products? Why are consumers susceptible to such ploys? What could be done to increase the accuracy of messages related to health care?

2. List several conditions (resulting from illness or accident) for which you don't need to seek medical help. When would you consider each condition to be bad enough to require medical attention? How would you decide to whom and where to go for treatment?

3. What are the pros and cons of group practices? Of non-profit and for-profit hospitals? If you had health insurance,

where do you believe you would get the best care? On what do you base your choice?

4. What are the inherent benefits and risks of managed care organizations?

5. Explain the differences between traditional indemnity insurance and managed health care. Which would you feel more comfortable with? Should insurance companies dictate rates for various medical tests and procedures in an attempt to keep prices down?

Application Exercise

Reread the What Do You Think? scenario at the beginning of the chapter, and answer the following questions.

1. What are the advantages of being able to choose your own health care treatment? Are there any disadvantages?

2. What, if any, alternatives are available to Leon? What would you advise him to do?

Accessing Your Health on the Internet `http`

Visit the following Internet sites to explore further topics and issues related to personal health. To visit an organization's website, go to the Companion Website for *Health: The Basics, Fifth Edition* at www.aw.com/donatelle, click on the book image, and select "Accessing Your Health on the Internet" from the navigation menu on the left.

1. ***National Committee for Quality Assurance.*** The NCQA assesses and reports on the quality of managed care plans, including health maintenance organizations.
2. ***Agency for Health Care Research and Quality (AHRQ).*** A gateway to consumer health information, providing links to sites that can address health care concerns and provide information on what questions to ask, what to look for, and what you should know when making critical decisions about personal care.
3. ***Food and Drug Administration (FDA).*** News on the latest government-approved generic drugs and investigations.
4. ***Health Touch.*** Search for prescription and over-the-counter drug uses and side effects, plus other health-related resources.
5. ***National Library of Medicine—General Information Center for Health-Related Research.*** Supports Medline/Pubmed information retrieval systems in addition to providing public health information for consumers.

Further Reading

Anders, G. *Health Against Wealth: HMOs and the Breakdown of Medical Trust.* Boston: Houghton Mifflin, 1997. *A series of cases that outlines some of the severe problems of managed care.*

Geyman, John. *Health Care In America: Can an Ailing System Be Healed?* 2001. Butterworth-Heinemann. ISBN 0750673222

Rowell, J., and M. Green, *Understanding Health Insurance: A Guide to Betting,* 2002. Delmar Publishers. ISBN 0766832066

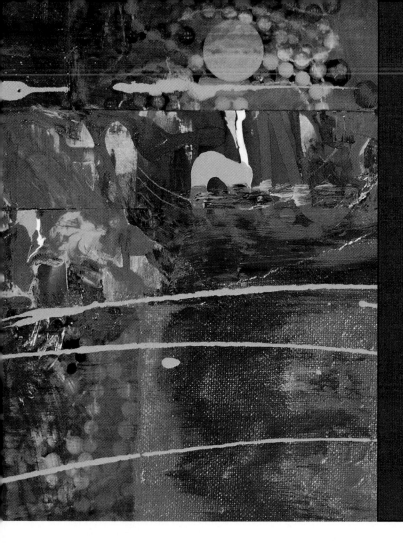

18

Complementary and Alternative Medicine

NEW CHOICES AND RESPONSIBILITIES FOR HEALTHWISE CONSUMERS

objectives

* Describe what complementary and alternative medicine (CAM) is, and identify its typical domains. Explain why it is growing in popularity in the United States and throughout the world, and who is most likely to use it.

* Describe the major types of complementary and alternative medicine providers, and list the common forms of treatment they offer.

* Discuss the various types of complementary and alternative medicines being used in America today, their patterns of use, and their potential benefits and risks.

* Describe why you must be cautious as you evaluate testimonials and claims

related to complementary and alternative products and services, and what you can do to ensure that you are getting reliable and accurate information and sound treatment.

* Discuss the challenges and opportunities related to complementary and alternative medicine in ensuring our health and wellness.

What do you think?

For over a year, Elena has suffered from chronic knee pain. She has just undergone an MRI scan to determine the source of the problem. She expects a diagnosis of torn cartilage, minor knee surgery, and a speedy recovery. She is surprised when the MRI reveals no structural damage to the knee. Her doctor recommends rest, over-the-counter anti-inflammatory medications, and four weeks of physical therapy. After four weeks, Elena is still in pain. Looking for another strategy, she visits a chiropractor, who tells her that she needs joint manipulation, acupuncture, and pain medication. Her best friend tells her to take chondroitin and glucosamine to rebuild cartilage. A quick check of the Internet yields long lists of herbal medications and exercises to help her knee. Meanwhile, her mother suggests that Elena should be eating functional foods to rebuild tissue. Elena doesn't know *what* to do.

What are Elena's options? ✷ *What are the potential risks and benefits of each option?* ✷ *Where can Elena get the most reliable information?* ✷ *How would you recommend that she proceed?*

Consumers today face an amazing array of choices when they consider taking action to improve their health. One of the newest movements toward self-care and health promotion focuses on *complementary and alternative medicine (CAM)*. Various foods, products, and services offer us a new range of health options and an opportunity for greater control over our own health care.

Complementary and Alternative Medicine (CAM): What Is It, and Who Uses It?

If you think that alternative medicine is just a fad, you are in for a surprise. Today, Americans and people from most other cultures of the world are much more likely to try therapies once considered exotic and strange. This trend is becoming stronger as more people from different regions and cultures of the world come to the United States and introduce others to their culturally based health practices. Many of these cultures have great diversity in their native therapies, having assimilated CAM techniques from the earliest human eras of history. Referred to as **complementary and alternative medicine (CAM),** these therapies are defined as "neither being taught widely in U.S. medical schools nor generally available in U.S. hospitals during the previous year."[1] They vary

widely in terms of nature of treatment, extent of therapy, and types of problems for which they offer help. Typically, CAM therapies are compared with the more traditional, allopathic treatments offered by individuals who graduate from U.S.-accredited schools of medicine or are licensed medical practitioners recognized by the American Medical Association and its governing board.[2] The list of practices that are considered CAM changes continually as CAM therapies that are proven safe and effective become accepted as "mainstream" health care practices.[3] CAM therapies, in general, serve as alternatives to an allopathic system that some people regard as too invasive, too high tech, and too toxic in terms of laboratory-produced medications.

CAM in the United States Today

In 1993, a landmark research study showed that one in three Americans sought some form of alternative care.[4] A follow-up study five years later found that these numbers had jumped to 47 percent, reflecting an unprecedented explosion in use. In fact, the study revealed that in recent years, people were actually more likely to seek out and use some form of alternative care than they were to seek out and use a form of what we've long regarded as traditional medicine. By the late 1990s, total out-of-pocket expenditures for alternative care were conservatively estimated at $27 billion, an amount that is comparable to out-of-pocket expenditures for all U.S. physician services. Additionally, an estimated 15 million Americans took prescription medications concurrently with herbal remedies or high-dose vitamins and supplements, which are not included in these estimates.[5]

Although it is widely assumed that increasing numbers of us are choosing alternative care, we have known little about the nature and extent of CAM use until fairly recently. According to the studies cited above, the following are the most frequently used alternatives to conventional medicine:

Complementary and alternative medicine (CAM)
Forms of treatment distinct from traditional allopathic medicine that until recently were neither taught widely in U.S. medical schools nor generally available in U.S. hospitals.

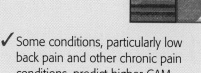
Who Seeks Alternative Medical Treatment?

People who decide to use complementary and alternative medicine tend not to make this decision on a whim. In fact, in many cases, they are more educated than people who rely solely on traditional health care. They are also more likely to be middle-aged and have a middle-class socioeconomic status. A randomized study of several thousand patients seeking care for low back pain, through traditional allopathic providers versus chiropractic providers, found that those opting for chiropractic help were more likely to question their providers about the nature and extent of recommended treatments. People who seek alternative care do so for one of three reasons:

✓ *Dissatisfaction.* Patients may be unhappy with ineffective treatment or treatment that has resulted in adverse effects, may find traditional allopathic medicine too impersonal and technologically oriented, or may find it too costly. Also, it appears that managed care may have pushed some people out of the allopathic system. Many began to distrust it after watching family members experience problems.

✓ *Need for personal control.* Patients view CAM therapies as less authoritarian and more empowering.

✓ *Philosophical congruence.* For some people, CAM is just a better fit. Referred to as *cultural creatives,* these CAM users tend to be committed to the environment; to feminism; to involvement with esoteric forms of spirituality and personal growth psychology, including self-actualization and self-expression; and to exploring anything foreign and exotic. They also identify with cultural change and innovation and are among those most likely to adopt alternative treatments.

Research has also revealed the following:

✓ CAM users didn't have a particularly negative attitude toward traditional medicine.
✓ Racial or ethnic status didn't predict CAM usage.
✓ Men and women were equally likely to use CAM.
✓ Those with poorer health status were more likely to use CAM.

✓ Some conditions, particularly low back pain and other chronic pain conditions, predict higher CAM usage.
✓ Those who had gone through a transformational experience that had changed their world view were more likely to use CAM.

Sources: J. Astin, "Why Patients Use Alternative Medicine: Results of a National Study," *Journal of the American Medical Association* 279 (1998): 1548–1552; D. Eisenberg, et al., "Trends in Alternative Medicine Use in the United States, 1990–1997: Results of a Follow-up National Study," *Journal of the American Medical Association* 280 (1998): 1569–1579; R. Donatelle, J. Nyiendo, and M. Haas, "Health Care Decision-Making Among Those Seeking Care for Low Back Pain from Traditional Medical and Chiropractic Physicians," paper presented at the American Public Health Association's annual meeting, 1998; R. H. Ray, "The Emerging Culture," *American Demographics* (1997) (see http://www.demographics.com).

- Relaxation techniques (16.9 percent of respondents)
- Chiropractic (31 percent)
- Massage (18 percent)
- Self-help (13 percent)
- Energy healing (6 percent)
- Other therapies (16 percent)

Major Domains of CAM

Today, the United States government not only has sanctioned the concept of CAM in prevention and treatment, but also has moved aggressively to create the Center for Complementary and Alternative Medicine (NCCAM) within the National Institutes of Health. This center serves as a form of clearinghouse for CAM information and a focal point for research initiatives, policy development, and general recommendations

for CAM use. NCCAM broadly groups CAM practices into five major domains: (1) alternative medical systems, (2) manipulative and body-based methods, (3) energy therapies, (4) mind–body interventions, and (5) biologically based treatments. Many of these alternatives are discussed in other parts of this book, but it would be impossible to do justice to all of them. As such, we focus on alternatives that have been the subject of increasing use and interest in recent years or that might be of particular interest to young adults.

Alternative Medical Systems

Alternative medical systems involve complete systems of theory and practice that have evolved independently of, and often prior to, the conventional biomedical approach that we tend to think of as a traditional health care system. In the

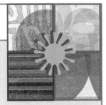

Consumer Fears Grow about Medical Treatment

Just when you thought you were in the capable hands of a hand-picked allopathic physician, you probably experienced a tinge of anxiety in November 1999, when the Institute of Medicine proclaimed to the world that if we were to count them, the numbers of deadly medical mistakes in the United States would surpass death rates for breast cancer, traffic accidents, and AIDS. By these calculations, medical error would come in as the eighth leading cause of death for Americans. In fact, the report indicated that "medical mistakes are a stunningly huge problem, causing between 44,000 and 98,000 deaths among hospital patients each year."

After making most of us more than a little concerned, the report went on to say that although "to err is human," patients who exercise their rights as consumers will have much better outcomes when nature necessitates a visit to the doctor. The report also recommended major changes in the national health care system that will set a minimum goal of a 50 percent reduction in medical mistakes within five years. This announcement prompted President Clinton to appoint a special task force to develop standards to help protect consumers from mistreatment. Congress has also passed legislation ordering the Agency for Health Care Policy and Research (AHCPR) to seek out strategies designed to reduce patient risk.

According to William Richardson, president of the W. K. Kellogg Foundation, and co-author of the Institute of Medicine report, "Errors can be prevented by designing systems that make it hard for people to do the wrong thing and easy for people to do the right thing." These "people" refer to both consumers and to the health care professionals charged with their care. As such, the Institute of Medicine report recommends the following actions:

- The establishment of a well-funded Federal Center for Patient Safety—$35 million to start and $100 million a year for research. (This represents just a fraction of the $8.8 billion spent per year as a result of medical mistakes.)
- Setting requirements that hospitals and eventually other health organizations report all serious mistakes to state agencies, so that experts can detect patterns of problems and take action. Currently, 20 states require error reporting, but the penalties levied vary greatly. In addition, little is being done to avoid cover-ups of potentially costly malpractice claims.
- The establishment of state licensing boards and medical accreditors who periodically reexamine health practitioners for competence, stressing safety practices. Standardized medical equipment and treatment guidelines can help doctors keep up with currently advised protocols.
- Change the "culture of secrecy" that surrounds medical mistakes, encouraging doctors to discuss errors as well as near-misses, so that problems can be fixed.

Other areas in need of improvement include the following:

- Reducing errors caused by the poor handwriting of doctors. Errors in dispensing drugs can be reduced significantly if doctors take the time to write legibly or use computerized labeling systems to write for them.
- Better training in new technology. Often, even superb doctors fumble to figure out how a machine works after attending short seminars taught by equipment specialists or sales personnel.
- Regular testing for retention of licenses. Is a physician practicing with knowledge and expertise learned 10 to 20 years ago? Is training needed to learn about today's technologically advanced techniques?
- Monitoring doctors' records across state lines. Today, changes in residence have been difficult to monitor. As a result, malpracticing physicians often can find lucrative employment in another state, without repercussions.

As a consumer, there are many things that you can do to protect yourself:

- *Know what is wrong with you.* Ask questions of and seek second opinions from physicians outside the health group that you routinely visit.
- *Learn about medications you are taking.* Review the contraindications and possible side effects listed in a current *Physician's Desk Reference (PDR).* Ask doctors why a certain drug has been prescribed and whether alternatives with fewer side effects exist.
- *Monitor all changes in your body while you are taking a prescription drug.* Moreover, monitor your body *prior to* going to the doctor, so that you can be as precise as possible when discussing what is wrong with you.
- *Know what lab tests are being requested, why they are being requested, and what possible alternatives exist.* Ask about the costs of the test and whether this is the best test possible. Know the risk of all tests and procedures. When you get lab results, ask that they be explained in detail.
- *Have a patient advocate with you at all times.* If you don't have one, hire one. When things are not going well, they must be assertive enough to force action by health care providers, either by bringing in another specialist, by making changes in medications and procedures, or through other actions.

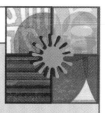

They should be willing to question the nurses and doctors about medications, and receive information about your vital signs and any problems while you are unconscious or unable to act for yourself.

- *Broaden your perspective.* Many alternatives are available today, both in terms of practitioners and medications. Don't be afraid to branch out and seek options from others, particularly those options that are less invasive and less

harmful. Read widely, seek different opinions, and question apparent successes. In short, be a responsible and active participant in your health care—seeking behaviors.

United States, the term *traditional* or *allopathic* has historically referred to a system that is directed by the American Medical Association guidelines for licensing and that most insurance plans cover as fairly standard and acceptable procedure. In contrast, *nonallopathic* medicine has been dubbed as "alternative." This situation is changing. In the past decade, some specialists in nonallopathic medicine have been accepted by professional groups, and their inclusion in mainstream medicine is growing daily. Many traditional medical schools are now offering coursework in CAM, and many traditional doctors refer patients to alternative providers, who are in turn reimbursed by the patients' health insurance plans. Modalities that have received the greatest degree of acceptance include chiropractic medicine, acupuncture, herbal and homeopathic medicine, and naturopathy. However, it is important to realize that there are many "other" *traditional* systems of medicine that have been practiced by various cultures throughout the world. Many come from several venerable Asian approaches.[6]

Traditional Oriental Medicine and Ayurveda

Two major systems that are at the root of much of our CAM thinking today are the Traditional Oriental medicine (TOM) system, and the Ayurvedic system, which is India's traditional system of medicine. **Traditional oriental medicine (TOM)** emphasizes the proper balance or disturbances of **qi** (pronounced "chi"), or vital energy in health and disease, respectively.[7] In TOM, diagnosis is based on history, on observation of the body (especially the tongue), on palpation, and on pulse diagnosis, an elaborate procedure requiring considerable skill and experience by the practitioner. Techniques such as acupuncture, herbal medicine, oriental massage, and *qi gong* (a form of energy therapy described in more detail later in this chapter) are among the TOM approaches to health and healing.

   Ayurveda (or **Ayurvedic medicine**) relates to the "science of life," which places equal emphasis on body, mind, and spirit and strives to restore the innate harmony of the individual. Ayurvedic practitioners diagnose mostly by observation and touch and assign patients to one of three major

body types and to a variety of subtypes. Once classified, patients are treated mostly through dietary modifications and herbal remedies that have been drawn from the vast botanical wealth of the Indian subcontinent. Treatments may also include animal and mineral ingredients, even powdered gemstones. Massage, steam baths, exposure to sunlight, and controlled breathing are among some of the more common forms of Ayurvedic treatments.[8]

Homeopathy and Naturopathy

Other alternative systems of medicine include **homeopathy** and **naturopathy**. *Homeopathic medicine* is an unconventional Western system that is based on the principle that "like cures like." According to this principle, the same substance that in large doses produces the symptoms of an illness will in very small doses cure the illness.[9] Essentially, homeopathic physicians use herbal medicine, minerals, and chemicals in extremely diluted forms as natural agents to kill or ward off illnesses that are caused by more potent forms or doses of the agents.

Traditional oriental medicine (TOM)   Comprehensive system of diagnosis and treatment in which dietary change, touch, massage, medicinal teas, and other herbal medicines are used extensively.

qi   Element of traditional oriental medicine that refers to the vital energy force that courses through the body. When qi is in balance, health is restored.

Ayurveda (Ayurvedic medicine)   A method of treatment derived largely from ancient India, in which practitioners diagnose by observation and touch and then assign a largely dietary treatment laced with herbal medicines.

Homeopathy   Unconventional western system of medicine based on principle that "like cures like."

Naturopathy   System of medicine that attempts to restore natural processes of body and promote healing through natural means.

Table 18.1
Popular Complementary Treatments

Energy healing	Different therapies are based on the philosophy that humans produce waves of energy that are disrupted during illness.
Food therapy	Treatment is based on the belief that many disorders are based on allergies and toxic synergism among food combinations. Naturopaths test for and treat food allergies and assign special diets designed to produce nutritional balance.
Hypnosis	The treatment of disease by suggestion while the patient is in a hypnotic trance.
Relaxation techniques	The goal is to remove stress and promote healing. Techniques include yoga, meditation, breathing and posture exercises, and visualization.
Megavitamins	Treatment with megavitamins promotes the consumption of large doses of common essential vitamins and minerals to prevent disease and heal illness.
Massage	Massage involves rubbing, stroking, kneading, or lightly pounding the body with the hands or other instruments.
Aromatherapy	Aromatherapists use scented materials to evoke sensations through the smell centers of the body. Treatment focuses on odors regarded as pleasurable.
Iridology	Therapy used to stimulate brain centers in order to promote peace and calmness or enlightenment and awakening.

Naturopathic medicine views disease as a manifestation of an alteration in the processes by which the body naturally heals itself. Disease results from the body's effort to ward off impurities and harmful substances from the environment. Working under this principle, naturopathic physicians emphasize restoring health rather than curing disease. They employ an array of healing practices, including diet and clinical nutrition; homeopathy; acupuncture; herbal medicine; hydrotherapy (the use of water in a range of temperatures and methods of applications); spinal and soft-tissue manipulation; physical therapies involving electric currents, ultrasound, and light therapy; therapeutic counseling; and pharmacology. Three major naturopathic schools in the United States and Canada provide thorough training, conferring the *naturopathic doctor (N.D.)* degree on students who have completed a four-year graduate program that emphasizes humanistically oriented family medicine.

While these systems of medical philosophy and patterns of treatment have exerted great influences on populations worldwide, other, more regionally limited, traditional medical systems are also noteworthy. Native American, Aboriginal, African, Middle Eastern, Tibetan, and South American cultures also have their own, unique alternative systems. International surveys of CAM outside the United States suggest that alternative therapies are popular throughout most of the world. Public opinion polls and consumer surveys in Europe and the United Kingdom suggest high CAM use in Italy, France, Denmark, Finland, and Australia, in addition to most Asian cultures.[10]

As the number of alternative therapists grow and as systems become intertwined, so do the number of health care options available to consumers. (See Table 18.1 for ex-

amples of some of them.) Before considering the practices of any medical system, wise consumers will use the most reliable resources to thoroughly evaluate risks, the scientific basis of claimed benefits, and any contraindications for using the CAM service or product. Avoid practitioners who promote their treatments as a cure-all for every health problem or who seem to promise remedies that have thus far defied the best scientific efforts of mainstream medicine. Asking questions, seeking reputable resources for information, and other strategies used by wise consumers of traditional medical care in the United States (see Chapter 17) should also be applied to CAM.

Manipulative and Body-Based Methods

Another category of CAM includes methods that are based on manipulation and/or movement of the body. For example, chiropractors focus on the relationship between the body's structures (primarily the spine) and function and on how that relationship affects the preservation and restoration of health. Chiropractors use manipulation as a key therapy.[11]

Chiropractic Medicine

Chiropractic medicine has been practiced for over 100 years. A century ago, allopathic medicine and chiropractic medicine were in direct competition.[12] Today, however, many managed care organizations work closely with chiropractors,

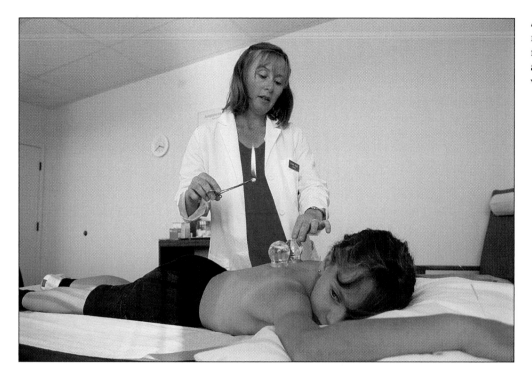

A popular form of Chinese medicine, moxabustion (use of moxa stick) warms certain acupuncture points to treat a variety of conditions.

and many insurance companies will pay for chiropractic treatment, particularly if it is recommended by a medical doctor. More than 20 million Americans now visit chiropractors each year.

Chiropractic medicine is based on the idea that a life-giving energy flows through the spine via the nervous system. If the spine is subluxated (partly misaligned or dislocated), that force is disrupted. Chiropractors use a variety of techniques to manipulate the spine back into proper alignment so that the life-giving energy can flow unimpeded. It has been established that their treatment can be effective for back pain, neck pain, and headaches. The average chiropractic training program requires four years of intensive courses in biochemistry, anatomy, physiology, diagnostics, pathology, nutrition, and related topics, combined with hands-on clinical training. Like allopathic physicians, chiropractors are licensed and regulated by the states in which they practice. You should investigate and question a chiropractor as carefully as you would any licensed medical doctor. As with many health professionals, you may note vast differences in technique among specialists. It is recommended that you choose a chiropractor who follows standard chiropractic regimens for treating musculoskeletal conditions.

Other Manipulation Therapies

There are other specialties that involve manipulation of the body. D.O.'s, or *doctors of osteopathy*, place particular emphasis on the musculoskeletal system. Osteopathic practitioners believe that all of the body's systems work together and that disturbances in one system may have an impact upon function elsewhere in the body.[13] As such, they specialize in body manipulation yet also have a more traditional form of medical school training.

Energy Therapies

Energy therapies focus either on energy fields originating with the body (biofields) or on fields from other sources (electromagnetic fields). Biofield therapies are intended to affect energy fields, whose existence is not experimentally proven, that surround and penetrate the human body. Some forms of energy therapy manipulate biofields by applying pressure and/or manipulating the body by placing the hands in, or through, these fields.[14] Examples include *qi gong, reiki,* and *therapeutic touch*. Qi gong is a component of traditional Chinese medicine that combines movement, meditation, and regulation of breathing to enhance the flow of vital energy (qi), improve blood circulation, and enhance immune function.[15] Reiki, whose name derives from the Japanese word representing "universal life energy," is based on the belief that by channeling spiritual energy through the practitioner, the spirit is healed, and it in turn heals the physical body.[16] Therapeutic touch is derived from the ancient technique of "laying on" of hands and is based on the premise that it is the healing force of the therapist that affects the patient's recovery and that healing is promoted when the body's energies are in balance. By passing the hands over the body, the healers identify body imbalances.[17]

Bioelectromagnetic-based therapies involve the unconventional use of electromagnetic fields, such as pulsed fields, magnetic fields, or alternating current or direct current fields to, for example, treat asthma, cancer, pain, and migraines. The energy field techniques mentioned above have little scientific documentation to support their claims at this point. However, there are two derivatives of energy therapy that have gained much wider acceptance in recent years: acupuncture and acupressure.

Acupuncture

Chinese medical treatments are growing in popularity and offer an important complement to Western biomedical care. Acupuncture, one of the more popular forms of Chinese medicine among Americans, is sought for a wide variety of health conditions, including musculoskeletal dysfunction, mood enhancement, and wellness promotion. Following acupuncture, most respondents report high satisfaction with the treatment, improved quality of life, improvement in or cure of the condition, and reduced reliance on prescription drugs and surgery.[18]

Acupuncturists in the United States are state licensed, and each state has specific requirements regarding training programs. Most acupuncturists have either completed a two-to three-year postgraduate program to obtain a master of traditional Oriental medicine (M.T.O.M.) degree or attended a shorter certification program in the United States or in Asia. They may be licensed in multiple areas—for example, the M.T.O.M. is also trained in the use of herbs and moxabustion

(the application of a heated herbal moxa stick). Some licensed M.D.s and chiropractors have trained in acupuncture and obtained certification to use this treatment.

Acupressure

Acupressure is similar to acupuncture, but it does not use needles. Instead, the practitioner applies pressure to points critical to balancing yin and yang. Practitioners must have the same basic understanding of energy pathways as do acupuncturists. Acupressure should not be applied by an untrained person to pregnant women or to anyone with a chronic condition.

What do you think?

Why do you think more and more people are opting for complementary and alternative treatments? ✳ *What are the potential benefits of these treatments?* ✳ *What are the potential risks?* ✳ *What types of controls are reasonable to regulate the quality and consistency of foreign-trained health care providers?*

Mind–Body Interventions

Mind–body interventions employ a variety of techniques designed to facilitate the mind's capacity to affect bodily function and symptoms.[19] Many therapies might fall under

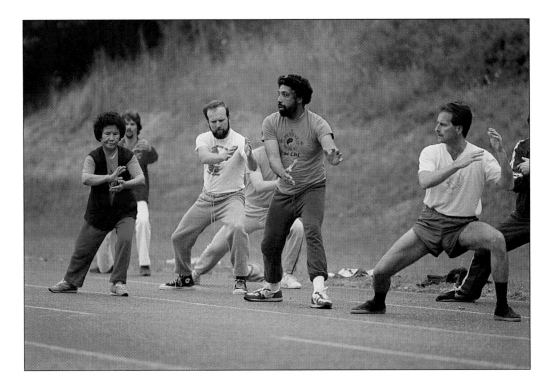

The practice of tai chi can improve balance and overall fitness.

this category, but some areas, such as biofeedback, patient education, and cognitive-behavioral techniques, have been so well investigated that they are no longer considered alternative therapies. However, meditation, yoga, Tai chi, certain uses of hypnosis, dance, music and art therapy, prayer and mental healing, and others are still categorized as complementary and alternative. (See Chapter 11.)

Body Work

Body work actually consists of several different forms of exercise. *Feldenkrais* work is a system of movements, floor exercises, and body work designed to retrain the central nervous system to help it find new pathways around areas of blockage or damage. It is gentle and effective in rehabilitating trauma victims. *Rolfing* is a more invasive form of body work, aimed at restructuring the musculoskeletal system by working on patterns of tension held in deep tissue. The therapist applies firm pressure to different areas of the body. (The pressure may be painful.) Rolfing can release repressed emotions as well as dissipate muscle tension. *Shiatsu* is a traditional healing art from Japan that makes use of firm finger pressure applied to specified points on the body and is intended to increase the circulation of vital energy. The client lies on the floor, with the therapist seated alongside. *Trager work,* one of the least invasive forms of body work, employs gentle rocking and bouncing motions to induce states of deep, pleasant relaxation.[20]

> ### What do you think?
> *Have you ever tried any of these CAM therapies?*
> ✳ *What role do CAM exercises have in your overall quest for physical fitness? Spiritual fitness?* ✳ *Which of these therapies are offered on your campus or in your community?*

Biologically Based Therapies

Biologically based therapy is perhaps one of the most controversial domains of CAM practice, largely because of the sheer numbers of options that are available and the myriad of claims that are made about the magic effects of these products and services. To date, many of these claims have not been thoroughly investigated, and regulation of this aspect of CAM has been relatively slow in coming. **Biologically based therapies** include natural and biologically based practices, interventions, and products, many of which overlap with conventional medicine's use of dietary supplements. Included are *herbal, special dietary, orthomolecular,* and *individual* biological therapies.

Herbs and plants have been part of medical practice for thousands of years. Poppy extract was used to quiet crying children in the time of the pharaohs, thousands of

years before the medical use of opiates. *Ephedra,* the main ingredient of some over-the-counter asthma treatments, has relieved breathing problems in China for 5,000 years. Even today, an estimated 25 percent of all modern pharmaceutical drugs are derived from herbs, including aspirin (white willow bark), the heart medication digitalis (foxglove), and the cancer treatment taxol (Pacific yew tree). Practitioners who base their therapies primarily on the medicinal qualities of plants and herbs are referred to as *herbalists.*

Although plants have been used for medicinal purposes for centuries and form the basis of many modern drugs, herbal remedies are not to be taken lightly. Just because something is natural does not necessarily mean that it is safe. Many plants are poisonous, and others can be toxic if ingested in high doses. Still others are dangerous when combined with other drugs and/or may disrupt the normal action of certain prescription medications. Properly-trained herbalists and homeopaths have received graduate-level training in special programs, such as herbal nutrition or traditional Chinese medicine. These practitioners are trained in diagnosis, mixing herbs, interactions with other drugs, titrations and dosages, and patient follow-up and side effects. Checking on the education and training of anyone who recommends or sells herbal medications is a part of intelligent consumerism as well as just plain good sense. Also, it is important to look at the research surrounding individual substances and remedies. Checking the NCCAM website to review summaries of recent research on products and services is a good place to start.

Herbal Remedies

Largely derived from Ayurvedic or traditional Chinese medicine, herbal medications are widely available in the United States. Fueled by mass advertising and promoted as part of multiple vitamin and mineral regimens by major drug manufacturers, herbal supplements represent the hottest trend in the health market.

Herbal remedies come in several different forms. **Tinctures** (extracts of fresh or dried plants) usually contain a high percentage of grain alcohol to prevent spoilage and are among the best herbal options. Freeze-dried extracts are very stable and offer good value for your money. Standardized extracts are also among the more reliable forms of herbal preparations. In general, herbal medicines tend to be milder than

---

Biologically based therapies Combination of natural and biologically based therapies and products used to restore health.

Tinctures Herbal extracts usually combined with grain alcohol to prevent spoilage.

Mixing Foods and Medicines

Did you know that certain foods can cause serious reactions when combined with some medications? According to a national consumer alert from the Food and Drug Administration, here are some combinations to avoid:

- Never drink grapefruit juice less than two hours before or five hours after taking heart drugs called calcium channel blockers, such as Procardia. This combination can kill.
- Grapefruit juice taken with cyclosporin, which fights organ rejection in transplant recipients, can cause confusion and trembling.

- Combining grapefruit juice with antihistamines, either prescription versions such as Claritin and Allegra, or over-the-counter types such as Benadryl, can cause serious heart problems.
- High doses of vitamin E thin the blood. If high doses of vitamin E are taken by heart patients along with the popular blood thinner Coumadin (generic name: warfarin), the risk of serious bleeding increases.
- Foods high in vitamin K, such as broccoli, spinach, and turnip greens, can reduce the effectiveness of Coumadin.
- Antidepressants called MAO inhibitors can cause a potentially fatal rise in blood pressure when taken with foods high in the chemical tyramine, such as cheese and sausage.

- Drinking coffee or colas with certain antibiotics, such as Cipro, or the ulcer drugs Tagamet, Zantac, and Pepcid, can increase caffeine levels, causing jitters and stomach irritation.
- Consuming bananas or potassium supplements along with heart drugs called ACE inhibitors, such as Capoten and Vasotec, can cause harmful potassium buildup if not monitored carefully.

Source: Food and Drug Administration, "Food and Drug Interactions" (1998). For a free copy, call (800)639-8140, or visit the Internet site: www.nclnet.org

---

chemical drugs and produce their effects more slowly; they also are much less likely to cause toxicity because they are diluted forms of drugs rather than concentrated forms.[21] But diluted or not, herbal products are still drugs. They should not be taken casually, any more than you would take over-the-counter or prescription drugs without really needing them or knowing their side effects. No matter how natural they are, they still contain many of the same chemicals as synthetic prescription drugs. Too much of an herb can cause problems, particularly herbs that come from nonstandardized extracts. Some herbs can interact with prescription drugs or cause unusual side effects. The following discussion gives an overview of some of the most common herbal supplements on the market.

Ginkgo Biloba   Ginkgo biloba is an extract from the leaves of a deciduous tree that lives up to 1,000 years. This tree is the world's oldest living tree species; it can be traced back more than 200 million years. The ginkgo was almost destroyed during the last Ice Age in all regions of the world except China, where it is considered a sacred tree with medicinal properties.[22] Today, ginkgo leaf extracts are among the leading prescription medicines in Germany and France, where they account for nearly 2 percent of total prescription sales.[23]

There are many purported benefits. Ginkgo biloba is used to treat depression; impotence; premenstrual syndrome; diseases of the eye, such as retinopathy and macular degeneration; and general vascular disease. In particular, ginkgo biloba has been shown to improve short-term memory and concentration for individuals with impaired blood flow to the brain due to narrowing of vessels or clogging of key arteries. A Harvard-based study of 202 men and women with mild to moderately severe dementia caused by stroke or Alzheimer's disease was among the first to promote ginkgo in the United States. After one year, the group receiving ginkgo experienced significant improvement in cognitive performance (memory, learning, reading) and social functioning (carrying on conversations, recognizing familiar faces) than those in the placebo group (those who did not receive ginkgo).[24] Much of this improvement was believed to be due to the antioxidant properties of the herb, as well as to the blood-thinning properties that seem to improve blood and oxygen flow to clogged blood vessels. Whether this herb will improve memory in people with normal blood flow remains largely unexplored.

Most nutritional experts and physicians recommend that people who are considering using ginkgo take a 40-milligram tablet three times a day for a month or so to determine whether there is any improvement. If there is none, continuing to take this supplement is largely unwarranted. Also, remember that disturbing memory loss or difficulty thinking, regardless of age, should be checked by a doctor to determine underlying causes. Because the main action of ginkgo appears to be as a blood thinner, it should not be taken with other blood-thinning agents, such as aspirin, vitamin E, garlic, ginger, the prescription drug warfarin (trade name: Coumadin), or any other medications that list thinning of the blood as a potential side effect.[25] Doing so could increase the risk of hemorrhage.

St. John's Wort The bright yellow, star-shaped flowers of St. John's wort (SJW) have a rich and varied history in Europe, Asia, and Africa. The name for this herb dates back to early Christian times and relates to the red oil that glands in the flowers secrete when they are pinched or cut. Christians believed that the flowers secreted this blood-red oil on August 29, the anniversary of the beheading of St. John the Baptist, and that they bloomed on June 24, St. John's birthday. The term *wort* is Old English for "plant." In addition, John the Baptist represents light, and the flowers themselves seemed to represent the bright yellow light of the sun.[26] Colonists to the United States brought SJW with them, only to find that Native Americans were already using it for everything from snake bite to a general health enhancer. In the United States, SJW grows in abundance in northern California and southern Oregon and is also referred to as *klammath weed*.[27]

Today, SJW enjoys global popularity. It is the favored therapy for depression in a number of countries, including Germany, actually surpassing most standard antidepressants as the first mode of treatment for clinical depression. German researchers report that it is decidedly better than placebos in medical trials and at least as good as some prescription antidepressants for treatment of mild depression. It is also cheaper and appears to cause fewer side effects than drugs such as Prozac®, Paxil®, and Zoloft®.[28] SJW is believed to have the following effects:

- Acts as a positive mood enhancer by helping maintain levels of serotonin, a natural neurotransmitter that helps brain function and calms the body[29]
- Helps as a sleep enhancer for those having difficulty sleeping[30]
- Supports immune functioning by suppressing the release of interleukin-6, a protein that controls certain aspects of the immune response[31]

A review of 23 well-designed clinical trials published in the *British Medical Journal* concluded that extracts of SJW "are more effective than placebo for the treatment of mild to moderately severe depressive disorders." This review also found evidence from eight other studies that SJW may work as well as some other drugs in countering mild depression. The research team called for more rigorously controlled studies with larger samples comparing this herb with prescription doses of Prozac®.[32] Like other plants, SJW contains a number of different chemicals, many of which are not clearly understood.

As with most antidepressants, SJW's benefits are not felt for about four weeks. The herb does have several side effects. Most are more bothersome than severe and range from slight gastrointestinal upset to fatigue, dry mouth, dizziness, skin rashes, and itching. Some people have noted sensitivity to sunlight. Most of these side effects are minor, however, when compared with those of major antidepressant medicines.

In spite of the positive news about SJW, consumers should proceed with caution when considering its use. Recent advisories put out by the Food and Drug administration and disturbing results from recent research trials indicate that there may be serious risks of drug interactions when SJW is taken with certain other drugs. In particular, SJW has been shown to decrease the effectiveness of protease inhibitors used to treat HIV infections and to interfere with medications given for heart disease, depression, and seizures.[33] Additionally, SJW may interfere with drugs given to treat cancer and drugs used to prevent organ transplant rejection, and it potentially may interfere with the effectiveness of oral contraceptives used for birth control.[34]

Because SJW is sold in the United States as a dietary supplement, not a drug, it is not regulated by the FDA and has not been rigorously tested. Anyone suffering from clinical depression should be under a psychologist's care, and SJW may not help severe depression.

In addition, SJW should never be taken in combination with prescription antidepressants. When combined with other serotonin-enhancing drugs, such as Prozac, SJW may result in serotonin overload, leading to tremors, agitation, or convulsions. SJW also should not be used by pregnant women or women who are nursing, by young children, or by the frail elderly, because the safety margins have not been established.

Echinacea Echinacea, or the *purple coneflower*, is found primarily in the Midwest and the prairie regions of the United States. Two of the nine species of echinacea in the United States are now on the federal endangered species list, a cause of growing concern for many environmentalists as the herb's popularity has grown. Believed to be used extensively by Native Americans for centuries, echinacea eventually gained widespread acceptance in the United States before being shipped to Europe, where its use grew gradually over the eighteenth and nineteenth centuries.

Today, echinacea is the best-selling herb in health and natural food stores in the United States and is widely used throughout most of the world. It is said to stimulate the immune system and increase the effectiveness of the white blood cells that attack bacteria and viruses. Many people believe it to be helpful in preventing and treating the symptoms of a cold or flu. However, echinacea remains controversial. Although many studies in Europe have provided preliminary evidence of its effectiveness, recent controlled trials in the United States indicate that echinacea is no more effective than a placebo in preventing a cold.[35]

As with many herbal treatments, little research has been conducted on the benefits and risks of echinacea. Because it can affect the immune system, people with autoimmune diseases such as arthritis should not take it. Other people who should avoid echinacea include pregnant women, people with diabetes or multiple sclerosis, and anyone allergic to the daisy family of plants. See Table 18.2 for other herbal remedies that are popular for treating common health conditions.

Table 18.2
Herbal Remedies for Common Conditions

CONDITION	HERBAL PRODUCT	DOSE	SIDE EFFECTS
Constipation	Aloe	20–30 mg hydroxyanthracene derivatives/day	Electrolyte and fluid imbalance
	Buckthorn	20–30 mg glycofrangulin per day	
	Cascara	20–30 mg cascaroside/day	
	Flaxseed	1 tbs. whole flaxseed with 8 oz water 2–3 times/day	None if taken as directed
	Manna	20–30 g/day	Nausea, flatulence
	Psyllium	12–40 g (seed) or 4–20 g (husk) daily with 8 oz water for every 5 g drug	Allergic reaction (rare)
	Senna leaf	20–30 mg sennoside per day	Electrolyte and fluid imbalance; can produce rebound constipation if used longer than 1–2 weeks
Dysmenorrhea (menstrual cramps)	Black cohosh	40–60% extract with alcohol	Occasionally, gastric discomfort
	Potentilla	4–6 g powdered herb	Aggravates any gastric discomforts
Leg cramps and swelling	Butcher's broom	7–11 mg ruscogenin in extract	Gastric disturbance, nausea in rare cases
	Horse chestnut	250–312.5 mg extract 2 times/day	Itching, nausea in rare cases
	Sweet clover	3–30 mg coumarin/day	May cause headache
Memory loss	Ginkgo biloba	60–80 mg extract 2–3 times/day	Rarely, headache, stomach upsets
Menopausal symptoms	Black cohosh	40–60% extract with alcohol	Occasionally, gastric discomfort
	Chaste tree fruit	30–40 mg in aqueous-alcohol extracts	May cause itching, rash
Premenstrual syndrome	Block cohosh	40–60% extract with alcohol	Occasionally, gastric discomfort
	Chaste tree fruit	30–40 mg in aqueous-alcohol extracts	May cause itching, rash
	Yarrow	4.5 g powder for infusion	None known
Sleep disturbances	Hops flower	0.5 g powder for infusion	None known
	Valerian root	2–3 g powder for infusion	None known

Source: "New Guides to Herbal Remedies: Examples of Herbs Approved by German Commission E," *Harvard Women's Health Watch* 6 (1999): 2–3.

Special Supplements

The Dietary Supplement Health and Education Act defines dietary supplements as "products (other than tobacco) that are intended to supplement or add to the diet and contain one or more of the following ingredients: vitamins, minerals, amino acids, herbs, or other substance that increases total dietary intake, and that is intended for ingestion in the form of a capsule, powder, soft gel, or gelcap, and is not represented as a conventional food or as a sole item." Typically, these supplements are taken to enhance health, prevent disease, or enhance mood. In recent years, reports on the health benefits of a number of vitamins and minerals have increased. When taken to increase work output or the potential for it, dietary supplements are labeled as **ergogenic aids.** Examples include bee pollen, caffeine, glycine, carnitine, lecithin, brewer's yeast, and gelatin. In recent years, a new generation of performance-enhancing ergogenic aids has hit the market. Many of these claim to increase muscular strength and performance, boost energy, and enhance resistance to disease.

Ergogenic aids Special dietary supplements taken to increase strength, energy, and the ability to work.

Muscle Enhancers In 1998, Mark McGwire made headline news for his home run records. At the same time, he also made news for his admission that he was a regular user of the diet supplement androstenedione, a substance that is found naturally in meat and some plants and is also produced in the human body by the adrenal glands and gonads. The synthetic version, sold in concentrated form, is known in locker room talk as "andro" and is a precursor to the human hormone testosterone (see Chapter 7 for more on andro). In other words, the body converts andro directly into testosterone, which enables an athlete to train harder and recover more quickly. Ironically, although the NCAA, the NFL, and the International Olympic Committee have banned andro, it is readily available over the counter.

The McGwire controversy has encouraged new research into the compound. Early results indicate that andro has a chemical structure that is very similar to anabolic steroids, which may result in long-term risks similar to those of the illegal androgens.[36]

Creatine is a naturally occurring compound found primarily in skeletal muscle that helps to optimize the muscles' energy levels. In recent years, the use of creatine supplements has increased dramatically because of claims that it increases muscle energy and allows a person to work harder with less muscle fatigue and build muscle mass with less effort. Reports of creatine's benefits, however, appear exaggerated. Over one-third of people taking creatine are unable to absorb it in the muscles and achieve no benefit. Side effects include muscle cramping, muscle strains, and possible liver and kidney damage.[37]

Ginseng   Grown commercially throughout many regions of the United States, ginseng is much prized for its reported sexual restorative value. It is believed that ginseng affects the pituitary gland, increasing resistance to stress, affecting metabolism, aiding skin and muscle tone, and providing the hormonal balance necessary for a healthy sex life. Other purported benefits include improved endurance, muscle strength, recovery from exercise, oxygen metabolism during exercise, auditory and visual reaction time, and mental concentration.[38] Studies of the effectiveness of ginseng, however, have raised questions about it: Primarily, what are appropriate dosages, and how long should it be taken to realize benefits? Because the potency of plants varies considerably, dosage is difficult to control, and side effects are fairly common. Noteworthy side effects of high doses of ginseng include nervousness, insomnia, high blood pressure, headaches, skin eruptions, chest pain, depression, and abnormal vaginal bleeding.[39]

Glucosamine   Glucosamine is a substance produced by the body that plays a key role in the growth and development of cartilage. When present in sufficient amounts, it stimulates the manufacture of substances necessary for proper joint function and joint repair. It is manufactured commercially and sold under a variety of different names, usually glucosamine sulfate. Glucosamine has been shown to be effective for treating osteoarthritis and related degenerative joint diseases and appears to relieve swelling and decrease pain.

Unlike many other herbal supplements, glucosamine sulfate has an excellent safety record with few noteworthy side effects.[40]

Chromium Picolinate   A few years ago, chromium picolinate was believed to be the new miracle for anyone interested in weight loss. Since then, at least two major studies at the U.S. Department of Agriculture Human Nutrition Research Center have shown no benefit.[41]

SAMe   SAMe (pronounced "Sammy") is the nickname for S-adenosyl-methionine, a compound produced biochemically in all humans to help perform some 40 functions in the body, ranging from bone preservation (hence its purported osteoarthritis benefits) to DNA replication.

SAMe has been reported to have a significant effect on mild-to-moderate depression without many of the typical side effects of prescription medications, such as sexual dysfunction, weight gain, and sleep disturbance. Scientists speculate that SAMe somehow affects brain levels of the neurotransmitters noradrenaline, serotonin, and, possibly, dopamine, all of which are related to the human stress response and the origins of depression in the body.[42]

Anyone interested in SAMe should consider these factors:[43]

- Although preliminary evidence suggests that SAMe may promote joint health and enhance mood, no large-scale, scientifically controlled studies in the United States have verified such claims.
- Many question the high cost of SAMe (between $15 and $35 or higher for 20 pills).
- Clinical depression requires more than self-treatment. Any depressed person should consult a physician to explore all options, including counseling as well as pharmaceutical and natural remedies.
- People with a family history of heart disease should not take SAMe; preliminary indications are that it may trigger coronary events.

Under no circumstances should SAMe be taken by anyone on prescription antidepressants, and the time lag between taking the prescription and beginning SAMe, and vice versa, should be carefully considered.[44]

Antioxidants   Although covered in depth in the chapter on nutrition, it should be noted that antioxidants are among the most sought-after supplements on the market. Primary antioxidants include beta-carotene, selenium, vitamin C, and vitamin E.

Creatine   A naturally occurring compound found primarily in skeletal muscle that helps optimize the muscles' energy levels.

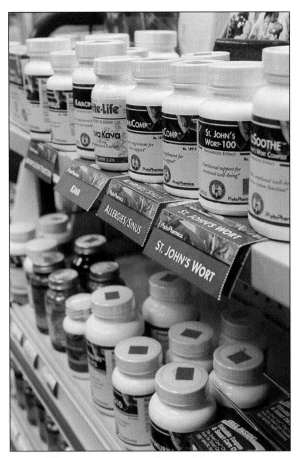

Buying herbal supplements can be confusing because so many brands exist and their manufacture is not strictly regulated for potency and quality.

Foods as Healing Agents

It has been widely documented that many Americans rely on *functional foods*—foods or supplements designed to improve some aspect of physical or mental functioning. Sometimes referred to as **nutraceuticals** for their combined nutritional and pharmaceutical benefit, several are believed to actually work in much the same way as pharmaceutical drugs in making a person well or bolstering the immune system.

Foods contain many "nonnutrient" active ingredients that can affect us in different ways. For example, chili peppers contain ingredients that make your eyes water and clear your sinuses. Many of these active ingredients, or constituents, can promote good health. A number of foods, such as sweet potatoes, tangerines, and red peppers, are recognized as excellent sources of antioxidants. Onion and garlic contain allium com-

Nutraceuticals Term often used interchangeably with *functional foods;* refers to the combined nutritional and pharmaceutical benefit derived through use of foods or food supplements.

pounds that reduce blood clotting. Other foods have natural anti-inflammatory properties or aid digestion. Some are known by the term *prebiotics,* foods that promote good bacteria in the body that may help fight off infection.[45]

Some of the most common healthful foods and their purported benefits include the following:

- *Plant stanol.* Can lower "bad" LDL cholesterol.
- *Oat fiber.* Can lower "bad" LDL cholesterol; serves as a natural soother of nerves; stabilizes blood sugar levels.
- *Sunflower.* Can lower risk of heart disease; may prevent angina.
- *Soy protein.* May lower heart disease risk; provides protective estrogen-like effect; may reduce risk from certain cancers.
- *Red meats and dark green, leafy vegetables.* Contain B vitamins (B_6, B_{12}, folate), which can lower levels of homocysteine, an amino acid associated with heart disease.
- *Garlic.* Lowers cholesterol and reduces clotting tendency of blood; lowers blood pressure; may serve as form of antibiotic.
- *Japanese green tea.* Lowers cholesterol; may have a role in fighting certain cancers.
- *Ginger.* Fights motion sickness, stomach pain, and upset; discourages blood clots; may relieve rheumatism.
- *Yogurt.* Untreated, nonpasteurized yogurt contains active, friendly bacteria that can fight off infections.

Table 18.3 lists other foods and supplements with their risks and benefits.

Many people purchase foods labeled *organic* because they expect these products to contain only health-promoting substances. But what does *organic* really mean? Today, when something is labeled as *organic,* it doesn't necessarily mean that it is free of anything. Even though the Organic Foods Production Act (OFPA) of 1990 established a national certification process to ensure consumer safety, few states consistently apply the standards defined in that legislation.

> **What do you think?**
> *Why do you think the government has not acted more aggressively to regulate or control herbal and other dietary supplements?* ✳ *Why are many CAM treatments not covered under typical insurance plans?*

Protecting Consumers and Regulating Claims

Although many CAM products appear promising, be aware that most of these products are not regulated in the United States as strictly as are foods and drugs. This situation is a sharp contrast to that in nations such as Germany, where the government holds companies to strict standards for ingredients and manufacturing. In the United States, nutritional supplements and genetically engineered and organic foods

Table 18.3
Common Herbal, Vitamin, and Mineral Supplements: Benefits vs. Risks

SUPPLEMENT	USE	CLAIMS OF BENEFITS	RISKS
Ephedra (*ma huang, epitonin,* and *sida cordifolia*)	Serves as a stimulant and bronchodilator	Natural source of ephedrine for use as bronchodilator in asthmatic attack	Numerous reports of side effects including heart palpitations and psychosis, heart attacks and strokes; banned in several states; TOXIC
Chaparral	Sold as teas and pills	Fights cancer and purifies blood	Linked to serious liver damage
Comfrey	Originated as a poultice to reduce swelling, but later used internally	Wound healing, infection control	Contains alkaloids toxic to the liver, and animal studies suggest it is carcinogenic
Melatonin	"Clock hormone"	Role in regulating circadian rhythms and sleep patterns	Anti-aging claims unfounded
DHEA	Hormone that turns into estrogen and testosterone in the body	Fights aging, boosts immunity, strengthens bones, and improves brain functioning	No anti-aging benefits proven; could increase cancer risk and lead to liver damage, even when taken briefly
Dieter's teas	Herbal blends containing senna, aloe, rhubarb root, buckthorn, cascara, and castor oil	Act as laxatives	Can disrupt potassium levels and cause heart arrhythmias; linked to diarrhea, vomiting, chronic constipation, fainting, and death
Pennyroyal (member of the mint family)		Soothing effect in teas	Pregnancy-related complications, heart arrhythmias, death
Sassafras	Once a flavoring in root beer; used in tonics and teas	No real claims	Shown to cause liver cancer in animals
Flax seeds	Produce linseed oil	Omega-3 fatty acid benefits	Delay absorption of medicine
Kava kava			Increases the effects of alcohol and other drugs
High-dose vitamin E	Antioxidants	Reduces risk of heart disease; better survivability after heart attack	Causes bleeding when taking blood thinners
Vitamin C	Antioxidant, manufactures collagen, wound repair, nerve transmission	Improves blood vessel relaxation in people with CVD, diabetes, hypertension, and other problems; can relieve pain of angina pectoris	
L-Carnitine	Amino acid	Improves metabolism in heart muscle, purported to increase fat burning enzymes	Heart palpitations, arrhythmias, sudden death; claims largely unsubtantiated
Licorice root		None proven	Speeds potassium loss
Niacin (vitamin B_3)	Reduces serum lipids, vasodilation, and increased blood flow		Skin flushing, gastrointestinal distress, stomach pain, nausea and vomiting
Chondroitin (shark cartilage or sea cucumber)		Improves osteoporosis and arthritis by improving cartilage function	Fewer benefits than glucosamine; benefits still unproven

have had a long history of unregulated growth, including an abundance of claims and testimonials about their health-enhancing attributes. With few regulatory controls in place, many get-rich-quick charlatans have jumped into the health food and CAM market.

Strategies to Protect for Health

The burgeoning popularity of nutraceuticals and functional foods concerns many scientists. According to National Institutes of Health (NIH) nutritional biochemist Dr. Terry Krakower,

> NIH does have some concerns about them and we are looking into them, especially the potential for interaction with other medications. We advise anyone who uses them to talk to their physician. [Functional foods] are so new we don't know yet if they are good, bad, or indifferent. [Much] of the herb content in these food products is so small that it's probably ineffective, and if it were included in large amounts, it could be harmful. Anyone taking these supplements, whether in pill form or in foods, should do their homework and thoroughly research them rather than rely on health claims made by manufacturers.[46]

By legal definition, herbal supplements and functional foods are neither prescription drugs nor over-the-counter medications. Instead, classified as food supplements, they can be sold without FDA approval. Because they are not regulated by the FDA, these products are not subject to the strict guidelines that govern the research and development of medications.

Consumer groups, members of the scientific community, and government officials are calling for action. Pressure is mounting to establish consistent standards for herbal supplements and functional foods similar to those used in Germany and other countries. Many scientists advocate a more stringent FDA approval process for virtually all supplements sold in the United States.

The German Commission E

The German Commission E is among the most noteworthy of the international groups attempting to regulate the sale of alternative medicines and supplements. Consisting of an expert panel established in 1970, its mission was to conduct a formal evaluation of the hundreds of herbal remedies that have been part of traditional German medicine for centuries.

Phytomedicines   Another name for medicinal herbs, many of which are sold over the counter in Europe.

Commission members carefully analyzed data from clinical trials, observational studies, biological experiments, and chemical analyses. Between 1983 and 1996, they evaluated 383 herbal remedies, approving almost two-thirds of them for use but discounting nearly another third, some of which continue to be sold in the United States.[47]

Essentially, the German Commission E analyzed a growing list of **phytomedicines,** another name for medicinal herbs, many of which are sold over the counter in Europe. Typically, phytomedicines are integrated into conventional medical practice and are prepared in several different ways, usually as tablets or ground into powders.[48] Many are sold in much the same way as over-the-counter remedies in the United States.

Looking to Science for More Answers

Even as CAM treatments gain credibility, this credibility must be tempered with good science. Although slow in coming, legislators have pushed for better science, increased funding, and an agency designed to help garner information useful to consumers.

In 1993, Congress established the Office of Alternative Medicine (OAM) at the NIH. Recently renamed the National Center for Complementary and Alternative Medicine (NC-CAM) and with a budget of nearly $50 million, it can fund its own projects and has established research centers at universities and other institutions throughout the United States, where many clinical trials are being conducted.[49] In addition, numerous other studies into alternative treatments for ailments from arthritis to depression to high blood cholesterol are taking place across the United States.

Healthy Living in the New Millennium

Clearly, CAM is here to stay. It appears to serve a very real need for consumers. While consumers are making the adjustment to CAM in record numbers, members of the health care delivery system seem slow to act. Although progress has been noted, there is still a long way to go before CAM becomes fully accepted in mainstream medical practice.

Enlisting Support from Insurers and Providers

More and more insurers are hiring alternative practitioners as staff or covering alternative care as a routine benefit, at least to some degree. This is especially true as criticisms of managed care increase and government agencies get involved.

In 1999, over 60 health maintenance groups throughout the United States covered some form of alternative care, nearly three times the number in 1994. In some cases, consumers are offered an optional "extra-cost" rider on their insurance policy, through which they may choose to see alternative practitioners for a higher premium and co-pay agreement. For many consumers, just knowing they have a choice seems to be worth the extra cost. Usually the cost of these added practitioners to the treatment pool adds $3 to $9 dollars per patient to the monthly premium.

Support from professional organizations, such as the American Medical Association (AMA), is also increasing, as more physician training programs require or offer electives in alternative treatment modalities. In some cases, medical schools are educating a new generation of medical doctors to be better prepared to advise patients about the pros and cons of alternative treatments, and more comprehensive studies are underway to compare the efficacy of alternative strategies to traditional treatments.[50]

> ### What do you think?
> *What can you do as a consumer to obtain the greatest benefit from CAM? ✳ How can you protect yourself from possible negative risks?*

Self-Care: Protecting Yourself

Like no other time in human history, today we are faced with an astounding array of possible health choices. With a few notable exceptions, much of what we read on the Internet about functional foods, herbal medicines, and CAM is, in general, unreliable at best—and strewn with potentially harmful and downright false information at worst.

When considering alternative treatments, do your homework, and protect yourself by remembering the following points:

- Consult only reliable sources—texts, journals, periodicals, and government resources. Start with the sites and sources listed at the end of this chapter.
- Remember that *natural* and *safe* are not necessarily synonyms. Many people have become seriously ill from seemingly harmless products. For example, some people have suffered serious liver damage from sipping teas brewed with comfrey, an herb used in poultices and ointments to treat sprains and bruises but that should not be taken internally. Pregnant women face special risks from herbs such as echinacea, senna, comfrey, and licorice.
- Realize that no one is closely monitoring the purity of herbal supplements. The FDA has verified industry reports that certain shipments of ginseng were contaminated with high levels of fungicides. Other problems with imported herbs have been noted.
- Recognize that dosage levels in many herbal products are not regulated. German manufacturers produce identical batches of herbal remedies as required by law. Look for reputable manufacturers.
- Tell your doctor if you are taking herbal medications. Several may interact with prescription medications.
- Remember that no herbal medicine is likely to work miracles. Monitor your health, and seek help if you notice any unusual side effects from herbal products.
- Always look for the word *standardized* on any herbal product you buy.

As we enter a new era of medicine, more than ever, you are being called upon to take responsibility for what goes into your body. This means you must educate yourself. CAM can offer new avenues toward better health, but it is up to you to make sure that you are on the right path.

Taking Charge

18 **18** **18**

Making Healthful Decisions about CAM

Based on the information in this chapter, you can see that you should not use CAM products and services lightly, just as you should not take decision making about the traditional, allopathic health care system lightly. Though the U.S. government has stepped up research and testing, we have addressed only the tip of the iceberg regarding information about the benefits and risks from CAM.

You need to constantly remain aware of the risks facing you in all of your decisions about health. As long as you are armed with the best sources of information, reading widely from reputable sources and questioning the basis of claims and testimonials, you are taking critical steps in reducing risks. Consider the following as you make decisions about using any health care product or service.

Checklist for Change

Making Personal Choices

✓ Find the most reputable sources for CAM-related information. Determine whether the information is current and whether it represents a single finding or one that is consistent with other research. Also, check the qualifications of the people who wrote the materials. Pay more heed to professionals with recognized credentials in specific areas, such as an M.D. or Ph.D. in a particular specialty. Find out whether such authors are conducting active research using randomized, controlled trials.

✓ Focus on websites sponsored by professional organizations such as the American Dietetic Association, the Centers for Disease Control and Prevention, the American Public Health Association, and the American Medical Association.

✓ Consider your current health status, the areas you would like to improve, and the wide array of options that may help. Ask questions of other people who have experienced similar conditions or situations. What worked for them? Consult people whose judgment and knowledge you

trust. Then itemize your options, and choose those that appear to offer the most benefit and the least risk.

✓ When shopping at health food stores or fitness centers that sell supplements and other purported health products, request the qualifications of those who are selling the products. Have they graduated with degrees in health education, nutrition, pharmacology, exercise physiology, or other reputable fields? Or have they simply attended a one- to two-week training program provided by their employer? Do they offer you choices and talk about risks and concerns, or are they primarily in "sell" mode?

✓ Does your student health center have anyone available to answer your questions? Is there a certified health educator on staff? A dietitian? Does your doctor have time to answer some of your questions? Prepare a list, and ask for advice from experts on your own campus. Also, ask where you can go for reputable, easy-to-understand information about a given topic.

✓ Consider a balance in all things. Just because CAM modalities are available, it doesn't mean that you should toss out all the op-

tions in the traditional health care system. Optimize your health by utilizing the most effective modalities from both systems of treatment.

Making Community Choices

✓ Assess CAM providers in your community. Support those that are reputable and offer products and services including appropriate scientific information for consumers. Report those who offer questionable products and services.

✓ Write to congressional leaders in support of insurance provisions that allow consumers to choose CAM therapies that have been shown through scientific evidence to be safe and effective.

✓ Review policies about CAM products and services on your campus. What is offered? Who is using the services? How aware are other students of these services?

✓ Act responsibly, and stay informed about CAM and traditional medicine practices. Whenever someone is treated unfairly or inappropriately, make your concerns known. Be an advocate for good information and ethical treatment of all health problems.

Summary

* Complementary and alternative medicine includes at least five major domains of products and services: (1) alternative systems, (2) mind–body interventions, (3) energy therapies, (4) biologically based systems (5) manipulative and body-based methods.

* People throughout the world are choosing complementary and alternative medicine options, and these numbers are growing exponentially. Much of the influence of these CAM strategies may be traced to other cultures, particularly those with traditional oriental medicine or ayurvedic roots.

* The National Center for Complementary and Alternative Medicine is a relatively new NIH center devoted to CAM research and information dissemination.

* Major types of CAM providers and treatment modalities include chiropractic medicine, acupuncture, herbal remedies, homeopathy, and naturopathy.

* Herbal remedies, largely derived from traditional oriental medicine, include ginkgo biloba, St. John's wort, and echinacea. Other herbal remedies have also received widespread attention as potential miracle drugs without having harmful side effects. Special supplements include muscle

enhancers, ginseng, glucosamine, chromium picolinate, SAMe, and antioxidants. A number of functional foods also serve as healing agents.

* Though many positive effects are associated with CAM, there are potential risks for consumers as with most health care options. The drive for profits and the lack of strict government regulation put increased responsibility for decision making on consumers. As a consumer, you must be aware of the risks and check reputable sources to ensure that the products and services you are considering are safe and effective and that they represent reasonable alternatives for some of the more widely accepted forms of treatment.

Discussion Questions

1. What are some of the potential benefits and risks of CAM? Why do you think these practices and products are growing in popularity so rapidly?
2. What are the major domains of CAM treatments? Have you tried any of them? Would you feel comfortable trying any new ones? Why or why not?
3. What are the major herbal remedies? Special supplements? What are some of the risks and benefits associated with each?
4. What can you do to ensure that you are receiving accurate information regarding CAM treatments or medicines? What is the name of the federal agency that oversees CAM in the United States?
5. What is being done in the United States to ensure continued growth of CAM?

Application Exercises

Reread the What Do You Think? scenario at the beginning of the chapter, and answer the following questions.

1. Why are there so many conflicting sources of information in today's health care system about even a seemingly simple problem? What could we do to streamline sources and give consumers access to the best information available?
2. Would you favor a government watchdog agency to monitor such a source of information? Why or why not?
3. What can consumers like Elena do to protect themselves from misleading information about important health concerns? How can they find answers to their questions?

Accessing Your Health on the Internet

Visit the following Internet sites to explore further topics and issues related to personal health. To visit an organization's website, go to the Companion Website for *Health: The Basics, Fifth Edition* at www.aw.com/donatelle, click on the book image, and select "Accessing Your Health on the Internet" from the navigation menu on the left.

1. **National Center for Complementary and Alternative Medicines (NCCAM).** A new division of the National Institutes of Health dedicated to providing the latest information on complementary and alternative practices, including NCCAM-funded centers of research on alternative medicine.

2. **National Institutes of Health, Office of Dietary Supplements.** An excellent resource for information on dietary supplements.
3. **Alternative Medicine Links.** Provides links to a number of the best alternative, complementary, and preventive health news pages.
4. **Acupuncture.com.** Provides resources for consumers regarding traditional Asian therapies, geared to students and practitioners.
5. **Complementary & Alternative Medicine Program at Stanford.** Stanford Center for Health Promotion, Research and Disease Prevention.

Further Reading

Blumenthal, M. (Ed.). *Complete German Commission E Monographs: Therapeutic Guide to Herbal Medicines.* Austin, TX: The American Botanical Council, 1998.
Overview of German E Commission findings and relevant information about supplement research for consumers.

Provides an interesting perspective on international herbal research, policies, recommendations, and future directions.

Cassileth, B. R. *The Alternative Medicine Handbook: The Complete Reference Guide to Alternative and Complementary*

Therapies. New York: W. W. Norton & Co., 1998.
A complete reference for patients and physicians alike on possible alternative treatments.

Jonas, W. B., and J. S. Levin, eds. *Essentials of Complementary and Alternative Medicine.* Philadelphia: Lippincott Williams & Wilkins, 1999.
Comprehensive text on the foundations of CAM and the safety of CAM products and practices.

Pelletier, Ken. *The Best Alternative Medicine: What Works? What Does Not?* Simon & Schuster. New York, 2000.
Excellent overview of commonly used CAM techniques with scientific information for consumers.

Turchaninov, R., and C. A. Cox. *Medical Massage.* Scottsdale, AZ: Stress Less Publishing and Phoenix: Aesculapius Books, 1998.
An in-depth review of therapeutic practices from around the world.

Uhlmann, P. *Flowing the Tai Chi Way: A Voyage of Discovery by a Tai Chi Master and His Student.* Powell River, BC, Canada: China Books and Periodicals, 1998.
Revealing autobiography of the author's spiritual search in tai chi.

Appendix
Injury Prevention
and Emergency Care

Unintentional injuries are one of the major public health problems facing the United States today. On an average day, more than a million people will suffer a nonfatal injury; 70,000 will die as a result of unintentional injuries. Unintentional injuries are the leading cause of death for Americans under the age of 44. In the United States, unintentional injuries are the fourth leading cause of death, after heart disease, cancer, and stroke.

Vehicle Safety

The risk of dying in an auto crash is related to age. Young drivers (16–24) have the highest death rate, owing to their inexperience and immaturity. Each year 41,000 Americans die in automobile crashes and another 1.6 million are disabled, 140,000 permanently. Most of these car crashes were avoidable. The best line of prevention against car crashes is to practice risk management driving, accident-avoidance techniques, and to be aware of safety technology when purchasing your car.

Risk Management Driving   Practicing risk driving management techniques when you drive helps reduce your chances of being involved in a collision. Techniques include:

- **Surround your car with a bubble space.** The rear bumper of the car ahead of you should be three seconds away. To measure your safety bubble, choose a roadside landmark such as a signpost or light pole as a reference point. When the car in front of you passes this point, count "one-one-thousand, two-one-thousand." Make sure you are not passing the reference point before you've finished saying "three-one-thousand."
- **Scan the road ahead of you and to both sides.**
- **Drive with your low beam headlights on.** Being seen is an important safety factor. Driving with your low beam headlights on *day or night* makes you more visible to other drivers.

In addition:

- Anticipate other drivers' actions.
- Drive refreshed.
- Drive sober.
- Obey all traffic laws.
- Use safety belts.

Accident-Avoidance Techniques   Sometimes when driving you need to react instantly to a situation. To avoid a more severe accident you may need to steer into another less severe collision. The point of accident evasion is to save lives. Here are AAA's rules for accident avoidance:

1. Generally veer to the right.
2. Steer, don't skid, off the road.
3. If you have to hit a vehicle, hit one moving in the same direction as your own.
4. If you have to hit a stationary object, try to hit a soft one (bushes, small trees, etc.) rather then a hard one (boulders, brick walls, giant oaks).
5. If you have to hit a hard object, hit it with a glancing blow.
6. Avoid hitting pedestrians, motorcyclists, and bicyclists at all costs.
7. Try never to be involved in a head-on collision.

Safety Technology   The last line of defense against a collision is the car itself. How a car is equipped can mean the difference between life and death. When purchasing a car, look for the following features:

- Does the car have airbags? Remember airbags do not eliminate the need for everyone to wear safety belts. Airbags inflate only in the case of frontal crashes.
- Does the car have antilock brakes? Antilock brakes help pump the brakes and prevent them from locking up and, hence, the car from skidding.
- Does the car have impact-absorbing crumple zones?
- Are there strengthened passenger compartment side walls?
- Is there a strong roof support? (The center door post on four-door models gives you an extra roof pillar.)

(Source: Insurance Institute for Highway Safety)

What should I do if my car breaks down?

- Try to get off the road as far as possible.
- Turn on your car's emergency flashers and raise the hood. Set out flares or reflective triangles.
- Stay in the car until a law enforcement officer arrives. If others stop to help, ask them to contact the police, sheriff's office, or the State Patrol.
- If you must leave your car, leave a note with the car explaining the problem (as best you can), the time and date,

your name, the direction in which you are walking, and what you are wearing. This information will help them look for you if necessary.
- Remove all valuables from the car if you must leave it.

Pedestrian Safety

Each year approximately 13 percent of all motor vehicle deaths involve pedestrians, and another 82,000 pedestrians are injured each year. The highest death rates involving pedestrians occur in the very young and elderly population. Pedestrian injuries occur most frequently after dark, in urban settings primarily in intersections where pedestrians may walk or dart into traffic. It is not uncommon for alcohol to play a role in the death or injury of a pedestrian. How can you protect yourself from being injured or becoming a fatality? AAA has the following suggestions for joggers and walkers:

- Carry or wear reflective material at night to help drivers see you.
- Cross only at crosswalks. Keep to the right in crosswalks.
- Before crossing, look both ways. Be sure the way is clear before you cross.
- Cross only on the proper signal.
- Watch for turning cars.
- Never go into the roadway from between parked cars.
- Where there is no sidewalk, and it is necessary to walk in a roadway, walk on the left side facing traffic.
- Don't wear headphones for a radio or tape player. These may interfere with your ability to hear sounds of motor vehicles.

Cycling Safety

Currently over 63 million Americans of all ages ride bicycles for transportation, recreation, and fitness. The Consumer Product Safety Commission reports about 800 deaths per year from cycling accidents. The biggest risk factors are failure to wear a helmet, being male, and riding after dark. Children age 10 to 14 also are at higher risk for injury. Motorists can't be blamed for many of these as approximately 87% of the collisions were due to cyclists' errors, usually failure to yield at intersections. Alcohol also plays a significant role in bicycle deaths and injuries. The following are suggestions cyclists should consider following to reduce their risk of injury or death.

- Wear a helmet. It should be ANSI or Snell approved. This can reduce head injuries by 85%.
- Don't drink and ride.
- Respect traffic.
- Wear light reflective clothing that is easily seen at night and during the day.
- Avoid riding after dark.
- Ride with the flow of traffic.

- Know and use proper hand signals.
- Maintain the operating condition of the bike.
- Use bike paths whenever possible.
- Stop at stop signs and traffic lights.

Water Safety

Drowning is the third most common cause of accidental death in the United States, according to the National Safety Council. About 85% of drowning victims are teenage males. Many drowned swimmers are strong swimmers. Alcohol plays a significant role in many drowning cases. Most drownings occur in unorganized or supervised facilities, such as ponds, or pools with no lifeguards present. Swimmers should take the following precautions:

- Don't drink alcohol before or while swimming.
- Don't enter the water unless you can swim at least fifty feet unassisted.
- Know your limitations; get out of the water as soon as you start to feel even slightly fatigued.
- Never swim alone, even if you are a skilled swimmer. You never know what might happen.
- Never leave a child unattended, even in extremely shallow water or wading pools.
- Before entering the water, check the depth. Most neck and back injuries result from diving into water that is too shallow.
- Never swim in muddy or dirty water that obstructs your view of the bottom.
- Never swim in a river with currents too swift for easy, relaxed swimming.

Alcohol Poisoning

Alcohol overdose is considered a medical emergency when one or both of the following occur: an irregular heartbeat or coma. The two immediate causes of death in such cases are cardiac arrhythmia and respiratory depression. The critical signs for alcohol poisoning are as follows:

- Mental confusion, stupor, coma, or a persona cannot be roused
- Vomiting
- Seizures
- Slow breathing (fewer than eight breaths per second)
- Irregular breathing (10 seconds or more between breaths)
- Hypothermia (low body temperature) bluish skin color, paleness

What to do when dealing with someone who has consumed a large amount of alcohol:

1. Stay calm. Assess the situation.
2. Speak in a clear, firm, reassuring manner.
3. Keep your distance. Before approaching or touching the person, explain what you intend to do.

4. Stay with the person if he or she is vomiting. When lying him or her down, turn the head to the side to prevent it from falling back. This helps keep the person from choking on vomit.
5. Monitor the person's breathing.

Don't be afraid to seek medical help for a friend that has had too much to drink.

Emergency Care

In certain situations, it may be necessary to administer first aid. Ideally, first-aid procedures should be performed by someone who has received formal training from the American Red Cross or some other reputable institution. If you do not have such training, contact your physician or call your local emergency medical service (EMS) by dialing 911 or your local emergency number. In life-threatening situations, however, you may not have time to call for outside assistance.

In cases of serious injury or sudden illness, you may need to begin first aid immediately and continue until help arrives. The remainder of this appendix contains basic information and general steps to follow for various emergency situations. Simply reading these directions, however, may not prepare you fully to handle these situations. For this reason, you may want to enroll in a first-aid course.

Calling for Emergency Assistance

When calling for emergency assistance, be prepared to give exact details. Be clear and thorough, and do not panic. Never hang up until the dispatcher has all the information needed. Be ready to answer the following question:

1. Where are you and the victim located? This is the most important information the EMS will need.
2. What is your phone number and name?
3. What has happened? Was there an accident or is the victim ill?
4. How many people need help?
5. What is the nature of the emergency? What is the victim's apparent condition?
6. Are there any life threatening situations that the EMS should know about (for example, fires, explosions, or fallen electrical lines)?
7. Is the victim wearing a medic-alert tag (a tag indicating a specific medical problem such as diabetes)?

Are You Liable?

According to the laws in most states, you are not required to administer first aid unless you have a special obligation to the victim. For example, parents must provide first aid for their children, and a lifeguard must provide aid to a swimmer.

Before administering first aid, you should obtain the victim's consent. If the victim refuses aid, you must respect that person's rights. However, you should make every reasonable effort to persuade the victim to accept your help. In emergency situations, consent is *implied* if the victim is unconscious.

Once you begin to administer first aid, you required by law to continue. You must remain with the victim until someone of equal or greater competence takes over.

Can you be held liable if you fail to provide adequate care or if the victim is further injured? To help protect people who render first aid, most states have "Good Samaritan" laws. These laws grant immunity (protection from civil liability) if you act in good faith to provide care to the best of your ability, according to your level of training. Because these laws vary from state, you should become familiar with the Good Samaritan laws in your state.

When Someone Stops Breathing

If someone has stopped breathing, you should perform mouth-to-mouth resuscitation. This involves the following steps:

1. Check for responsiveness by gently tapping or shaking the victim. Ask loudly, "Are you OK?"
2. Call the local EMS for help (usually 911).
3. Gently roll the victim onto his or her back.
4. Open the airway by tilting the victim's head back; placing your hand nearest the victim's head on the victim's forehead, and applying backward pressure to tilt head back and lift the chin.
5. Check for breathing (3 to 5 seconds): look, listen, and feel for breathing.
6. Give 2 slow breaths

- Keep victim's head tilted back.
- Pinch the victim's nose shut.
- Seal your lips tightly around the victim's mouth.
- Give 2 slow breaths, each lasting $1\frac{1}{2}$ to 2 seconds.

7. Check for pulse at side of neck; feel for pulse for 5 to 10 seconds.
8. Begin rescue breathing.

- Keep victim's head tilted back.
- Pinch the victim's nose shut.
- Give 1 breath every 5 to 6 seconds.
- Look, listen, and feel for breathing between breaths.

9. Recheck pulse every minute.

- Keep victim's head tilted back.
- Feel for pulse for 5 to 10 seconds.
- If the victim has a pulse but is not breathing, continue rescue breathing. If there is no pulse, begin CPR.

There are some variations when performing this procedure on infants and children. For children ages 1 to 8, at step

8, give one slow breath every 4 seconds. For infants, you should not pinch the nose. Instead, seal you lips tightly around the infant's nose and mouth. Also, at step 8, you should give one slow breath every 3 seconds.

In cases in which the victim has no pulse, cardiopulmonary resuscitation (CPR) should be performed. This technique involves a combination of artificial respiration and chest compressions. You should not perform CPR unless you have received training in it. You cannot learn CPR simply by reading directions, and without training, you could cause further injury to the victim. The American Red Cross offers courses in mouth-to-mouth resuscitation and CPR as well as general first aid. If you have taken a CPR course in the past, you should be aware that certain changes have been made in the procedure. You should, therefore, consider taking a refresher course.

When Someone Is Choking

Choking occurs when an object obstructs the trachea (windpipe), thus preventing normal breathing. Failure to expel the object and restore breathing can lead to death within 6 minutes. The universal signal of distress related to choking is the clasping of the throat with one or both hands. Other signs of choking include not being able to talk and/or noisy and difficult breathing. If a victim can cough or speak, do not interfere. The most effective method for assisting choking victims is the Heimlich maneuver, which involves the application of pressure to the victim's abdominal area to expel the foreign object.

The Heimlich maneuver involves the following steps: If the victim is standing or seated:

1. Recognize that the victim is choking.
2. Wrap your arms around the victim's waist, making a fist with one hand.
3. Place the thumb side of the fist on the middle of the victim's abdomen, just above the navel and well below the tip of the sternum.
4. Cover your fist with your other hand.
5. Press fist into victim's abdomen, with up to 5 quick upward thrusts.
6. After every 5 abdominal thrusts, check the victim and your technique.
7. If the victim becomes unconscious, gently lower him or her to the ground.
8. Try to clear the airway by using your finger to sweep the object from the victim's mouth or throat.
9. Give 2 rescue breaths. If the passage is still blocked and air will not go in, proceed with the Heimlich maneuver.

If the victim is lying down:

10. Facing the person, kneel with your legs astride the victim's hips. Place the heel of one hand against the abdomen, slightly above the navel and well below the tip of the sternum. Put the other hand on top of the first hand.

11. Press inward and upward using both hands with up to 5 quick abdominal thrusts.
12. Repeat the following steps in this sequence until the airway becomes clear or the EMS arrives:
    a. Finger sweep.
    b. Give 2 rescue breaths.
    c. Do up to 5 abdominal thrusts.

Controlling Bleeding

External Bleeding   Control of external bleeding is an important part of emergency care. Survival is threatened by the loss of 1 quart of blood or more. There are three major procedures for the control of external bleeding.

Direct pressure. The best method is to apply firm pressure by covering the wound with a sterile dressing, bandage, or clean cloth. Wearing disposable latex gloves or an equally protective barrier, apply pressure for 5 to 10 minutes to stop bleeding.

Elevation. Elevate the wounded section of the body to slow bleeding. For example, a wounded arm or leg should be raised above the level of the victim's heart.

Pressure points. Pressure points are sites where an artery that is close to the body's surface lies directly over a bone. Pressing the artery against the bone can limit the flow of blood to the injury. This technique should be used only as a last resort when direct pressure and elevation have failed to stop bleeding.

Knowing where to apply pressure to stop bleeding is critical (see Figure 1). For serious wounds, seek medical attention immediately.

Internal Bleeding   Although internal bleeding may not be immediately obvious, you should be aware of the following signs and symptoms:

- Symptoms of shock (discussed later in this appendix)
- Coughing up or vomiting blood
- Bruises or contusions of the skin
- Bruises on chest or fractured ribs
- Black, tarlike stools
- Abdominal discomfort or pain (rigidity or spasms)

In some cases, a person who has suffered an injury (such as a blow to the head, chest, or abdomen) that does not cause external bleeding may experience internal bleeding. If you suspect that someone is suffering from internal bleeding, follow these steps:

1. Have the person lie on a flat surface with knees bent.
2. Treat for shock. Keep the victim warm. Cover the person with a blanket, if possible.
3. Expect vomiting. If vomiting occurs, keep the victim on his or her side for drainage, to prevent inhalation of vomit, and to prevent expulsion of vomit from the stomach.

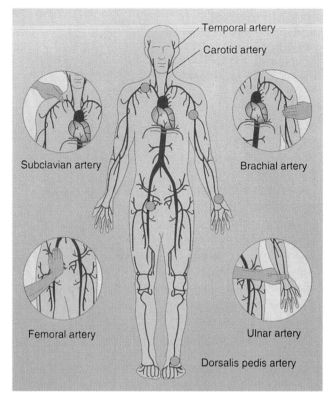

Figure 1
This figure shows pressure points; the points at which pressure can be applied to stop bleeding. Unless absolutely necessary, you should avoid applying pressure to the carotid arteries, which supply blood to the brain. Also, never apply pressure to both carotid arteries at the same time.

4. Do *not* give the victim any medications or fluids.
5. Send someone to call for emergency medical help immediately.

Nose Bleeds   To control a nosebleed, follow these steps:

1. Have the victim sit down and lean slightly forward to prevent blood from running into the throat. If you do not suspect a fracture, pinch the person's nose firmly closed using the thumb and forefinger. Keep the nose pinched for at least 5 minutes.
2. While the nose is pinched, apply a cold compress to the surrounding area.
3. If pinching does not work, gently pack the nostril with gauze or a clean strip of cloth. Do not use absorbent cotton, which will stick. Be sure that the ends of the gauze or cloth hang out so that it can be easily removed later. Once the nose is packed with gauze, pinch it closed again for another 5 minutes.
4. If the bleeding persists, seek medical attention.

Treatment for Burns

Minor Burns   For minor burns caused by fire or scalding water, apply running cold water or cold compresses for 20 to 30 minutes. Never put butter, grease, salt water, aloe vera, or topical burn ointments or sprays on burned skin. If the burned area is dirty, gently wash it with soap and water and blot it dry with a sterile dressing.

Major Burns   For major burn injuries, call for help immediately. Wrap the victim in a dry sheet. Do not clean the burns or try to remove any clothing attached to burned skin. Remove jewelry near the burned skin immediately, if possible. Keep the victim lying down and calm.

Chemical Burns   Remove clothing surrounding the burn. Wash skin that has been burned by chemicals by flushing with water for at least 20 minutes. Seek medical assistance as soon as possible.

Shock

Shock is a condition in which the cardiovascular system fails to provide sufficient blood circulation to all parts of the body. Victims of shock display the following symptoms:

- Dilated pupils
- Cool, moist skin
- Weak, rapid pulse
- Vomiting
- Delayed or unrelated responses to questions

All injuries result in some degree of shock. Therefore, treatment for shock should be given after every major injury. The following are basic steps for treating shock:

1. Have the victim life flat with his or her feet elevated approximately 8 to 12 inches. (In the case of chest injuries, difficulty breathing, or severe pain, the victim's head should be slightly elevated if there is no sign of spinal injury.)
2. Keep the victim warm. If possible, wrap him or her in blankets or other material. Also, keep the victim calm and reassured.
3. Seek medical help.

Electrical Shock

Do not touch a victim of electrical shock until the power source has been turned off. Approach the scene carefully, avoiding any live wires or electrical power lines. Pay attention to the following:

1. If the victim is holding on to the live electrical wire, do not remove it unless the power has been shut off at the plug, circuit breaker, or fuse box.

2. Check the victim's breathing and pulse. Electrical current can paralyze the nerves and muscles that control breathing and heartbeat. If necessary, give mouth-to-mouth resuscitation. If there is no pulse, CPR might be necessary. (Remember that only trained people should perform CPR.)
3. Keep the victim warm and treat for shock. Once the person is breathing and stable, seek medical help or send someone else for help.

Poisoning

Of the 1 million cases of poisoning reported in the United States each year, about 75 percent occur in children under age 5, and the majority are caused by household products. Most cases of poisoning involving adults are attempted suicides or attempted murders.

You should have emergency telephone numbers for the poison control center and the local EMS ready. Many people keep these numbers on labels on their telephones. Check the front of your telephone book for these numbers. The National Safety Council recommends that you be prepared to give the following information when calling for help:

- What was ingested? Have the container of the product and the remaining contents ready so you can describe it. You should also bring the container to the emergency room with you.
- When was the substance taken?
- How much was taken?
- Has vomiting occurred? If the person has vomited, save a sample to take to the hospital.
- Are there any other symptoms?
- How long will it take to get to the nearest emergency room?

When caring for a person who has ingested a poison, keep these basic principles in mind:

1. Maintain an open airway. Make sure the person is breathing.
2. Call the local poison control center. Follow their advice for neutralizing the poison.
3. If the poison control center or another medical authority advises inducing vomiting, then do so.
4. If a corrosive or caustic (i.e., acid or alkali) substance was swallowed, immediately dilute it by having the victim drink at least one or two 8-ounce glasses of cold water or milk.
5. Place the victim on his or her left side. This position will delay advancement of the poison into the small intestine, where absorption into the victim's circulatory system is faster.

Injuries of Joints, Muscles, and Bones

Sprains   Sprains result when ligaments and other tissues around a joint are stretched or torn. The following steps should be taken to treat sprains:

1. Elevate the injured joint to a comfortable position.
2. Apply an ice pack or cold compress to reduce pain and swelling.
3. Wrap the joint firmly with a (roller) bandage.
4. Check the fingers or toes periodically to ensure that blood circulation has not been obstructed. If the bandage is too tight, loosen it.
5. Keep the injured area elevated, and continue ice treatment for 24 hours.
6. Apply heat to the injury after 48 hours if there is no further swelling.
7. If pain and swelling continue or if a fracture is suspected, seek medical attention.

Fractures   Any deformity of an injured body part usually indicates a fracture. A fracture is any break in a bone, including chips, cracks, splinters, and complete breaks. Minor fractures (such as hairline cracks) might be difficult to detect and might be confused with sprains. If there is doubt, treat the injury as a fracture until X-rays have been taken.

Do not move the victim if a fracture of the neck or back is suspected because this could result in a spinal cord injury. If the victim must be moved, splints should be applied to immobilize the fracture, to prevent further damage, and to decrease pain. Following are some basic steps for treating fractures and applying splints to broken limbs:

1. If the person is bleeding, apply direct pressure above the site of the wound.
2. If a broken bone is exposed, do not try to move it back into the wound. This can cause contamination and further injury.
3. Do not try to straighten out a broken limb. Splint the limb as it lies.
4. The following materials are needed for splinting:

- Splint: wooden board, pillow, or rolled up magazines and newspapers
- Padding: towels, blankets, socks, or cloth
- Ties: cloth, rope, or tape

5. Place splints and padding above and below the joint. Never put padding directly over the break. Padding should protect bony areas and the soft tissue of the limb.
6. Tie splints and padding into place.
7. Check the tightness of the splints periodically. Pay attention to the skin color, temperature, and pulse below the fracture to make sure the blood flow is adequate.
8. Elevate the fracture and apply ice packs to prevent swelling and reduce pain.

Head Injuries

A head injury can result from an auto accident, a fall, an assault, or a blow from a blunt object. All head injuries can potentially lead to brain damage, which may result in a cessation of breathing and pulse.

For minor head injuries:

1. For a minor bump on the head resulting in a bruise without bleeding, apply ice to decrease the swelling.
2. If there is bleeding, apply even, moderate pressure. Because there is always the danger that the skull may be fractured, excessive pressure should not be used.
3. Observe the victim for a change in consciousness. Observe the size of pupils and not signs of inability to think clearly. Check for any signs of numbness or paralysis. Allow the victim to sleep, but wake him or her periodically to check for awareness.

For severe head injuries:

1. If the victim is unconscious, check the airway for breathing. If necessary, perform mouth-to-mouth resuscitation.
2. If the victim is breathing, check the pulse. If it is less than 55 or more than 125 beats per minute, the victim may be in danger.
3. Check for bleeding. If fluid is flowing from the ears or nose, do not stop it.
4. Do not remove any objects embedded in the victim's skull.
5. Cover the victim with blankets to maintain body temperature, but guard against overheating.
6. Seek medical help as soon as possible.

Temperature-Related Emergencies

Frostbite   Frostbite is damage to body tissues caused by intense cold. Frostbite generally occurs at temperatures below 32°F. The body parts most likely to suffer frostbite are the toes, ears, fingers, nose, and cheeks. When skin is exposed to the cold, ice crystals form beneath the skin. Avoid rubbing frostbitten tissue, because the ice crystals can scrape and break blood vessels.

To treat frostbite, follow these steps:

1. Bring the victim to a health facility as soon as possible.
2. Cover and protect the frostbitten area. If possible, apply a steady source of external warmth, such as a warm compress. The victim should avoid walking if the feet are frostbitten.
3. If the victim cannot be transported, you must rewarm the body part by immersing it in warm water (100°F to 105°F). Continue to rewarm until the frostbitten area is warm to the touch when removed from the bath. Do not allow the body part to touch the sides or bottom of the water container. After rewarming, dry gently and wrap the body part in bandages to protect from refreezing.

Hypothermia   Hypothermia is a temperature-related emergency that can be prevented with proper precautions. Hypothermia is a condition of generalized cooling of the body resulting from exposure to cold temperatures or immersion in cold water. It can occur at any temperature below 65°F and can be made more severe by wind chill and moisture. The following are key symptoms of hypothermia:

- Shivering
- Vague, slow, slurred speech
- Poor judgment
- A cool abdomen
- Lethargy, or extreme exhaustion
- Slowed breathing and heartbeat
- Numbness and loss of feeling in extremities

After contacting EMS, you should take the following steps to provide first aid to a victim of hypothermia:

1. Get the victim out of the cold.
2. Keep the victim in a flat position. Do not raise the legs.
3. Squeeze as much water from wet clothing, and layer dry clothing over wet clothing. Removal of clothing may jostle victim and lead to other problems.
4. Give the victim warm drinks only if he or she is able to swallow. Do not give the victim alcohol or caffeinated beverage, and do not allow the victim to smoke.
5. Do not allow the victim to exercise.

Temperature-related problems common in the summer months include heatstroke, heat exhaustion, and heat cramps. These conditions result from prolonged exertion or exposure to high temperatures and humidity.

Heatstroke   Heatstroke, the most serious heat-related disorder, results from the failure of the brain's heat regulating mechanism (the hypothalamus) to cool the body. The following are signs and symptoms of heatstroke:

- Rapid pulse
- Hot, dry, flushed skin (absence of sweating)
- Disorientation leading to unconsciousness
- High body temperature

As soon as these symptoms are noticed, the body temperature should be reduced as quickly as possible. The victim should be immersed in a cool bath, lake, or stream. If there is no water nearby, a fan should be used to help lower the victim's body temperature.

Heat Exhaustion   Heat exhaustion results from excessive loss of salt and water. The onset is gradual, with the following symptoms:

- Fatigue and weakness
- Anxiety
- Nausea
- Profuse sweating
- Clammy skin
- Normal body temperature

To treat heat exhaustion, move the victim to a cool place. Have the victim lie down flat, with feet elevated 8 to 12 inches. Replace lost fluids slowly and steadily. Sponge or fan victim.

Heat Cramps   Heat cramps result from excessive sweating, resulting in an excessive loss of salt and water. Although heat cramps are the least serious heat-related emergency, they are the most painful. The symptoms include muscle cramps, usually starting in the arms and legs. To relieve symptoms, the victim should drink electrolyte-rich beverages or a light salt-water solution or eat salty foods.

First-Aid Supplies

Every home, car, or boat should be supplied with a basic first-aid kit. In order to respond effectively to emergencies, you must have the basic equipment. This kit should be stored in a convenient place, but it should be kept out of the reach of children. Following is a list of supplies that should be included:

- Bandages, including triangular bandages (36 inches by 36 inches), butterfly bandages, a roller bandage, rolled white gauze bandages (2- and 3-inch width), adhesive bandages

- Sterile gauze pads and absorbent pads
- Adhesive tape (2- and 3-inch widths)
- Cotton-tip applicators
- Scissors
- Thermometer
- Antibiotic ointments
- Syrup of Ipecac (to induce vomiting)
- Aspirin
- Calamine lotion
- Antiseptic cream or petroleum jelly
- Safety pins
- Tweezers
- Flashlight
- Paper cups
- Blanket

You cannot be prepared for every medical emergency. Yet these essential tools and a knowledge of basic first aid will help you cope with many emergency situations.

References

CHAPTER 1

1. S. Cummings, K. Goodrick, and J. Foreyt, "Position of the American Dietetic Association: Weight Management," *Journal of the American Dietetic Association* 97 (1997): 71–114.
2. J. Seidell, "Dietary Fat and Obesity: An Epidemiological Perspective," *American Journal of Clinical Nutrition* 67 (1998): 546–552.
3. U.S. Department of Health and Human Services, Centers for Disease Control and Prevention (2000) (see http://www.cdc.gov/).
4. National Institute for Mental Health (2000) (see http://www.nimh.nih.gov/).
5. National Center for Health Statistics (2000) (see http://www.cdc.gov/nchs/search/search.htm).
6. Agency for Healthcare Research and Quality (AHRQ) (2000) (see http://www.ahcpr.gov/).
7. World Health Organization, "Constitution of the World Health Organization," *Chronicles of the World Health Organization* (Geneva, Switzerland, 1947).
8. R. Dubos, *So Human the Animal* (New York: Scribners, 1968), 15.
9. National Center for Health Statistics. About Healthy People 2010. NCHS http://www.cdc.gov/nchs
10. Centers for Disease Control and Prevention, Best Practices for Comprehensive Tobacco Programs—August 1999. Atlanta, GA: U.S. Department of Health and Human Services, Centers for Disease Control and Prevention, National Center for Chronic Disease Prevention, Office on Smoking and Health, August 1999. Reprinted with corrections
11. R. Donatelle and S. Prows, *The Use of Financial Incentives and Social Support to Motivate Smoking Cessation Among High-Risk Pregnant Smokers,* technical report submitted to R. W. Johnson, Smoke-Free Families Office, Birmingham, AL.
12. Adapted from "Ten Great Public Health Achievements—United States, 1900–1999," *MMWR Weekly,* 48 (12) (April, 1999): 241–243; Centers for Disease Control and Prevention. Poliomyelitis prevention in the United States. Updated recommendations of the Advisory Committee on Immunization Practices. Morbidity and Mortality Weekly Report 2000; 49 (RR-5)
13. L. Miller, "Medical Schools Put women in Curricula," *Wall Street Journal* (May 24, 1994): B1, B7.
14. E. Austin, "Women in Focus," *Shape* (September 1994): 46–47.
15. C. Tavris, *The Mismeasure of Woman* (New York: Touchstone, 1992), 99.
16. National Heart, Blood, and Lung Institute. Facts about the Women's Health Initiative. NHBLI website, http://www.nhlbi.nih.gov.
17. K. Glanz, F. Lewis, and B. Rimer, *Health Behavior and Health Education* (San Francisco: Jossey Bass, 1997), Chapter 4.
18. E. P. Sarafino, *Health Psychology* (New York: Wiley, 1990), 189–191.
19. G. D. Bishop, *Health Psychology* (Boston: Allyn and Bacon, 1994), 84–86.
20. Glanz et al., op. cit., Chapters 8 and 9.
21. Ibid.
22. R. Donatelle, S. Prows, D. Champeau, and D. Hudson, "Randomized Controlled Trial Using Social Support and Financial Incentives for High-Risk Pregnant Smokers: Significant Other Supporter (SOS) Program," *Tobacco Control* 9 Suppl. III (2000): iii, 67–69; S. Higgins et al. "Participation of Significant Others in Outpatient Behavioral Treatment Predicts Greater Cocaine Abstinence," *American Journal of Drug and Alcohol Abuse* (1994): 2047.
23. A. Ellis and M. Bernard, *Clinical Application of Rational Emotive Therapy* (New York: Plenum, 1985).
24. P. Watson and R. Tharp, *Self-Directed Behavior: Self-Modification for Personal Adjustment* (Pacific Grove, CA: Brooks/Cole, 1993), 13.

CHAPTER 2

1. National Mental Health Association, *Mental Health* (Alexandria, VA: National Mental Health Association, 1988), 3–4; W. Menninger, "Emotional Maturity," in *A Psychiatrist for a Troubled World: Selected Papers of William Menninger,* ed. B. H. Hall (New York: Viking, 1967), 789–807.
2. R. Lazarus, *Emotion and Adaptation* (New York: Oxford Press, 1991).
3. C. Ritter, "Social Supports, Social Networks, and Health Behaviors," in *Health Behavior: Emerging Research Perspectives,* ed. D. Gochman (New York: Plenum, 1988); S. Kashubeck and S. Christensen, "Parental Alcohol Use, Family Relationships Quality, Self-Esteem, and Depression in College Students," *Journal of College Health* 36 (1995): 431–445.
4. Patrick McGuire, "Seligman Touts the Art of Arguing with Yourself." American Psychological Association: T*he APA Monitor Online,* Volume 29 No. 10, October 1998.
5. M. Seligman, *Learned Optimism* (New York: Knopf, 1990).
6. Steve Proffit, "Pursuing Happiness with a Positive Outlook, not a Pill." Los Angeles Times, January, 24, 1999, http://www.apa.org/releases/pursuing.html. "Learned Optimism Yields Health Benefits" APA HelpCenter: Mind/Body Connection.
7. P. Zimbardo, A. Weber, and R. Johnson, *Psychology* (Boston: Allyn and Bacon, 2000), 403.
8. G. Wilson, P. Nathan, K. O'Leary, and L. E. Clark, *Abnormal Psychology* (Boston: Allyn and Bacon, 1996), 137.
9. Excerpted by permission from the *University of California at Berkeley Wellness Letter,* July 1992, 3–4. © Health Letter Associates, 1992.
10. S. Hawks, M. Hull, R. Thalman, and P. Richins, "Review of Spiritual Health: Definition, Role, and Intervention Strategies in Health Promotion," *American Journal of Health Promotion* 9 (5) (1995): 371–378.
11. A. Scandurra, "Everyday Spirituality: A Core Unit in Health Education and Lifetime Wellness," *Journal of Health Education* 30 (2) (1999): 104–109.
12. Ibid., 106.
13. L. Chapman, "Developing a Useful Perspective on Spiritual Health: Love, Joy, Peace and Fulfillment," *American Journal of Health Promotion* 2 (1987): 121–127.
14. Ibid., 122.
15. Ibid., 124.
16. R. Sloan, E. Bagiella, and T. Powell, "Religion, Spirituality, and Medicine," *The Lancet* 353-9153 (1999): 664–672.
17. D. Elkins, *Beyond Religion—A Personal Program for Building a Spiritual Life Outside the Walls of Traditional Religion,* (Wheaton, IL: Quest Books, 1998).
18. Ibid.
19. Ibid.
20. D. Elkins, "Spirituality: It's What's Missing in Mental Health," *Psychology Today* (September/October, 1999), 48.
21. D. G. Myers and E. Diener, "Who Is Happy?" *Psychological Science* 6 (1995): 10–19.

22. Ibid.
23. Ibid.
24. B. Fredrickson, "Cultivating Positive Emotions to Optimize Health and Well-Being." American Psychological Association: Prevention and Treatment, Volume 3, Article 0001a (March 7, 2000).
25. P. Doskoch, "Happily Ever Laughter," *Psychology Today* 29 (1996): 32–34.
26. B. Fredrickson, op cit.
27. D. Grady, "Think Right, Stay Well," *American Health* xi (1992): 50–54.
28. B. Siegel, *Love, Medicine, and Miracles* (New York: HarperCollins, 1988).
29. L. A. Lefton, *Psychology* 7th ed. (Boston: Allyn and Bacon, 2000).
30. R. Hirshchfeld et al., "The National Depressive and Manic Depressive Association Consensus Statement on the Undertreatment of Depression. *Journal of the American Medical Association* 277 (4) (1997): 333–340.
31. Lefton, op. cit., 540.
32. National Institute for Mental Health (2000) (see http://www.nimh.nih.gov/); Lefton, op. cit., 541.
33. I. Levav, R. Kohn, J. Golding, and M. Weissman, "Vulnerability of Jews to Affective Disorders," *American Journal of Psychiatry* 154 (1997): 941–947.
34. S. Wood and E. Wood, *The World of Psychology* (Boston: Allyn and Bacon, 1999), 513.
35. S. Banks and R. Kerns, "Explaining High Rates of Depression in Chronic Pain: A Diathesis–Stress Framework," *Psychological Bulletin* 119 (1996): 995–110.
36. Lefton, op. cit., 543.
37. Adapted by permission of the author from Kathryn Rose Gertz, "Mood Probe: Pinpointing the Crucial Differences between Emotional Lows and the Gridlock of Depression," *Self* (November 1990): 165–168, 204.
38. R. G. Gladstone and L. Koenig, "Sex Differences in Depression Across the High School to College Transition," *Journal of Youth and Adolescence* 23 (1994): 643–669.
39. S. Scott, "Biology and Mental Health: Why Do Women Suffer More Depression and Anxiety?" *Maclean's* (January 12, 1998): 62–64.
40. L. Rabasca, "Psychotherapy May Be as Useful as Drugs in Treating Depression, Study Suggests." American Psychological Association: The APA Monitor Online, Volume 30 No. 8, September 1999.
41. NIMH, op. cit.
42. Ibid., 13
43. "Anxiety Disorders," *USA Weekend* (October 12, 2000): 12.
44. Zimbardo et al., op. cit., 505.
45. Ibid., 506.
46. G. Wilson, P. Nathan, K. O'Leary, and L. Clark, *Abnormal Psychology* (Boston: Allyn and Bacon, 1996), 147.
47. Ibid., 147.
48. R. Saltus, "The PMS Debate," *Boston Globe Magazine* (July 25, 1999): 8–9.
49. U.S. Health Centers for Disease Control and Prevention (2000) (see http://www.cdc.gov).
50. K. Kendler and C. Gardner, "Boundaries of Major Depression: An Evaluation of DSM-IV Criteria," *American Journal of Psychiatry* 155 (1998): 172–176.
51. Lefton, op. cit., 542.

CHAPTER 3

1. H. Selye, *Stress Without Distress* (New York: Lippincott, 1974), 28–29.
2. W. Schafer, *Stress Management for Wellness,* 2nd ed. (New York: Harcourt Brace, Jovanovich, 1992).
3. R. Ader and S. Cohen, "Psychoneuroimmunology: Conditioning and Stress," *Annual Review of Psychology* 44 (1993): 53–85.

4. M. D. Jeremko, "Stress Inoculation Training: A Generic Approach for the Prevention of Stress-Related Disorders," *The Personal and Guidance Journal* 62 (1984): 544–550; H. S. Freidman, and S. Booth-Kewley, "The Disease-Prone Personality: A Meta-analytic View of the Construct." *American Psychologist* 42 (1987): 539–555.
5. G. E. Vaillant, *Adaptation to Life* (Boston: Little, Brown, 1977).
6. S. A. Lyness, "Predictions of Differences Between Type A and B Individuals in Heart Rate and Blood Pressure Reactivity," *Psychological Bulletin* 114 (1993): 266–295; J. C. Barefoot and M. Schroll, "Symptoms of Depression, Acute Myocardial Infraction, and Total Mortality in a Community Sample, 1976–1980," *Circulation* 93 (1996); Schiraldi, G. T. Spalding, and C. Holford, "Expanding Health Educators' Roles to Meet Critical Needs in Stress Management and Mental Health," *Journal of Health Education* (1998): 70.
7. R. Glaser, B. Rabin, M. Chesney, S. Cohen, and B. Natelson, "Updates Linking Evidence and Experience: Stress-Induced Immunomodulation," *Journal of the American Medical Association* 281 (24) (1999): 2268–2270.
8. B. Rabin, *Stress, Immune Function, and Health: The Connection.* (New York: Wiley-Liss, 1999).
9. D. Padgett, J. Sheridan, J. Dome, G. Berntson, J. Candelora, and R. Glaser, "Social Stress and the Reactivation of Latent Herpes Simplex Virus-Type 1," *Proceedings of the National Academy of Sciences, USA* 9 (1998): 7231–7235.
10. J. Kiecolt-Glaser, R. Glaser, S. Gravenstein, W. Malarkey, and J. Sheridan, "Chronic Stress Alters the Immune Response to Influenza Virus Vaccines in Older Adults," *Proceedings of the National Academy of Sciences, USA* 93 (1996): 3043–3047.
11. R. Glaser, J. Kiecolt-Glaser, W. Malarkey, and J. Sheridan, "The Influence of Psychological Stress on the Immune Response to Vaccines," *Annals of the N.Y. Academy of Sciences* 840 (1998): 649–655.
12. S. Cohen, E. Frank, W. Doyle, D. Skoner, B. Rabin, and J. Gwaltney, "Types of Stressors That Increase Susceptibility to the Common Cold in Adults." *Health Psychology* 17 (1998): 214–223.
13. S. Cohen, W. Doyle, D. Skoner, B. Rabin, and J. Gwaltney, "Social Ties and Susceptibility to the Common Cold," *Journal of the American Medical Association* 277 (1997): 1940–1944.
14. R. Kessler, "The Effects of Stressful Life Events on Depression," *Annual Reviews of Psychology* 48 (1997): 191–214.
15. Schiraldi et al., op cit., 69.
16. T. Holmes and R. Rahe, "The Social Readjustment Rating Scale," *Journal of Psychosocial Research* (1967): 213–217.
17. Ibid., 214.
18. R. Lazarus, "The Trivialization of Distress," in *Preventing Health Risk Behaviors and Promoting Coping with Illness,* ed. J. Rosen and L. Solomon (Hanover, NH: University Press of New England, 1985), 279–298.
19. L. Lefton, *Psychology* (Boston: Allyn and Bacon, 1994), 471.
20. M. Kenny and K. Rice, "Attachment to Parents and Adjustment in College Students: Current Status, Applications, and Future Considerations," *Counseling-Psychologist* 23 (1995): 433–456.
21. R. C. Kessler, K. S. Kendler, A. C. Heath, M. C. Neale, and L. J. Eaves, "Social Support, Depressed Mood, and Adjustment to Stress: A Genetic Epidemiological Investigation," *Journal of Personality and Social Psychology* 62 (1992): 257–272.
22. M. Friedman and R. H. Rosenman, *Type A Behavior and Your Heart* (New York: Knopf, 1974).
23. R. Ragland and R. Brand, "Distrust, Rage May Be Toxic Cores That Put Type A Person at Risk," *Journal of the American Medical Association* 261 (1989): 813, 814.
24. P. L. Rice, *Stress and Health* (Monterey, CA: Brooks/Cole, 1992), 471.
25. Ibid.
26. L. Towbes and L. Cohen, "Chronic Stress in the Lives of College Students: Scale Development and Prospective Prediction of Distress," *Journal of Youth and Adolescence* 25 (1996): 206–217.

27. C. Crandell, J. Preisler, and J. Ausspring, "Measuring Life Event Stress in the Lives of College Students: The Undergraduate Stress Questionnaire (USQ)," *Journal of Behavioral Medicine* 15 (1992): 627–642.

28. "Hearts and Minds," *Harvard Mental Health Letter,* 14 (1997): 1-4.

29. Towbes and Cohen, op. cit., 209.

CHAPTER 4

1. D. Zucchio, "Today's Violent Crime Is an Old Story with a New Twist," *San Jose Mercury News* (November 21, 1994), transmitted via America Online.

2. Bureau of Justice Statistics, "Expenditures and Employment Report: 1997" (Washington, D.C.: U.S. Department of Justice, 1998) (http://www.ojp.usdoj.gov/bjs/).

3. L. Cohen and S. Swift, "A Public Health Approach to the Violence Epidemic in the United States," *Environment and Urbanization* (October 1993): 1–12; L. Lamberg, "Prediction of Violence Both Art And Science," *Journal of the American Medical Association* 275 (1996): 1712–1715; D. Elliot, op. cit.; D. P. Barash, *Understanding Violence* (Boston: Allyn and Bacon, 2001), 118–122.

4. M. Leeds, Violence Prevention Conference (1996), Linnfield Community College, McMinnville, OR.

5. Ibid.

6. Ibid.

7. Lamberg, op. cit., 1713.

8. Leeds, op. cit.

9. Ibid.

10. Ibid.

11. F. Rivera, B. Mueller, G. Somas, Mendosa, and C. N. Rushfork, "Alcohol and Illicit Drugs and the Risk of Violent Death in the Home," *Journal of the American Medical Association* 278 (1997): 569–572.

12. "Substance Abuse: A Significant Characteristic in Domestic Violence Assailants," *Brown University Digest of Addiction Theory and Application* 16: 1–3.

13. M. Swartz, J. Swanson, et al., "Violence and Severe Mental Illness: The Effects of Substance Abuse and Non-Adherence to Medication," *American Journal of Psychiatry* 155 (1998): 226.

14. Rivera et al., op. cit., 571.

15. U. S. Center for Health Statistics, "Health, United States, 2000, (Atlanta, GA: Centers for Disease Control and Prevention, 2000).

16. Ibid.

17. Ibid., 44.

18. Ibid., 46.

19. R. Lacyo, "Still Under the Gun?" *Time* (July 6, 1998): 32–56.

20. FBI, *Crime in the United States—1998* (Washington, DC: Government Printing Office, 1999).

21. R. Fenske and L. Gordon, "Reducing Racial and Ethnic Hate Crimes on Campus: The Need for Community," in *Violence on Campus: Defining the Problems, Strategies for Action,* ed. A. Hoffman et al. (Gaithersburg, MD: Aspen, 1998).

22. Ibid.

23. Ibid.

24. National Center for Domestic Violence and Abuse. Fact Sheet (2000).

25. Ibid.

26. J. Barley et al., "Risk Factors for Violent Death in the Home," *Archives of Internal Medicine* 157 (1997): 786.

27. D. Brookkoff, K. Obrien, C. Cook, T. Thompson, and C. Williams, "Characteristics of Participants in Domestic Violence: Assessment at the Scene of Domestic Violence," *Journal of the American Medical Association* 277 (1997): 1369.

28. "Injury and Domestic Violence Prevention," *Nurse Practitioner* 22 (1997): 122.

29. F. Trevino, S. Walker, and G. Ramirez, "Violent Crime in American Society," in *Violence on Campus: Defining the Problems,* *Strategies for Action,* ed. A. Hoffman et al. (Gaithersburg, MD: Aspen, 1998); Federal Bureau of Investigation, *Uniform Crime Report* (Washington DC: U.S. Department of Justice, 1997).

30. A. Joerger and L. McClellan, "Why Men Batter: Why Women Stay," *Community Safety Quarterly* 5 (1992): 22–23.

31. N. West, "Crimes Against Women," *Community Safety Quarterly* 5 (1992): 3.

32. M. A. Straus and R. Gelles, eds., *Physical Violence in American Families: Risk Factors and Adaptations to Violence in 8,145 Families* (New Brunswick, NJ: Transaction, 1993), 101–201.

33. H. Pan, P. Neidig, and K. O'Leary, "Physical Aggression in Early Marriage: Pre-relationship and Relationship Effects," *Journal of Consulting and Clinical Psychology.*

34. G. T. Wilson, P. Nathan, K. D. O'Leary, and L. A. Clark, *Abnormal Psychology* (Boston: Allyn and Bacon, 1996).

35. Ibid.

36. Ibid.

37. E. Newberger, "Child Sexual Abuse," in *Violence in America: A Public Health Approach,* ed. M. Rosenberg and M. Fenley (New York: Oxford University Press, 1991), 85.

38. M. Whittaker, "The Continuum of Violence Against Women: Psychological and Physical Consequences," *Journal of American College Health* 40 (1992): 155.

39. D. Finkelhor, "Child Sexual Abuse," in *Violence in America: A Public Health Approach,* ed. M. Rosenberg and M. Fenley (New York: Oxford University Press, 1991), 25.

40. N. West, "Children: The Invisible Victims of Domestic Violence," *Community Safety Quarterly* 5 (1992): 20.

41. Whittaker, op. cit., 152.

42. K. Hunnicutt, "Women and Violence on Campus," in *Violence on Campus: Defining the Problems, Strategies for Action,* ed. A. Hoffman et al. (Gaithersburg, MD: Aspen, 1998), 150.

43. Ibid., 149.

44. A. Berkowitz, "College Men as Perpetrators of Acquaintance Rape and Sexual Assault: A Review of Recent Literature," *Journal of American College Health* 40 (1992): 175.

45. J. Lenssen, "Update on Violence Statistics for Young Adults," Violence Prevention Summer Institute (2000), Corvallis, OR.

46. N. Neft and A. Levine, *Where Women Stand—An International Report on the Status of Women in 140 Countries,* 1997–1998 (New York: Random House, 1997).

47. A. Hoffman, J. Schuh, and R. Fenske, *Violence on Campus* (Gaithersburg, MD: Aspen, 1998), 149–168.

48. D. Benson, C. Charlton, and F. Goohart, "Acquaintance Rape on Campus: A Literature Review," *Journal of American College Health* (1992): 157.

49. Benson et al., op. cit., 158.

50. M. W. Leidig, "The Continuum of Violence Against Women: Psychological and Physical Consequences," *Journal of American College Health* 40 (1992): 151. Reprinted with permission of the Helen Dwight Reid Education Foundation. Published by Heldref Publications, 1319 Eighteenth Street NW, Washington, DC 20036-1802. Copyright © 1992.

51. Berkowitz, op. cit., 177.

52. Ibid., 175.

53. Whittaker, op. cit., 153–154.

54. Berkowitz, op. cit., 718.

55. Ibid., 175.

56. Ibid., 176.

57. Hoffman et al., op. cit., 1–40.

58. Ibid., 175.

59. Ibid., 183.

60. J. Baier, M. Rosenzweig, and E. Shipple, "Patterns of Sexual Behavior, Coercion, and Victimization of University Students," *Journal of College Student Development* 32 (1991): 178.

61. M. Koss, "Rape: Scope, Impact, Interventions, and Public Policy Responses," *American Psychologist* 48 (1993): 1062–1069.

62. Hoffman et al., op. cit., 242.

63. E. Dersinger, C. Cychosz, and L. Jaeger, "Strategies for Dealing with Campus Violence," in *Violence on Campus: Defining the Problems, Strategies for Action,* ed. A. Hoffman et al. (Gaithersburg, MD: Aspen, 1998).

64. A. Matthews, "Campus Crime 101," *Eugene Register Guard* (March 1993): 4B.

65. Dersinger et al., op. cit., 248.

66. B. Moyers, "What Can We Do About Violence?" Public Broadcasting Service, January 1995.

67. "National Census of Fatal Occupational Injuries, 1997." Bureau of Labor Statistics, U.S. Department of Labor.

68. "National Census of Fatal Occupational Injuries, 1999." Bureau of Labor Statistics. US. Dept. of Labor.

CHAPTER 5

1. G. Goenthals, S. Worchel, and L. Heatherington, *Pathways to Personal Growth: Adjustments in Today's World* (Boston: Allyn and Bacon, 1999), 480.

2. Living Longer. Healthy Links: Invest in Relationships." MayoClinic.com. Copyright 2001 Mayo Foundation for Medical Education and Research (MFMER). http://www.mayohealth.org/.

3. Gudy Kunst, W.B.; Nishida, T. Anxiety, uncertainty, and perceives effectiveness of communication across relationship and cultures. International Journal of Incultural Relations. Jan. 2001. Vol. 25 (1) Pp 55–71.

4. D. Tannen, You Just Don't Understand: Women and Men in Conversation (New York: William Morrow, 1990).

5. S. L. Michaud and R. M. Warner, "Gender Differences in Self-Reported Response in Troubles Talk," *Sex Roles: A Journal of Research,* 37 (1997): 527–541: D. J. Canary and M. J. Cody, *Interpersonal Communication* (New York: St. Martin's 1994), 528.

6. C. Snapp and M. Leary, Hurt feelings among new acquaintances: moderating effects of interpersonal familiarity. Journal of Social and Personal Relationships. June 2001. (Vol. 18, 3), p 1344–1350.

7. Manusov, Valerie, and J. Harvey, Attributors, communication behavior and relationships. 2001. Cambridge University Press. New York, New York.

8. S. S. Brehm, *Intimate Relationships* (New York: McGraw Hill, 1992), 4–5.

9. L. Lefton, *Psychology* (Boston: Allyn and Bacon, 2000), 480.

10. Ibid., 481.

11. C. Weiskopf, "Real Friends," *Current Health* 24 (1998): 16–18.

12. J. Turner and L. Rubinson, *Contemporary Human Sexuality* (Englewood Cliffs, NJ: Prentice Hall, 1993), 457.

13. Ibid., 457.

14. G. Levinger, "Can We Picture Love?" in *The Psychology of Love,* ed. R. J. Sternberg and M. Barnes (New Haven: Yale University Press, 1988), 139–159.

15. E. Hatfield, "Passionate and Companionate Love," in *Psychology of Love,* ed. R. J. Sternberg and M. Barnes (New Haven: Yale University Press, 1988), 191–217.

16. R. A. Baron and D. Byrne, *Social Psychology* (Boston: Allyn and Bacon, 1997), 290–295.

17. E. Hatfield and G. W. Walster, *A New Look at Love* (Reading, MA: Addison Wesley, 1981).

18. Sternberg, R. "The Triangular Theory of Love," 1986.

19. A. Toufexis and P. Gray, "What Is Love? The Right Chemistry," *Time* (1993), 47–52.

20. Ibid., 51.

21. Ibid., 49.

22. H. Fisher, *Anatomy of Love: The Natural History of Monogamy, Adultery, and Divorce* (New York: Norton, 1993).

23. E. Hatfield, *Love, Sex, and Intimacy: Their Psychology, Biology, and History* (Reading, MA: Addison-Wesley, 1993).

24. D. Tannen, *You Just Don't Understand: Women and Men in Conversation* (New York: William Morrow, 1990).

25. Machaud and Warner, op. cit., 528; Kay Palsey, Jennifer Kerpelman, Doug Guilbert. Gender conflict; identity disruption and marital instability. Expanding Gottman's model/ Journal of Social and Personal Relationships. Feb. 2001, vol. 18, No. 1, p. 1107-1114; Linda C. Gallo and timothy W. Smith. Attachment style in marriage: adjustments and responses to interaction. Journal of Social and Personal Relationships. April 2001, vol. 18, No. 2, p.1231–1237; Manusov, Valerie and John Harvey (eds.). Attribution, communication behavior and close relationships. 2001. Cambridge University Press. New York.

26. M. McGill, *The McGill Report on Male Intimacy* (New York: Holt, Rinehart and Winston, 1985), 87–88.

27. C. Morris, *Understanding Psychology* (Englewood Cliffs, NJ: Prentice Hall, 1993).

28. McGill, op. cit., 87–88.

29. M. Klausner and B. Hasselbring, *Aching for Love: The Sexual Drama of the Adult Child* (New York: Harper and Row, 1990).

30. Brehm, op. cit., 263.

31. B. Strong, C. DeVaul, and B. Sayad, *Human Sexuality* (Mountain View, CA: Mayfield Publishing, 1999), 219.

32. U.S. Census Bureau, U.S. Department of Commerce. World Almanac & Book of Facts. U.S. Median Age at First Marriage 2001, p.876.

33. A.P. Greeff and H.L., Malherbe, "Intimacy and Marital Satisfaction in Spouses," *Journal of Sex and Marital Therapy* 27 (May-June 2001, Special Issue): 247–257; "IS Your Love Life Making You Sick?" *Ebony* (July 2001): 38–41; L. Waite and M. Gallagher, *The Case for Marriage: Why Married People Are Healthier, Happier, and Better Off Financially* (New York: Doubleday, 2000).

34. M. Young, G Denny, T. Young, and R. Tuquis, "Sexual Satisfaction Among Married Women," *American Journal of Health Studies* 16 (2) (2000): 73-78.

35. R. Alsop, "As Same-Sex Households Grow More Mainstream, Businesses Take Note," *Wall Street Journal* August 8, 2001, B1, B4.

36. Ibid.

37. Ibid.

38. Centers of Disease Control and Prevention, Advanced Data, "First Marriages Dissolution, Divorce, and Remarriage, United States.," May 31, 2001, 323.

39. Alsop, op. cit.

40. National Vital Statistics Report. Vol. 49 no. 6, August 2001. Centers for Disease Control.

41. National Center for Health Statistics and U.S. Census Bureau. 2001. http://www.cdc.gov/nchs/fastats/divroce.htm

42. H. Marano, "Love Lessons: 6 New Moves to Improve Your Relationship," *Psychology Today* (March/April 1997): 42–49.

43. A. H. Slyper, "Childhood Obesity, Adipose Tissue Distribution, and the Pediatric Practitioner," *Pediatrics* 102 (1998): 4.

44. Mayo Foundation for Medical Education and Research, "HRT: A Risk/Benefit Analysis" (2000) (see www.mayohealth.org/mayo/0003/htm/hrt.htm).

45. American Psychological Association (see http://www.apa.org/monitor/oct97/conversion.html/).

46. D. J. Bem, "Exotic Becomes Erotic: A Developmental Theory of Sexual Orientation," *Psychological Review* 103 (2) (1996): 320–335; J. P. DeCecco and D. A. Parker, "The Biology of Homosexuality: Sexual Orientation or Sexual Preference?" *Journal of Homosexuality* 28 (1995): 1–28; G. Haumann, "Homosexuality, Biology, and Ideology," *Journal of Homosexuality* 28 (1) (1995): 57–77; S. LeVay, *Queer Science: The Use and Abuse of Research into Homosexuality* (Cambridge, MA: MIT Press, 1996).

47. G. M. Herek, J. Roy Gillis, and J. C. Cogan, "Psychological Sequelae of Hate-Crime Victimization Among Lesbian, Gay, and Bisexual Adults," *Journal of Consulting and Clinical Psychology* 67 (6) (1999): 945–951.

48. G. F. Kelly, "Sexual Individuality and Sexual Values," in *Sexuality Today: The Human Perspective* Dubuque, IA: McGraw Hill, 1998), 203–206.

49. Ibid.
50. R. T. Michael, J. H. Gagnon, E. O. Laumann, and G. Kolata, *Sex in America: A Definitive Survey* (Boston: Little, Brown, 1994).
51. Ibid.
52. J. G. Beck, "Hypoactive Sexual Desire Disorder: An Overview" *Journal of Consulting and Clinical Psychology* 36 (6) (1995): 919–927.
53. B. Handy, "The Potency Pill," *Time* (May 4, 1998): 50–57.
54. Arnot Ogden Medical Center, "Frequently Asked Questions" (1998) http://www.aomc.org/HOD2/general/ViagraFAQ.html.
55. S. A. Lyman, C. Hughes-McLain, and G. Thompson, " 'Date-Rape Drugs': A Growing Concern," *Journal of Health Education* 29 (5) (1998): 271–274.

CHAPTER 6

1. Centers for Disease Control, Contraceptive Options: Increasing Your Awareness (Washington, D.C.: NAACOG, 1990).
2. University of Southern California School of Medicine, "Non-contraceptive Health Benefits," *Dialogues in Contraception* 3 (1990): 2.
3. National Center for Health Statistics, "Fertility, Family Planning, and Women's Health," 23 (1997): 7.
4. K.N. Anderson, *Mosby's Medical, Nursing & Allied Health Dictionary* (W.B. Saunders Co., 2002).
5. "FDA Approves Emergency Contraceptive Kit," College Health Report 1 (1998): 8.
6. Boston Women's Health Collective, *Our Bodies Ourselves for the New Century: A Book by Women and for Women* (New York: Simon and Schuster, 1998).
7. P. Gober, "The Role of Access in Explaining State Abortion Rates," *Social Science and Medicine* 44 (1997): 7.
8. Allan Guttmacher Institute, "Facts in Brief: Induced Abortion" (2000) (see www.agi-usa.org).
9. J. Gans Epner, H. Jonas, and D. Seckinger, "Late Term Abortion," *Journal of the American Medical Association* 280 (1998): 726.
10. Ibid., 728.
11. D. A. Grimes and R. J. Cook, "Mifepristone (RU-486)—An Abortifacient to Prevent Abortion?" *New England Journal of Medicine,* 8 October 1992, 1041–1044.
12. C. O. Byer, L. W. Shainberg, and G. Galliano, *Dimensions of Human Sexuality* (Boston: McGraw-Hill College, 1999), 489.
13. K. Schmidt, "The Dark Legacy of Fatherhood," U.S. News and World Report (December 14, 1992): 94–95.
14. "USDA Report Estimates Child Born in 1999 will Cost $160,140 to Raise," Press Release No. 0138.00, U.S. Department of Agriculture, (see www.usda.gov/cnpp).
15. Baby Center Website "College Savings Calculator," (2000) (see http://www.babycenter.com/live/calculator.html).
16. U.S. Department of Health and Human Services, *The Health Benefits of Smoking Cessation: A Report of the Surgeon General* (Washington, DC: Government Printing Office, 1990).
17. Centers for Disease Control & Prevention. Women and Smoking: A Report of the Surgeon General, 2001. "Cigarette Smoking Among Pregnant Women." CDC.gov/tobacco.
18. National Center for Health Statistics, op. cit., 19.
19. National Down Syndrome Society (1998): (http://www.ndss.org/).
20. M. Avery, L. Duckett, J. Dodgson, K. Savik, and S. Henly, "Factors Associated with Very Early Weaning Among Primiparas Intending to Breastfeed," *Maternal and Child Health Journal* 2 (1998): 167–179.
21. E. Nagourney, "New Guidelines for Reducing Caesareans," *New York Times* (September 5, 2000): 8.
22. R. Hatcher, J. Trussell, F. Stewart, W. Cates, G. Stewart, F. Guess, and D. Kowal, *Contraceptive Technology,* 17th rev. ed. (New York: Ardent Media, Inc., 1998), 204.
23. Boyer et. Al., op. cit., 196.

CHAPTER 7

1. U.S. Department of Health and Human Services, Substance Abuse and Mental Health Services Administration (SAMHSA), "Substance Abuse: A National Health Challenge," October 4, 2001, http://www.samhsa.gov/oas/oas.html/.
2. Ibid.
3. H.F. Doweiko, *Concepts of Chemical Dependency* (Pacific Grove, CA: Brooks/cole,1993), 9.
4. C. Nakken, *The Addictive Personality* (Center City, MN: Hazelden, 1996), 24.
5. J Shuster, "Insomnia: Understanding Its Pharmacological Treatment Options," *Pharmacy Times* 62 (1996): 67–76.
6. Food & Drug Administration, "Phenylpropanolamine (PPA) Information Page," http://www.fda.gov/cder/drug/infopage/ppa/default.htm.
7. U.S. Department of Health and Human Services, "National Household Survey on Drug Abuse Main Findings 1998" (Washington, D.C.: Author, 2000).
8. Ibid.
9. National Institute of Health, Substance Abuse and Mental Health Services Administration (SAMHSA), "National Household Survey on Drug Abuse," 2000, http://www.samhsa.gov/oas.html, October, 2001 document as part of the "Monitoring of the Future."
10. Ibid.
11. M. Fishman and C. Johanson, "Cocaine," in *Pharmacological Aspects of Drug Dependence: Towards an Integrated Neurobehavior Approach (Handbook of Experimental Pharmacology),* ed. C. Schuster and M. Kuhar (Hamburg: Springer Verlag, 1996), 159–195.
12. Ibid.
13. National Institute on Drug Abuse, *Capsules* (1996).
14. National Institute on Drug Abuse, "Methamphetamines, 016," *Infofax* (1998): 1.
15. L. Morrow, "Kids and Pot," *Time* (December 9, 1996): 36.
16. "Your Health: Marijuana as Medicine," *Consumer Reports* (May 1997): 1–4.
17. American Academy of Ophthalmology, Medical Library, Medical Library, "The Use of Marijuana in the Treatment of Glaucoma," http://www.medem.com/MedLB/article_detaillb.cfm?article_ID = ZZZXIEOMH4C&sub_cat-1.
18. R. Mathias, "Marijuana Impairs Driving-Related Skills and Workplace Performance," *NIDA Notes* 11 (1) (January/February 1996): 6.
19. National Institute on Drug Abuse, "Heroin, 0–12," *Infofax* (1998): 1.
20. National Institute on Drug Abuse, "National Survey Results on Drug Use, 1975–1999," op. cit.
21. National Institute on Drug Abuse, "NIDA Launches Initiative to Combat Club Drugs," *NIDA Notes* 14 (2) (2000).
22. U. S. Department of Justice, Drug Enforcement Administration, Drug Abuse Warning Network (DAWN), 2000, http://www.usdoj.gov/dea/concern/mdma.htm.
23. National Institute on Drug Abuse, "Anabolic Steroid Abuse," *NIDA Research Report Series* (2000).
24. National Institute on Drug Abuse, "Costs to Society," *NIDA Infofax* (1998).
25. National Institute on Drug Abuse, "Worker Drug Use and Workplace Policies and Programs: Results from the 1994 and 1997 National Household Survey on Drug Abuse" (1999).
26. Ibid.

CHAPTER 8

1. L. D. Johnson, P. M. O'Malley, and J. G. Bachman, *The Monitoring the Future Study, 1975–1999,* vol. 2 (Rockville, MD: NIDA, 2000), 71.
2. A. Cohen, "Battle of the Binge," *Time* (September 8, 1997).
3. H. Wechsler et al., "College Binge Drinking in the 1990s: A Continuing Problem," *Journal of American College Health* 28 (2000): 202.
4. Johnson et al., op. cit., 19.
5. H. Wechsler et al., op. cit.

6. Ibid., 201.

7. National Institute on Alcohol Abuse and Alcoholism, "Apparent Per Capita Alcohol Consumption: National, State, and Regional Trends, 1997–98." *Surveillance Report* 55 (December 2000).

8. T. Katsouyanni et al., "Ethanol and Breast Cancer: An Association That May Be Both Confounded and Causal," *International Journal of Cancer* 58 (3):(1994) 356–361.

9. C. Ikonomidou et al., "Ethanol-Induced Apoptotic Neurodegeneration and the Fetal Alcohol Syndrome," *Science* 287 (2000): 1056–1060.

10. National Highway Traffic Safety Administration, "Traffic Safety Facts," 1998, 1999.

11. H. Wechsler et al., "Changes in Binge Drinking and Related Problems Among American College Students Between 1993 and 1997," *Journal of American College Health* 47 (2) (1998): 57–68.

12. National Highway Traffic Safety Administration, "Traffic Safety Facts" 1996, Alcohol, Washington, DC: National Center for Statistics and Analysis, 1997.

13. National Highway Traffic Safety Administration, "Traffic Safety Facts," 1998, 1999.

14. Ibid.

15. Insurance Institute for Highway Safety. "Fatality Facts: Alcohol." October, 2000.

16. F. K. Goodwin and E. M. Gause, "Alcohol, Drug Abuse, and Mental Health Administration," *Prevention Pipeline* 3 (1990): 19.

17. Shockit, Marc A., "New Findings on Genetics of Alcoholism," *Journal of American Medical Association,* 281 (20) (1999): 1875-1976.

18. "Adult Children of Alcoholics," *Alcohol Issues and Solutions* 6 (2) (2000): 6.

19. B. F. Grant, "Estimates of U. S. Children Exposed to Alcohol Abuse and Dependence in the Family," *American Journal of Public Health,* 90 (1) (2000).

20. U.S. Department of Health and Human Services, *Ninth Special Report to the U.S. Congress on Alcohol and Health* (1997): 261.

21. E. Gomberg, "Women and Alcohol: Issues for Prevention Research," *National Institute on Alcohol Abuse and Alcohol Research Monograph* 32 (1996): 185–214.

22. Ibid.

23. J. M. McGinnis and W. H. Foege, "Actual Causes of Death in the United States," *Journal of the American Medical Association* 270 (1993): 2207–2212.

24. American Lung Association, "Trends in Cigarette Smoking," March 1999.

25. Centers for Disease Control and Prevention, "Trends in Cigarette Smoking Among High School Students—United States, 1991–1999," *Morbidity and Mortality Weekly* 49 (2000): 755–758.

26. U.S. Department of Health and Human Services, "Targeting Tobacco Use: The Nation's Leading Cause of Death," Centers for Disease Control and Prevention, 1998, 2.

27. N. Rigotti, J. Lee, and H. Wechsler, "U.S. College Students' Use of Tobacco Products," *Journal of the American Medical Association* 284 (2000): 699–705.

28. Everett, et. Al., "Smoking Initiation and Smoking Patterns Among U. S. College Students," *Journal of American College Health,* 48 (1999): 55.

29. American Cancer Society, Tobacco Information: Cigar Smoking and Cancer, 1998.

30. American Lung Association, op. cit.

31. S. Hansen, The University of Iowa Student Health Service Website, downloaded August 21, 2000.

32. National Institutes of Health, *Smokeless Tobacco or Health,* Monograph 2 (May 1993): 3

33. American Cancer Society, "Cancer Facts and Figures" (2000), 18.

34. American Cancer Society, op. cit.

35. "Study Links Smoking to Pancreatic Cancer," *Science News* (October 22, 1994): 261.

36. WHO Collaborative Study of Cardiovascular Disease and Steroid Hormone Contraception, "Acute Myocardial Infraction and Combined Oral Contraceptives: Results of an International Multicentre Case-Control Study," *Lancet* (April 26, 1997): 1202–1209.

37. American Cancer Society, op. cit.

38. NIDA Notes, "Nicotine Conference Highlights Research Accomplishments and Challenges" (September/October 1995): 11–12.

39. American Lung Association Website, "Secondhand Smoke" (see http://ala.org.).

40. K. Steenland, "Passive Smoking and the Risk of Heart Disease," *Journal of the American Medical Association* 267 (1992): 94–99.

41. P. Hilts, "Wide Peril Is Seen in Passive Smoking, *New York Times* (May 9, 1990): A25.

42. American Lung Association Website, op. cit.

43. D. Mannino, "Children Exposed to ETS Miss More School," *Tobacco Control* (May 1996).

44. The State Tobacco Information Center at http://stic.neu.edu. National Association of Attorneys General, "Multistate Settlement with Tobacco Industry." Downloaded August 23, 2000.

45. "Nicotine Patches Seen to Help Smokers Quit," *Boston Globe* (June 23, 1994): 3.

46. "Grounds for Breaking the Coffee Habit," *Tufts University Diet and Nutrition Newsletter* 7 (1990): 4.

47. "Fetal Loss Associated with Caffeine," *Fact and Comparisons Drug Newsletter* 13 (March 1994): 39.

CHAPTER 9

1. Oregon Dairy Council, Nutrition Education Services, "Quotable Nutrition: It's All About You," news press release, 1998.

2. J. Beary and R. Donatelle, unpublished doctoral dissertation, 1994, Oregon State University.

3. C. Georgiou et al., "Among Young Adults, College Students and Graduates Practiced More Healthful Habits and Made More Healthful Food Choices Than Did Non-Students," *Journal of the American Dietetic Association* 97 (1997): 754–762.

4. E. Whitney and S. Rolfes, *Understanding Nutrition,* 8th ed. (San Francisco: Wadsworth, 1999), 3–4.

5. National Center for Health Statistics, *Prevalence of Overweight and Obesity Among Adults: United States* (1999) (see http://www.cdc.gov/nchs/products/pubs/pubd/hestats/obese/obse99.htm).

6. Ludwig, D., Obesity: A New Dietary Treatment for a Major Public Health Threat. Linus Pauling. Institute International Conference. Diet & Optimum Health. May 2001. Portland OR

7. International Conference on Diet and Optimum Health: The Linus Pauling Institute, Portland Oregon. May, 2001. Willett, Walter, *Eat, Drink, and Be Healthy,* (Simon and Schuster, 2001).

8. "Proteins," Harvard Women's Health Watch, 5 (1998): 4.

9. Ibid., 4.

10. J. W. White and M. Wolraich, "Effect of Sugar on Behavior or Cognition in Children: A Meta-Analysis," *Journal of the American Medical Association* 274 (1995): 1617–1621.

11. Food, Nutrition, and the Prevention of Cancer: A Global Perspective (World Cancer Research Fund and the American Institute for Cancer Research, 1997); C. Fuchs et al., "Dietary Fiber and the Risk of Colorectal Cancer and Adenoma in Women," *New England Journal of Medicine* 340 (1999): 169–176.

12. Ibid., 170.

13. R. Mensink and M. Katan, "Effect of Dietary Trans-Fatty Acids on High-Density and Low-Density Lipoprotein and Cholesterol Levels in Healthy Subject," *New England Journal of Medicine* (August 16, 1990).

14. G. Ruoff, "Reducing Fat Intake with Fat Substitutes," *American Family Physician* 43 (1991): 1235–1242.

15. *Food, Nutrition and the Prevention of Cancer,* op. cit., 532.

16. W. Willet and A. Ascherio, "Health Effects of Trans-Fatty Acids," *American Journal of Clinical Nutrition* 66 (1997): 1006S–1010S.

17. Whitney and Rolfes, op. cit., 144.

18. American Heart Association, Nutrition Advisory Committee, News Release, on trans-fatty acids, May 13, 1994.
19. Willet and Ascherio, op. cit., 1997.
20. Whitney and Rolfes, op. cit., 144.
21. J. Midgley, A. Matthew, C. Greenwood, and A. Logan, "Effects of Reduced Dietary Sodium on Blood Pressure: A Meta-Analysis of Randomized Controlled Trials," *Journal of the American Medical Association* 275 (1996): 1590–1598.
22. Whitney and Rolfes, op. cit., 412.
23. A. C. Looker et al., "Prevalence of Iron Deficiency in the United States, *Journal of the American Medical Association* 277 (1997): 973–976; "Recommendations to Prevent and Control Iron Deficiency in the United States," *Morbidity and Mortality Weekly Report* 47 (1998 supplement).
24. G. T. Sempos, A. C. Looker, and R. E. Gillum, "Iron and Heart Disease: the Epidemiological Data," *Nutrition Reviews* 54 (1996): 73–84.
25. Whitney and Rolfes, op. cit., 412.
26. "Food as Medicine," *Harvard Women's Health Watch* 5 (1998): 4–5.
27. Blumber, J., Changing Vitamin Requirements. Paper presented at the Linus Pauling Institute's Diet & Optimum Health Conference.; Kolonel, L., Overview of Diet and Cancer Epidemiology 2001. Paper presented at the Linus Pauling Institute's Diet & Optimum Health Conference 2001.; Gould, M., The Anticancer Effects of Plant Monoterpenes 2001. Paper presented at the Linus Pauling Institute's Diet & Optimum Health Conference 2001.; Potter, J., Diet and Colorectal Cancer, 2001. Paper presented at the Linus Pauling Institute's Diet & Optimum Health Conference 2001.
28. "Food as Medicine," op. cit., 5.
29. J. Smythies, *Every Person's Guide to Antioxidants* (Newark, NJ: Rutgers University Press, 1998).
30. Ibid.
31. Frie, op. cit.
32. Ibid.
33. Ibid.
34. Balz, F., Closing Remarks-Summary. 2001. Paper presented at the Linus Pauling Institute's Diet & Optimum Health Conference, May, 2001.
35. Malinow, R., Hompcysteine, Folic Acid and CVD, 2001. Linus Pauling Institute's Diet & Optimum Health Conference, May, 2001.
36. Frie, op. cit.
37. Malinow, R., op. cit.
38. U.S. Department of Agriculture, "Dietary Guidelines, 1998," available from the Superintendent of Documents, Consumer Information Center, Department 378-C, Pueblo, CO.
39. Loft, S., Diet, Osxidative DNA Damage and Cancer, 2001. Linus Pauling Institute's Diet & Optimum Health Conference, May, 2001.
40. Kolonel, L., Overview of Diet and Cancer Epidemiology, 2001. Linus Pauling Institute's Diet & Optimum Health Conference, May, 2001.
41. J. Stephenson, "Public Health Experts Take Aim at a Moving Target: Food-Borne Infections," *Journal of the American Medical Association* 277 (1997): 97–102.
42. Ibid., 97.
43. Ibid., 98.
44. Ibid.
45. Ibid., 99.
46. P. Morris, Y. Motarjemi, and F. Kaferstein, "Emerging Food-Borne Diseases," *World Health* 50 (1997): 16–22. Also see CDC website indicated in this chapter.
47. "Special Report: Irradiation Plants Geared to 'Zap' Meat and Poultry—Is it Safe?" *Tufts University Health and Nutrition Letter* 18 (1) (2000): 4–7.
48. Ibid., 5.

CHAPTER 10

1. National Center for Health Statistics, *Prevalence of Overweight and Obesity Among Adults, 1999* (Hyattsville, MD: NCHS, 2000) (see www.cdc.gov/nchs/products/pubs/pubd/hestats/obese/obse99.htm).
2. G. Cowley, "Generation XXL," *Newsweek* (July 3, 2000): 40–46.
3. Ibid., 42.
4. Ibid.
5. S. St. Jeor, "New Trends in Weight Management," *Journal of the American Dietetic Association* 97 (1997): 2000.
6. National Institute of Diabetes & Digestive & Kidney Diseases of the National Institute of Health (NIDDK), Weight Control Information Network. Statistics Relating to Overweight and Obesity. http://www.niddk.nih.gov/health/nutrit/pubs/statobes.htm; December 10, 2001
7. National Center for Health Status (www.cdc.gov/nchs/products/pubs/hestats/obese/obse99.htm).
8. Ibid.
9. Ibid.
10. NIDDK, op. cit.
11. ADA Position adopted by the House of Delegates, October 20, 1996. ADA headquarters at 800-877-1600, ext. 4896.
12. S. Cummings, K. Goodrick, and J. Foreyt, "Position of the American Diabetes Association: Weight Management 97," (1997): 71–75.
13. J. G. Meisler and S. St. Jeor, "Summary and Recommendations from the American Health Foundation's Expert Panel on Healthy Weight," *American Journal of Clinical Nutrition* 63 (1996): 474S–477S.
14. S. Cummings, et al., op. cit.
15. U.S. Department of Health and Human Services, 2001. Surgeon General Launches Effort to develop action plan to combat overweight, obesity. http://www.surgeongeneral.gov/todo/pressreleases/obesitypressrelease.htm.; National Task Force on Prevention and Treatment of Obesity. Towards Prevention of Obesity: Research Directions. Obes. Res., 2, 571–584.
16. Nestle, M. and Jacobson, M.F. (2000). Halting the obesity epidemic: a Public Health policy approach. Public Health Reports. 115. 12.24.; Flegal, K.M., Carroll, M.D. Kuczmarski, R.J. amd Johnsomn, C.L. 1998. Overweight and Obesity in the United States: Prevalance and Trends, 1960–1996-Int. J. Obes Related Metabolic Disorders. 22, 39–47.
17. French, S.A. Story, M., and Jeffrey, R.W. 2001. Environmental Influences on eating and Physical activity. Annual Review Public Health. 22. 309-335.
18. Ibid, p.312 & 320.
19. Gillman, M.W., Rifas-Shiman, S.L., Camargo, C.A., Berkey, C.Sl., Frazier, A.L., Rockett, H.R. Fields, A.E. and Colditz, G.A. 2001. Risk of Overweight among adolescents who were breastfed as infants. Journal of the American Medical Association 285, 2461–2467; Hediger, M.L., Overpeck, M.D., Kuczmarski, R.J. and Ruan, W.J. 2001. Association between infant breastfeeding and overweight in young children. Journal of the American Medical Association 285. 2453–2460.
20. National Center Health Statistics. Prevalence of overweight and obesity among adults; United States, 2000.
21. Crespo, C.J., Smit, E., Troianao, R.P., Bartlett, S.J., Macera, C.A. and Anderson, R.E. 2001. Television watvhing, energy intake and obesity in U.S. children: results from the thirs National Health and Nutrition Examination Survey. Arch. Pediatr. Adolesc. Med., 155, 360–365.; Dietz, W.H. 2001. The obesity epidemic in young children. Reduce television viewing and promote playing. BMJ. 322, 313–324.
22. Dowda, M., Ainsworth, B.E., Addy, C.L., Saunders, R., Riner, W. 2001. Environmental influences, physical activity and weight status in 8–12 year olds. Arch Pediatr. Adolesc. Med., 155, 711–717.
23. Ibid, p. 715.
24. "Special Report: Weight Control," from *Women's HealthSource* (Mayo Clinic, 1997), 3.

25. A. Stunkard et al., "The Body Mass Index of Twins Who Have Been Raised Apart," *New England Journal of Medicine* 322 (1990): 1477–1482.
26. C. Bouchard et al., "The Response to Long-Term Overfeeding in Identical Twins," *New England Journal of Medicine* 322 (1990): 1483–1487.
27. Ibid.
28. Cummings et al., op. cit., 73.
29. P. Jaret, "The Way to Lose Weight," *Health* (January/February 1995): 52–59.
30. A. Novitt-Morena, "Obesity: What's the Genetic Connection?" *Current Health* 24 (1998): 18–23.
31. "Genes and Appetite," *Harvard Women's Health Watch,* January 1996; L. Tartaglia et al., "Identification and Expression Cloning of a Leptin Receptor," *Cell* 83 (1995): 1263–1271.
32. M. Turton, D. O'Shea, I. Gunn, et al., "A Role for Glucagon-like Peptide 1 in the Central Regulation of Feeding," *Nature* 379 (1996): 69–72.
33. F. Katch and W. McArdle, *Introduction to Nutrition, Exercise, and Health,* 4th ed. (Philadelphia: Lea and Febiger, 1992), 53.
34. Special Report: Weight Control, op. cit., 4.
35. K. Brownell, "Comments on the Latest Study on Yo-Yo Diets by Steven Blair of the Institute for Aerobics Research" (paper originally presented in 1993, newer report at paper presented at Oregon State University by Steven Blair, Fall, 1998).
36. National Center for Health Statistics, "Prevalence of Sedentary Leisure-Time Behavior Among Adults in the United States," December 2000 (see http://www.cdc.gov/nchs/products/pubs/pubd/hestats/3and4/sedentary.htm).
37. Ibid.
38. Ibid
39. Special Report: Weight Control, op. cit., 4.
40. N. Diehl, C. Johnson, and R. Rogers, "Social Physique Anxiety and Disordered Eating: What's the Connection?" *Addictive Behaviors* 23 (1998): 1–16.
41. Special Report: Weight Control, op. cit., 4.
42. G. K. Goodrick and J. P. Foreyt, "Why Treatments for Obesity Don't Last," *Journal of the American Dietetic Association* 91 (1991): 1243–1247.
43. C. F. Telch and W. S. Agras, "The Effects of Very Low Calorie Diet on Binge Eating," *Behavior Therapy* 24 (1993): 177–193.
44. *USA TODAY Weekend* (July 14–16, 2000): 6.
45. Cummings et al., op. cit., 75.
46. "Eating Disorders," *Harvard Mental Health Letter* 14 (1997): 4.

CHAPTER 11
1. U.S. Department of Health and Human Services, *Physical Activity and Health: A Report of the Surgeon General* (Atlanta, GA: U.S. Department of Health and Human Services, Centers for Disease Control and Prevention, National Center for Chronic Disease Prevention and Health Promotion, 1996).
2. F. Booth and S. Gordon, "Advocacy Is Needed to Promote Research into Diseases of Physical Inactivity," *Exercise and Sport Sciences Reviews* 28 (4) (2000): 145–147.
3. U.S. Department of Health and Human Services, *Physical Activity and Health: A Report of the Surgeon General,* op. cit.
4. R. Gates, "Fitness Is Changing the World: For Women," *IDEA Today* (July–August 1992): 58.
5. U. S. Department of Health and Human Services, Healthy People 2000: National Health Promotion and Disease Prevention Objectives (DHHS [PHS] Publication no. 91-50213. Washington, D. C.: Government Printing Office, 1991).
6. C. J. Caspersen, K. E. Powell, and G. M. Christianson, "Physical Activity, Exercise, and Physical Fitness: Definitions and Distinctions for Health-Related Research," *Public Health Report* 100 (1985): 126–131.
7. L. J. Ransdell and C. L. Wells, "Physical Activity in Urban, African-American, and Mexican-American Women," *Medicine and Science in Sports and Exercise* 30 (1998): 1608–1615.
8. T. Baranowski et al., "Assessment, Prevalence, and Cardiovascular Benefits of Physical Activity and Fitness in Youth," *Medicine and Science in Sports and Exercise* 24 (6) Supplement (1992): S237–S247.
9. M. Artal and C. Sherman, "Exercise Against Depression," *The Physician and Sportsmedicine* 26 (1998): 55–60; S. J. Petruzello et al., "Effects of Exercise on Anxiety and Mood," *Sports Medicine* 11 (1991): 143–182.
10. L. Bernstein et al., "Adolescent Exercise Reduces Risk of Breast Cancer in Younger Women," *Journal of the National Cancer Institute,* September 1994.
11. U.S. Department of Health and Human Services, *Physical Activity and Health: A Report of the Surgeon General,* op. cit.
12. C. B. Corbin and R. Lindsey, *Concepts in Physical Education with Laboratories,* 8th ed. (Dubuque, IA: Times Mirror, 1994).
13. U.S. Department of Health and Human Services, *Physical Activity and Health: A Report of the Surgeon General,* op. cit.
14. W. L. Haskell et al., "Cardiovascular Benefits and Assessment of Physical Activity and Physical Fitness in Adults," *Medicine and Science in Sports and Exercise* 24 (6) Supplement (1992): S201–S220.
15. C. Christmas, "Fitness for Reducing Osteoporosis," *The Physician and Sports Medicine,* 28 (October, 2000): 33–34.
16. C.M. Snow, J.M. Shaw, and C.C. Matkin, "Physical Activity and Risks for Osteoporosis," *Osteoporosis,* eds. R. Marcus, D. Feldman, J. Kelsy (San Diego: Academic Press, 1996), 511–528.
17. American College of Sports Medicine, *ACSM's Guidelines for Exercise Testing and Prescription,* 6th ed. (Baltimore: Lippincott, Williams and Wilkins, 2000).
18. R. Ross, J. A. Freeman, and I. Janssen, "Exercise Alone Is an Effective Strategy for Reducing Obesity and Related Comorbidities," *Exercise and Sport Sciences Reviews* 28 (4) (2000): 165–170.
19. Ibid.
20. National Institutes of Health, "Consensus Development Conference Statement on Diet and Exercise in Non-Insulin-Dependent Diabetes Mellitus," *Diabetes Care* 10 (1987): 639–644.
21. S. P. Helmrich, D. R. Ragland, and R. S. Paffenbarger, Jr., "Prevention of Non-Insulin-Dependent Diabetes Mellitus with Physical Activity," *Medicine and Science in Sports and Exercise* 26 (1994): 824–830.
22. S. N. Blair et al., "Physical Fitness and All-Cause Mortality: A Prospective Study of Healthy Men and Women," *Journal of the American Medical Association* 262 (1989): 2395–2401.
23. E. R. Eichner, "Infection, Immunity, and Exercise: What To Tell Patients?" *The Physician and Sportsmedicine* 21 (January 1993): 125–135.
24. W. A. Primos, Jr., "Sports and Exercise During Acute Illness: Recommending the Right Course for Patients," *The Physician and Sportsmedicine* 24 (January 1996): 44–53.
25. D. C. Nieman et al., "Infectious Episodes in Runners Before and After the Los Angeles Marathon," *Journal of Sports Medicine and Physical Fitness* 30 (1990): 316–328.
26. Eichner, op. cit.
27. Ibid.
28. R. Gates, "Fitness Is Changing the World: For women," *IDEA Today,* (July–August 1992):58.
29. E. T. Howley and D. B. Franks, *Health Fitness Instructor's Handbook,* 2nd ed. (Champaign, IL: Human Kinetics Books, 1992).
30. U.S. Department of Health and Human Services, *Physical Activity and Health: A Report of the Surgeon General,* op. cit.
31. B. Stamford, "Tracking Your Heart Rate for Fitness," *The Physician and Sportsmedicine* 21 (March 1993): 227–228.
32. U.S. Centers for Disease Control and Prevention and American College of Sports Medicine, "Summary Statement: Workshop on Physical Activity and Public Health," *Sports Medicine Bulletin* 28 (4) (1993): 7.

33. G. A. Klug and J. Lettunich, *Wellness: Exercise and Physical Fitness* (Guilford, CT: Dushkin Publishing Group, 1992).

34. P. D. Wood, "Physical Activity, Diet, and Health: Independent and Interactive Effects." *Medicine and Science in Sports and Exercise* 26 (1994): 838–843.

35. American College of Sports Medicine, "ACSM Position Stand on the Recommended Quantity and Quality of Exercise for Developing and Maintaining Cardiorespiratory and Muscular Fitness, and Flexibility in Adults," op. cit.

36. American College of Sports Medicine, "ACSM Position Stand on the Recommended Quantity and Quality of Exercise for Developing and Maintaining Cardiorespiratory and Muscular Fitness, and Flexibility in Adults," op. cit.

37. M. Cyphers, "Flexibility," in *Personal Trainer Manual,* 2nd ed. (San Diego: American Council on Exercise, 1996), 291–308.

38. P. A. Sienna, *One Rep Max: A Guide to Beginning Weight Training* (Indianapolis: Benchmark Press, 1989).

39. H. G. Knuttgen and W. J. Kraemer, "Terminology and Measurement in Exercise Performance," *Journal of Applied Sport Science Research* 1 (1987): 1–10.

40. M. S. Feigenbaum and M. L. Pollock, "Prescription of Resistance Training for Health and Disease," *Medicine and Science in Sports and Exercise* 31 (1999): 38–45.

41. M. L. Pollock and W. J. Evans, "Resistance Training for Health and Disease: Introduction," *Medicine and Science in Sports and Exercise* 31 (1999): 10–11.

42. American College of Sports Medicine, "ACSM Position Stand on the Recommended Quantity and Quality of Exercise for Developing and Maintaining Cardiorespiratory and Muscular Fitness, and Flexibility in Adults," op. cit.

43. C. L. Wells, *Women, Sport, and Performance: A Physiological Perspective,* 2nd ed. (Champaign, IL: Human Kinetics, 1991).

44. American College of Sports Medicine, "ACSM Position Stand on the Recommended Quantity and Quality of Exercise for Developing and Maintaining Cardiorespiratory and Muscular Fitness, and Flexibility in Adults," op. cit.

45. W. C. Whiting and R. F. Zernicke, *Biomechanics of Musculoskeletal Injury* (Champaign, IL: Human Kinetics, 1998).

46. D. M. Brody, "Running Injuries: Prevention and Management," *Clinical Symposia* 39 (1987).

47. J. C. Erie, "Eye Injuries: Prevention, Evaluation, and Treatment," *The Physician and Sportsmedicine* 19 (November 1991): 108–122.

48. R. C. Wasserman and R. V. Buccini, "Helmet Protection from Head Injuries Among Recreational Bicyclists," *American Journal of Sports Medicine* 18 (1990): 96–97.

49. S. M. Simons, "Foot Injuries of the Recreational Athlete," *The Physician and Sportsmedicine* 27: (January 1999): 57–70.

50. J. Andrish and J. A. Work, "How I Manage Shin Splints," *The Physician and Sportsmedicine* 18 (December 1990): 113–114.

51. E. A. Arendt, "Common Musculoskeletal Injuries in Women," *The Physician and Sportsmedicine* 24 (July 1996): 39–48.

52. American Academy of Orthopaedic Surgeons, *Athletic Training and Sports Medicine,* 3rd ed., (Park Ridge, IL: AAOS, 2000).

53. J. J. Mistovich, B. Q. Hafen, and K. J. Karren, *Prehospital Emergency Care,* 6th ed. (Upper Saddle River, NJ: Prentice-Hall, 2000).

54. American College of Sports Medicine, "Position Stand—Heat and Cold Illnesses During Distance Running," *Medicine and Science in Sports and Exercise* 28 (December 1996): i–x.

55. American College of Sports Medicine, "Position Stand—Exercise and Fluid Replacement," *Medicine and Science in Sports and Exercise* 28 (January 1996): i–vii.

56. P. R. Below, P. Mora-Rodriguez, J. Gonzalez-Alonso, and F. F. Coyle, "Fluid and Carbohydrate Ingestion Independently Improve Performance During 1 Hr of Intense Exercise," *Medicine and Science in Sports and Exercise* 27 (1995): 200–210.

57. D. J. Casa et al., "National Athletic Trainers' Association Position Statement: Fluid Replacement for Athletes," *Journal of Athletic Training* 35 (2) (2000): 212–224.

58. J. S. Thornton, "Hypothermia Shouldn't Freeze Out Cold-Weather Athletes," *The Physician and Sportsmedicine* 18 (January 1990): 109–113.

59. American College of Sports Medicine, "Position Stand: Heat and Cold Illnesses During Distance Running," op. cit.

CHAPTER 12

1. American Heart Association, "2001 Heart and Stroke Statistical Update" (Dallas, TX: American Heart Association, 2001).

2. Ibid., 4.

3. Ibid.

4. Ibid., 5.

5. Ibid.

6. American Heart Association. Heart Stroke Statistical Update. 2001. http://www.americanheart.org or http://www.strokeassociation.org.

7. Ibid.

8. American Heart Association, "2001 Heart and Stroke Statistical Update," p. 7.

9. Ibid.

10. R. Ross, "Atherosclerosis—an Inflammatory Disease," *New England Journal of Medicine* 340 (1999): 115–126.

11. C. Napoli, E. P. D'Armiento, F. P. Mancini, et al., "Fatty Streak Formation Occurs in Human Fetal Aortas and Is Greatly Enhanced by Maternal Hypercholesterolemia: Intimal Accumulation of Low-Density Lipoprotein and Its Oxidative Precede Monocyte Recruitment into Early Atherosclerotic Lesions," *Journal of Clinical Investigation* 100 (1997): 2680–2690.

12. J. L. Breslow, "Cardiovascular Disease Burden Increases, NIH Funding Decreases," *Nature Medicine* 3 (1997): 6000–6009.

13. Ross, op. cit., 115.

14. J. Danesh, R. Collins, and R. Peto, "Chronic Infections and Coronary Heart Disease: Is There a Link?" *Lancet* 350 (1997): 430–436.

15. E. Braunwald, "Cardiovascular Medicine at the Turn of the Millennium: Triumphs, Concerns, and Opportunities," *New England Journal of Medicine* 337 (1997): 1360–1369.

16. Ross, op cit., 122.

17. A. Forman, "The Threat of Insulin Resistance to Your Heart," *Environmental Nutrition* 23 (8) (2000): 4–6.

18. American Heart Association, "2001 Heart and Stroke Statistical Update," 11.

19. Ibid., 13.

20. Ibid., 19.

21. Ibid., 20.

22. Ibid., 19–20.

23. Ibid., 14.

24. Ibid.

25. American Heart Association. Heart Stroke Statistical Update. 2001. http://www.americanheart.org or http://www.strokeassociation.org.

26. American Heart Association, "2001 Heart and Stroke Statistical Update," 22.

27. Ibid., 24

28. Ibid.,

29. National Heart, Lung and Blood Institute: Third Report of the National Cholesterol Education Program (NCEP) Expert Panel on Detection, Evaluation and Treatment of High Blood Cholesterol in Adults, (Adult Treatment Panel III). May, 2001. http://www.hin.nhlbi.nih.gov

30. Ibid.

31. American Heart Association, "2001 Heart and Stroke Statistical Update."

32. National Heart, Lung and Blood Institute, op. cit.

33. Ibid.

34. Ibid.

35. Ibid., 15. Center for Science in the Public Interest, op. cit., 6.

36. U.S. Department of Health and Human Services, *Surgeon General's Report on Physical Activity* (1996); American Heart Association, "2001 Heart and Stroke Statistical Update," 11.

37. American Heart Association, '2001 Heart and Stroke Statistical Update," op. cit.

38. Ibid, 17.

39. Ross, op. cit., 117.

40. R. Eliot, "Changing Behavior: A New Comprehensive and Quantitative Approach" (keynote address at the annual meeting of the American College of Cardiology on stress and the heart, Jackson Hole, Wyoming, July 3, 1987).

41. American Heart Association, "2001 Heart and Stroke Facts," 2.

42. A. G. Boston et al., "Elevated Plasma Lipoprotein(a) and Coronary Heart Disease in Men Aged 55 Years and Younger: A Prospective Study," *Journal of the American Medical Association* 276 (1996): 555–558.

43. Ibid., 555.

44. Ibid., 556.

45. National Heart, Lung, and Blood Institute, "Heart Memo: The Cardiovascular Health of Women" (1995): 5.

46. Ibid., 5.

47. American Heart Association, "2001 Heart and Stroke Facts," 25.

48. J. E. Willard, R. A. Lange, and D. L. Hillis, "The Use of Aspirin in Ischemic Heart Disease," *New England Journal of Medicine* 327 (1992): 175–179.

49. Agency for Health Care Policy and Research, "Cardiac Rehabilitation: Exercise, Training, Education, Counseling, and Behavioral Interventions," Publication #96-0672 (1996).

CHAPTER 13

1. American Cancer Society, *Cancer Facts and Figures, 2001*. National Program Office, 1559 Clifton Road NE, Atlanta, GA. p.4, http://www.cancer.org.

2. Ibid.

3. American Cancer Society, *Cancer Facts and Figures, 2000*. American Cancer Society, 2000, Atlanta, GA., http://www.cancer.org/cancerinfo/.

4. American Cancer Society. *Cancer Facts and Figures, 2001.*, op. cit.

5. Ibid.

6. Ibid., 4, 31.

7. Peto, Julian. "Cancer Epidemiology in the Last Century and Next Decade," *Nature*. 2001, 411, 390–395.

8. Ibid.

9. L. Remennick, "The Cancer Problem in the Context of Modernity, Sociology, Demography and Politics," *Current Sociology*, 46 (1998): 144.

10. American Cancer Society, *Cancer Facts and Figures 2001*, op. cit., 3.

11. Ibid.

12. M. Osborne, P. Boyle, and M. Lipkin, "Cancer Prevention," *The Lancet* 349 (1997): 1–8 (special oncology supplement).

13. Peto, J., op.cit.

14. Ibid., p. 393.

15. Ibid.

16. Josefson, D. "Obesity and Inactivity fuel Global Cance Epidemic." B. Med J. 2001. 322, 945–953.

17. American Cancer Society, *Cancer Facts and Figures, 2001*, op. cit

18. Ibid.

19. M. Osborne, et al., op. cit.

20. IARC. Hormonal Contraception and Post-Menopausal Hormonal Therapy (IARC Monographs on the Evalutaion of Carcinogenic Risks to Humans, 72) (IARC, Lyon, 1999)

21. Peto, J. *Nature*. P.394.

22. American Cancer Society, op. cit.

23. Osborne et al., op. cit.

24. Peto, J., op. cit.

25. American Cancer Society, op. cit.

26. Ibid.

27. Ibid.

28. Ibid.

29. American Cancer Society, *Cancer Facts and Figures, 2001*, op. cit.

30. Ibid.

31. Ibid.

32. Ibid.

33. Peto, J., op. cit.

34. Ibid.

35. Bergstrom, A., Pisani, P., Tenet, V., Wolk, A., and Adamis, O., "Overweight as an Avoidable Cause of Cancer in Europe," Int. J. Cancer (2001) 91, 421–430.

36. American Cancer Society. *Cancer Facts and Figures, 2001*, p. 12.

37. Janne, P.A. and Mayer, R.J. "Chemoprevention of Colorectal Cancer." New England Journal of Medicine. 2000. 342, p.1960–1968.

38. American Cancer Society. *Cancer Facts and Figures, 2001*, p. 16.

39. Ibid.

40. Ibid.

41. Ibid.

42. Ibid.

43. Ibid.

44. Artunian, J. "Here Comes the Sun," *Current Health* 2 (April 1995) vol. 21, no. 8, p. 26; Munsun, M., and Yeykal, T., "Dark Dangers" *Prevention* (September 1995) vol. 47, no. 9, p. 40.

45. American Cancer Society, op. cit.

46. Ibid.

47. American Cancer Society. *Cancer Facts and Figures, 2001*, op. cit.

48. American Cancer Society, op. cit.

49. A. Harvey, M. J. Risch, L. D. Marrett, and G. R. Howe, "Dietary Fat Intake and Risk of Epithelial Ovarian Cancer," *Journal of the National Cancer Institute* 86 (1994): 21.

50. American Cancer Society, *Cancer Facts and Figures, 2001*, op. cit, p. 15.

51. American Cancer Society. *Cancer Facts and Figures, 2001*, op. cit., p. 19. 52. Ibid.

53. Ibid.

54. Ibid.

55. Ibid., p. 15.

56. American Cancer Society, op. cit.

57. Ibid.

58. American Cancer Society. Cancer Facts and Figures, p. 13.

CHAPTER 14

1. K. Nelson, C. Williams, and N. Graham, *Infectious Disease Epidemiology: Theory and Practice* (Gaithersburg, MD: Aspen, 2001), 17–39.

2. "Group B Streptococcal Infections," Respiratory Disease Branch, Division of Bacterial and Mycotic Diseases, National Center for Infectious Diseases, Centers for Disease Control and Prevention (CDC), 2000 (see http://www.cdc.gov/ncidod/diseases/bacter/strep_b.htm).

3. Ibid.

4. "Preventing Emerging Infectious Diseases: A Strategy for the 21st Century," U.S. Department of Health and Human Services (Atlanta, GA: CDC, 1998).

5. A. Evans and P. Brachman, *Bacterial Infections of Humans: Epidemiology and Control*, 3rd ed. (Atlanta, GA: Plenum, 1998).

6. Nelson et al., op. cit., 431

7. Global Tuberculosis Program, "Tuberculosis Fact Sheet No. 104" (see http://wwwwho.int/inffs/en/fact104.html; accessed January 2000).

8. Ibid.

9. A. Evans and R. Kaslow, *Viral Infections in Humans: Epidemiology and Control*, fourth edition. (New York: Plenum, 1997), 6–11.

10. National Institute of Allergy and Infectious Diseases. National Institute of Health, March 2001., Fact Sheet: The Common Cold. http://www./NIAID.nih.gov/factsheets/cold.htm.

11. Ibid.

12. Ibid.

13. National Institutes of Health, "Promote Prevention: Hepatitis—Education and Information for Patients and Professionals (National Digestive Diseases Information Clearinghouse, 2000) (see http://www.niddk.nih.gov/health/digest/digest.htm).
14. Ibid.
15. Ibid.
16. Ibid.
17. Nelson et al., op. cit., 17–39.
18. National Center for Infectious Disease-Centers for Disease Control and Prevention, January 2002, http://www.cdc.gov/ncidod/diseases/cjd.cjd.htm.
19. Ibid.
20. Nelson et al., op. cit., 315–318.
21. Ibid.
22. R. Fenner, *The History of Smallpox and Its Spread Around the World* (Geneva, Switzerland: World Health Organization, 1988).
23. T. J. Torok, R. V. Tauxe, and R. P. Wise, "A Large Community Outbreak of Salmonellosis Carried by Intentional Contamination of Restaurant Salad Bars" *Journal of the American Medical Association* 279 (1997): 389–395.
24. Centers for Disease Control and Prevention, Division of Sexually Transmitted Diseases, *1999 Annual Report* (Atlanta, GA: CDC, 2000).
25. K. Painter, "STI Rate Higher than Previously Believed," *USA Today* (December 3, 1998): DI (taken from CDC December 1998 report).
26. "Chlamydia Fact Sheet," National Institute of Allergy and Infectious Diseases, National Institutes of Health, November 2000 (see http://www.niaid.nih.gov).
27. "Pelvic Inflammatory Disease," National Institute of Allergy and Infectious Diseases, National Institutes of Health, November 2000 (see http://www.niaid.nih.gov).
28. "PID: Guidelines for Prevention, Detection, and Management," *Clinical Courier* 10 (1992): 1–5
29. "Gonorrhea Fact Sheet," National Institute of Allergy and Infectious Diseases, National Institutes of Health, October 2000 (see http://www.niaid.nih.gov).
30. Ibid.
31. Evans and Brachman, op. cit., 285.
32. "Genital Herpes Fact Sheet," National Institute of Allergy and Infectious Diseases, National Institutes of Health, March 2000 (see http://www.niaid.nih.gov).
33. Ibid.
34. G. Stine, *AIDS Update* 2000 (Upper Saddle River, NJ: Prentice Hall, 2000), 349.
35. Centers for Disease Control. National Center for HIV, STD, and TB Prevention: of HIV/AIDS Prevention, Basic Statistics, http://www.cdc.gov/hiv/stats.htm.
36. "CDC Update: Critical Need to Pay Attention to HIV Prevention for Women" (CDC, July 24, 1998); Stine, op. cit.
37. Ibid, 343–349; Society for the Advancement of Women's Health Research, "Some Ailments Found Guilty of Sex Bias," *New York Times* (November 11, 1998): D12: B. M. Branson, "Home Sample Collection Tests for HIV Infection," *Journal of the American Medical Association* 280 (1998): 1699–1701.
38. Centers for Disease Control, Revised Recommendations for HIV Screening of Pregnant Women, MMWR: November, 9 2001, 50 (RR19): 59-86, http://www.cdc.gov/mmwr/review.
39. Centers for Disease Control, National Center for HIV, STD, and TB Prevention: Division of HIV/AIDS Prevention, January, 2002, http://www.cdc.gov/pubs/facts.htm.
40. Ibid. http://www.cdc.gov/hiv/stats.htm
41. F. Cox, *The AIDS Booklet* 6th ed. (Boston: McGraw Hill Higher Education, 2000), 27–30.
42. R. Brownson, P. Remington, and J. Davis, eds., *Chronic Disease Epidemiology and Control* (Washington, DC: American Public Health Association, 1998), 379–382.
43. American Academy of Allergy, Asthma, and Immunology, accessed February 2001 (see http://www.aaaai.org).
44. Brownson et al., op. cit., 389.
45. American Lung Association, accessed January 2001 (see http://www.lungusa.org).
46. Ibid., 516.
47. J. Adler and A. Rogers, "The New War Against Migraines," *Newsweek* (January 11, 1999): 46–55.
48. Ibid., 48.
49. Ibid., 49.
50. Adler and Rogers, op. cit., 52.
51. J. Adler and C. Kalb, "An American Epidemic: Diabetes," *Newsweek,* (September 4, 2000): 40–48: Centers for Disease Control and Prevention, accessed January 2001 (see http://www.cdc.gov).
52. Brownson, et al., op. cit., 424.
53. Adler and Kalb, op. cit., 42.
54. Brownson, et al., op. cit., 424.
55. "Prevalence of Low Back Pain in the United States: New Estimates," *The Back Letter,* 1998, Philadelphia: Lippincott, Williams, and Wilkins.
56. N. Hadler and T. Carey, "Low Back Pain: An Intermittent Predicament in Life," *Annals of the Rheumatic Diseases* 57 (1998): 1–3.
57. K. Nelson, C. Williams, and N. Graham, *Infectious Disease Epidemiology* (Gaithersburg, MD: Aspen, 2001), 348–349.

CHAPTER 15

1. J. Kavenaugh, *Adult Development and Aging* (Pacific Grove, CA: BrooksCole/ITP, 1996), 45.
2. W. Madar, "Life Stories as Well as Theory Needed to Understand Aging," *Center for the Humanities Newsletter* (Consortium of Humanities Centers and Institutes, Oregon State University, spring 2000), 8.
3. Federal Interagency Forum on Aging-Related Statistics, "Older Americans 2000: Key Indicators of Well-Being," (December 27, 2000) (see http://www.agingstats.gov/chartbook2000/population.html).
4. Ibid.
5. Ibid.
6. Department of Health and Human Services, Administration on Aging, A Profile of Older Americans: 2001, January, 2002
7. Ibid.
8. Ibid.
9. Ibid.
10. National Institutes of Health, Osteoporosis and Related Bone Diseases National Resource Center (December 2000) (see http://www.osteo.org/osteo.html).
11. T. Hickey, M. Speers, and T. Prochaska, *Public Health and Aging* (Baltimore: Johns Hopkins University Press, 1997), 69–71.
12. Ibid., 137–138.
13. National Council on Aging, press release, "Half of Older Americans Report They Are Sexually Active, 4 in 10 Want More Sex, Says New Survey" (September 28, 1998) (see http://ncoa.org/news/archieves/sexsurvey.htm).
14. National Institute of Mental Health, Older Adults: Depression and Suicide Facts, Jan. 2002, http://www.nimh.nih.gov/publicat/elderlydepsuicide.cfm
15. National Institute on Aging and National Institutes of Health. 2000 Progress Report on Alzheimer's Disease: "Taking the Next Step," January, 2002.
16. Ibid.
17. Ibid.
18. Ibid.
19. Ibid.
20. Ibid.
21. National Institute of Alcohol and Alcohol Abuse, National Institute of Health, Frequently Asked Questions, January, 2002, http://www.niaa.nih.gov/faq/faq.htm.
22. Ibid.
23. Ibid.

24. *Oxford English Dictionary* (Oxford, UK: Oxford University Press, 1969), 72, 334, 735.

25. President's Commission for the Study of Ethical Problems in Medicine and Biomedical and Behavioral Research, *Deciding to Forgo Life-Sustaining Treatment* (New York: Concern for Dying, 1983), 9.

26. Ad Hoc Committee of the Harvard Medical School to Examine the Definition of Brain Death, "A Definition of Irreversible Coma," *Journal of the American Medical Association* 205 (1968): 377.

27. L. R. Aiken, *Dying, Death, and Bereavement,* 3rd ed. (Boston: Allyn and Bacon, 1994), 4.

28. *Civilization,* 6 (6) (2000): 30, 33–34.

29. E. Kübler-Ross, *On Death and Dying* (New York: Macmillan, 1969), 113.

30. R. J. Kastenbaum, *Death, Society, and Human Experience,* 6th ed. (Boston: Allyn and Bacon, 1998), 95.

31. Kastenbaum, op.cit., 336–337.

32. K. J. Doka (ed.), *Disenfranchised Grief: Recognizing Hidden Sorrow* (Lexington, MA: Lexington Books, 1989).

33. "Last Rights: Why a 'Living Will' Is not Enough," *Consumer Reports on Health* (September 1993): 5, 9.

34. J. G. Bachman, K. H. Alcser, D. J. Doukas, R. L. Lichtenstein, A. D. Corning, and H. Brody, "Attitudes of Michigan Physicians and the Public Toward Legalizing Physician-Assisted Suicide and Voluntary Euthanasia," *New England Journal of Medicine* 334 (1996): 303.

35. M. A. Lee, H. D. Nelxon, V. P. Tilden, L. Ganzini, T. A. Schmidt, and S. W. Tolle, "Legalizing Assisted Suicide: Views of Physicians in Oregon," *New England Journal of Medicine* 334 (1996): 310–315.

CHAPTER 16

1. M. Renner, "Economic Features," *Vital Signs 1997: The Environmental Trends that Are Shaping our Future* (New York: W. W. Norton & Co., 1997).

2. R. Caplan, *Our Earth, Ourselves* (New York: Bantam, 1990), 247.

3. United Nations, *Global Population Policy Database* (New York: UN Population Division, 1995).

4. J. Abramovitz and S. Dunn, "Record Year for Weather-Related Disasters," in *Vital Signs Brief 98-5* (Washington, DC: Worldwatch Institute, 1998).

5. L. R. Brown, M. Renner, and C. Flavin, *Vital Signs 1998: The Environmental Trends That Are Shaping Our Future* (New York: W. W. Norton & Co., 1998).

6. Brown, et. al., op. cit

7. L. Gordon, "Environmental Health and Protection: Century 21 Challenges," *Journal of Environmental Health,* 57 (1995): 28–34.

8. L. R. Brown, G. Gardner, and B. Halweil, *Beyond Malthus: Sixteen Dimensions of the Population Problem* (Washington, DC: Worldwatch Institute, 1998).

9. Ibid.

10. J. Schwartz, "Health Effects of Particulate Air Pollution," *The Center for Environmental Health Newsletter* 7 (1998) (University of Connecticut, College of Agriculture & Natural Resources).

11. National Center for Environmental Health, *Screening Young Children for Lead Poisoning: Guidance for State and Local Public Health Officials.* (Atlanta: Centers for Disease Control and Prevention, U.S. Public Health Service, 1997).

12. L. Brown, "A New Era Unfolds," in *State of the World, 1993,* Lester Brown, ed. (New York: W. W. Norton Co., 1993), 107.

13. Environmental Protection Agency, "The INSIDE STORY: A Guide to Indoor Air Quality," EPA Document #402-K-93-007, January, 2002, http://epa.gov.iaq/pubs/insidest.html.

14. Ibid

15. K. E. Warner, D. Mendez, and P. N. Courant, "Toward a More Realistic Appraisal of the Lung Cancer Risk from Radon," *American Journal of Public Health* 86 (1996): 1222–1227.

16. Environmental Protection Agency, "The INSIDE STORY: A Guide to Indoor Air Quality," op. cit.

17. B. Condor, "Alternative Watch: Clearing the Air in Classrooms," *Chicago Tribune,* 2000.

18. N. Carpenter, "'Sick' Buildings Can Be Root of Work-Related Maladies," *Boston Business Journal* 20 (2000): 36–37.

19. U.S. Environmental Protection Agency, *Questions and Answers on Ozone Depletion* (Washington, DC: Stratospheric Protection Division, 1998).

20. Brown et al., op. cit.

21. J. Abramovitz, *Taking a Stand: Cultivating a New Relationship with the World's Forests* (Washington, DC: Worldwatch Institute, 1998).

22. Ibid.

22. Ibid.

23. U. S. Environmental Protection Agency, "Water on Tap: A Consumer's Guide to the Nation's Drinking Water" (Washington, D. C.: Safe Drinking Water Information System, 1997).

24. Ibid.

25. Ibid.

26. Brown et al., op. cit.

27. A. Hoyer, "Organochlorine Exposure and Risk of Breast Cancer," *Lancet* 352 (1998): 1816–1831.

28. B. L. Johnson and C. T. DeRosa, "The Toxicologic Hazard of Superfund Hazardous Waste Sites," *Environmental Health* 12 (1997): 235–251.

29. Ibid., 242.

30. Ibid., 243.

31. U.S. Environmental Protection Agency, *Meeting the Environmental Challenge: EPA's Review of Progress and New Directions in Environmental Protection* (EPA Publication No. 21K-2001, 1990), 4.

32. Environmental News Network (see http://www.enn.com).

CHAPTER 17

1. L. C. Baker and L. S. Baker, "Excess Cost of Emergency Department Visits for Nonurgent Care," *Health Affairs* (winter 1994): 162–180.

2. Hospital Health Network, "Emergency Care: The Number of Visits to U.S. Hospital Emergency Departments Has Declined," *Hospital Health Network* 70 (1996): 14.

3. R. M. Williams, "The Costs of Visits to Emergency Departments," *New England Journal of Medicine* 334 (1996): 642–646.

4. J. Schmittdiel, J. V. Selby, K. Grumbach, and C. P. Quesenberry, "Choice of a Personal Physician and Patient Satisfaction in a Health Maintenance Organization," *Journal of the American Medical Association* 278 (1997): 1596–1599.

5. G. Annas, *The Rights of Patients: The Basic ACLU Guide to Patient Rights,* 2nd ed. (Chicago: Southern Illinois University Press, 1989), 105.

6. Pennsylvania Medicine, "Use of Non-Physician Practitioners," *Pennsylvania Medicine* 101 (1998): 17–19.

7. C. Hafner-Eaton, "Patterns of Hospital and Physician Utilization Among the Uninsured," *Journal of Health Care for the Poor and Underserved* 5 (1994): 297–315.

8. Agency for Healthcare Research and Quality (AHRQ): New Data About Health Care Costs. Press Reslease-July 10, 2000. Percent of Population with Health Expenses-PDF File-http://www.ahcpr.gov/news/press/pr2000/meps96pr.htm

9. K. Levit et al., "Healthy Spending in 1998: Signals of Change," *Health Affairs* 19 (11) (2000): 124–132.

10. Institute of Medicine – Report on Medical Errors, Publication No. OM00-0004, http://www.ahrqpubs@ahrq.gov

11. Ibid.

12. Ibid.

13. Ibid.

14. Zhan, G. et al. Potentially Inappropriate Medications in the Community Dwelling Elderly. Journal of the American Medical Association. De. 12, 2001.

15. Institute of Medicine—Report on Medical Errors, op. cit.

16. The Uninsured American: MEPS-Medical Expenditure Panel Survey, 2000, Agency for Health Care Research and Quality, AHRQ Publication No. 00-P056, http://www.ahrg.gov/data/quesmeos.htm.
17. Centers for Disease Control and Prevention, *Morbidity and Mortality Weekly Report* 47 (1998): 529–532.
18. *Medical Group Practice Digest: Managed Care Digest Series 1998* (Kansas City: Hoechst Marion Roussel, Inc., 1998).
19. Ibid.
20. Ibid.
21. Ibid.
22. Ibid.

CHAPTER 18

1. E. Eisenberg et al., "Trends in Alternative Medicine Use in the United States, 1990–97: Results of a Follow-up National Study," *Journal of the American Medical Association* 280 (1998): 1569–1579.
2. L. C. Paramore, "Use of Alternative Therapies," *Journal of Pain and Symptom Management* 13 (1997): 83–89; Landmark Healthcare, *The Landmark Report on Public Perceptions of Alternative Care* (Sacramento, CA: Landmark Healthcare, 1998).
3. National Institute of Health, National Center for Complementary and Alternative Medicine (NCCAM), for Consumers and Practitioners, http://www.nccam.nih.gov/fcp/classify/.
4. D. M. Eisenberg, R. C. Kessler, C. Foster, et al., "Unconventional Medicine in the United States," *New England Journal of Medicine* 328 (1993): 246–252.
5. Eisenberg, op. cit., 247: Eisenberg et al., op. cit., 1570.
6. National Institute of Health, National Center for Complementary and Alternative Medicine (NCCAM), op. cit.
7. Ibid.
8. A. Weil, *Spontaneous Healing* (New York: Fawcett Columbine, 1995), 233.
9. National Institute of Health, National Center for Complementary and Alternative Medicine (NCCAM), op. cit.
10. N. Rasmussen and J. Morgall, "The Use of Alternative Treatments in the Danish Adult Population," *Complementary Medicine Research* 4 (1990): 16–22; A. MacLennan, D. Wilson, and A. Taylor, "Prevalence and Cost of Alternative Medicine in Australia," *The Lancet* 347 (1996): 569–573; P. Fisher and A. Ward, "Complementary Medicine in Europe," *British Medical Journal* 309 (1994): 107–111; W. Miller, "Use of Alternative Health Care Practitioners by Canadians, *Canadian Journal of Public Health* 88 (1997): 154–158.
11. National Institute of Health, National Center for Complementary and Alternative Medicine (NCCAM), op. cit.
12. M. Angell and J. P. Kassirer, "Alternative Medicine—The Risks of Untested and Unregulated Remedies," *New England Journal of Medicine* 339 (1998): 839–841.
13. National Institute of Health, National Center for Complementary and Alternative Medicine (NCCAM), op. cit.
14. Ibid.
15. Ibid.
16. Ibid.
17. Ibid.
18. J. Greenwald, "Herbal Healing," *Time* (November 23, 1998): 63–65.
19. National Institute of Health, National Center for Complementary and Alternative Medicine (NCCAM), op. cit.
20. A. Weil, *Spontaneous Healing* (New York: Fawcett Columbine, 1995), 233.
21. Ibid., 241.
22. J. Kleignene and P. Knipschild, "Ginkgo Biloba," *The Lancet* 340 (1992): 1136–1139.

23. M. Murray, "Ginkgo Biloba Extract and Ginkgo Phytosome," Ask the Doctor, Vital Communication, 1998.
24. P. L. LeBars et al., "A Placebo-Controlled, Double Blind, Randomized Trial of an Extract of Ginkgo Biloba for Dementia," *Journal of the American Medical Association* 278 (1997): 1327–1332.
25. "The Pill That Helps You Think?" *Tufts University Health and Nutrition Letter* 15 (1997): 8–10.
26. "St. John's Wort," Nature's Life Brochure, 1998.
27. H. Schultz, "St. John's Wort for Depression," *British Medical Journal* 7052 (1996): 313–319.
28. K. D. Hansgen et al., "Multicenter Double Blind Study Examing the Anti-Depressant Effectiveness of the Huypericum Extract L1160," *Journal of Psychiatric Neurology,* Supplement 1 (October 7, 1994): x15–18; H. Schultz et al. "Effects of Hypericum Extract on the Sleep EEG in Older Volunteers," *American Journal of Geriatric Psychiatry,* Supplement 1 (1994): x65–68.
29. Schultz et al., op. cit., 66
30. Ibid.
31. H. Martin, "St. John's Wort vs. Tricyclic Antidepressants," *American Journal of Naturopathic Medicine* 2 (1995): 42.
32. Schultz, op. cit., 314.
33. Henney, J., "Risk of Drug Interactions with St. John's Wort" (JAMA) April 5, 2000, Volume 283, No 13.
34. U.S. Food and Drug Administration, Center for Drug Evaluation and Research, Public Health Advisory, http://www.fda.gov/cder/drug/advisory/sjwort.htm.
35. J. Blair, "Echinacea—New Wonder Drug? *Archives of Family Medicine* (November 24, 1998): 1332–1339.
36. "New Guides in Herbal Remedies," *Harvard Women's Health Watch* 41 (1999): 6–8.
37. P. A. DeSmet, "Health Risks of Herbal Remedies," *Drug Safety* 13 (1996): 81–93.
38. E. Ernst, "Harmless Herbs," *American Journal of Medicine* 104 (1998): 170–178.
39. "New Guides in Herbal Remedies," op. cit., 7.
40. Ernst, op. cit., 172.
41. Ibid., 173
42. J. Astin, "Why Patients Use Alternative Medicine: Results of a National Study," *Journal of the American Medical Association* 279 (1998): 1553.
43. C. Marwick, "Medical News and Perspectives: Alternatives Are Ahead of the OAM," *Journal of the American Medical Association* 280 (1998): 1553–1554; D. Wilson, "Health Food Masquerade," *Corvallis Gazette Times* (August 11, 1999): C-4.
44. "The Pill that Helps You Think," op. cit.
45. Marwick, op. cit., 1553–1554.
46. Wilson, op. cit.
47. Greenwald, op. cit., 64.
48. Ibid., 65.
49. Marwick, op. cit.
50. M. Angell and J. P. Kassirer, op. cit., 839–841; "CAM Centers of Research: Overview of the Specialty Centers," National Center for Complementary and Alternative Medicine (2000) (see http://nccam.nih.gov/nccam/research/centers.html); Astin, op. cit., 1550; D. Eskinazi, "Policy Perspectives: Factors That Shape Alternative Medicine" 280 (18) (1998): 1621; National Institutes of Health, Office of Alternative Medicine, 1997 Practice and Policy Guidelines Panel, "Clinical Practice Guidelines in Complementary and Alternative Medicine: An Analysis of Opportunities and Obstacles," *Archives of Family Medicine* 6 (1997): 149–154; D. M. Studdert, D. M. Eisenberg, E. H. Miller, et al., "Medical Malpractice Implications of Alternative Medicine," *Journal of the American Medical Association* 280 (1998): 1610–1615.

Photo Credits

Index

Note: Boldface page numbers indicate definitions. A *t* following a page number indicates tabular material and a *f* indicates a figure.

failure rate, 130*t*
  protection against STIs, 131*t*
Cervical mucus method, **139**
Cervical sponge, failure rate, 130*t*
Cervix, **115**
Cesarean section (C-section), **153**
CFCs (chlorofluorocarbons), **411**, 411*f*
CFS (chronic fatigue syndrome), 378
Chancre, **361**
Chemicals, household, 410–411, 410*t*
Chemotherapy, **341**
Chewing tobacco, 207
CHF (congestive heart failure), **303**
Child abuse
  in domestic violence, 85–87
  sexual, 87
Childbirth, 151–155, 152*f*
  birthing alternatives, 152–153
  complications, 153–155
  labor and delivery, 151–152, 152*f*
Childbirth Without Fear method, 153
Childrearing, cost of, 144
Children
  alcoholism's effect on, 200–201
  deciding to have, 111, 112*t*
  percentage in various types of families, 112*t*
Chiropractic medicine, 446–447
Chlamydia, **357**, 359–360
Chloride, 237–238*t*
Chlorofluorocarbons (CFCs), **411**, 411*f*
Chloroform, health effects of exposure to, 410*t*
Cholera, 356
Cholesterol, **233**
  drugs to reduce, 308, 309*t*
  heart disease risk and, 304–309
  levels by race and age, 312
  physical activity and, 278
  recommended levels, 308*t*
  Tangier disease and, 317
Chorionic villus sampling (CVS), 151
Chromium, 237–238*t*, 240
Chromium picolinate, 453
Chronic fatigue syndrome (CFS), 378
Chronic lung disease, 15*t*, 370–372
Chronic mood disorder, **40–41**
Chronic obstructive pulmonary disease (COPD), 370
Cigarettes. *See* Smoking
Cigars, 207
Circadian rhythms, 36
Circulation, collateral, **302**
Circumcision
  pharaonic, 117
  risk *vs.* benefit, 119
Cirrhosis, **196**
Clinical/psychiatric social workers, **49**
Clitoridectomy, 117
Clitoris, **115**, 115*f*, 117
Clove cigarettes, 206
Club (designer) drugs, **181–182**
Cocaine, **170–174**, 172*f*
  pregnancy and, 172–173
Codeine, **177**
Codependence, 171
Cognitive coping strategies, 63–64
Cognitive stress system, **61**

Cognitive therapy, 43
Cohabitation, **108**
Colds, 350
Colitis, ulcerative, **376**
Collateral circulation, **302**
College students
  alcohol drinking, 189–191, 191*t*
  drug use patterns, 169–170, 170*t*
  eating habits, 244–245
  hate crimes among, 81
  sexual assault on campus, 90–91
  smoking and, 205
  stress levels of, 60, 62
  unhealthy relationships and, 112
Colon/rectal cancers
  assess yourself, 325–327
  diet to decrease risk, 332*t*
  early detection recommendations, 336*t*
  incidence, 335
  treatment, 335
Communication
  assertive (assess yourself), 101
  improving, 100–101
  in relationships, 99–101
  listening skills, 100–101
Comorbidity, **393**
Companionate, *vs.* passionate love, 104
Complementary and alternative medicine (CAM), 441–460, **442**
  acupressure/acupuncture, 448
  Ayurveda, 445
  chiropractic, 446–447
  dietary supplements, 452–454, 455*t*
  energy therapies, 447–448
  herbal remedies, 449–452, 452*t*
  homeopathy, 445–446
  mind-body interventions, 448–449
  naturopathy, 445–446
  osteopathy, 447
  popular treatments, 446*t*
  regulating claims, 454, 456
  self-care and, 457
  traditional oriental medicine, 445
  who uses and why, 442–443
Compulsion, **164**
Computer dating, 106
Computerized axial tomography (CAT) scan, **341**
Concentric muscle action, **287**, 287*f*
Conception, **129**
Condom, **131–132**, 131*f*
  costs, 138*t*
  failure rate, 130*t*
  female, 131*t*, **133**, 138*t*
  protection against STIs, 131*t*
Congeners, **195**
Congenital heart disease, **303**, 317
Congestive heart failure (CHF), **303**
Conjunctivitis, **360**
Consequences of behavior, 22
  negative, **164–165**
Consumable reinforcers, 21
Consumerism. *See* Health care consumers
Contraception, 128–138, **129**
  access to, 12
  barrier methods, 129, 131–132
  comfort/confidence scale (assess yourself), 132

failure rates, 129, 130*t*
  future methods, 139
  hormonal methods, 134–135
  implants, 139
  male pill, 139
  oral contraceptives, 134–135
  patches, 139
  protection against STIs, 131*t*
  surgical methods, 136
  vaginal rings, 139
Controlled substances, 170–184
  schedules for, 170, 172*t*
COPD (chronic obstructive pulmonary disease), **370**
Copper, 237–238*t*
Coronary artery disease, 301
Coronary bypass surgery, **316**
Coronary heart disease (CHD), 301–302
Coronary thrombosis, **301–302**
Cortisol, **56**
Counselors, **49**
Couples/partners, 103
  childrearing and, 111, 112*t*
  selecting, 105
Cowper's glands, 118*f*, **119**
Crack cocaine, **173**
Creatine, **453**
Criminal justice system, 77
Cross-tolerance, drug, **169**
Cryptosporidium, 356
C-section (cesarean section), **153**
Cultural beliefs
  perceived health risks and, 19
  regarding death, 396
  violence related to, 77, 81
Cunnilingus, **122**
Cystic fibrosis, 378*t*

Dance therapy, 449
Date rape, 88
Date rape drugs, 124–125
Dating, computer, 106
Death, **394–400**. *See also* Dying
  attitude toward, 394
  coping with loss, 396–398
  customs worldwide, 396
  funeral practices, 400
  leading causes of, 15*t*, 80*t*
  right-to-die issues, 398–399
Decision making
  for behavior change, 16–20, 22
  regarding health, 3
Dehydration, **195**, **228**
Delirium tremens (DTs), **202**
Dementia, **390–391**
Dengue hemorrhagic fever, **356**
Dengue virus, **356**
Denial, **165**
Dentist, **430**
Depo-Provera, **135**
  costs, 138*t*
  failure rate, 130*t*
  protection against STIs, 131*t*
Depression, 40–43
  facts/fallacies about, 41–42
  in older adults, 390
  risks for, 41
  signs/symptoms, 41*t*